T0270868

The Science of Mental Health

of Mental Health

Volume 2
Autism

Series Content

The Science
of Mental Health

Volume 2
Autism

Edited with introductions by

Steven Hyman
National Institute of Mental Health

ROUTLEDGE
New York/London

Published in 2001 by

Routledge
711 Third Avenue
New York, NY 10017

Published in Great Britain by
Routledge
2 Park Square, Milton Park
Abingdon, Oxon OX14 4RN

Routledge is an Imprint of Taylor & Francis Books, Inc.

Library of Congress Cataloging-in-Publication Data

The science of mental health / edited with introductions by Steven Hyman.
    p. cm.
Includes bibliographical references.
  ISBN 0-8153-3743-4 (set)
  1. Mental health. I. Hyman, Steven E.
RA790 .S435 2002
616.89--dc21
                              2001048491

POD ISBN: 9780415532525
Set ISBN: 9780815337430
Vol 1:   9780815337447
Vol 2:   9780815337454
Vol 3:   9780815337461
Vol 4:   9780815337478
Vol 5:   9780815337485
Vol 6:   9780815337492
Vol 7:   9780815337508
Vol 8:   9780815337515
Vol 9:   9780815337522
Vol 10:   9780815337539

Contents

Neurobiology of Disease

Treatment

Introduction

Autism and the autism-spectrum disorders are serious developmental disorders characterized by marked impairment in social interaction and communication. Children with autism typically will not make eye contact with others and will not engage others with other nonverbal signals such as facial expressions. Children with autism fail to form peer relationships at a developmentally appropriate level and do not seek to share their interests, observations, or concerns with others. They have little involvement with others and seem to lack a sense of empathy. There is delay in the development of spoken language; in severe cases, spoken language may not develop at all. Use of language is characterized by stereotyped and repetitive words or sounds. Children with autism exhibit restricted and often stereotyped patterns of interests and behavior. For example, they may be preoccupied with a narrow range of interests and may adhere to inflexible and specific routines and rituals. They may also exhibit stereotyped, repetitive body movements such as hand flapping. In addition to these core features of autism, there is a high incidence of mental retardation and of seizure disorders (Tuchman et al., 1991). Autism begins prior to the age of three with two major patterns: the failure to develop; or the beginning of normal development and then regression, which involves the loss of any developmental progress that has been made.

Autism appears to be the most severe expression of a spectrum of developmental disorders. At the milder end is Asperger's syndrome, in which there are features of autism but normal early language development and normal intelligence. There is speculation that the spectrum disorders may result from a smaller number of autism risk genes, partial penetrance of these genes, or attenuation of environmental risk factors. In addition to the autism spectrum, there are a number of independent, rare genetic disorders in which autistic features may be prominent. One such disorder is Rett syndrome. In this disorder, development proceeds in apparently normal fashion through the first five months of life. After that time, there is loss of social engagement and many other symptoms, such as slowing of head growth, loss of previously acquired purposeful hand movements, deterioration in motor coordination, and mental retardation.

Until the 1990s little study was done on the science of autism. This deficit was due in part to views of autism that held sway until the early 1980s in which it was seen as a purely psychogenic disorder resulting from pathological mother-child interactions. Our current understanding of autism makes these all-too-recent formulations seem extraordinarily strange. The frequent co-occurrence of mental retardation and epilepsy with autism should have suggested the neural origins of this disorder even prior to the development of modern neurobiology. Ironically, autism appears to be the mental disorder in which genes have the greatest aggregate influence, the diametric opposite of the radical environmental determinism of the past.

This volume follows the plan of others in this series. It begins with an overview presentation of a case (Rapin, 2001) and a recent consensus description of diagnostic instruments for autistic-spectrum disorders (Filipek et al., 1999). This is followed by recent epidemiologic data (Bryson and Smith, 1998; Fombonne, 1999). Epidemiology has an enhanced prominence in studies of autism because there is an unresolved controversy about the incidence of new cases of autism. In some surveys the incidence of autism appears to be increasing, and the controversy is over whether this is a true observation or whether greater diagnostic awareness is leading to the apparent increase. Clearly, the conflicting data must be resolved because if autism is indeed on the rise, there must be a new, significant environmental risk factor, which has to be identified with a view to prevention.

As already mentioned, there is a substantial genetic component of risk for autism. This is well established, based on family (Spiker et al., 1994) and twin (Bailey, 1995) studies. The concordance of monozygotic (identical) twins for autism is extremely high. Even more striking is that the concordance among dizygotic twins (fraternal) is relatively low. This lopsided ratio, along with the study of patterns of inheritance in families, suggests that autism is an illness in which multiple genes interact to create risk. Given this complexity, it is not surprising that discovering the genes that produce risk of autism remains extremely difficult, as it does for other genetically complex disorders described in this series. One early study that requires replication is included here because it provides an example, still heuristic, of the types of genes that may be involved in risk of autism. In particular, a gene, *wnt2,* that plays an important role in brain development has been preliminarily linked to autism (Wassink et al., 2001). While the search for the genetic risk factors for autism proceeds, much can potentially be learned from the genetics of diseases with some similar features. As already noted, Rett syndrome is a genetic disorder in which there is social disengagement. It is caused by a single gene, and current technologies have made it possible to identify that gene (Amir et al., 1999). The gene in which certain mutations cause Rett syndrome encodes a protein that is involved in controlling gene expression (by binding to modified nucleotide bases within the DNA). The Rett-causing mutation within the human gene has been inserted into the germ line of mice, creating a transgenic mouse model that has abnormalities reminiscent of Rett syndrome (Guy et al., 2001). This animal model will permit detailed study of the effects of the mutation on brain development and can be used to test possible drug therapies. This rapid application of human genetics to the production of animal models is an important example for a host of neurologic and psychiatric disorders.

Like that of the genetics of autism, the understanding of the neurobiology of autism is in the early stages. There have been several major approaches. These include general studies of the neural basis of emotion and empathy as well as autism-focused studies based either on pathological examination of postmortem brain specimens from people with autism or on noninvasive neuroimaging studies.

Studies of emotion have included human subjects with brain damage that has altered their social functioning. Such studies have pointed to the amygdala and orbital prefrontal cortex as playing critical roles in social judgments (Adolphs et al., 1998). Overall, circuits involving the amygdala and the prefrontal cerebral cortex appear to be important candidates for involvement in autism. The information from postmortem studies has not yet converged on a clear set of brain abnormalities. Rather, the existing studies can be seen as an initial survey of brain abnormalities in autism that will lead to a more refined focus in the future (Bailey et al., 1998; Kemper and Bauman, 1998). Studies using noninvasive neuroimaging have examined brain structure and more recently have incorporated cognitive neuroscience approaches to perturb brain function and observe brain activity in healthy and affected individuals with autism or Asperger's syndrome. Studies included here describe differential responses to observation of the human face, a critical aspect of social interaction (Schultz et al., 2000; Adolphs et al., 2001). The combination of cognitive science and imaging is leading to the elaboration of hypotheses about the nature of the deficits in autism (Stone et al., 1998; Happe et al., 1996). The pathogenesis and the neural circuitry involved in autism and autism-spectrum disorders need to be understood in order to develop better diagnostic tools and treatments. Moreover, given the fundamental nature of the problem in autism— serious abnormalities of social interaction— studies of autism will also teach us profound lessons about normal human brain function.

In many conditions, the pathogenesis remains obscure, but treatments have been discovered serendipitously that prove useful. Unfortunately for individuals with autism and for their families, treatment lags behind that of many other mental disorders. At the present time labor-intensive, individualized psychosocial treatments are the best interventions. Indeed, these have shown good efficacy when intensive and when begun early in life (Rogers, 1998; McEachern et al., 1993). The use of medication remains focused on symptom control, which is not to be belittled, but as yet there are no pharmacologic treatments that affect the core deficits of autism (McDougle et al., 1999).

An 8-Year-Old Boy With Autism

Isabelle Rapin, MD, Discussant

DR PARKER: AUSTIN IS AN 8-YEAR-OLD BOY DIAGNOSED AS HAVing autism at age 2½ years. He has improved substantially in cognition and speech but still struggles with social interactions. This is his first year in a public school with his peers, and his parents wonder what the future holds. They live in a suburb of Boston, and Austin's medical care is covered by managed care insurance.

Austin weighed 8 lb 10 oz at birth, after a normal pregnancy and delivery. He appeared alert and normal in all respects. The parents noted normal early development, but at 12 months Austin began to box his ears at loud noises and cry for no apparent reason. Friends and family told the parents not to worry. At 18 months, Austin spoke only a few words (eg, "Mama, Daddy, juice"), yet these few words soon disappeared from his speech. The pediatrician reassured the concerned parents and advised them not to compare Austin with his older sibling.

A day care program teacher noted Austin's paucity of speech, lack of napping, and biting of children and staff when frustrated. Consequently, at age 2½ years, Austin participated in a full-day evaluation at Children's Hospital and his speech and language were noted to be at the 8- to 15-month level. Psychological assessment revealed diminished attention, preference for solitary play, perseveration, and limited social interacting. Physical examination findings were normal, and the diagnosis of autism was made.

Austin received interventional services focusing on speech development and sensory integration. He showed improvement in both receptive and expressive language abilities, but still echoed other people's language. Hitting, kicking, and biting behaviors diminished as his speech improved. Eye contact improved, and Austin liked being with other children but did not play with them reciprocally. At a second evaluation at age 3 years 4 months, his language skills remained at the 8- to 15-month developmental range. The psychologist described him as quiet and even-tempered with a generally sunny affect. His attention was highly distractible and wandering. He talked gibberish to himself in the mirror and produced humming, grunting, screeching, and beeping noises. At age 3½ years Austin received methylphenidate hydrochloride, which worsened his aggressive behaviors. Consequently, the medication was discontinued.

At age 5 years, Austin participated in a school program for children with pervasive developmental disorder (PDD).

He showed steady improvement and, in the fall of his seventh year, entered a public school classroom with an adult aide. He also received speech therapy and consultation from a behavioral specialist.

Austin now can read, write, and speak in sentences, and he interacts more with children. A recent videotape reveals intermittent rhythmic, repetitive movements of the head and entire body, and his parents wonder about the significance of that behavior. He currently takes fluvoxamine maleate, 25 mg twice daily, which seems to help with social skills. The addition of trazodone hydrochloride, 50 mg at bedtime, seemed to improve his sleeping and general focus. Chromosomal analysis was normal, fragile X testing was negative, and electroencephalography (EEG) following sleep deprivation was normal.

By age 8 years, many behaviors continued to improve. Austin seems happy and smiles often. He enjoys riding his bicycle, bowling with his father, and playing with his mother. His parents wonder if there are any new effective medications for symptoms of autism and if there will ever be a cure.

MR D, AUSTIN'S FATHER: HIS VIEW

At about 18 months or so, he lost the few words he knew. He didn't say anything. He would go to the refrigerator if he wanted something to drink. Or if he wanted a toy, he would walk to the toy and just stand there. He wouldn't even point at it. You just had to read his mind.

I knew that something was different about him. My wife and I were very nervous about bringing him to the evaluation at Children's Hospital. If you asked me what the doctor said to me after the word *autism* came out of her mouth, I cannot tell you. My first thoughts were of 10 or 20 years from now: What does this mean about later? About now—I couldn't think about now. I wondered, will he ever ride a bike? Will he ever go to school? Get married? Drive a car?

This conference took place at the Medicine Grand Rounds of Children's Hospital, Boston, Mass, on December 20, 2000.
Author Affiliation: Dr Rapin is Professor of Neurology and Pediatrics, Attending Neurologist and Child Neurologist, Albert Einstein College of Medicine, Bronx, NY.
Corresponding Author: Isabelle Rapin, MD, Professor of Neurology and Pediatrics, Albert Einstein College of Medicine, Kennedy Center Room 807, 1410 Pelham Pkwy S, Bronx, NY 10461 (e-mail: rapin@aecom.yu.edu).
Reprints: Erin E. Hartman, MS, Division of General Medicine and Primary Care, Beth Israel Deaconess Medical Center, 330 Brookline Ave, LY318, Boston, MA 02215.
Clinical Crossroads at Beth Israel Deaconess Medical Center is produced and edited by Tom Delbanco, MD, Richard A. Parker, MD, and Risa B. Burns, MD; Erin E. Hartman, MS, is managing editor.
Clinical Crossroads Section Editor: Margaret A. Winker, MD, Deputy Editor.

Table 1. *DSM-IV* Diagnostic Criteria for Autistic Disorder*

A. A total of 6 (or more) items from (1), (2), and (3) with at least 2 items from (1), and 1 each from (2) and (3).

1. Qualitative impairment in social interaction, manifested by at least 2 of the following:
   (a) Marked impairment in the use of multiple nonverbal behaviors such as eye-to-eye gaze, facial expression, body postures, and gestures to regulate social interaction
   (b) Failure to develop peer relationships appropriate to developmental level
   (c) A lack of spontaneous seeking to share enjoyment, interests, or achievements with other people (eg, by a lack of showing, bringing, or pointing out objects of interest)
   (d) Lack of social or emotional reciprocity

2. Qualitative impairment in communication as manifested by at least 1 of the following:
   (a) Delay in, or total lack of, the development of spoken language (not accompanied by attempts to compensate through alternative modes of communication such as gestures or mime)
   (b) In individuals with adequate speech, marked impairment in ability to initiate or sustain a conversation with others
   (c) Stereotyped and repetitive use of language or idiosyncratic language
   (d) Lack of varied, spontaneous make-believe play or social imitative play appropriate to developmental level

3. Restricted repetitive and stereotyped patterns of behavior, interests, and activities, as manifested by at least 1 of the following:
   (a) Encompassing preoccupation with 1 or more stereotyped and restricted patterns of interest that is abnormal either in intensity or focus
   (b) Apparently inflexible adherence to specific, nonfunctional routines or rituals
   (c) Stereotyped and repetitive motor mannerisms (eg, hand or finger flapping or twisting, or complex whole-body movements)
   (d) Persistent preoccupation with parts of objects

B. Delays or abnormal functioning in at least 1 of the following areas, with onset prior to age 3 years: (1) social interaction, (2) language as used in social communication, or (3) symbolic or imaginative play

C. The disturbance is not better accounted for by Rett disorder or childhood disintegrative disorder

*Reprinted with permission from the American Psychiatric Association. *Diagnostic and Statistical Manual of Mental Disorders, Fourth Edition, Text Revision.* Washington, DC: American Psychiatric Association: 2000:69-84.

It was difficult then. But now I find myself saying—you know, my son is different. But he's my son. At this point, I really wish that he didn't have autism, because he's extremely smart and there's no telling where he could go with his life without that saddled on him. But he's come so far. He's really done many things that I was unsure that he would ever be able to do. So we've been very lucky.

I think that the program in school has been very good. The kids are very welcoming. But I do fear that there will come a day when he does know that he's different.

AT THE CROSSROADS: QUESTIONS TO DR RAPIN

What are autism and PDD and what are the possible etiologies? How does an affected child manifest abnormalities of sociability, language and play, behavior, sleep, cognition, and creativity? What is the appropriate diagnostic evaluation for a child on the autistic spectrum and what are the possible treatments? What is on the horizon for understanding and treating this group of disorders?

DR RAPIN: According to the *Diagnostic and Statistical Manual of Mental Disorders, Fourth Edition* (*DSM-IV-TR*)[1] and *International Classification of Diseases, 10th Edition* (*ICD-10*),[2] PDD, or as I prefer to call it, "the autistic spectrum," or, more simply, "autism," refers to 5 behaviorally defined disorders of early life with a wide range of severity and associated deficits. These lifelong disorders have in common impairments in social skills and verbal and nonverbal communication and imaginative play, with narrow, rigid, repetitive interests and behaviors. Both *DSM-IV* and *ICD-10* list 4 descriptors for behaviors in each of these 3 domains; these provide the principal basis for subtyping individuals with PDD (TABLE 1).

Although the majority of individuals on the autistic spectrum have cognitive deficits, level of intelligence is not a defining criterion. Substantial confusion surrounds the terminology applied to individuals with PDD. The term *PDD* applies to the entire spectrum of autistic disorders and does not mean mild autism, or "rule out" autism.

Autistic disorder refers to the classic, early childhood subtype described by Kanner in 1943.[3] A few individuals with autistic disorder are bright and may improve so much with early, intensive, appropriate intervention that they may achieve independence as adults, although the majority do not. Children with *Asperger disorder* speak at the expected age, their IQ is above 70 and may range to giftedness, but they are socially inept. Often rigid and pedantic, they have narrow interests, and some are clumsy. The term *PDD not otherwise specified* (PDD-NOS) applies to individuals on the autistic spectrum who do not fulfill criteria for another subtype of PDD. The fourth subtype, which is mercifully much rarer than the others, is *disintegrative disorder*. Sometime between 2 and 10 years, these previously sociable intelligent children whose development was completely normal, including speaking in sentences, undergo a massive regression of sociability, cognition, language, self-help skills, and behavior and are left severely and, usually, permanently demented.[4,5] Its etiology is undefined and probably diverse; its relationship, if any, to the much more common autistic regression discussed later is unclear. *Rett syndrome*, the fifth subtype, is a specific etiology for PDD with an identified gene defect on the X chromosome.[6,7] It affects virtually only girls whose brains do not grow adequately after birth; they have severe mental retardation, are generally nonverbal and nonambulatory, have prominent hand stereotypies, epilepsy, and other handicaps, and, like most of those with disintegrative disorder, will remain totally dependent for life. Subtyping of PDD has been based on plentiful descriptions of behavioral symptomatology, but only in the past dozen years has multidisciplinary research on its biological basis provided much evidence-based information on its causes, pathology, medical therapies, and the efficacy of early educational/behavioral interventions.

2

Onset and Symptoms

Austin's history is typical in every way of autism, which presents in infants or toddlers—by definition before age 3 years. The parents' complaint is generally inadequate language, although questioning often reveals that social skills, such as responses to greeting and cuddling, were already blunted in infancy. Children may act deaf, yet cover their ears or scream to particular sounds. Aloofness and inadequate peer relations may improve but persist. Toddlers may drag an adult by the hand to what they want because of failure to discover that pointing provides power to influence another's behavior. Older children fail to imagine the impact of their behavior on others or on what others may be thinking, so-called "theory of mind."[8] Impoverished play and tolerance for monotony may take the form of rolling a toy car back and forth or lining up toys rather than playing imaginatively with them. Insistence on clutching a prop like a string, eating very few types of foods, demanding to wear one particular shirt, or accepting no deviation in a bedtime ritual or route to school exemplify inflexibility. Switching activities or changing routines may result in such fearful temper tantrums that parents capitulate; the outcome is that the child becomes a tyrant and the arbiter of all family activities.

Like Austin, most children without severe mental retardation have no apparent physical anomalies, except for the minority whose head circumferences may be slightly larger than average,[9] yet most have motor signs, notably stereotypies. Explanations for these repetitive purposeless movements range from "habits" to be discouraged because they may be stigmatizing, to a means for pleasurable self-stimulation or, conversely, for self-soothing. The most common stereotypy is flapping the hands, but rocking, pacing, jumping, twiddling the fingers, shaking a string, and many others are frequent. Normal in infancy, some stereotypies may be difficult to differentiate, as in Austin, from the tics of Tourette syndrome, now viewed as a movement disorder of basal ganglia origin under strong genetic influence.[10] Like tics, autistic stereotypies increase with stress or excitement; they tend to become smaller and less conspicuous with age, especially in more able individuals, but they rarely disappear entirely. Other motor signs include toe walking, again normal in infancy but often persistent in autism, and hypotonia or joint laxity.[9,11] Weakness is not a feature of autism, but clumsiness and, especially, apraxia—difficulty programming or imitating complex motor acts—are.

Among sensory deficits, the co-occurrence of apparent deafness with intolerance to sound, as when Austin boxed his ears, is puzzling. Squinting, looking out of the corner of the eyes, gaze aversion, staring at the shadows of waving fingers, smelling food and people, gagging on chocolate pudding, and craving pretzels are other paradoxical sensory responses. It is not clear whether infants who stiffen and arch their backs when you want to cuddle them are demonstrating heightened tactile sensitivity or social aversion.[12]

Table 2. Inadequate Language Features Suggesting Autism

At any age
- Regression of language or communicative gestures
- Lack of reliable orienting to speech, turning to name
- Concern about language comprehension
- Persistent mutism unpredictably interrupted by rare isolated clear words or sentences

In toddlers
- No pointing by 1 year; dragging by the hand
- No words by 12-14 months
- Less than a dozen words by 18 months
- No 2-word phrases by 2 years or sentences by 3 years
- Very delayed or absent head shaking or nodding to signify no/yes

In preschoolers and older children
- Failure to answer questions or responding beside the point
- Inability to use language conversationally, "talking to talk" rather than to communicate (request, show, etc)
- Frequent, persistent verbatim repetition (echolalia)
- Persistent pronoun inversion (you/me confusion), referring to self by name
- Verbatim repetition of overlearned expressions (delayed echolalia, formulaic speech) rather than self-generated expressions
- Inability to recount an event or tell a coherent story
- Perseveration on a favorite topic
- Overuse of pedantic words or expressions
- High-pitched, sing-song, or uninflected robotic speech

Austin's history illustrates an unfortunate but all too frequent mistake of toddlers' physicians: insensitivity to language regression as an ominous and unequivocal sign of trouble. In toddlers it is likely to signal autism[13] and in older children, acquired epileptic aphasia or Landau-Kleffner syndrome, which manifests with loss of speech production and comprehension associated with clinical or subclinical epilepsy.[14,15] Austin's parents reported that the 3 words he spoke at 18 months disappeared, whereas most children have at least a dozen words at that age (TABLE 2).[16,17] If queried, parents of one third of children with autism report language and behavioral regression at a mean age of 21 months, which is before the emergence of full sentences.[18] This explains why physicians may be unimpressed in contrast to alarmed at language loss in the fully verbal child with disintegrative disorder or Landau-Kleffner syndrome. Autistic regression almost never denotes a degenerative disease of the brain, as its usual course is improvement after a prolonged plateau—sometimes with fluctuations—that may last weeks or months. Full recovery is unusual.[4] My experience indicates that language regression is the harbinger of autism in 90% of toddlers, as opposed to older children in whom it is much more likely to be associated with clinical or subclinical epilepsy with epileptiform EEG findings.[13,19]

Cognitive abilities vary widely in children on the autistic spectrum, most of whom are moderately impaired. Most of these children exhibit a ragged profile, with peaks in abilities such as rote memory and valleys in reasoning, planning, and common sense.[20] Some autistic hyperlexic preschoolers are so fascinated with letters that they may learn to "read," ie, decode written language with minimal or no comprehension. Early fascination with letters and numbers does not necessarily predict brilliance, although it does rule out severe mental retardation.[21] Attention to minute details and tolerance for monotony are assets for certain occupational niches, provided social skills are adequate.

3

Prevalence and Etiologies

A major controversy is whether autistic disorders are on the increase or whether less severe cases are increasingly identified. Earlier estimates suggested a prevalence of 4:10000,[22] whereas more recent epidemiologic studies suggest 1-1.3: 1000,[23-25] and figures increase to 1-2:500 if mildly affected children are included.[26]

The physician must consider genetic or environmentally determined etiologies, although today they are found in at most 20% of cases.[27,28] The rubella epidemic of 1964 left in its wake many children with autism, in addition to the profoundly deaf or blind[29]; follow-up showed that the less severely affected fared reasonably well.[30] Cytomegalovirus infection may account for an occasional case.[31,32] Early bilateral mesial temporal lobe lesions due to herpes simplex infection or anoxic or ischemic damage may cause severe autism with mental retardation.[33-35] Thalidomide exposure between 20 and 24 days of gestation may be responsible for autism as well as major malformations, which yields information on the timing of this toxin on brain development.[36,37] Very low birth weight accounts for a few cases,[38] especially if associated with retinopathy of prematurity.[39] Many parents attribute their child's unexplained autism to acquired events such as perinatal asphyxia, trauma, encephalitis, and many other alleged postnatal insults. Evidence for such causation is weak when no other evidence of brain damage exists, unless the timing association is very strong.

What is now clear is that genetics plays the major etiologic role.[40] The strong preponderance of boys over girls, some 4:1, should have indicated this, but it took twin studies to prove it. Among monozygotic (identical) twins without known etiology for their autism, concordance for an autistic spectrum disorder is 90% or more, but concordance for severity is lower.[41] These figures imply nongenetic as well as genetic influences.[42,43] Concordance (for diagnosis but again not severity) in same-sex dizygotic twins and in siblings is less than 10%,[44-46] which illustrates the rarity of causal single-gene defects. Parents of children with autism of unknown etiology need to be informed of their low (<10%) but real risk of having 2 or more children on the autistic spectrum.[47]

A large number of genetic, cytogenetic, and syndromic conditions may be associated with autism.[26] One of the better known genetic disorders is tuberous sclerosis, especially when associated with infantile spasms in infancy.[34,48] Untreated phenylketonuria (PKU), now rare, typically causes severe mental retardation with autism.[49] The best known associated cytogenetic abnormality is fragile X, a prevalent cause of mental retardation in males.[50] Yet most individuals with fragile X syndrome are not autistic, and fragile X accounts for only 1% to 2.5% of persons on the autistic spectrum.[51] Angelman[52] and de Lange[53] syndromes and other chromosomal microdeletions, translocations, and inversions account for occasional cases of autism.[54]

That all children with medical disorders statistically associated with autism are not autistic points to complex causation. Phenotypic variability within families with members who have language, learning, obsessive, or bipolar disorders suggests polygenic interaction.[45,55] Heightened susceptibility to some usually innocuous environmental factor may be inherited.[43,56] The search for possible genetic-immunologic[57,58] or environmental causes for autism is feverish. Any number of speculative factors such as minute amounts of mercury preservative in vaccines, yeast infection of the gastrointestinal tract, allergy to gluten and casein, and others are widely and uncritically accepted despite lack of convincing scientific proof.

The report of increased prevalence of epilepsy in autism in the 1970s[19] helped overturn the prevailing belief that autism was a child's emotional response to inept parenting. In a retrospective study of some 300 children with autism, Tuchman et al[19] found that by adolescence one third had had at least 2 unprovoked seizures—the definition of epilepsy. They also found that those with motor and cognitive evidence of brain damage had the highest risk for epilepsy, with all types of seizures seen. In contrast, children like Austin whose intelligence and motor function were normal or near normal were not at risk for seizures after early childhood. It is not yet known whether epilepsy causes autism and the severe language disorder,[59] or whether some underlying brain dysfunction is responsible for both the autism and the language deficit.[60] Appearance of communicative language in preschool is a favorable prognostic sign.[26(p112)]

Diagnosis and Evaluation

Clues to a PDD diagnosis in a toddler or preschooler like Austin include delayed speech and, especially, poor language comprehension, language regression or stagnation, frequent stereotypies such as hand flapping or twirling, indifference or rejection of social overtures, solitary and repetitive play, lack of attention to activities introduced by others, tantrums, and unprovoked aggression. In intelligent school-aged children and adolescents, rigidity, lack of friends, anxiety, and stilted speech with a narrow repetitive focus are suggestive. An evidence-based consensus on the importance of early detection and evaluation was reached independently by the American Academy of Child and Adolescent Psychiatry,[61,62] New York State's Guideline for Early Intervention,[63] and in the algorithm (FIGURE) published jointly by the American Academy of Neurology and Child Neurology Society.[64] Although concordance among experienced clinicians for a diagnosis of an autistic spectrum disorder is high,[65] practice parameters (evidence-based guidelines for good practice) encourage the use of questionnaires[66-69] and observation schedules[70,71] to foster uniformity, especially for research. Multidisciplinary evaluation in a tertiary care center is desirable but not mandated if the diagnosis is clear to an experienced clinician capable of making the appropriate diagnostic and educational referrals. The justification for early psychological and language tests is to help develop each child's individual educational plan, not for predictive purposes.

4

In brief, the neurologic practice parameter[64,72] recommends taking a complete history (including family history) and performing a physical examination and a definitive test of hearing for all children who do not speak clearly and well.[73,74] Further biological testing is based on what was learned from the preliminary findings, since no omnibus approach is suitable for all children. Tests for fragile X are recommended for families with undiagnosed members with retardation, blood lead levels for children with pica, a urine test for PKU if earlier results are unavailable, and prolonged EEG monitoring in deep sleep, especially for children with a history of language loss or poor language. Brain imaging is not required in the absence of a neurologic indication, even if the head is mildly enlarged.[9,75] Extensive metabolic testing is not recommended unless clues point to a potential metabolic condition. Although research on the causes of autism calls for much more probing biological testing, testing outside of a research protocol is wasteful, expensive, and stressful for the child and family.

It is essential to diagnose autism spectrum disorders promptly so as not to jeopardize early intervention. Parents need to know that, early on, prognosis is almost always undefined and that, as in Austin, substantial improvement is possible. Beating around the bush to spare parents' feelings is an error and confuses them. If the diagnosis is not clear to me, I tell the parents that I am uncertain of the diagnosis but that I am considering the possibility of an autistic spectrum disorder. Parents weep, some are angry, but many thank me for having provided them with a road map of what to do to help their child.

Educational Interventions

There is no cure for autism, but substantial—albeit uncontrolled—evidence indicates that early, intensive, individualized education alters outcome for all children, even those who have severe retardation.[76,77] Unfortunately, estimates of future cognitive ability are unreliable at preschool age because scores describe only current functional level. The federal government mandates early intervention for any child younger than 5 years suspected to have developmental impairment.[78] New York State's thorough literature review concluded that subtyping of developmentally impaired children younger than 3 years on the spectrum is unreliable, which makes all of them potentially eligible for intensive services.[63] The recommendation of up to 20 hours per week of individual intervention for these toddlers, more than for any other developmental disorder, highlights the position that intensive early intervention is key. In the review, evidence on the efficacy of early intervention was limited to applied behavior analysis (ABA),[79] which is quite effective in getting children to attend to activities introduced by trainers who reward them systematically for progressive compliance with the required task, including speech. The original one-on-one classic conditioning (Lovaas version) was applied 40 hours per week in the home by a series of train-

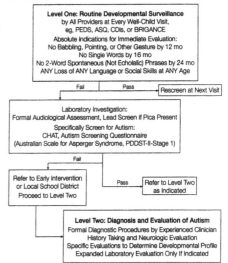

Figure. Algorithm for the Detection and Evaluation of Autism

Level One: Routine Developmental Surveillance
by All Providers at Every Well-Child Visit,
eg, PEDS, ASQ, CDIs, or BRIGANCE
Absolute Indications for Immediate Evaluation:
No Babbling, Pointing, or Other Gesture by 12 mo
No Single Words by 16 mo
No 2-Word Spontaneous (Not Echolalic) Phrases by 24 mo
ANY Loss of ANY Language or Social Skills at ANY Age

Fail — Pass → Rescreen at Next Visit

Laboratory Investigation:
Formal Audiological Assessment, Lead Screen if Pica Present
Specifically Screen for Autism:
CHAT, Autism Screening Questionnaire
(Australian Scale for Asperger Syndrome, PDDST-II-Stage 1)

Fail

Refer to Early Intervention or Local School District Proceed to Level Two — Pass → Refer to Level Two as Indicated

Level Two: Diagnosis and Evaluation of Autism
Formal Diagnostic Procedures by Experienced Clinician
History Taking and Neurologic Evaluation
Specific Evaluations to Determine Developmental Profile
Expanded Laboratory Evaluation Only If Indicated

Adapted with permission from Filipek et al.[72] Copyright 1999, Kluwer Academic/Plenum Publishers.
PEDS indicates Parents' Evaluations of Developmental Status; ASQ, Ages and Stages Questionnaire; CDIs, Child Development Inventories; CHAT, Checklist for Autism in Toddlers; and PDDST, Pervasive Developmental Disorders Screening Test. Educational and skill assessment materials authored by Albert H. Brigance are published and distributed by Curriculum Associates Inc (Maryville, Tenn) as the BRIGANCE System.

ers to 19 children, 9 of whom (47%) were attending regular schools on follow-up, although the other 10 (53%) did not benefit as much.[80] Less intensive and rigid conditioning has been found effective and is widely used in preschool settings providing more eclectic remediation approaches.[76,81,82]

All modern intervention programs for children with autism share a high degree of structure and predictability and an intensive individual approach to each child's specific language and behavioral requirements. The TEACCH method (Treatment and Education of Autistic and Related Communication Handicapped Children),[83] introduced in North Carolina and widely practiced in that state because of its effectiveness, is school-based but addresses the needs of the entire family. Training the parents in effective behavioral methods is often missing in educational programs for autistic children. Other options include well-structured therapeutic nurseries that require children to participate in group activities. In older, relatively well functioning intelligent children, the goal, achieved with Austin at 7 years, is mainstreaming in a regular classroom for part of or the

5

entire day, often with the help of an individual or shared aide to keep the child focused on the task at hand. Teenagers may profit from social skills training groups to help them cope more effectively with increasingly complex social demands. The common denominator in autism interventions is ongoing individualized education that addresses each child's changing needs sensitively but firmly.

The choice and intensity of educational approaches is an educational, not medical, decision. Therefore, it is inappropriate for physicians to prescribe the details of programs, although they need to be informed since parents are sure to ask for advice. For nonverbal children, language therapy that focuses on using gestures, pictures, or reading to supplement speech is essential. Occupational therapy that addresses problems with dyspraxia and clumsiness is valuable, with sensory desensitization reserved for children with troublesome hypersensitivity, although not every child on the autistic spectrum needs occupational or physical therapy.

Medical and Other Interventions

Medications may alleviate troublesome behaviors but do not cure the underlying disorder. Some children require no medication at all, whereas others with extremely troublesome behaviors, like self-injury or aggression, may respond best to a combination of behavioral management and medication. Austin's condition responded to a selective serotonin reuptake inhibitor, a class of drugs used widely in PDD,[84] and another antidepressant, trazodone. Psychotropic drugs also are in wide use, though with few controlled studies in autistic children. Weinberg and colleagues[85] provide a comprehensive review of most of these drugs, together with algorithms for their use. A systematic therapeutic trial is often required to select the appropriate medication. The choice of monotherapy vs polytherapy is controversial. Because most physicians are not familiar with the many potentially effective drugs targeted to specific behavioral issues, consulting a child psychiatrist familiar with psychopharmacology can be helpful.

Anticonvulsants are prescribed by psychiatrists to stabilize mood and by neurologists to control epilepsy. What to do for children who have clearly epileptiform EEG findings without clinical seizures is unresolved.[86] Anecdotal reports suggest efficacy of corticotropin, prednisone, valproic acid, and even carbamazepine in small numbers of children with language regression, usually with, but occasionally without, epileptiform EEG findings.[26] At this time, since there are no reliable guidelines, all physicians can offer is individualized therapeutic decision making involving the parents.

Parents often ask about elimination diets and other dietary, vitamin, and many other unproved treatments anecdotally reported to improve autism.[87-91] My answer is that, if they think it helps, I have no problem with these nonspecific treatments, but I cannot prescribe them because I am unconvinced of their efficacy.[63]

Social and Family Issues

Austin's parents were fortunate to receive a clear, relatively early diagnosis and appropriate ongoing services. Siblings also need a frank explanation because they may receive less parental attention than the affected child. Siblings are often effective advocates and protectors, and younger siblings can be steadfast playmates. It is easy, however, for parents to make the autistic child's siblings surrogate guardians. This situation should be avoided during childhood when arrangements for respite care are essential to provide relief for both parents and siblings. Parents who are advancing in age need to find guardians other than themselves for their incompetent adult autistic offspring. At some point, Austin will need to learn his diagnosis and be told that his differentness is not his fault. This generally helps self-esteem and facilitates acceptance of interventions. Adolescents should receive sex and contraceptive information. Children and adolescents who may innocently engage in socially unacceptable behaviors need the protection of wearing a MediAlert identification.

Children with autism place extreme demands on their families, who may have to adopt very rigid schedules. Parents need training in behavior management techniques, not once in a while, but intensively. Nurseries that require parents or other caregivers to attend school with the child to learn how to handle difficult behaviors efficiently train both the child and the family; this model deserves wider dissemination.[92] Severely affected children may need constant supervision. Worse, some are destructive, aggressive, endlessly demanding, and unpredictable. As a result, parents may be so stressed that those who do not have a strong supportive relationship fight over management issues or divorce. Clearly, the entire family needs support services and counseling, in-home help, and respite care. The parents of severely affected children, adolescents, and adults may need help accepting the need for residential arrangements. What will enable intelligent children on the autistic spectrum, like Austin, to achieve independence as adults is the adequacy of their social skills, which may require repeated training tailored to their advancing age. This may enable them to be educated in regular schools and other educational establishments commensurate with their cognitive abilities and tastes. Insightful vocational counseling may be needed to identify a unique occupation for which their quirks will not disqualify them and that will capitalize on their special strengths.[93] Few autistic adults marry but some achieve meaningful lives, seem content, and maintain strong and loyal ties with supportive families and one or a few friends with shared interests.

Future Research Directions

Clarifying etiologies of autism may help with prenatal diagnosis, genetic counseling, and avoidance of environmental triggers. Better understanding of the pathophysiology of autism will spur more specific pharmacologic interventions. Identifying 1 or more "autism genes" is unlikely to

6

lead to a cure for a disorder that neuroscientific evidence suggests is, in most cases, the result of a very early, lifelong alteration in brain development.[94] On the other hand, it has been only a decade since autism has been seen as worthy of the intensive research lavished on Alzheimer disease and other dementias.[95]

Urgent needs for autism research include tissue donation and rigorous evaluation of the many pharmacologic or educational treatments, some without definitive evidence of efficacy, currently offered to individuals with autism. Autism is extremely expensive to society and to families who pay for individual treatments not covered by insurance. Maybe children need only a fraction of the many services offered them or, maybe, if focused services were made available earlier, a greater proportion would be able to attend regular schools. Many more might be spared idle, dependent, deprived adult lives. That alone would result in spectacular savings, let alone decrease their families' lifelong heartache.

QUESTIONS AND DISCUSSION

MR D: As a parent, should I investigate any neurologic tests for my child?

DR RAPIN: Neuroimaging is not indicated in every case. A study done at the NIH[96] did MRI [magnetic resonance imaging] on 1000 healthy controls and found that 15% had unsuspected abnormalities that nobody knew what to do with and only 3% warranted referral, none immediate. I've seen this repeatedly in autistic children. Even though some autistic children tend to have large heads, it is not an indication for MRI, especially if they have no related symptoms. At this point, in an 8-year-old verbal child who had no seizures, EEG is not important. I also do not recommend extensive metabolic testing, because without symptoms, the probability of finding a medically treatable disorder is minimal.

A PHYSICIAN: Could you comment on the more successful behavioral approaches for treating these kids, specifically in applied behavioral analysis?

DR RAPIN: In autism at the moment, the treatment in vogue is applied behavior analysis known as ABA or Lovaas.[79,80] It is basically Skinnerian training. I believe that this is a useful approach for young children who cannot follow verbal directions. The TEACCH approach[83] is a less rigid method that has been successful. We have a nursery school where the parent is required to attend school with the child for half the day, every day and learn behavioral management techniques.[92] This program has been extremely successful in less severely cognitively impaired children. Dr Greenspan discusses the "floor method," in which you have to be "in a child's face," and not allow the child to float around doing nothing.[97] Another is picture exchange,[98] which uses visual presentation of materials to help children express their needs. I believe that treatment should be eclectic and tailored to each child's specific needs and that families as well as affected children need help.[92] I don't think any one method works for every kid.

Funding/Support: Clinical Crossroads is made possible by a grant from The Robert Wood Johnson Foundation.
Acknowledgment: We thank the patient's father for sharing his son's story in person and in print.

REFERENCES

1. American Psychiatric Association. Diagnostic and Statistical Manual of Mental Disorders, Fourth Edition, Text Revision (DSM IV-TR). Washington, DC: American Psychiatric Association; 2000:69-84.
2. World Health Organization. The ICD-10 Classification of Mental and Behavioural Disorders—Diagnostic Criteria for Research. 10th ed. Geneva, Switzerland: World Health Organization; 1993:147-150.
3. Kanner L. Autistic disturbances of affective contact. Nervous Child. 1943;2:217-250.
4. Kurita H, Kita M, Miyake Y. A comparative study of development and symptoms among disintegrative psychosis and infantile autism with and without speech loss. J Autism Dev Disord. 1992;22:175-188.
5. Volkmar FR, Klin A, Marans W, Cohen DJ. Childhood disintegrative disorder. In: Cohen DJ, Volkmar FR, eds. Handbook of Autism and Pervasive Developmental Disorders. New York, NY: John Wiley & Sons; 1997:47-59.
6. Amir RE, van den Veyver IB, Wan M, Tran CQ, Francke U, Zoghbi HY. Rett syndrome is caused by mutations in x-linked MECP2, encoding methyl-CpG-binding protein. Nat Genet. 1999;23:185-188.
7. Hagberg B, ed. Rett Syndrome—Clinical and Biological Aspects. London, England: Mac Keith Press; 1993.
8. Baron-Cohen S, Swettenham J. Theory of mind in autism: its relationship to executive function and general coherence. In: Cohen DJ, Volkmar FR, eds. Handbook of Autism and Pervasive Developmental Disorders. New York, NY: John Wiley & Sons; 1997:880-893.
9. Rapin I. Neurological examination. In: Rapin I, ed. Preschool Children With Inadequate Communication: Developmental Language Disorder, Autism, Low IQ. London, England: Mac Keith Press; 1996:98-122.
10. Rapin I. Autistic spectrum disorders: relevance to Tourette syndrome. In: Cohen DJ, Jankovic J, Goetz C, eds. Tourette Syndrome. Philadelphia, Pa: Lippincott Williams & Wilkins; 2001:89-101.
11. Bauman ML. Motor dysfunction in autism. In: Joseph AB, Young RR, eds. Movement Disorders in Neurology and Neuropsychiatry. Boston, Mass: Blackwell; 1992:660-663.
12. Kientz MA, Dunn W. A comparison of the performance of children with and without autism on the Sensory Profile. Am J Occup Ther. 1997;51:530-537.
13. Shinnar S, Rapin I, Arnold S, et al. Language regression in childhood. Pediatr Neurol. In press.
14. Landau WM, Kleffner FR. Syndrome of acquired aphasia with convulsive disorder in children. Neurology. 1957;7:523-530.
15. Rapin I, Mattis S, Rowan AJ, Golden GS. Verbal auditory agnosia in children. Dev Med Child Neurol. 1977;19:197-207.
16. Fenson L, Dale PS, Reznick JS, et al. The MacArthur Communicative Development Inventories: User's Guide and Technical Manual. San Diego, Calif: Singular Publishing Group; 1993.
17. Coplan J, Gleason JR. Quantifying language development from birth to 3 years using the Early Language Milestone Scale. Pediatrics. 1990;86:963-971.
18. Tuchman RF, Rapin I, Shinnar S. Autistic and dysphasic children, I: clinical characteristics. Pediatrics. 1991;88:1211-1218.
19. Tuchman RF, Rapin I, Shinnar S. Autistic and dysphasic children, II: epilepsy. Pediatrics. 1991;88:1219-1225.
20. Bishop DVM. Comprehension of English syntax by profoundly deaf children. J Child Psychol Psychiatry. 1983;24:415-434.
21. Burd L, Fisher W, Knowlton D, Kerbeshian J. Hyperlexia: a marker for improvement in children with pervasive developmental disorder? J Am Acad Child Adolesc Psychiatry. 1987;26:407-412.
22. Lotter V. Epidemiology of autistic conditions in young children. Social Psychiatry. 1966;1:124-137.
23. Sugiyama T, Abe A. The prevalence of autism in Nagoya, Japan: a total population study. J Autism Dev Disord. 1989;19:87-96.
24. Bryson SE, Clark BS, Smith IM. First report of a Canadian epidemiological study of autistic syndromes. J Child Psychol Psychiatry. 1988;29:433-445.
25. Bryson SE, Smith IM. Epidemiology of autism: prevalence, associated characteristics, and implications for research and service delivery. Ment Retard Dev Disabil Res Rev. 1998;4:97-103.
26. Gillberg C, Coleman M. The Biology of the Autistic Syndromes. 3rd ed. London, England: Mac Keith Press; 2000.
27. Gillberg C, Coleman M. Autism and medical disorders: a review of the literature. Dev Med Child Neurol. 1996;38:191-202.
28. Rutter M, Bailey A, Bolton P, LeCouteur A. Autism and known medical conditions: myth and substance. J Child Psychol Psychiatry. 1994;2:311-322.
29. Chess S, Korn SJ, Fernandez PB. Psychiatric Disorders of Children With Congenital Rubella. New York, NY: Brunner/Mazel; 1971.

7

30. Chess S. Follow-up report on autism in congenital rubella. *J Autism Child Schizophr.* 1977;7:69-81.

31. Ivarsson SA, Bjerre I, Vegfors P, Ahlfors K. Autism as one of several disabilities in two children with congenital cytomegalovirus infection. *Neuropediatrics.* 1990;21:102-103.

32. Stubbs EG, Ash E, Williams CPS. Autism and congenital cytomegalovirus. *J Autism Dev Disord.* 1984;14:183-189.

33. DeLong GR, Heinz ER. The clinical syndrome of early-life bilateral hippocampal sclerosis. *Ann Neurol.* 1997;42:11-17.

34. Chugani HT, Da Silva E, Chugani DC. Infantile spasms, III: prognostic implications of bitemporal hypometabolism on positron emission tomography. *Ann Neurol.* 1996;39:643-649.

35. Bolton PF, Griffiths PD. Association of tuberous sclerosis of temporal lobes with autism and atypical autism. *Lancet.* 1997;349:392-395.

36. DeLong GR. Autism: new data suggest a new hypothesis. *Neurology.* 1999; 52:911-916.

37. Rodier PM, Ingram JL, Tisdale B, Croog VJ. Linking etiologies in humans and animal models: studies of autism. *Reprod Toxicol.* 1997;11:417-422.

38. Halsey CL, Collin MF, Anderson CL. Extremely low-birth-weight children and their peers: a comparison of school-age outcomes. *Arch Pediatr Adolesc Med.* 1996; 150:790-794.

39. Chase JB. *Retrolental Fibroplasia and Autistic Symptomatology.* New York, NY: American Foundation for the Blind; 1972.

40. Cook EH Jr. Genetics of autism. *Ment Retard Dev Disabil Res Rev.* 1998;4: 113-120.

41. Bailey A, LeCouteur A, Gottesman I, et al. Autism as a strongly genetic disorder: evidence from a British twin study. *Psychol Med.* 1995;25:63-77.

42. Nanson JL. Autism in fetal alcohol syndrome: a report of six cases. *Alcohol Clin Exp Res.* 1992;16:558-565.

43. Rodier PM, Hyman SL. Early environmental factors in autism. *Ment Retard Dev Disabil Res Rev.* 1998;4:121-128.

44. Ritvo ER, Freeman BJ, Mason-Brothers A, Mo A, Ritvo AM. Concordance for the syndrome of autism in 40 pairs of afflicted twins. *Am J Psychiatry.* 1985;142: 74-77.

45. Rutter M, Bailey A, Simonoff E, Pickles A. Genetic influences and autism. In: Cohen DJ, Volkmar FR, eds. *Handbook of Autism and Pervasive Developmental Disorders.* New York, NY: John Wiley & Sons; 1997:370-387.

46. Trottier G, Srivastava L, Walker CD. Etiology of infantile autism: a review of recent advances in genetic and neurobiological research. *J Psychiatry Neurosci.* 1999;24:103-115.

47. Spiker D, Lotspeich L, Kraemer HC, et al. Genetics of autism: characteristics of affected and unaffected children from 37 multiplex families. *Am J Med Genet.* 1994;54:27-35.

48. Smalley SL, Tanguay PE, Smith M, Gutierrez G. Autism and tuberous sclerosis. *J Autism Dev Disord.* 1992;22:339-355.

49. Lowe TL, Tanaka K, Seashore MR, Young JG, Cohen DJ. Detection of phenylketonuria in autistic and psychotic children. *JAMA.* 1980;243:126-128.

50. Laxova R. Fragile X syndrome. *Adv Pediatr.* 1994;41:305-342.

51. Bailey A, Bolton P, Butler L, et al. Prevalence of the fragile-X anomaly amongst twins and singletons. *J Child Psychol Psychiatry.* 1993;34:673-678.

52. Steffenburg S, Gillberg CL, Steffenburg U, Kyllerman M. Autism in Angelman syndrome: a population-based study. *Pediatr Neurol.* 1996;14:131-136.

53. Berney TP, Ireland M, Burn J. Behavioural phenotype of Cornelia de Lange syndrome. *Arch Dis Child.* 1999;81:333-336.

54. Gillberg C. Chromosomal disorders and autism. *J Autism Dev Disord.* 1998; 28:415-425.

55. Risch N, Spiker D, Lotspeich L, et al. A genomic screen of autism: evidence for a multilocus etiology. *Am J Hum Genet.* 1999;65:493-507.

56. Tanoue Y, Oda S. Weaning time of children with infantile autism. *J Autism Dev Disord.* 1989;19:425-434.

57. van Gent T, Heijnen CJ, Treffers PD. Autism and the immune system. *J Child Psychol Psychiatry.* 1997;38:337-349.

58. Burger RA, Warren RP. Possible immunogenetic basis for autism. *Ment Retard Dev Disabil Res Rev.* 1998;4:137-141.

59. Deonna T. Developmental consequences of epilepsies in infancy. In: Nehlig A, Motte J, Moshe SL, Plouin P, eds. *Childhood Epilepsies and Brain Development.* London, England: John Libbey; 1999:113-122.

60. Holmes GL, McKeever M, Saunders Z. Epileptiform activity in aphasia of childhood: an epiphenomenon? *Epilepsia.* 1981;22:631-639.

61. Volkmar F, Cook EH Jr, Pomeroy J, Realmuto G, Tanguay P. Practice parameters for the assessment and treatment of children, adolescents, and adults with autism and other pervasive developmental disorders. *J Am Acad Child Adolesc Psychiatry.* 1999;38(suppl):32S-54S.

62. Volkmar F, Cook E Jr, Pomeroy J, Realmuto G, Tanguay P. Summary of the Practice Parameters for the Assessment and Treatment of Children, Adolescents, and Adults with Autism and other Pervasive Developmental Disorders. *J Am Acad Child Adolesc Psychiatry.* 1999;38:1611-1616.

63. New York State Department of Health Early Intervention Program. *Clinical Practice Guideline for Autism/Pervasive Developmental Disorders: Assessment and Intervention for Young Children (Age 0-3 Years).* Albany: NY State Dept of Health; 1999.

64. Filipek PA, Accardo PJ, Ashwal S, et al. Practice parameter: screening and diagnosis of autism: report of the Quality Standards Subcommittee of the American Academy of Neurology and the Child Neurology Society. *Neurology.* 2000;55: 468-479.

65. Volkmar FR, Klin A, Siegel B, et al. Field trial for autistic disorder in DSM-IV. *Am J Psychiatry.* 1994;151:1361-1367.

66. Baron-Cohen S, Allen J, Gillberg C. Can autism be detected at 18 months? the needle, the haystack, and the CHAT. *Br J Psychiatry.* 1992;161:839-843.

67. Baron-Cohen S, Cox A, Baird G, et al. Psychological markers in the detection of autism in infancy in a large population. *Br J Psychiatry.* 1996;168:158-163.

68. Berument SK, Rutter M, Lord C, Pickles A, Bailey A. Autism screening questionnaire: diagnostic validity. *Br J Psychiatry.* 1999;175:444-451.

69. Lord C, Rutter M, LeCouteur A. Autism Diagnostic Interview-Revised: a revised version of a diagnostic interview for caregivers of individuals with possible pervasive developmental disorders. *J Autism Dev Disord.* 1994;24:659-684.

70. Schopler E, Reichler RJ, Renner BR. *The Childhood Autism Rating Scale (CARS) for Diagnostic Screening and Classification in Autism.* New York, NY: Irvington Publishers; 1986.

71. Lord C, Risi S, Lambrecht L, et al. The Autism Observation Schedule-Generic: a standard measure of social and communication deficits associated with spectrum of autism. *J Autism Dev Disord.* 2000;30:205-223.

72. Filipek PA, Accardo PJ, Baranek GT, et al. The screening and diagnosis of autistic spectrum disorders. *J Autism Dev Disord.* 1999;29:439-482.

73. Stapells DR, Oates P. Estimation of the pure-tone audiogram by the auditory brainstem response: a review. *Audiol Neurootol.* 1997;2:257-280.

74. Grewe TS, Danhauer JL, Danhauer KJ, Thornton AR. Clinical use of otoacoustic emissions in children with autism. *Int J Pediatr Otorhinolaryngol.* 1994;30:123-132.

75. Woodhouse W, Bailey A, Rutter M, Bolton P, Baird G, LeCouteur A. Head circumference in autism and other pervasive developmental disorders. *J Child Psychol Psychiatry.* 1996;37:665-671.

76. Cohen S. *Targeting Autism: What We Know, Don't Know, and Can Do to Help Young Children With Autism and Related Disorders.* Berkeley: University of California Press; 1998.

77. Rogers SJ. Neuropsychology of autism in young children and its implications for early intervention. *Ment Retard Dev Disabil Res Rev.* 1998;4:104-112.

78. Individuals with Disabilities Education Act, USC §1400, Pub L No. 94-142 (1975).

79. Lovaas OI. Behavioral treatment and normal educational and intellectual functioning in young autistic children. *J Consult Clin Psychol.* 1987;55:3-9.

80. McEachin JJ, Smith T, Lovaas OI. Long-term outcome for children with autism who received early intensive behavioral treatment. *Am J Ment Retard.* 1993; 97:359-372.

81. Rogers SJ. Empirically supported comprehensive treatments for young children with autism. *J Clin Child Psychol.* 1998;27:168-179.

82. Sheinkopf SJ, Siegel B. Home-based behavioral treatment of young children with autism. *J Autism Dev Disord.* 1998;28:15-23.

83. Schopler E. Implementation of TEACCH philosophy. In: Cohen DJ, Volkmar FR, eds. *Handbook of Autism and Pervasive Developmental Disorders.* New York, NY: John Wiley & Sons; 1997:767-795.

84. McDougle CJ. Psychopharmacology. In: Cohen DJ, Volkmar FR, eds. *Handbook of Autism and Pervasive Developmental Disorders.* New York, NY: John Wiley & Sons; 1997:707-729.

85. Weinberg WA, Schraufnagel CD, Chudnow RS, et al. Neuropsychopharmacology II: antidepressants, mood stabilizers, neuroleptics (antipsychotics), and anxiolytics. In: Coffey CE, Brumback RA, eds. *Textbook of Pediatric Neuropsychiatry.* Washington, DC: American Psychiatric Press; 1998:1287-1349.

86. Tuchman RF, Rapin I. Regression in pervasive developmental disorders: seizures and epileptiform EEG correlates. *Pediatrics.* 1997;99:560-566.

87. Sandler AD, Sutton KA, DeWeese J, Girardi MA, Sheppard V, Bodfish JW. Lack of benefit of a single dose of synthetic human secretin in the treatment of autism and pervasive developmental disorder. *N Engl J Med.* 1999;341:1801-1806.

88. Findling RL, Maxwell K, Scotese-Wojtila L, Huang J, Yamashita T, Wiznitzer M. High-dose pyridoxine and magnesium administration in children with autistic disorder: an absence of salutary effects in a double-blind, placebo-controlled study. *J Autism Dev Disord.* 1997;27:467-478.

89. Pfeiffer SI, Norton J, Nelson L, Shott S. Efficacy of vitamin B6 and magnesium in the treatment of autism: a methodology review and summary of outcomes. *J Autism Dev Disord.* 1995;25:481-493.

90. Gravel JS. Auditory integration training: placing the burden of proof. *Am J Speech Lang Pathol.* May 1994:25-29.

91. Eberlin M, McConnachie G. Facilitated communication: a failure to replicate the phenomenon. *J Autism Dev Disord.* 1993;23:507-530.

92. Allen DA, Mendelson L. Parent-child, and professional: meeting the needs of young autistic children and their families in a multidisciplinary therapeutic nursery model. *Psychoanal Inquiry.* 2000;20:704-731.

93. Van Bourgondien ME, Woods AV. Vocational possibilities for high-functioning

8

adults with autism. In: Schopler E, Mesibov GB, eds. *High-Functioning Individuals With Autism*. New York, NY: Plenum Press; 1992:227-239.

94. Kemper TL, Bauman M. Neuropathology of infantile autism. *J Neuropathol Exp Neurol*. 1998;57:645-652.

95. Rapin I, Katzman R. Neurobiology of autism. *Ann Neurol*. 1998;43:7-14.

96. Katzman GL, Dagher AP, Patronas NJ. Incidental findings on brain magnetic reso-nance imaging from 1000 asymptomatic volunteers. *JAMA*. 1999;282:36-39.

97. Greenspan SI, Wieder S, Simons R. *The Child With Special Needs: Encour-aging Intellectual and Emotional Growth*. Reading, Mass: Addison-Wesley; 1998.

98. Bondy AS, Frost LA. The picture exchange communication system. *Semin Speech Lang*. 1998;19:373-388.

9

Journal of Autism and Developmental Disorders Vol. 29, No. 6, 1999

The Screening and Diagnosis of Autistic Spectrum Disorders[1]

Pauline A. Filipek,[2,17] Pasquale J. Accardo,[3] Grace T. Baranek,[4] Edwin H. Cook, Jr.,[5] Geraldine Dawson,[6] Barry Gordon,[7] Judith S. Gravel,[8] Chris P. Johnson,[9] Ronald J. Kallen,[5] Susan E. Levy,[10] Nancy J. Minshew,[11] Barry M. Prizant,[12] Isabelle Rapin,[8] Sally J. Rogers,[13] Wendy L. Stone,[14] Stuart Teplin,[4] Roberto F. Tuchman,[15] and Fred R. Volkmar[16]

The Child Neurology Society and American Academy of Neurology recently proposed to formulate Practice Parameters for the Diagnosis and Evaluation of Autism for their memberships. This endeavor was expanded to include representatives from nine professional organizations and four parent organizations, with liaisons from the National Institutes of Health. This document was written by this multidisciplinary Consensus Panel after systematic analysis of over 2,500 relevant scientific articles in the literature. The Panel concluded that appropriate diagnosis of autism requires a dual-level approach: (a) routine developmental surveillance, and (b) diagnosis and evaluation of autism. Specific detailed recommendations for each level have been established in this document, which are intended to improve the rate of early suspicion and diagnosis of, and therefore early intervention for, autism.

KEY WORDS: Practice parameters diagnosis and evaluation of autism; dual-level approach.

INTRODUCTION

The synonymous terms *Autistic Spectrum Disorders* and *Pervasive Developmental Disorders* refer to a wide continuum of associated cognitive and neurobehavioral disorders, including, but not limited to, three core-defining features: impairments in socialization, impairments in verbal and nonverbal communication, and restricted and repetitive patterns of behaviors (American Psychiatric Association [APA], 1994). Many terms have been used over the years to refer to these disorders, (e.g., infantile autism, pervasive developmental disorder- residual type, childhood schizophrenia, and autistic psychoses). Although autism was

---

Portions of this manuscript were reproduced with permission from Filipek, P. A. (1999). The autistic spectrum disorders. In K. F. Swaiman & S. Ashwal (Eds.). *Pediatric neurology. Principles and practice* (3rd ed., pp. 606–628). St. Louis, MO: Mosby

[1] With the exception of the first author, all authors are listed in alphabetical order.
[2] University of California, Irvine, Irvine, California 92717.
[3] New York Medical College, Valhalla, New York 10595.
[4] University of North Carolina at Chapel Hill, Chapel Hill, North Carolina 27599.
[5] University of Chicago, Chicago, Illinois 60637-1513.
[6] University of Washington, Seattle, Washington 98195.
[7] Johns Hopkins University School of Medicine, Baltimore, Maryland 21218.
[8] Albert Einstein College of Medicine, Bronx, New York.
[9] University of Texas Health Science Center at San Antonio, San Antonio, Texas 78284-8200.

[10] University of Pennsylvania School of Medicine, Philadelphia, Pennsylvania.
[11] University of Pittsburgh School of Medicine, Pittsburgh, Pennsylvania.
[12] Brown University, Providence, Rhode Island 02912.
[13] University of Colorado Health Science Center, Denver, Colorado 80262.
[14] Vanderbilt University Medical Center, Nashville, Tennessee.
[15] University of Miami School of Medicine, Coral Gables, Florida.
[16] Yale University, New Haven, Connecticut 06520.
[17] Address all correspondence to Pauline A. Filipek, Departments of Pediatrics and Neurology, University of California, Irvine, College of Medicine, UCI Medical Center, Route 81-4482, 101 City Drive South, Orange, California 92868-3298; e-mail: filipek@uci.edu.

439

0162-3257/99/1200-0439$16.00/0 © 1999 Plenum Publishing Corporation

11

first described over 50 years ago by Kanner (1943), our improved understanding of this complex disorder has emerged over the past two decades, and, despite the recent intense focus on autism, it continues to be an art and science in rapid evolution.

The terms *autism, autistic,* and *autistic spectrum disorders* are used interchangeably throughout this paper and refer to the broader umbrella of pervasive developmental disorders (PDD), whereas the specific term *Autistic Disorder* is used in reference to the more restricted criteria as defined by the *Diagnostic and Statistical Manual of Mental Disorders, 4th Edition* (DSM-IV; APA, 1994). The complexity and wide variability of symptoms within the autistic spectrum point to multiple etiologies which are currently grouped together under this diagnostic umbrella because of the similar core behavioral symptomatology.

The autistic spectrum disorders are not rare disorders, but instead are more prevalent in the pediatric population than cancer, diabetes, spina bifida, and Down syndrome. The earliest epidemiology studies noted a prevalence of Infantile Autism of 4–5 per 10,000 which is approximately 1 in every 2,000 people (Lotter, 1966). With the broader clinical phenotype and improved clinical recognition, the prevalence estimates have increased to 10–20 per 10,000, or one in every 500 to 1,000 people (Bryson, 1996; Bryson, Clark, & Smith, 1988a; Ehlers & Gillberg, 1993; Gillberg, Steffenburg, & Schaumann, 1991; Ishii & Takahasi, 1983; Sugiyama & Abe, 1989; Wing & Gould, 1979). Recent statistical analyses by the Commonwealth of Massachusetts Department of Public Health indicate a prevalence rate in the Zero-to-Three Early Intervention Program of 1 in 500 children (Tracey Osbahr, Massachusetts DPH, personal communication, March 1999). These higher prevalence rates imply that there are between 60,000 and 115,000 children under 15 years of age in the United States who meet diagnostic criteria for autism (Rapin, 1997). Most recently, Baird *et al.* (1999) found a prevalence rate of 30.8 cases per 10,000 of Autistic Disorder (1 in 333 children), with 27.1 additional cases per 10,000 for the autistic spectrum disorders. These prevalence rates are significantly higher than those noted in previous reports and require reconfimation in a future study. However, the notion of these markedly increasing prevalence rates further affirms the need for improved early screening and diagnosis.

The overall ratio of males to females with autism has traditionally been reported at approximately 3:1 to 4:1 (Lotter, 1966; Wing & Gould, 1979). However, the ratio seems to vary with IQ, ranging from 2:1 with severe dysfunction to more than 4:1 in those with average IQ (Bryson, 1997; Ehlers & Gillberg, 1993; Wing & Gould, 1979). Some feel that fewer females with normal IQ are diagnosed with autism because they may be more socially adept than males with similar IQ (McLennan, Lord, & Schopler, 1993; Volkmar, Szatmari, & Sparrow, 1993b).

Every health care or educational agency serving young children can expect to see children with autism. Although symptoms of autism may be present in the first year of life in children who are diagnosed later, and symptoms are virtually always present before the age of 3 years, autism is often not diagnosed until 2 to 3 years after symptoms appear. Individuals with autism also often remain undiagnosed or inaccurately diagnosed. Many clinicians hesitate to discuss the possibility of a diagnosis of autism with parents of young children even when some symptoms are present, due to concerns about family distress, the possible adverse effects of labeling a child, the possibility of being incorrect, or the hope that the symptoms will reverse over time. However, it is believed that the positive outcomes of *accurate* diagnosis far outweigh the negative effects, and families universally express the desire to be informed as early as possible (Marcus & Stone, 1993).

In actuality, the advantages of early diagnosis of autism are many and include earlier educational planning and treatment, provision for family supports and education, reduction of family stress and anguish, and delivery of appropriate medical care to the child (Cox *et al.*, 1999). Screening activities are crucial to early diagnosis. The purpose of screening is to identify children at risk for autism as soon as possible so that they can be rapidly referred for full diagnostic assessment and needed interventions. The press for early identification comes from evidence gathered over the past 10 years that intensive early intervention in optimal educational settings results in improved outcomes in most young children with autism, including speech in 75% or more and significant increases in rates of developmental progress and intellectual performance (Dawson & Osterling, 1997; Rogers, 1996, 1998). However, these kinds of outcomes have been documented only for children who receive 2 years or more of intensive intervention services *during the preschool years* (Anderson, Avery, Dipietro, Edwards, & Christian, 1987; Anderson, Campbell, & Cannon, 1994; Fenske, Zalenski, Krantz, & McClannahan, 1985; Hoyson, Jamieson, & Strain, 1984; Lovaas, 1987; McEachin, Smith, & Lovaas, 1993; Ozonoff & Cathcart, 1998). Thus, early screening and early identification are crucial for improving outcomes of children with autism (Hoyson *et al.*, 1984; McEachin *et al.*, 1993; Rogers, 1996, 1998, in press; Rogers & Lewis, 1989; Sheinkopf & Siegel, 1998).

Howlin and Moore (1997) described the diagnostic experiences of almost 1,300 families with children with autism from the United Kingdom. The average age at diagnosis in this study was not until 6 years (while in the U.S. the average is 3 to 4 years of age), despite the fact that most if not all parents of children with autism had a sense that something was wrong by 18 months of age on average and usually first sought medical assistance by 2 years of age. The U.K. parents reported that despite concerns in at least three different developmental areas, fewer than 10% were given a diagnosis at initial presentation. About 90% were referred to another professional (at a mean age of 40 months). Twenty-five percent were nonetheless told "not to worry." In the remaining 10%, over half were told to return if their worries persisted, and the rest were told that their child "would grow out of it." Of those families referred to a second professional, only 40% were given a formal diagnosis and 25% were referred to yet a third or fourth professional. Almost 25% of the families were either reassured by the second professional and told not to worry, or their concern was acknowledged but no further action was taken. Almost 20% reported that they either had to exert considerable pressure to obtain the referrals or pay privately. Over 30% of parents referred to subsequent professionals reported that no help was offered (e.g., with education, therapy, or referrals to parent support groups), and only about 10% reported that a professional explained their child's problems. Almost half of the families reported that the school system and other parents were the major source of assistance over time, rather than the medical health care community.

Howlin and Moore (1997) concluded that (a) early parental concerns about a child's development should be taken more seriously by both primary care and specialist professionals, with speedy referrals to appropriate facilities, (b) labels such as "autistic tendencies" or "features" should be avoided if one is unable to give a specific diagnosis of autism, and that (c) diagnosis in itself may be a critical step but will not improve prognosis unless combined with practical help and support to assist parents in obtaining treatment for the child, in order to develop skills and strategies applicable throughout the child's life.

DESCRIPTION OF THE ANALYTICAL PROCESS

Selection of Consensus Panel

Filipek was named by the American Academy of Neurology to chair a committee to determine practice parameters for screening and diagnosis of autism. Nominations were then sought from the American Academy of Audiology, American Academy of Child and Ado-

lescent Psychiatry, American Academy of Family Physicians, American Academy of Neurology, American Academy of Pediatrics, American Occupational Therapy Association, American Psychological Association, American Psychological Society, American Speech-Language Hearing Association, Child Neurology Society, Society for Developmental and Behavioral Pediatrics, and the Society for Developmental Pediatrics for representative(s) from each organization with the requisite expertise in the screening and diagnosis of autism, whether by clinical research or clinical practice.

Final representatives include Judith S. Gravel (American Academy of Audiology); Edwin H. Cook Jr. and Fred R. Volkmar (American Academy of Child and Adolescent Psychiatry); Isabelle Rapin and Barry Gordon (American Academy of Neurology); Stuart Teplin, Ronald J. Kallen, and Chris Plauche Johnson (American Academy of Pediatrics); Grace T. Baranek (American Occupational Therapy Association); Sally J. Rogers and Wendy L. Stone (American Psychological Association); Geraldine Dawson (American Psychological Society); Barry M. Prizant (American Speech-Language Hearing Association); Nancy J. Minshew and Roberto F. Tuchman (Child Neurology Society); Susan E. Levy (Society for Developmental and Behavioral Pediatrics); and Pasquale J. Accardo (Society for Developmental Pediatrics). Representatives were named from the following associations: Barbara Cutler and Susan Goodman (Autism National Committee), Cheryl Trepagnier (Autism Society of America), Daniel H. Geschwind (Cure Autism Now), and Charles T. Gordon (National Alliance for Autism Research). The National Institutes of Health also named liaisons to serve on this committee, including Marie Bristol-Power (National Institute of Child Health and Human Development), Judith Cooper (National Institute of Deafness and Communication Disorders), Judith Rumsey (National Institute of Mental Health), and Giovanna Spinella (National Institute of Neurological Disorders and Stroke).

Consensus was reached by group discussion in all cases, either including the entire panel, or within subgroups by specialities.

Literature Review

Comprehensive computerized literature searches of *Medline* (National Library of Medicine) and *PsychINFO* (American Psychological Association) in all languages using the terms "(autistic OR autism OR pervasive) NOT treatment" produced over 4,000 documents. The focus was on literature published since 1990 that reported scientific research, but older sources and less stringent studies were included when relevant. A bibliography of over 2,750 references was developed for this review; article abstracts were initially reviewed, followed by the relevant articles in entirety. The review process was expedited by the many review papers and meta-analyses developed for DSM-IV (APA, 1994), the research overview resulting from the *National Institutes of Health State of the Science Conference on Autism* in 1995 (see Bristol *et al.,* 1996, and accompanying articles) and current review articles, book chapters and books (Bailey, Phillips, & Rutter, 1996; Bauer, 1995a, 1995b; D. J. Cohen & Volkmar, 1997; Filipek, 1999; Minshew, 1996a; Minshew, Sweeney, & Bauman, 1997; Rapin, 1997; Rutter, 1996).

HISTORICAL PERSPECTIVE

Autism from 1943 to 1980

Kanner (1943) first described a syndrome of "autistic disturbances" with case histories of 11 children who presented between the ages of 2 and 8 years and who shared "unique" and previously unreported patterns of behavior including social remoteness, obsessiveness, stereotypy, and echolalia. After its initial description, autism was poorly ascertained during the middle decades of the 20th century. In DSM-I (APA, 1952) and DSM-II (APA, 1968), "psychotic reactions in children, manifesting primarily autism," were classified under the terms "schizophrenic reaction or schizophrenia, childhood type" (p. 28).

Despite this early but persisting view of autism as a psychosis, several prominent research groups formulated the first set of diagnostic criteria for this disorder by the 1970s (Ritvo & Freeman, 1978; Rutter & Hersov, 1977). With DSM-III (APA, 1980), the term *Pervasive Developmental Disorders* (PDD) was first used to describe disorders

> characterized by *distortions* in the development of multiple basic psychological functions that are involved in the development of social skills and language, such as attention, perception, reality testing, and motor movement . . . The term Pervasive Developmental Disorder was selected because it describes most accurately the core clinical disturbance: many basic areas of psychological development are affected at the same time and to a severe degree. (p. 86)

Under this new PDD umbrella, the possible diagnoses included, for the first time, the term *Infantile Autism* (with onset prior to age 30 months) as well as Childhood Onset Pervasive Developmental Disorder (with onset after age 30 months), each further subclassified into "Full Syndrome Present" or "Residual State," and Atypical

Pervasive Developmental Disorder. In DSM-III, autism was also clearly differentiated from childhood schizophrenia and other psychoses for the first time, and the *absence* of psychotic symptoms, such as delusions and hallucinations, became one of the six diagnostic criteria. The revised DSM-III-R (APA, 1987) broadened the PDD spectrum and narrowed the possible diagnoses to two, Autistic Disorder and Pervasive Developmental DisorderNot Otherwise Specified (PDD-NOS).

Currently, DSM-IV (APA, 1994) includes five possible diagnoses under the PDD umbrella (Table I) which are concordant with the *International Classification of Disease,* 10th edition (ICD-10), used primarily abroad (World Health Organization [WHO], 1992).

The Broader Phenotype

Although Allen first coined the phrase "autistic spectrum disorder" (1988), the same year that Wing wrote about the "autistic continuum" (1988), controversy still surrounds this concept of a broader clinical phenotype. DSM-III (APA, 1980) acknowledged that such a continuum existed, and labeled it PDD; the term Autistic Disorder was reserved only for those with classical signs and symptoms presenting before 30 months of age. Over the past 10 years, however, there has been a slowly growing clinical consensus that the umbrella of "pervasive developmental disorders" does actually represent an "autistic spectrum" (Wing, 1997). For the first time, DSM-IV criteria included the term *qualitative* to describe the impairments within the major criteria, defining a *range of impairments* rather than the *absolute presence or absence* of a particular behavior as sufficient to meet a criterion for diagnosis.

Table I. The Pervasive Developmental (Autistic Spectrum) Disorders

DSM-IV Diagnoses (APA, 1994)	ICD-10 Diagnoses (WHO, 1992, 1993)
Autistic disorder	Childhood autism
Asperger disorder	Asperger syndrome
Childhood disintegrative disorder	Other childhood disintegrative disorder
Rett disorder	Rett syndrome
PDD-NOS[a]	Atypical autism
Atypical autism	Other PDD
	PDD, unspecified
(no corresponding DSM-IV diagnosis)	Overactive disorder with mental retardation with stereotyped movements

[a] PDD-NOS = Pervasive Developmental Disorder-Not Otherwise Specified.

The currently recognized clinical phenotype includes children with milder, but nonetheless unequivocal, social, communication, and behavioral deficits. Many high-functioning autistic children are diagnosed after presentation to clinics specializing in learning disabilities or Attention-Deficit/Hyperactivity Disorder (ADHD) (Porter, Goldstein, Galil, & Carel, 1992). Almost 15% of previously undiagnosed children receiving special education services met criteria for DSM-III-R Autistic Disorder in one series (Deb & Prasad, 1994). Autistic "traits" were also retrospectively found in almost one quarter of 2,201 adults previously diagnosed with various learning disabilities (Bhaumik, Branford, McGrother, & Thorp, 1997). Questionnaires devised to specifically diagnose ADHD will not identify autistic symptomatology, and 74% of children with high-functioning autism in another series had erroneously been previously diagnosed with ADHD despite clear differences in their social competence, cognitive development, and restricted range of activities (Jensen, Larrieu, & Mack, 1997).

PRESENTING SIGNS AND SYMPTOMS OF THE AUTISTIC SPECTRUM DISORDERS

All children on the autistic spectrum demonstrate the same core deficits, in (a) reciprocal social interactions and (b) verbal and nonverbal communication, with (c) restricted and repetitive behaviors or interests (APA, 1994). There is, nonetheless, marked variability in the severity of symptomatology across patients, and level of intellectual function can range from profound mental retardation through the superior range on conventional IQ tests. The DSM-IV criteria for Autistic Disorder are presented in Table II and are described below for each neurobehavioral domain. The symptoms and signs represent a summary of clinical features which are discussed in greater detail in the DSM-IV (APA, 1994), in the monograph edited by Rapin (1996c), in the *Wing Autistic Disorders Interview Checklist- Revised* (Wing, 1996), and in numerous additional publications describing the clinical presentation of the Autistic Spectrum Disorders (Allen, 1991; Bauman, Filipek, & Kemper, 1997; D. J. Cohen & Volkmar, 1997; Filipek, 1999; Lord & Paul, 1997; Minshew, 1996a; Rapin, 1997).

Autistic Disorder

(DSM-IV A1). Qualitative Impairment in Social Interactions

It is important to understand that these criteria refer to a *qualitative impairment* in reciprocal social interac-

tions, and *not* to the absolute lack of social behaviors. The behaviors under this rubric range from total lack of awareness of another person, to eye contact which is present but not used to modulate social interactions. The outline for this section follows the DSM-IV outline for the criteria for Autistic Disorder (Table II) (APA, 1994).

Table II. Diagnostic Criteria for 299.00 Autistic Disorder (APA, 1994)[a]

A. A total of six (or more) items from (1), (2), and (3), with two from (1), and at least one each from (2) and (3):
  (1) qualitative impairment in social interaction, manifest by at least two of the following:
    a) marked impairment in the use of multiple nonverbal behaviors, such as eye-to-eye gaze, facial expression, body postures, and gestures, to regulate social interaction;
    b) failure to develop peer relationships appropriate to developmental level;
    c) a lack of spontaneous seeking to share enjoyment, interests, or achievements with other people (e.g., by lack of showing, bringing or pointing out objects of interest);
    d) lack of social or emotional reciprocity
  (2) qualitative impairment in communication, as manifest by at least one of the following:
    a) delay in, or total lack of, the development of spoken language (not accompanied by an attempt to compensate through alternative modes of communication such as gesture or mime);
    b) in individuals with adequate speech, marked impairment in the ability to initiate or sustain a conversation with others;
    c) stereotyped and repetitive use of language, or idiosyncratic language;
    d) lack of varied, spontaneous make-believe, or social imitative play appropriate to developmental level.
  (3) restrictive repetitive and stereotypic patterns of behavior, interests, and activities, as manifested by at least one of the following:
    a) encompassing preoccupation with one or more stereotyped and restricted patterns of interest that is abnormal either in intensity or focus;
    b) apparently inflexible adherence to specific nonfunctional routines or rituals;
    c) stereotyped and repetitive motor mannerisms (e.g., hand or finger flapping or twisting, or complex whole-body movements);
    d) persistent preoccupation with parts of objects.
B. Delays or abnormal functioning in at least one of the following areas, with onset prior to age 3 years: (1) social interaction, (2) language as used in social communication, or (3) symbolic or imaginative play.
C. The disturbance is not better accounted for by Rett's Disorder or Childhood Disintegrative Disorder.

[a] Reprinted with permission from the *Diagnostic and Statistical Manual of Mental Disorders* (4th ed., pp. 70–71 Washington, DC: American Psychiatric Association, 1994.

(A1a). Marked Impairment in the Use of Multiple Nonverbal Behaviors, Such As Eye-to-Eye Gaze, Facial Expression, Body Posture, and Gestures to Regulate Social Interaction. As infants, some children with autism do not lift up their arms or change posture in anticipation of being held. They may not or may cuddle or stiffen when held, and often do not look or smile when making a social approach. Some children do make eye contact, often only in brief glances, but the eye contact is usually not used to direct attention to objects or events of interest. Other children make inappropriate eye contact, by turning someone else's head to gaze into their eyes. Autistic children often ignore a familiar or unfamiliar person because of a lack of social interest. Some children do make social approaches, although their conversational turn-taking or modulation of eye contact is often grossly impaired. At the opposite extreme of social interactions, some children may make indiscriminate approaches to strangers (e.g., may climb into the examiner's lap before the parent has even entered the room, or be unaware of psychological barriers, or be described as a child who continuously and inappropriately "gets into your face" in an intrusive manner).

(A1b). Failure to Develop Peer Relationships Appropriate to Developmental Level. Younger children may demonstrate lack of interest, or even apparent lack of awareness of peers or other children. Some children with autism have no age-appropriate friends, and often older children may be teased or bullied. A child may want "friends" but usually does not understand the concept of the reciprocity and sharing of interests and ideas inherent in friendship. For example, they might refer to all classmates as "friends." One telling example is the child who said without compunction, "Oh, I have many, many, twenty-nine friends, but none of them like me." Verbal children may have one "friend" but the relationship may be very limited or may focus only on a similar circumscribed interest, such as a particular computer game. Often, children gravitate to adults or to older peers, in which case they play the role of a follower, or to much younger peers, where they become the director. In either case, the demands on social reciprocity are much less compared to interactions with age-appropriate peers.

(A1c). A Lack of Spontaneous Seeking to Share Enjoyment, Interests, or Achievements with Other People (e.g., by a Lack of Showing, Bringing, or Pointing Out Objects of Interest). As infants, some children with autism do not reciprocate in lap play, but rather either hold the parent's arms as the parent performs the game in a mechanical fashion, or insist that the parent watch the child perform the game. Regardless, the characteristic give-and-take in lap play that is seen in typically

developing children by the end of the first year is often missing. They often do not point things out or use eye contact to share the pleasure of seeing something with another person, which is called *joint attention.*

(A1d). Lack of Social or Emotional Reciprocity. Some children with autism show no interest in other children or adults, and tend to play alone by themselves away from others. Others play with adults nearby, or sit on the outskirts of other children's play and either engage in parallel play or simply watch the other children. Some children involve other children in designated, often repetitive play, but often only as "assistants" without heeding any suggestions from the other children. Some tend to serve in the passive role in other children's play, for example as the baby in a game of "house," and simply follow others' directions. Other children may seek out one specific child with whom there is a limited solitary interest that dominates the entire relationship.

(A2). Qualitative Impairment in Communication

The communication impairments seen in the autistic spectrum are far more complex than presumed by simple speech delay and share some similarities with the deficits seen in children with developmental language disorders or specific language impairments (Allen & Rapin, 1992). Expressive language function across the autistic spectrum ranges from complete mutism to verbal fluency, although fluency is often accompanied by many semantic (word meaning) and verbal pragmatic (use of language to communicate) errors. Young autistic children, even if verbal, almost universally have comprehension deficits, in particular deficits in understanding higher order complex questions. Deficits in pragmatics, the use of language to communicate effectively, are also almost universally present. Some children with autism do not respond to their names when called by a parent or other favored caretaker, and often they are initially presumed to be severely hearing-impaired. This syndrome, *verbal auditory agnosia* (VAA), is similar to adult-onset *acquired word deafness,* with one very important exception: adults with *acquired word deafness* remain fluent because their language has been overlearned, whereas children with autism with either developmental VAA or acquired VAA with an epileptiform aphasia usually are mute (Rapin & Allen, 1987).

(A2a). Delay in, or Total Lack of, the Development of Spoken Language (Not Accompanied by an Attempt to Compensate Through Alternative Modes of Communication Such As Gesture or Mime). In early infancy, some children with autism do not babble or use any

other communicative vocalizations, and are described as very quiet babies. Some children have absolutely no spoken language when speech should be developing, and also fail to compensate with facial expressions or gestures. A typically developing infant or toddler may pull his mother over to a desired object, but then will clearly point to the object while looking at the mother's face. In contrast, a characteristic behavior of many children with autism is to mechanically use *another person's hand to indicate the desired object*, often called "hand over hand pointing." Some children even throw another's arm up towards the desired object that is out of reach, without any communicative pointing, gesturing, or vocalizations. Other "independent" children make no demands or requests of the parents, but rather learn to climb at a young age and acquire the desired object for themselves.

(A2b). In Individuals with Adequate Speech, Marked Impairment in the Ability to Initiate or Sustain a Conversation with Others. Some children with autism speak relatively fluently, but are unable to engage in a conversation, defined as two or more parties communicating in a give-and-take fashion on a mutually agreed upon topic. In a conversation, Partner A makes a statement in turn on the given topic that is directed at Partner B, who then makes another statement directed back at Partner A, which is continued over more than one cycle of turn-taking. Questions may be included, but they are obviously not the dominant sentence structure used in conversation. A hallmark of verbally fluent autistic children is their inability to initiate or sustain a conversation on a topic of mutual interest, although they may be able to respond relatively well to, or ask a myriad of questions, or talk "at" another person in a monologue or soliloquy about their favorite topic.

(A2c). Stereotyped and Repetitive Use of Language, or Idiosyncratic Language. A hallmark of autistic speech is *immediate* or *delayed echolalia.* Immediate echolalia refers to immediate repetition of words or phrases spoken by another—the children are simply repeating exactly what was heard without formulating their own language. It is important to realize that immediate echolalia is a very crucial aspect of normal language development in infants under the age of 2 years. It becomes pathologic when it is still present as the *sole and predominant expressive language* after the age of about 24 months, and can often be present throughout the preschool or school-age years in children with autism. It is imperative to differentiate speech that consists predominantly of immediate echolalia from the more classic picture of immediate echolalia progressing rapidly to spontaneous phrase speech in typically developing toddlers. *Delayed*

echolalia or *scripts* refer to the use of ritualized phrases that have been memorized (e.g., from videos, television, commercials, or prior overheard conversations). The origin of this stereotypic language does not necessarily have to be clearly identifiable. Many older children with autism incorporate the scripts in appropriate conversational context, which can give much of their speech a "rehearsed" and often more fluent quality relative to the rest of their spoken language. Children also show difficulties with pronouns or other words that change in meaning with context, and often reverse pronouns or refer to themselves in the third person or by name. Others may use literal idiosyncratic phrases or neologisms. Verbal children with autism may speak in very detailed and grammatically correct phrases, which are nonetheless repetitive, concrete, and pedantic. If a child's answers to questions seem to "miss the point," further history and conversation should be elicited with the child, as this is also a hallmark of autistic language deficits. These children typically answer factual questions correctly and appropriately, but when asked a question that requires understanding concepts or concept formation, they give details that are often only tangentially related to the actual question.

(A2d). Lack of Varied, Spontaneous Make-Believe, or Social Imitative Play Appropriate to Developmental Level. Some children with autism do not use miniature objects, animals, or dolls appropriately in pretend play. Others use the miniatures in a repetitive mechanical fashion without evidence of flexible representational play. Some highly verbal children may invent a fantasy world which becomes the sole focus of repetitive play. A classic example of the lack of appropriate play is the verbal autistic preschooler who "plays" by repeatedly reciting a soliloquy of the old witch scene *verbatim* from *Beauty and the Beast* while manipulating dollhouse characters in sequence precisely according to *the script.* When given the same miniature figures and dollhouse, but instructed to play something other than *Beauty and the Beast*, this same child is incapable of creating any other play scenario.

(A3). Restricted, Repetitive, and Stereotypic Patterns of Behaviors, Interests, and Activities

Again, this category of stereotyped behaviors and interests, like the previous ones, encompasses qualitative deficits in several behaviors.

(A3a). Encompassing Preoccupation with One or More Stereotypic and Restricted Patterns of Interest That Is Abnormal in Intensity or Focus. Some verbal children with autism ask the same question repeatedly, regardless of what reply is given, or engage in highly

repetitive perseverative play. Others are preoccupied with unusual special interests. For example, many children are fascinated with dinosaurs, but children with autism may not only amass exhaustive facts about every conceivable type of dinosaur, but also about which museums house which particular fossils, and so forth; these children will often repeatedly "share" their knowledge with others regardless of the others' interest or suggestions to the contrary. Some autistic preschoolers are zealous fans of *Wheel of Fortune* or *Jeopardy*, even when still preverbal or minimally verbal; this unusual interest in a preschool child is considered by many to be a hallmark of autism (Allen, 1991).

(A3b). Apparently Inflexible Adherence to Specific Nonfunctional Routines or Rituals. Many children with autism are so preoccupied with "sameness" in their home and school environments or with routines, that little can be changed without prompting a tantrum or other emotional disturbance. Some may, for example, insist that all home furnishings remain in the same position, or that all clothing be of a particular color, or that only one specific set of favored sheets be on the bed. Others may eat only from a specific plate when sitting in a specific chair in a specific room, which may not necessarily be the kitchen or dining room. Some children may insist on being naked while in the home, but insist on wearing shoes to the dinner table. This inflexibility may also extend to familiar routines, for example, taking only a certain route to school, or entering the grocery store only by one specific door, or never stopping or turning around once the car starts moving. Many parents may either not be aware that they are following certain rituals to avoid an emotional upheaval, or may be aware but too embarrassed to volunteer such information. Within this context, some children have distinct behavioral repertoires that they self-impose to sustain sameness, even when not imposed externally. By adulthood, many of these rituals may evolve to more classic obsessive-compulsive symptoms, including hoarding unusable or broken objects, or repetitively whispering words or phrases to themselves.

(A3c). Stereotyped and Repetitive Motor Mannerisms (e.g., *Hand or Finger Flapping or Twisting or Complex Whole-Body Movements*). Some children will have obvious stereotypic motor movements, such as hand clapping or arm flapping whenever excited or upset, which is pathologic if it occurs after the age of about 2 years. Running aimlessly, rocking, spinning, bruxism, toe-walking, or other odd postures are commonly seen in children with autism. Others may simply repetitively tap the back of their hand in a less obtrusive manner. It has been noted that, in higher functioning youngsters, the stereotypic movements may become "miniaturized" as they get older into more socially acceptable behaviors, such as pill-rolling (Bauman, 1992a; Rapin, 1996c). It is also important to realize that not all children with autism have repetitive motor movements.

(A3d). Persistent Preoccupation with Parts of Objects. Many children demonstrate the classic behavior of lining up their toys, videotapes, or other favored objects, but others may simply collect "things" for no apparent purpose. Many engage in repetitive actions, such as opening and closing doors, drawers, or flip-top trash cans, or turning light switches off and on. Others are fascinated and repetitively flick strings, elastic bands, measuring tapes, or electric cords. Younger children with autism are often particularly fascinated with water, and they especially enjoy transferring water repetitively from one vessel into another. Some may taste or smell items. Others love spinning objects, and may either spend long periods spinning the wheels of a toy car or watching ceiling fans, or spinning themselves until they fall from dizziness. Some children will often look at objects out of the corner of their eyes.

Asperger Disorder

Unbeknownst to each other, the year after Kanner's (1943) first description of autism, a pediatrician named Asperger (1991/1944) also described four children with "autistic psychopathy," who had presumably milder autistic behaviors and normal IQ. This report written in German was not widely known until the 1980s (Wing, 1981b). The diagnostic term was included for the first time in DSM-IV (APA, 1994), and the criteria for the qualitative impairments in social interaction, and restrictive and repetitive patterns of behaviors and activities are identical to those for Autistic Disorder. This diagnostic category is clearly in evolution and, as discussed in Schopler, Mesibov, and Kunce (1998), it is unclear whether it will remain a valid syndrome separate from autism.

In contrast to the Autistic Disorder criteria which include deficits in verbal and nonverbal communication and play, Asperger criteria currently state that there is no evidence of "clinically significant" language delay, such that the child used single words by age 2 years, and communicative phrases by age 3 years (APA, 1994). (Note that those criteria for language delay are much laxer than those recommended for referral in the current guidelines.) Normal or near-normal IQ is also the rule, including self-help skills, "adaptive behavior (other than in social interaction), and curiosity about the environment in childhood." The lack of clear language deviance usually leads to later clinical recognition than with other autistic spectrum disorders, which is presumably due to the normal or near-normal adaptive behavior early in life (Volkmar & Cohen, 1991). Yet, the language in Asperger's is clearly not typical or normal. Individuals with Asperger disorder usually have pedantic and poorly modulated speech, poor nonverbal pragmatic or communication skills, and intense preoccupations with circumscribed topics such as the weather or railway timetables (Ghaziuddin & Gerstein, 1996; Klin, Volkmar, Sparrow, Cicchetti, & Rourke, 1995; Wing, 1981a). Their speech is often concrete and literal, and their answers often "miss the point." Some clinicians have mislabeled individuals with this speech pattern as having a *Semantic-Pragmatic Language Disorder* rather than Asperger's or autism (Bishop, Hartley, & Weir, 1994; Bishop, 1989; Gagnon, Mottron, & Joanette, 1997). However, this diagnosis of a language disorder is not an appropriate substitution for the diagnosis of autism, as it does not account for the social deficits and restrictive, repetitive interests.

Socially, individuals with Asperger disorder are usually unable to form friendships. Because of their naive, inappropriate one-sided social interactions, they are also often ridiculed by their peers. Often they cease their attempts because of the cruel ridicule, and remain extremely socially isolated. Yet, they honestly desire success in interpersonal relationships, and are often quite puzzled when they do not succeed (Bonnet & Gao, 1996). They often have both fine and gross motor deficits, including clumsy and uncoordinated movements and odd postures (Asperger, 1991/1944; Klin et al., 1995; Wing, 1981a). However, motor apraxia is an inconsistent finding, as formal tests of motor abilities do not differentiate high-functioning autism from Asperger disorder (Ghaziuddin, Butler, Tsai, & Ghaziuddin, 1994; Manjiviona & Prior, 1995).

The validity of Asperger disorder as a discrete diagnostic entity distinct from high-functioning (verbal) autism remains controversial (Kurita, 1997; Schopler, 1996; Schopler et al., 1998; Volkmar et al., 1996). Clinically, the diagnosis of Asperger disorder is often given as an alternative, more acceptable, "A-word" to high-functioning children with autism (Bishop, 1989). There are multiple partially overlapping clinical criteria currently in use around the world for the diagnosis of Asperger disorder, which adds to the confusion (APA, 1994; Attwood, 1998; Gillberg & Gillberg, 1989; 1995; Szatmari, Bremner, & Nagy, 1989; Wing, 1981a; WHO, 1992, 1993). The similarity and overlap of signs and symptoms of Asperger's with the Syndrome of Nonverbal Learning Disabilities further expands the spectrum of these developmental disorders (Harnadek & Rourke,

1994; Klin et al., 1995; Rourke, 1989a, 1989b; Voeller, 1986). However, again, a diagnosis of a learning disability is not an appropriate substitution for a diagnosis of autism, as all too often it does not account for the social deficits and restrictive, repetitive interests. To add to the confusion, a recent retrospective review of the original four Asperger cases (1991/1944) reported that these children actually meet current DSM-IV (APA 1994) criteria for Autistic Disorder (Miller & Ozonoff, 1997). As DSM-IV is now written, if criteria for Autistic Disorder are met, this precludes a diagnosis of Asperger disorder.

Childhood Disintegrative Disorder

Childhood Disintegrative Disorder (CDD) refers to the rare occurrence of normal early development until at least age 24 months, followed by a rapid neurodevelopmental regression that results most often in autistic symptomatology. CDD, previously called *Heller's syndrome, dementia infantilis* or *disintegrative psychosis*, usually occurs between 36 and 48 months of age but may occur up to 10 years of age. There have been only a hundred or so reports of CDD in the literature (Volkmar, Klin, Marans, & Cohen, 1997; Volkmar & Rutter, 1995). The hallmark signs include the loss of previously normal language, social, play, or motor skills, and frequently include the onset of restrictive repetitive behaviors, all typical of autism (APA, 1994). CDD is usually associated with more severe autistic symptoms than is early-onset autism, including profound loss of cognitive skills resulting in mental retardation (Catalano, 1998; Evans-Jones & Rosenbloom, 1978; Hoshino et al., 1987; Short & Schopler, 1988; Tuchman & Rapin, 1997; Volkmar & Rutter, 1995). A recent review of CDD noted a 4:1 male predominance, mean age of onset of 29 ± 16 months, with over 95% showing symptoms of speech loss, social disturbances, stereotyped behaviors, resistance to change, anxiety and deterioration of self-help skills (Volkmar, 1992, 1994).

In children with autism, it is also well recognized that clinical regression can and often does occur *as early as 15 months of age*, with a mean age of 21 months (Tuchman, 1996). The relationship between autism with an early regressive course (before 36 months), CDD (after 36 months), Landau-Kleffner syndrome (Landau & Kleffner, 1957; Landau & Kleffner, 1998), and electrical status epilepticus during slow wave sleep (ESES) is currently poorly understood, as is the underlying etiology and pathophysiology (Bristol et al., 1996; Tuchman & Rapin, 1997). Estimates of the rates of regression in children with autism range from 10 to over 50% (Hoshino et al., 1987; Tuchman & Rapin, 1997), with total loss of expressive language occurring in between 20 and 40% (Kurita, 1985, 1996; Kurita, Kita, & Miyake, 1992; Rutter & Lord, 1987). Between 36 and 55% of parents of children with autism note problems in the first year of life, but likely only retrospectively (Short & Schopler, 1988; Volkmar, Stier, & Cohen, 1985). Some children had autistic symptoms quite early, but did not receive a medical referral or assessment until 2 or 3 years of age. Either parents failed to recognize the insidious problems or the physician or others discounted the parental concerns. Acute or subacute loss of language is more likely to motivate parents to seek medical help than is the onset of social abnormalities (Rogers & DiLalla, 1990). One of the most troubling problems hindering a better understanding of autistic regression and CDD involves the disentangling of "age at onset" from "age at recognition" (Volkmar *et al.*, 1985). Retrospective evaluation of home movies and videotapes is now a well-accepted research strategy for identifying autistic symptoms by as early as 12 months of age (Adrien *et al.*, 1992; Baranek, 1999; Osterling & Dawson, 1994).

Autism with regression and CDD have both been associated with seizures or epileptiform electroencephalograms (EEG) (Rapin, 1997; Tuchman, 1995; Tuchman & Rapin, 1997; Tuchman, Rapin, & Shinnar, 1991a, 1991b). In a recent study of children with autism with a history of regression (Tuchman & Rapin, 1997), there were almost twice as many children in the sample with epileptiform EEGs (21%) as there were with clinical epilepsy (11%), which indexes a significant portion of children with autism with subclinical epileptiform activity. These investigators suggested that regression has a significant association with an epileptiform EEG, even in the face of a lack of clinical seizure activity (19% in those with regression vs. 10% in those without). The majority of the epileptiform EEGs were localized to the centrotemporal regions. It is noteworthy that seizures or epileptiform EEGs were more prevalent in those children with regression who also demonstrated a significant cognitive deficit (Tuchman & Rapin, 1997).

Atypical Autism/ PDD Not Otherwise Specified (PDD-NOS)

These diagnoses are used when clinically significant autistic symptomatology is present, including deficits in reciprocal social interactions, verbal or nonverbal communication, or stereotyped behavior, interests, and activities, but full criteria are not met for an alternative specific diagnosis under the autistic spectrum or PDD umbrella; for example, in a child who does not meet the required total of 6 of the possible 12 criteria

for the diagnosis of Autistic Disorder, or who had symptom onset after age 36 months. Also, children whose symptoms are atypical or not as severe would be coded under this diagnosis (APA, 1994).

Atypical autism/ PDDNOS is not a distinct clinical entity with a specific definition, although individuals given this diagnosis are traditionally thought to have milder symptoms. PDDNOS is a diagnosis by exclusion of the other autistic spectrum disorders (Towbin, 1997). It is often used as a "default" or "wastebasket" diagnosis when either insufficient or unreliable information is available, or when the practitioner is hesitant to use the term "autism." Indeed, when 176 children diagnosed by DSM-III-R criteria (APA, 1987) with Autistic Disorder were compared with 18 children diagnosed with PDDNOS, no significant differences were noted on any neuropsychological or behavioral measures when covaried for nonverbal IQ (Rapin *et al.*, 1996). Screening and diagnostic procedures for atypical autism/PDDNOS is the same as for the other autistic spectrum disorders, as is management.

Rett Syndrome

Rett syndrome, a neurodegenerative disorder essentially limited to girls, becomes manifest after a period of normal function after birth. Although it was first described by Rett in 1966, clinical awareness of the syndrome did not occur until Hagberg *et al.* (1983) reported 35 additional cases. The girl with Rett syndrome initially presents as early as age 6 to 8 months, after a normal birth, a normal newborn head circumference, and normal early developmental milestones, with a decelerating head circumference growth rate. This is eventually followed by microcephaly (i.e., head circumference less than the second percentile) and by the loss of purposeful hand skills. Subsequently, stereotypic hand movements such as wringing, washing, licking, or clapping, and poor truncal or gait coordination develop, with loss of social engagement and severely impaired receptive and expressive language development and cognitive skills (Armstrong, 1997; Hagberg *et al.*, 1983; Naidu, 1997; Percy, Gillberg, Hagberg, & Witt-Engerstrom, 1990). Almost all the children have abnormal EEGs with slow background activity and spikes, but clinical seizures occur in only about one third of cases (Armstrong, 1997; Naidu, 1997; Percy *et al.*, 1990). There is general agreement that Rett syndrome is a developmental disorder, although its classification in DSM-IV and ICD-10 as a PDD remains controversial (Burd, Fisher, & Kerbeshian, 1989; Gillberg, 1994; Tsai, 1992). However, it was classified under the PDD umbrella so that a misdiagnosis of autism would not be given in lieu of the correct diagnosis of Rett syndrome.

SCREENING AND DIAGNOSIS OF AUTISM: "SCREEN, PROBE, EVALUATE"

Screening for autism calls for two different levels of investigation, each answering a different question (Siegel, 1998). *Level 1* screening should be performed on all children and involves identifying children at risk for any type of atypical development. *Level 2* involves a more in-depth investigation of children already identified to be at risk for a developmental disorder, differentiates autism from other kinds of developmental difficulties, and includes evaluations by autism specialists aimed at determining the best means of intervention based on the child's profile of strengths and weaknesses. Please refer to the Algorithm (Fig. 1) for an overview of this process. Although the process itself has been separated into two levels of evaluation, this does not necessarily indicate separate independent levels of professional involvement, as a given single professional may well perform both sequential stages.

Since we currently have no biological marker for autism, screening must focus on behavior. Furthermore, in most cases, autism appears to have a gradual onset, often without clear evidence of sensorimotor impairment. Children with autism typically sit, crawl, and walk at the expected age. Many even produce a few words at developmentally appropriate times, although these words seldom develop into useful early language. Symptoms that may be present during infancy (a serious expression, increased irritability, sleep and eating difficulties, and placidity) are behaviors commonly seen in otherwise typically developing children.

At the present time, specific behaviors that distinguish infants with autism from others at 12 months of age have been identified in studies using observations based on home videotapes (Osterling & Dawson, 1994). Using home videotapes of first birthday parties in infants with autism versus typical development, these investigators found that four behaviors correctly identified over 90% of the autistic and typical infants. These behaviors, which were replicated in a subsequent study (Mars, Mauk, & Dowrick, 1998), were eye contact, orienting to name being called, pointing, and showing. A more recent study of home videotapes of first birthdays (Osterling & Dawson, 1999) found that these 1-year-olds with autism could also be distinguished from 1-year-olds with idiopathic mental retardation. One-year-old infants with autism used less eye contact and oriented to their names less frequently than those with mental retardation and those with typical development. Furthermore, these same behaviors distinguished these same infants with autism at 8 to 10 months from those with typical development (Brown, Dawson, Osterling, & Dinno, 1998). Baranek (1999) similarly used retrospective video analysis with 9- to 12-month-old infants and found that a pattern of nine behaviors differentiated between autism, developmental disabilities and typical development with 94% accuracy. The autistic pattern included greater problems with responsiveness to social stimuli (e.g., delayed responding to name; social touch aversion) as well as other nonsocial aspects of sensory responsiveness. Although the long-range stability and predictive utility of these findings remains to be determined, these results suggest that autism will eventually be reliably detected as early as 1 year of age, or even younger (Baranek, 1999; Teitelbaum, Teitelbaum, Nye, Fryman, & Maurer, 1998).

Autism can be diagnosed reliably in children by or before the age of 3 years. Recent studies have demonstrated that symptoms of autism are measurable by 18 months of age, and that these symptoms are stable

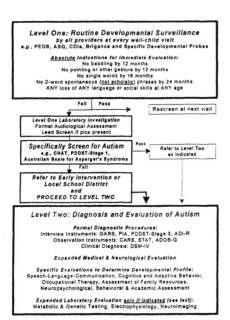

Level One: Routine Developmental Surveillance
by all providers at every well-child visit
e.g., PEDS, ASQ, CDIs, Brigance and Specific Developmental Probes

Absolute Indications for Immediate Evaluation:
No babbling by 12 months
No pointing or other gesture by 12 months
No single words by 16 months
No 2-word spontaneous (not echolalic) phrases by 24 months
ANY loss of ANY language or social skills at ANY age

Fail | Pass → Rescreen at next visit

Level One Laboratory Investigation
Formal Audiological Assessment
Lead Screen if pica present

Specifically Screen for Autism
e.g., CHAT, PDDST-Stage 1,
Australian Scale for Asperger's Syndrome
Pass → Refer to Level Two as indicated
Fail

Refer to Early Intervention or Local School District and PROCEED TO LEVEL TWO

Level Two: Diagnosis and Evaluation of Autism

Formal Diagnostic Procedures:
Interview Instruments: GARS, PIA, PDDST-Stage 3, ADI-R
Observation Instruments: CARS, STAT, ADOS-G
Clinical Diagnosis: DSM-IV

Expanded Medical & Neurological Evaluation

Specific Evaluations to Determine Developmental Profile:
Speech-Language-Communication, Cognitive and Adaptive Behavior,
Occupational Therapy, Assessment of Family Resources,
Neuropsychological, Behavioral & Academic Assessment

Expanded Laboratory Evaluation only if indicated (see text):
Metabolic & Genetic Testing, Electrophysiology, Neuroimaging

Fig. 1. Algorithm.

21

from toddler age through the preschool age (Charman *et al.*, 1997; Cox *et al.*, 1999; Lord, 1995; Stone *et al.*, 1999). Furthermore, these studies have identified the main characteristics that differentiate autism from other developmental disorders in the 20-month to 36-month age range, characteristics that early screening tools need to target. These involve negative symptoms, or behavioral deficits, in the following areas: eye contact, orienting to one's name, joint attention behaviors (e.g., pointing, showing), pretend play, imitation, nonverbal communication, and language development. There is some indication that socially directed emotional behavior may also differentiate the groups; neither sensory-perceptual nor positive symptoms such as repetitive behaviors or behavioral outbursts appear to consistently differentiate between autistic and nonautistic groups early on.

Screening for autism may not identify children with milder variants of the disorder (without mental retardation or obvious language delay). These children's difficulties often go undiagnosed for years, causing them increasing difficulty as they try to meet the demands of elementary education without needed supports. Their difficulties cause great stress for their families, who recognize the child's challenges but have difficulty convincing others that their child has a disability. These children and their families will benefit greatly from improved screening efforts and the increased opportunity for effective intervention that screening activities can yield. However, this screening also needs to target the symptoms of verbal individuals with high-functioning autism and Asperger disorder, and must focus on older children, adolescents, and young adults (Garnett & Attwood, 1998). Such screens are also relevant for educational settings, where these older children may also be recognized.

Level 1: Routine Developmental Surveillance and Screening Specifically for Autism

It is the consensus of this Panel that primary care providers must change their approach to well-child care, so as to perform proactive screening for developmental disorders. It has been estimated that almost 25% of children in any practice demonstrate developmental issues at some point. Therefore, developmental screening must become an absolutely essential routine of each and every well-child visit throughout infancy, toddler, and preschool years, and even beyond early school-age if concerns are raised. The additional use of Specific Developmental Probes will increase the sensitivity and specificity of the screening process for autism.

Unfortunately, fewer than 30% of primary care providers conduct standardized screening tests (in the rigid manner for which they were intended) at well-child appointments (Dworkin, 1989, 1992; Majnemer & Rosenblatt, 1994; Rapin, 1995). Additionally, the American Academy of Pediatrics (AAP) is stressing the importance of developmental *surveillance* at every well-child visit: a flexible, continuous process that is broader than screening and includes eliciting and valuing parental concerns, specific probing regarding age-appropriate skills in each developmental domain, and skilled observations (American Academy of Pediatrics Committee on Children with Disabilities, 1994; Johnson & Blasco, 1997). Implementation of the developmental surveillance process at every well-child visit and the acquisition of the necessary skills to make it happen will only be accomplished with training at the preservice and in-service levels. Additionally, current managed-care policy, which allows only a few minutes for well-child appointments, must change if clinicians are to implement the training they receive (Glascoe, Foster, & Wolraich, 1997). A high degree of advocacy on the part of parents, health care professionals, and managed care administrators is essential if the recommendations of this Practice Parameter are to be appropriately implemented.

It is important to realize that parents *usually are correct* in their concerns about their child's development (Glascoe, 1994, 1997, 1998; Glascoe & Dworkin, 1995). They may not be as accurate regarding the qualitative and quantitative parameters surrounding the developmental abnormality, but almost always, if there is a concern, there is indeed a problem in some aspect of the child's development. Any developmental concern on Chief Complaint must be valued and lead to further investigation.

Although a positive parental concern strongly suggests an underlying developmental problem, the lack of concern does not imply normal development. Lack of parenting experience, cultural influences, denial, time constraints in the presence of more pressing medical issues, all contribute to parental reluctance to bring up developmental issues. Even when the parents express no concerns, a child's development should be monitored closely by using one of the available parental questionnaire instruments. Some clinics utilize well-child clinic forms with preprinted developmental milestones that are appropriate for each routine visit. The information on these forms should be taken from valid milestone charts and cover each developmental domain.

General Developmental Screening: Parental Questionnaires

Traditional Instruments. The *Denver-II* (DDST-II, formerly the *Denver Developmental Screening Test-*

Revised; Frankenburg, Dodds, Archer, Shapiro, & Bresnick, 1992) has been the traditional tool used for developmental screening in primary care practices. It is designed for children from birth to 6 years of age, and samples receptive and expressive language, articulation, fine motor-adaptive, personal-social, and gross motor skills. It yields a single score (abnormal, questionable, untestable, normal, or advanced). Easy to administer and score, the test can be completed in 25 minutes or less. However, the validity of the test has not been studied. In addition, subsequent research found that the measure was significantly insensitive (meaning that the instrument missed a significant number of delayed children—many missed true positives) and lacked specificity (meaning that a significant number of normal children—true negatives—were misclassified as delayed) (Glascoe *et al.,* 1992). The *Revised Denver Pre-Screening Developmental Questionnaire* (R-DPDQ; Frankenburg, 1986), in contrast, is designed to identify a subset of children who need further screening. It uses parental report and presents 10 to 15 items, sampling the various domains, in the age range of birth to 6 years. R-DPDQ items were drawn from the Denver Developmental Screening Test (the very popular predecessor of the Denver-II) which detected only 30% of children with language impairments and 50% of children with mental retardation (Borowitz & Glascoe, 1986; Glascoe *et al.,* 1992; Greer, Bauchner, & Zuckerman, 1989). Many other comprehensive studies also document the lack of sensitivity and specificity of this instrument (Cadman *et al.,* 1984; Camp, van Doorninck, Frankenburg, & Lampe, 1977; Diamond, 1987; Grant & Gittelsohn, 1972; Harper & Wacker, 1983; Lindquist, 1982; Sciarillo, Brown, Robinson, Bennett, & Sells, 1986; Sturner, Green, & Funk, 1985). Because of the lack of sensitivity and specificity of both the DDST-II and R-DPDQ, an alternative instrument must be used for appropriate *Level 1* primary-care screening at every well-child visit.

Standardized Developmental Screening Instruments. Examples of Level 1 parent questionnaires with acceptable psychometric properties include: (a) *The Ages and Stages Questionnaire, Second Edition* (ASQ; Bricker & Squires, 1994; Bricker & Squires, 1999; Squires, Bricker, & Potter, 1997) uses parental report for children from birth to 3 years, and provides clear drawings and directions for eliciting thoughtful responses. Separate forms of 10 to 15 items for each age range are tied to the well-child visit schedule. Modifications are available for screening children at other particular ages. Well-standardized and validated, the ASQ has good sensitivity and excellent specificity and provides pass–fail scores. Because it is difficult to use the single outcome score to make referrals and because of the ASQ's brevity, it appears especially useful as a prescreening tool. (b) *The BRIGANCE® Screens* (Brigance, 1986; Glascoe, 1996) consist of seven separate forms, one for each 12-month age range from 21 to 90 months of age. It taps key developmental and early academic skills, including speech-language, fine and gross motor, graphomotor development, and general knowledge at younger ages and also reading and math at older ages. It uses direct elicitation and observation, and takes in approximately 10 minutes to administer. It is available in English or Spanish. It is well standardized and validated, and has been in use for over 10 years. The Screens produce cutoff and age-equivalent scores for motor, language, and readiness, and an overall cutoff score. The Screens also have good sensitivity and specificity to giftedness. (c) *The Child Development Inventories* (CDIs; Ireton, 1992; Ireton & Glascoe, 1995) include three separate measures with 60 items each (the Infant Development Inventory, birth to 21 months of age; Early Child Development Inventory, 15 to 36 months of age; and the Preschool Development Inventory, 36 to 72 months of age). All are completed by parental report in about 5 to 10 minutes. The CDIs can be self-administered in waiting or exam rooms or mailed to families. For parents with limited English, items can be directly administered to children. The CDIs screen for language, motor, cognitive, preacademic, social, self-help, behavior, and health problems. Forms for the older two age groups produce a single cutoff score equivalent to 1.5 standard deviations below the population mean. Clinicians must then analyze errors to determine the domains in which children are having the most difficulty in order to make appropriate referrals (e.g., fine motor deficits might dictate an occupational therapy referral whereas global deficits dictate the need for comprehensive assessment). Although the CDIs were standardized exclusively in St. Paul, MN, a number of validity studies support the instruments' effectiveness in other geographic locations, with minorities and with groups with lower socioeconomic status (Chaffee, Cunningham, Secord-Gilbat, Elbard, & Richards, 1990; Guerin & Gottfried, 1987; Ireton & Glascoe, 1995; Sturner, Funk, Thomas, & Green, 1982). These also showed the measures to have excellent sensitivity and good specificity. The parent instrument to the CDIs, the *Child Development Inventory,* is more of an assessment than a screening tool for children 15 to 72 months of age. (d) *The Parents' Evaluation of Developmental Status* (PEDS, Glascoe, 1998) helps providers carefully elicit and interpret parents' concerns. PEDS assigns probabilities of delays and disabilities to the various types of concerns, thus enabling clinicians to make evidence-based decisions, provide in-office counseling, encourage suggestions, and give reassurance. To use PEDS, parents must answer 10 questions. These are written at the fifth-grade level in English and in Spanish, and more than 90% of parents can complete the questionnaire in writing while they wait for their appointment. Clinicians or office staff can score and interpret the results in about 2 minutes. PEDS was validated and standardized on 971 children around the country in four separate validation studies (Glascoe, 1991, 1994; Glascoe, Altemeier, & MacLean, 1989; Glascoe, MacLean, & Stone, 1991). Its accuracy in the detection of disabilities meets conventional standards for screening tests (sensitivity to developmental problems and specificity to normal development of 70 to 80%). Research on PEDS shows that parents are likely to be accurate, regardless of their level of education or parenting experience.

Chief Complaints and Specific Probes Regarding Developmental Concerns

There are at least three general concerns with which young children and their parents present to the primary care provider at a well-child visit: speech or language delay; problems with social development with or without similar concerns in speech or language; and the development of a younger sibling of a child with known or suspected autism. Any child whose parents are concerned in these areas should be further evaluated through *Levels 1 and 2*, as appropriate. Any concern that implies "regression" or loss of skills in language or social skills should be a serious red flag.

The Child Whose Parents Are Concerned about Speech or Language Delay. Chief complaints about "isolated" speech deficits are the most common concerns raised by parents in children between the ages of 1 and 5 years. Most of the time these concerns relate to delayed expressive language, because parents are not usually as knowledgeable about their child's receptive language skills. There are several classic parental concerns, as well as absolute language milestone misses, either of which should immediately prompt further investigation (Table III). When these or other language concerns are voiced, the *Level 1* provider should probe with questions to the parent regarding social skills and behavior, as well as communication, in an effort to determine whether there are any problems in addition to language (Table IV).

The Child with a Suspected Problem in Social Development or Behavior (with or without Similar Concerns in Speech or Language). Any concerns regarding problems with social development should always be taken seriously, as seriously as an older child's com-

Table III. Parental Concerns that are RED FLAGS for Autism

Communication Concerns
  Does not respond to his/her name
  Cannot tell me what (s)he wants
  Language is delayed
  Doesn't follow directions
  Appears deaf at times
  Seems to hear sometimes but not others
  Doesn't point or wave bye-bye
  Used to say a few words, but now he doesn't

Social Concerns
  Doesn't smile socially
  Seems to prefer to play alone
  Gets things for himself
  Is very independent
  Does things "early"
  Has poor eye contact
  Is in his own world
  Tunes us out
  Is not interested in other children

Behavioral Concerns
  Tantrums
  Is hyperactive/uncooperative or oppositional
  Doesn't know how to play with toys
  Gets stuck on things over and over
  Toe walks
  Has unusual attachments to toys (e.g., always is holding a
    certain object)
  Lines things up
  Is oversensitive to certain textures or sounds
  Has odd movement patterns

Absolute indications for immediate further evaluation
  No babbling by 12 months
  No gesturing (pointing, waving bye-bye, etc) by 12 months
  No single words by 16 months
  No 2-word spontaneous (*not just echolalic*) phrases by
    24 months
  ANY Loss of ANY Language or Social Skills at ANY Age

plaint of back or chest pain. Unlike "stomachaches" and "headaches" which are common, self-limiting, and can often be treated symptomatically without a diagnostic workup, a complaint of back or chest pain is rare and deserves investigation. Similarly, parents rarely complain of social delays or problems, so any and all such concerns should be immediately investigated. In addition, complaints about behavioral concerns that coexist with any other concerns of social or communication development should be immediately investigated (see Tables III and IV). It is even more significant when parents voice additional concerns in the communication and behavior areas as well as in socialization.

The Younger Sibling of an Older Child with Known or Suspected Autism. The younger sibling(s) of an autistic child deserves special attention whether or

Table IV. Ask Specific Development Probes:
"Does (s)he . . ." or "Is there . . ."

Socialization
  . . . cuddle like other children?
  . . . look at you when you are talking or playing?
  . . . smile in response to a smile from others?
  . . . engage in reciprocal, back-and-forth play?
  . . . play simple imitation games, such as pat-a-cake or
      peek-a-boo?
  . . . show interest in other children?

Communication
  . . . point with his finger?
  . . . gesture? nod yes and no?
  . . . direct your attention by holding up objects for you to see?
  . . . anything odd about his/her speech?
  . . . show things to people?
  . . . lead an adult by the hand?
  . . . give inconsistent responses to name? . . . to commands?
  . . . use rote, repetitive, or echolalic speech?
  . . . memorize strings of words or scripts?

Behavior
  . . . have repetitive, stereotyped, or odd motor behavior?
  . . . have preoccupations or a narrow range of interests?
  . . . attend more to parts of objects (e.g., wheels)?
  . . . have limited or absent pretend play?
  . . . imitate other people's actions?
  . . . play with toys in the same exact way each time?
  . . . strongly attached to a specific unusual objects(s)?

not the parents have concerns about this child's development. Siblings constitute an important autism-risk group: their development needs to be monitored very carefully not only for autism-related symptoms but also for language delays and early anxiety symptoms. While some parents may be overly vigilant regarding the presence of "autistic features" and overreact, other parents may not realize that their younger child demonstrates milder autistic symptoms, because the severity of the older child overshadows the subtle abnormalities in the younger. The main advantage of identifying young children with autism as soon as possible is to provide them with early treatment in high quality autism intervention programs. Additionally, it is important to note that a younger sibling may mimic their older autistic sibling even when s/he has no innate autistic characteristics of her/his own. When the parents do have a concern, *Level 1* screening should proceed directly to the autism-specific questionnaires. When the parents have no concerns, screening should both probe for autistic behaviors and monitor all developmental domains at each and every well-child visit. Because there are no pathognomonic signs or diagnostic tests for autism, the history is one of the most important tools used to determine whether or not the child is at risk

for a diagnosis of autism. *Level 1* professionals must learn what questions to ask and how to interpret the answers in the context of normal child development (see Tables III and IV).

Level 1 Laboratory Investigations

Formal Audiologic Evaluation

All children with developmental delays, especially those with delays in social and language development, should undergo a formal audiologic hearing evaluation. This may become a moot point as the standard of pediatric care moves toward universal screening. Until such time, any child with delayed language or at risk for autism should be provided with a referral for audiologic testing on the same day that a concern is identified.

Parent or practitioner concern regarding a speech, language, or hearing problem (loss of sensitivity, inconsistent responses, no response, or unusual responses to sounds or sound sources) should result in an immediate referral for audiologic assessment. Comprehensive hearing tests should be provided by an audiologist with experience in the assessment of very young children and difficult-to-test populations. This referral should occur regardless of the child having "passed" a neonatal hearing screen. Integrity of hearing cannot be determined by informal observations of behavioral responses to environmental sounds or by parent-caregiver report. Hearing loss (conductive, sensorineural, or mixed) can co-occur with autism; children with autism may be incorrectly thought to have peripheral hearing loss (Adkins & Ainsa, 1979; Jure, Rapin, & Tuchman, 1991; Klin, 1993; Smith, Miller, Stewart, Walter, & McConnell, 1988). Audiologic assessment should occur early in the differential diagnostic process and include a battery of tests including behavioral audiometric measures, assessment of middle-ear function and electrophysiologic procedures (American Speech-Language-Hearing Association, 1991).

The goal of audiologic assessment is to delineate the type, degree, configuration, and symmetry of any existing hearing loss or to confirm the presence of normal peripheral hearing sensitivity. Two broad categories of hearing assessment methods are available: behavioral and electrophysiologic. Behavioral audiologic assessment should include measures of hearing that are appropriate for the child's developmental level. Unconditioned behavioral response procedures (behavioral observation audiometry or BOA) are of limited use in characterizing hearing sensitivity as a function of fre-

Visual Reinforcement Audiometry or Conditioned Play Audiometry) are useful in audiologic assessment of children beginning at the developmental age of 6 months. Reliable, accurate, frequency-specific threshold information may be obtained using this simple, pleasant, and cost-effective method. The audiologic assessment of children with autism may present challenges for the audiologist requiring modifications of traditional test techniques and test environments. Limited reports and clinical experience suggest that many children with autism may be assessed using operant test procedures (Gravel, Kurtzberg, Stapells, Vaughan, & Wallace, 1989; Verpoorten & Emmen, 1995).

Electrophysiologic procedures are useful for estimating hearing sensitivity and for examining middle ear, cochlear, and VIIIth nerve or auditory brainstem pathway integrity (Gorga, Kaminski, Beauchaine, Jesteadt, & Neely, 1989; Stapells, Gravel, & Martin, 1995). These methods require no behavioral response from the child, although a child must be quiet (usually, in natural or sedated sleep) for varying amounts of time depending upon the procedure. Acoustic immittance procedures, specifically tympanometry, are useful for quantifying middle-ear function, and acoustic reflex threshold assessment can be used as a cross-check of auditory function. Evoked otoacoustic emissions are useful for examining cochlear (sensory) function. This measure is frequency-specific, and time- and cost-efficient. Evoked otoacoustic emissions are absent with hearing losses greater than 30 to 40 dB (Prieve, 1992; Robinette, 1992) and the technique has been used in children with autism (Grewe, Danhauer, Danhauer, & Thornton, 1994). The frequency-specific Auditory Brainstem Response (ABR) is the single most useful electrophysiologic procedure for use in estimating hearing thresholds and has been demonstrated to be highly correlated with behavioral hearing thresholds in children who hear normally and in children who have sensorineural hearing loss (Stapells *et al.,* 1995).

Audiologic assessment should not be delayed in the differential diagnosis of autism. It is recommended that audiologic assessment be completed at centers that have qualified and experienced professional personnel (pediatric audiologists) who have current test methods and technologies readily available. It is recommended that facilities without these components enter consortial arrangements with centers that are able to provide this type of comprehensive assessment of children with autism.

When hearing loss (conductive or sensorineural) is detected, the child should be referred to an otolaryngologist, but concerns raised at the *Level 1* screen regarding other developmental indicators ('red flags") for autism (e.g., lack of social relationships, unusual behaviors) must not be ignored. The audiologist, speech-language pathologist, and medical practitioner's follow-up of the child should include surveillance for indicators of autism. When appropriate, in-depth assessment (psychological, sensorimotor) should be recommended in order to address the potential co-occurrence of autism and hearing loss.

Transient, fluctuant conductive hearing loss associated with otitis media with effusion can co-occur in children with autism. Audiologic and medical follow-up for conductive hearing loss associated with recurrent otitis media is important in the long-term management of children with autism.

Lead Screening

Children with developmental delays who spend an extended period in the oral–motor stage of play (where everything "goes into their mouths") are at increased risk for lead toxicity especially in certain environments. The prevalence of pica in this group can result in high rates of substantial and often recurrent exposure to lead and, quite possibly, other metals (Shannon & Graef, 1997). Several studies report the neurobehavioral effects and behavioral toxicity of lead and its potential clinical relevance in patients with autism. Mean blood lead concentration was notably higher in 18 children with autism than in 16 nonautistic children or in 10 normal siblings; 44% of the autistic and psychotic children had blood lead levels greater than 2 standard deviations above the mean for normal controls (Cohen, Johnson, & Caparulo, 1976). In three of six reported cases of lead poisoning in children with autism, developmental deviance seemed to have been present before the possible impact of lead toxicity, while in two, the lead poisoning may have contributed to the onset or acceleration of developmental symptomatology (Accardo, Whitman, Caul, & Rolfe, 1988). A more recent chart review found that 17 children with autism were treated for plumbism over a 6-year period from 1987 to 1992. When compared to a randomly selected group of 30 children without autism who were treated during the same interval, the children with autism were significantly older at diagnosis, had a longer period of elevated blood lead levels during treatment, and 75% were subsequently reexposed despite close monitoring, environmental inspection, and either lead hazard reduction or alternative housing (Shannon & Graef, 1997). Therefore, all children with delays or who are at risk for autism should have a periodic lead screen until the pica disappears (Centers for Disease Control and Prevention, 1997; Shannon & Graef, 1997).

Specific Screening for Autism

All professionals involved in early child care (pediatricians, neurologists, psychiatrists, psychologists, audiologists, language pathologists, occupational therapists, and physical therapists) should be sufficiently familiar with the signs and symptoms of autism to recognize possible indicators (social, communicative, and behavioral) of the need for further diagnostic evaluation. It is important to be aware that children with autism often are referred for a variety of concerns, such as language delays, regulatory behavior problems in infancy, motor or sensory problems, social and behavioral problems, emotional disturbance, and learning problems.

There are new screening instruments in the field that focus on children with autism: the *Checklist for Autism in Toddlers* (CHAT; Baron-Cohen, Allen, & Gillberg, 1992; Baron-Cohen *et al.*, 1996), the *Pervasive Developmental Disorders Screening Test* (PDDST., Siegel, 1998), and for undiagnosed older verbal children, the *Australian Scale for Asperger's Syndrome* (Garnett & Attwood, 1998).

Checklist for Autism in Toddlers (CHAT; Baron-Cohen *et al.*, 1992; 1996) is designed to screen for autism at 18 months of age, and is also aimed at the primary care setting. The first section consists of a series of nine questions to be asked of the parent, such as whether the child ever demonstrates any pretend play. The second section consists of a series of five items to be observed or administered to the child by the provider during the visit, such as seeing whether the child looks where you point (joint attention), has any interest in pretend play, or is able to follow a command. Strengths of the CHAT include its ease of administration and its demonstrated specificity to symptoms of autism in 18-month-old infants. From both the initial study of siblings of children with Autistic Disorder and from the larger epidemiological study involving a population study of 16,000 18-month-old infants, virtually all the children failing the five-item criterion on the CHAT administered twice (1 month apart) were found to have Autistic Disorder when diagnosed at 20 and 42 months (Baron-Cohen *et al.*, 1992, 1996; Charman *et al.*, 1998; Cox *et al.*, 1999). However, the epidemiological study has indicated that the CHAT was less sensitive to milder symptoms of autism, as children later diagnosed with PDDNOS, Asperger, or atypical autism did not routinely fail the CHAT at 18 months. As a tool for identifying 18-month-olds at risk of autism from a normal population, the CHAT appears to be a useful tool, but not an entirely sufficient tool, for identifying the majority of children who will fall within the autistic spectrum.

An unpublished variation on the CHAT is *The Developmental Checklist*, currently under development, which expands the CHAT into a 30-item checklist that a parent alone can fill out in about 10 minutes (Robins, Fein, Barton, & Liss, 1999).

Pervasive Developmental Disorders Screening Test-Stage 1 (PDDST; Siegel, 1998) is a clinically derived parent questionnaire, divided into three Stages, each of which is targeted at a different level of screening. PDDST-Stage 1 is aimed for use in the primary care setting, with items aimed incrementally from birth to 36 months of age. Unlike the CHAT, this instrument rates positive as well as negative symptoms, and includes a number of questions concerning regression. In addition to sampling similar areas as other scales, the PDDST also samples temperament, sensory responses, motor stereotypies, attention, attachment, and peer interest. Parental report of stereotypic behaviors is probably more accurate than observation, due to the greater length of observation and varied environments. The tool was developed in several steps, beginning with a review of clinical records of a large number of children with autism. Test–retest and interrater (between parents) reliabilities were then used to identify problematic items. Follow-up clinical diagnosis at age 5 was used to determine the accuracy of screening. Finally, the instrument was administered to a large number of children with mixed diagnoses to set cutoff scores and algorithms; this work is ongoing. A significant cutoff of three affirmative answers in PDDST-Stage 1 has been established for further diagnostic consideration of an Autistic Spectrum Disorder. This instrument has not yet been published but is available (see Appendix).

Australian Scale for Asperger's Syndrome (Garnett & Attwood, 1998) is a parent or teacher rating scale for high-functioning older children on the autistic spectrum who remain undetected at school age. It consists of 24 questions rated with a score from 1 to 6, plus a checklist of 10 additional yes or no behavioral characteristics. If the answer is yes to the majority of questions in the scale and most of the ratings are between 2 and 6, a referral for a diagnostic assessment of autism should be made.

Referral to Early Intervention or Local School District

As mandated by Public Law 99-457, and reauthorized as Public Law 105-17: Individuals with Disabilities Education Act- IDEA (1997), referral for early intervention must be initiated by the *Level 1* professional. Children less than 36 months of age should be referred to the zero-to-three service system in their community; children ages 36 months and older should be referred to the local school district.

Level 2: Diagnosis and Evaluation of Autism

Once a child screens positive, he/she then should be referred for an appropriate assessment by an experienced clinician, one with expertise in the diagnosis of developmental disorders. Although numerous studies show that autism can be reliably diagnosed in preschool children, experienced clinicians are usually necessary for accurate and appropriate diagnosis (Gillberg, 1990; Lord, Storoschuk, Rutter, & Pickles, 1993; Volkmar *et al.*, 1994). Many children who screen positive and enter into more comprehensive assessments may NOT, in the end, necessarily be considered to have autism but may have a range of other disorders—any of which may merit intervention in their own right. Accordingly, it is important that evaluators have a range of experience in the diagnosis and assessment of developmental disabilities. In some cases children may not come to diagnosis in the preschool years and it is important that screening encompass children in the older school-age group as well.

It is therefore the consensus of this Panel that *Level 2* evaluations should be performed only by professionals who have specific expertise in the evaluation and treatment of autism.

At the present time no biological marker or simple laboratory test or procedure exists for the diagnosis of autism and related conditions. Clinicians must, accordingly, rely on their clinical judgment, aided by guides to diagnosis such as DSM-IV and ICD-10, as well as by the results of various assessment instruments, rating scales, or checklists. The latter instruments do NOT substitute for the diagnosis by an experienced clinician.

Interdisciplinary collaboration and consultation are indicated in the diagnosis and assessment of children with autism and related difficulties. The needs for service from the various providers will vary depending on the needs of the child, family, symptomatic presentation, clinical context, and so forth (Volkmar, Cook, Pomeroy, Realmuto, & Tanguay, in press). The efforts may involve numerous specialists, including psychologists, neurologists, speech pathologists and audiologists, pediatricians, child psychiatrists, occupational therapists, and physical therapists as well as educators or special educators. When assessments are interdisciplinary in nature, it is critical that the service providers coordinate their work to avoid duplication of effort and maximize efficient use of time. It also is essential that one provider assume a major role as the "Coordinator of the Assessment."

Research from many studies suggests that the autistic spectrum disorders are not qualitatively different from Autistic Disorder, but differ primarily in terms of severity or the presence of repetitive or sensory behaviors. This distinction is often confounded by higher verbal skills in individuals with autistic spectrum disorders other than Autistic Disorder. It is important to insure that any individual with an autistic spectrum disorder receive adequate assessments and appropriate diagnoses. Factors that are not specific to autism, including degree of language impairment, mental handicap, and presence of nonspecific behavior disorders such as overactivity and aggression, significantly affect outcome and treatment of individuals with autism. Diagnostic evaluations must address these issues and provide continued monitoring of nonspecific as well as autism-related impairments across development.

In addition to its important role in diagnosis, a comprehensive assessment has an essential role in treatment planning. Although the focus of this paper is on screening and diagnosis, the other important functions of assessment and treatment are essential. As a practical matter, the assessment should be concerned not only with diagnosis as such but with obtaining information on patterns of strengths and weaknesses important to intervention. Indeed the results of the formal assessments are often not as important as the less formal, but clinically informative, observations of the child during the assessment. Parents should be intimately involved in this process. The assessment should also be careful to note areas of strength as well as weakness.

Expanded Medical and Neurological Evaluation

Birth, Medical, Developmental, and Family Histories

This evaluation would expand on that already performed at *Level 1*. Besides delineating social, communication, and behavior characteristics, the focus should be on the search for acquired brain injury, comorbid conditions, or other medical or neurologic difficulties common to autism.

Birth History. An increase of only *mild* obstetrical complications was noted in the deliveries of autistic individuals, which was independent of maternal age or parity, making a causal relationship unlikely (Bolton *et al.*, 1997). Specifically, no association was found between autism and gestational age or occurrence of vaginal bleeding, infection, diabetes, toxemia, maternal age, or prior abortions (Bolton *et al.*, 1997; Cryan, Byrne, O'Donovan, & O'Callaghan, 1996; Ghaziuddin, Shakal, & Tsai, 1995; Piven *et al.*, 1993; Rapin, 1996a). There was also no association between autism and birth weight, induction of labor, breech presentation, forceps or cesarian delivery, prolonged labor, neonatal depression, need for intensive care or mechanical ventilation, neonatal seizures, or prolonged neonatal hospitalization (Bolton et al., 1997; Fein et al., 1997; Piven et al., 1993; Rapin, 1996a). Although several prior studies indicated a possible association between autism and increased obstetrical risk factors, although mild, these have not been borne out (Bryson, Smith, & Eastwood, 1988b; Deykin & MacMahon, 1980; Finegan & Quarrington, 1979; Folstein & Rutter, 1977a; Folstein & Rutter, 1977b; Gillberg & Gillberg, 1983; Levy, Zoltak, & Saelens, 1988; Lord, Mulloy, Wendelboe, & Schopler, 1991; Mason-Brothers et al., 1987, 1990; Nelson, 1991; Tsai, 1987). Many of these studies did not correct for the strong influence of maternal parity (e.g., reproductive stoppage effect), which accounted for the differences in at least two studies (Lord et al., 1991; Piven et al., 1993).

Medical and Developmental History. Detailed history should be aimed at determining developmental milestones, developmental regression at any age, identifying any encephalopathic events, history of attention deficit disorder, seizure disorder, depression, mania, troublesome behaviors such as irritability, self-injury, sleep or eating disturbances, and pica for possible lead exposure.

Family History. Autism, mental retardation, fragile X syndrome, and tuberous sclerosis should specifically be inquired about in nuclear and extended family because of their implications regarding the need for chromosomal or genetic evaluation. In addition, the presence of affective disorder and anxiety disorder should be investigated, as these disorders have been shown to be increased in families of autistic individuals and increase the burden to the family (Bolton et al., 1994; DeLong, 1994; DeLong & Nohria, 1994; Fombonne, Bolton, Prior, Jordan, & Rutter, 1997; Piven et al., 1990, 1994).

Autism: Family studies have shown that there is a 50- to 100-fold increase in the rate of autism in first-degree relatives (Rutter, Bailey, Simonoff, & Pickles, 1997; Simonoff, 1998). Recent family studies have shown that first-degree relatives of autistic probands have elevated rates of social difficulties, characterized by social withdrawal or awkwardness, and have a higher incidence of cognitive and executive function deficits, anxiety, and affective disorders (Bailey, Palferman, Heavey, & Le Couteur, 1998b; DeLong, 1994; DeLong &, Nohria, 1994; Hughes, Leboyer, & Bouvard, 1997; Piven et al., 1990, 1991a, 1994, 1997). Extended relatives in both simplex and multiplex families (i.e., those with more than one autistic child) had a higher rate of social and communication deficits and stereotyped behaviors than did

relatives of children with Down syndrome (Bolton et al., 1994; Piven, Palmer, Jacobi, Childress, & Arndt, 1997a). These impairments were milder but qualitatively very similar to autism, with relatively normal intellectual function (IQ). In addition, first-degree relatives demonstrated higher verbal than nonverbal IQ scores, with significant discrepancies noted between the scores (Fombonne et al., 1997). The first twin study of 11 monozygotic (MZ) pairs reported a concordance rate of over 36% for Infantile Autism, with no concordance in 10 dizygotic (DZ) twin pairs (Folstein & Rutter, 1977a, 1977b). However, a total of 82% of these MZ and 10% of the DZ twin pairs were concordant for some form of cognitive, social, or language deficits. A recent study of 28 MZ twin pairs (including the original 11 pairs) showed a concordance rate of 60% for DSM-IV Autistic Disorder, 71% for the broader spectrum of PDD or Atypical Autism, and 92% for an even broader phenotype of social and communication deficits with stereotyped behaviors that nonetheless were clearly differentiated from normal (Bailey et al., 1995; Le Couteur et al., 1996).

Fragile X: Numerous early reports noted a highly significant association between fragile X (FraX) and autism, in up to 25% of autistic individuals (Blomquist et al., 1985; Brown et al., 1986; Gillberg & Wahlstrom, 1985; Wahlstrom, Gillberg, Gustavson, & Holmgren, 1986), although this association was and remains controversial (I. L. Cohen et al., 1991). While other studies report a much lower incidence of FraX (3–7%) in patients with autism (Bailey et al., 1993a; Bolton & Rutter, 1990; Piven, Gayle, Landa, Wzorek, & Folstein, 1991b), another study found no evidence of FraX using cytogenetic (not DNA analysis) techniques (Hashimoto, Shimizu, & Kawasaki, 1993). Molecular genetic analyses of a large cohort of autistic individuals found FraX in only three siblings: one girl with Autistic Disorder, her brother with Atypical Autism, and a second brother without autistic features but with a learning disability (Klauck et al., 1997). Because the presence of FraX genotype did not correlate with the autism phenotype, they concluded that the association between autism and fragile X does not exist. Therefore, although few children with autism have fragile X syndrome, children with fragile X syndrome often have autistic symptomatology (Feinstein & Reiss, 1998).

Tuberous Sclerosis Complex: Tuberous sclerosis complex (TSC) is a neurocutaneous disorder that also affects other organ systems, including the heart and kidneys. TSC has been linked to two distinct gene loci: TSC1 to chromosome 9 (9q34) and TSC2 to chromosome 16 (16p13.3) (OMIM™, 1997). The phenotypes of TSC1 and TSC2 have been considered identical; how-

29

ever, a recent study noted that mental handicap and sporadic rather than familial occurrence may be more frequently associated with the TSC2 genotype (Jones *et al.*, 1997; OMIM™, 1997), although this finding may also represent an ascertainment bias. Depigmented macules (shaped like an ash-leaf (Fitzpatrick, 1991)) are usually the first visible sign of the disease. They are often visualized only with the use of an ultraviolet light (Wood's lamp). Facial angiofibroma, formerly called adenoma sebaceum, and shagreen patches over the lower back are also characteristic, but often do not appear until late childhood or early adolescence (Webb, Clarke, Fryer, & Osborne, 1996). The major intracerebral lesions are the tubers which consist of histiogenic malformations of both neuronal and glial elements with giant heterotopic cells. They are characteristically located in the subependymal regions and in the cortex, predominantly in the frontal lobes (Braffman & Naidich, 1994; Harrison & Bolton, 1997; Truhan & Filipek, 1993). TSC has been strongly associated with autism. Estimates suggest that 17% to over 60% of mentally retarded individuals with TSC are also autistic, most commonly co-occurring with epilepsy (Curatolo *et al.*, 1991; Dykens & Volkmar, 1997; Gillberg, Gillberg, & Ahlsen, 1994; Harrison & Bolton, 1997; Hunt & Shepherd, 1993; Riikonen & Simell, 1990; Smalley, Smith, & Tanguay, 1991; Smalley, Tanguay, Smith, & Gutierrez, 1992). In contrast, the number of autistic individuals with TSC has been estimated to be between 0.4 and 3% in epidemiological studies (Dykens & Volkmar, 1997; Gillberg *et al.*, 1991; Lotter, 1967; Olsson, Steffenburg, & Gillberg, 1988; Ritvo *et al.*, 1990; Smalley *et al.*, 1992). This rate increased to 8 to 14% in autistic subjects with epilepsy (Gillberg, 1991; Riikonen & Amnell, 1981). A recent report noted an inverse correlation between IQ and the number of tubers identified on MRI in a small cohort of individuals with TSC; those individuals with both TSC and autism not only had the most tubers, but also had tubers located in the temporal lobes, a finding not seen in nonautistic subjects with TSC (Bolton & Griffiths, 1997).

Pertinent Positives on the Physical and Neurological Examination

Examination of persons with autism may require more time because of the likelihood of poor cooperation by a patient with impaired communication and behavioral problems. Severe unexplained behavioral changes may be due to an undiagnosed intercurrent illness (e.g., dental abscess, gastric ulcer, or ear infection) or an unrecognized injury. In some individuals, an adequate medical or dental examination may require sedation.

Head Circumference. The head circumference in children with autism is larger on average than in typically developing children (Bailey *et al.*, 1995; Bolton *et al.*, 1994; Davidovitch, Patterson, & Gartside, 1996; Lainhart *et al.*, 1997; Woodhouse *et al.*, 1996). The same has been noted with postmortem brain weights (Bailey *et al.*, 1993b, 1998a; Bauman, 1992b, 1996; Bauman & Kemper, 1994, 1997; Courchesne, Muller, & Saitoh, 1999). Only a small proportion of children with autism have frank macrocephaly with head circumferences above the 98th percentile, but the distribution of the measures is clearly shifted upward with the mean in autism falling at about the 75th percentile (Bailey *et. al.*, 1995; Bolton *et al.*, 1994; Davidovitch *et al.*, 1996; Filipek *et al.*, 1992b; Lainhart *et al.*, 1997; Rapin, 1996b; Woodhouse et al., 1996). It also appears that a large head size may not necessarily be present at birth, but may appear in early to mid-childhood due to an increased rate of brain growth (Lainhart *et al.*, 1997; Mason-Brothers *et al.*, 1987, 1990). The phenomenon of a larger head size without frank neuropathology in children with autism is widely acknowledged (Bailey *et al.*, 1995; Bolton *et al.*, 1994; Davidovitch *et al.*, 1996; Lainhart *et al.*, 1997; Rapin, 1996b; Woodhouse *et al.*, 1996). Barring lateralizing signs on the remainder of the examination, routine neuroimaging for the sole finding of a head circumference greater than the 98th percentile in an autistic individual is not warranted (Filipek, 1996, 1999; Filipek, Kennedy, & Caviness, 1992a; Minshew, 1996b; Minshew & Dombrowski, 1994).

General Examination. Given the high prevalence of autism in TSC, an examination using a hand-held ultraviolet light (Wood's lamp) should be performed on every child presenting with possible autism as an initial screen for tuberous sclerosis (Reich, Lenoir, Malvy, Perrot, & Sauvage, 1997; Smalley *et al.*, 1992). Also, unusual or dysmorphic features (of facies, limb, stature, etc) should be noted, for, if present, they suggest the need for consultation with a geneticist.

Mental Status Examination. The mental status examination should include the evaluation of social interactions, play, language, and communicative function. Social interactions should be queried if observation in the office proves inconclusive. Probes should be included for age-appropriate friendships, who initiates contact with the friends (child or parent), interest in other children, and the role within the friendship (e.g., leader of much younger peers or follower of much older peers with little or no same-aged peers). Deficient play skills are a hallmark of autism, independent of IQ (Rapin, 1996b). An adequate period of observation of the child's use of age-appropriate miniature toys in the examination room is essential to discriminate between simple manipulative (banging or mouthing) or stereotypic (lining up) use of toys, and actual functional or symbolic (using one item to represent another) pretend play (Sigman & Ungerer, 1984; Stone, Lemanek, Fishel, Fernandez, & Altemeier, 1990). For example, classifying or sorting miniature figures, which may be subtle, is a typical stereotypic behavior of higher functioning children with autism which may be mistaken for appropriate play if only given a brief glance.

Cranial Nerve Examination. Clinical cranial nerve abnormalities were only infrequently noted in a large sample of children with autism (Bauman, 1992a; Rapin, 1996b).

Motor Examination. Impairments of gross and fine motor function have been reported in autistic individuals, and are more severe in those with lower IQ (Rapin, 1996b). Hypotonia was found in about 25% of 176 children with autism and in 33% of 110 nonautistic mentally retarded children, whereas spasticity was found in less than 5% of either group (exclusionary criteria for this sample included the presence of lateralizing gross motor findings). Limb apraxia was noted in almost 30% of autistic children with normal IQ, in 75% of retarded autistic children, and in 56% of the nonautistic retarded control group. A third significant finding was the presence of observed motor stereotypies in over 40% of children with autism (in contrast to a much higher prevalence by parental report), and in over 60% of those with low IQ, but in only 13% of the nonautistic control group.

Autism Diagnostic Tools

The diagnosis of autism as distinct from other developmental disabilities requires a comprehensive multidisciplinary approach. The evaluation should include measures of parental report, child observation and interactions, and clinical judgment. Assessments should include cognitive, adaptive behavior, and diagnostic measures.

Diagnostic Parental Interviews/Questionnaires

The *Gilliam Autism Rating Scale* (GARS; Gilliam, 1995) is a checklist designed to be used by parents, teachers, and professionals to help both identify and estimate the severity of symptoms of autism in individuals age 3 to 22 years. Items are based on DSM-IV (APA, 1994) and are grouped into four subtests (a) stereotyped behaviors (b) communication, (c) social interaction, and (d) an optional subtest which describes development in the first 3 years of life. This tool provides a global rating of autistic symptomatology.

The *Parent Interview for Autism* (PIA; Stone & Hogan, 1993) is a structured interview designed to gather diagnostically relevant information from parents of young children suspected of having autism. The PIA consists of 118 items, organized into 11 dimensions assessing various aspects of social behavior, communicative functioning, repetitive activities, and sensory behaviors. Items are phrased as questions about specific observable behaviors, and ratings of the frequency of occurrence are obtained. Internal consistency and test–retest reliability were adequate, and concurrent validity with the DSM (APA, 1994) and the Childhood Autism Rating Scale (CARS; Schopler, Reichler, & Rochen-Renner, 1988) was demonstrated. Significant group differences between young children with autism and young children with developmental delays or mental retardation were obtained for the total score as well as the dimensions of Relating, Imitation, Peer Interactions, Imaginative Play, Language Understanding, and Nonverbal Communication. The PIA takes about 45 minutes to administer.

The *Pervasive Developmental Disorders Screening Test- Stage 2* (PDDST; Siegel, 1998). The PDDST is a clinically derived parent questionnaire divided into three Stages, each of which is targeted at a different level of screening. Further details on this instrument were included earlier under Level 1 Screening. PDDST-Stage 2 was developed for Developmental Disorders Clinics, and PDDST-Stage 3 for Autism or PDD Clinics. Significant cutoffs have been established for further diagnostic consideration of an Autistic Spectrum Disorder: four affirmative answers in PDDST-Stage 2, and six affirmative answers in PDDST-Stage 3. This instrument has not yet been published but is available (see Appendix).

The *Autism Diagnostic Interview-Revised* (ADI-R); Le Couteur *et al.*, 1989; Lord *et al.*, 1993, 1997; Lord, Rutter, & Le Couteur, 1994) is a comprehensive structured parent interview that probes for autistic symptoms in the spheres of social relatedness, communication, and ritualistic or perseverative behaviors. It permits DSM-IV (APA, 1994) and ICD-10 (WHO, 1992, 1993) diagnoses within the autistic spectrum, with definitive threshold scores for the diagnosis of Autistic Disorder. The ADI-R (and ADOS-G) are currently the "gold standard" diagnostic instruments in all appropriate autism research protocols. Because administration of the ADI-R takes approximately 1 hour and requires specific training and validation procedures, its utility to primary care or clinical specialty professionals is probably less than its import in the research community.

Diagnostic Observation Instruments

The Childhood Autism Rating Scale (CARS; Schopler et al., 1988) is a 15-item structured interview and observation instrument which is suitable for use with any child over 24 months of age. Each of the 15 items uses a 7-point rating scale to indicate the degree to which the child's behavior deviates from an age-appropriate norm; in addition, it distinguishes mild-to-moderate from severe autism. The CARS is widely recognized and used as a reliable instrument for the diagnosis of autism, and takes approximately 30 to 45 minutes to administer (Schopler, Reichler, DeVellis, & Daly, 1980).

The Screening Tool for Autism in Two-Year-Olds (STAT; Stone, 1998a, 1998b) is a theoretically and empirically derived, interactive measure to be administered to children ages 24 to 35 months by various early childhood professionals. The STAT, still in development, is designed to differentiate autism from other developmental disorders, thus it is a Level 2 screening instrument. In a 20-minute play interaction involving 12 activities, the tool samples three areas: play (both pretend and reciprocal social play), motor imitation, and nonverbal communicative development. The tasks used on the STAT were those that best differentiated between children with autism and those with other developmental disorders in studies of matched groups of two-year-olds on a wide range of measures. There is a manual with clear instructions for administration and scoring. In a pilot study involving 40 children, the tool correctly classified 100% of children with autism (n = 8) and 97% of children with other developmental delays (n = 32) using a criterion of failure on two of the three areas. Thus, demonstrating very strong sensitivity and specificity. Current work on the tool is focused on the empirical determination of best cutoffs and algorithm scoring.

The Autism Diagnostic Observation Schedule-Generic (ADOS-G; DiLavore, Lord, & Rutter, 1995; Lord, 1998; Lord *et al.*, 1989) is a semi-structured observational assessment in four modules that includes investigator-directed activities to evaluate communication, reciprocal social interaction, play, stereotypic behavior, restricted interests, and other abnormal behaviors, in autistic individuals ranging from nonverbal preschool children to verbal autistic adults. It takes approximately 30 to 45 minutes to administer. It also permits DSM-1V (APA, 1994) and ICD-10 (WHO, 1992, 1993) diagnoses within the autistic spectrum, with definitive threshold scores for the diagnosis of Autistic Disorder. As with the ADI-R, administration of the ADOS-G requires specific training and validation procedures. As mentioned earlier, the ADOS-G and ADI-R are the two "gold standard" diagnostic instruments in all appropriate autism research protocols. Because administration of the ADOS-G takes less time than the ADI-R, many autism specialty professionals are using this instrument in their clinical practices; albeit predominantly abroad where clinical time is not as limited as with managed care in the US.

Differential Diagnosis of Autistic Spectrum Disorders

The differentiation of autism from other developmental disorders is accomplished during *Level 2*. Using the data collected from the various evaluations, professionals must also determine the possible existence of comorbid disorders. The differential diagnosis of autism includes consideration of mental retardation not associated with autism, specific developmental disorders (e.g., of language), and other psychiatric conditions (Volkmar *et al.*, in press).

Mental retardation or *borderline intelligence* often coexists with autism. Individuals with severe and profound mental retardation may exhibit various characteristics that are often associated with autism, particularly stereotyped movements.

Specific developmental disorders, particularly developmental language disorders, may mimic autism and related conditions. Usually in children with language disorders, the primary deficits are in the area of language or communication, and social skills are typically well-preserved.

Schizophrenia occasionally has its onset in early childhood. Usually there is a history of previously relatively normal development with the onset of characteristic hallucinations and delusions typical of schizophrenia. However, a lack of typical social development is often part of the premorbid history.

Selective mutism sometimes is confused with autism and related conditions. In selective mutism the child's ability to speak in some situations is preserved, but the child is mute in other situations. The history and presentation are quite different from that of autism. Although it is the case that children with autism are often mute, their mutism is never "selective" nature.

Stereotyped movement disorder is characterized by motor mannerisms (stereotypies) and the presence of mental retardation. A diagnosis of stereotyped movement disorder is not made if the child meets criteria for one of the pervasive developmental disorders.

Dementia occasionally has its onset in childhood. In some cases the child will fulfill criteria for childhood disintegrative disorder, in which case that diagnosis as well as the specific medical diagnosis causing the dementia can be made. The typical pattern of dementia of childhood onset is one of progressive deterioration in mental and motor functioning.

Obsessive compulsive disorder (OCD) presents in some children with unusual interests and behaviors. However, social skills are preserved, as are language and communication skills. When social skill deficits or communication deficits are present in OCD, they are qualitatively different from those found in autism.

Schizoid personality disorder is characterized by relative isolation, with the ability to relate normally in some contexts. However, personality disorders are not diagnosed before the age of 18 years by current DSM-IV standards (APA, 1994).

Avoidant personality disorder is characterized by anxiety in dealing with social situations.

Reactive attachment disorder usually presents with a history of very severe neglect or abuse; the social deficits of reactive attachment disorder tend to remit dramatically in response to a more appropriate environment.

Specific Evaluations to Determine the Developmental Profile

Speech–Language–Communication Evaluation

Language pathologists are independent health care providers who have responsibilities at the levels of screening *(Level 1)*, diagnosis and evaluation *(Level 2)* of autism. Evaluation at both levels may be accomplished in a single session rather than in discrete segments. Standardized speech, language, and communication assessments conducted in formal testing situations may provide important information about specific parameters of speech and language functioning. However, such assessments may provide only limited information about social-pragmatic abilities (i.e., use of language and communicative abilities in social contexts), which are characteristically limited in the autistic spectrum disorders (Allen, 1989; Allen & Rapin, 1992; Lord & Paul, 1997; Stone, Ousley, Yoder, Hogan, & Hepburn, 1997; Wetherby, Prizant, & Hutchinson, 1998; Wetherby, Schuler, & Prizant, 1997; Wetherby, Yonclas, & Bryan, 1989). Therefore, a variety of strategies should be used, including direct assessment, naturalistic observation, and interviewing significant others, including parents and educators, who can be invaluable sources of information (Prizant & Wetherby, 1993; Stone & Caro-Martinez, 1990). Each of these strategies has the potential to provide qualitatively different information about a child's speech, language, and communicative abilities

that may ultimately be integrated to develop a profile for differential diagnosis and intervention planning. Observations should include a child's interactions with a variety of persons including family members and peers, as well as professionals, because variability in communicative functioning across persons and settings is to be expected (Wetherby *et al.*, 1997). Specific domains should be addressed in a comprehensive assessment for both preverbal and verbal individuals, taking into account their age, cognitive level, and socioemotional abilities (Wetherby *et al.*, 1998).

Receptive Language and Communication. Clinical experience suggests that caregivers or professionals often assume that a child understands others' communicative signals and may interpret a lack of response to gestures or speech as noncompliant or uncooperative behavior. Children's ability to respond to and use communicative gestures and vocalizations should be documented, with and without the support of situational cues. True linguistic comprehension is evidenced when children can comprehend words without situational or nonverbal cues, especially when words refer to persons, objects, and events outside of the immediate environment. At higher levels of ability, assessment should address comprehension of different simple and complex sentence types (e.g., negatives, questions, causal, conditional), of ongoing discourse (e.g., ability to understand a story or sequence of events), and of nonliteral language (i.e., idioms, sarcasm). Guidelines and procedures for more in-depth assessment of comprehension for preverbal and verbal individuals are available (Lund & Duchan, 1993; Miller & Paul, 1995).

Expressive Language and Communication. The primary focus in this domain is documentation of (a) communicative means, the behaviors by which a child expresses intentions, emotions, and physiological states, and (b) communicative functions, the purposes for which a child communicates (Prizant & Wetherby, 1993).

Communicative means in preintentional children may include a variety of nonverbal and vocal behaviors such as body posture and movement, facial expression, directed gaze and gaze aversion, and vocalizations. In developmentally more advanced children, intentional use of idiosyncratic (e.g., physically leading others) and conventional (e.g., pointing, nodding, waving) gestures, as well as vocalizations and emerging word forms should be documented (Schuler, Prizant, & Wetherby, 1997). Children with autism have been found to have a limited repertoire of conventional gestures and vocalizations (Stone *et al.*, 1997; Wetherby *et al.*, 1998), even when compared to children with other developmental language disorders.

Communicative functions expressed preverbally or verbally may include communicating for relatively nonsocial purposes to have immediate needs met (e.g., requesting objects or actions, protesting), or for more social purposes such as to bring attention to oneself (e.g., requesting social routines, greeting, calling) and communicating to bring others' attention to interesting objects or events (e.g., pointing to or commenting on interesting events). Young children with autism communicate primarily for relatively nonsocial purposes when compared to children with developmental language disorders (Mundy, Sigman, & Kasari, 1990; Wetherby *et al.*, 1989, 1998). In addition, the rate of communicative acts and a child's ability to persist in repairing communication breakdowns should also be documented. Assessment should also document forms and functions of unconventional nonverbal (e.g., disruptive behaviors) and verbal (e.g., immediate and delayed echolalia, perseverative speech, incessant questioning) communicative behavior (Carr & Durand, 1985; Prizant & Rydell, 1993).

For verbal children able to engage in conversation, collection and analysis of spontaneous language samples supplement scores on formal language tests (see below). It provides information about a child's narrative and conversational discourse, including ability to initiate, maintain, and terminate conversational interactions following acceptable conventions of discourse, the ability to maintain topic and follow topics introduced by others, and to take the perspective of others by providing sufficient, but not excessive, amounts of background or known information (Prizant, Wetherby, Schuler, & Rydell, 1997).

Voice and Speech Production. Some young children with autism may not be able to acquire and use speech as a primary mode of communication, due to severity of cognitive impairment, severe to profound hearing loss, or severe language comprehension disorders. Less frequently, specific neuromotor speech disorders are involved, including developmental verbal dyspraxia, a dysfunction in the ability to plan the coordinated movements to produce intelligible sequences of speech sounds, or dysarthria, a weakness or lack of control of the oral musculature. For nonspeaking individuals, or for those with speech of limited intelligibility, assessment should address quality and variety of communicative vocalizations and oral–motor abilities (e.g., chewing, swallowing). Other aspects of speech to evaluate in more verbal individuals include prosody, volume, and fluency of speech production, especially when disturbance in these parameters negatively impact on communicative competence.

It is recommended that tests be used for speech–language–communication assessments (Crais, 1995;

Wetherby & Prizant, 1992) that (1) focus on functions of communication; (2) analyze preverbal communication (gestures, gaze, vocalizations); (3) assess social-affective signaling; (4) profile social, communicative and symbolic abilities; (5) directly assess the child, not only rely on parental report; (6) permit observation of initiated and spontaneous communication, and (7) directly involve caregivers during the assessment (Wetherby & Prizant, 1992). The most widely used tests for children with language and communication disorders are listed in Table V, which was adapted from Wetherby and Prizant (1992) and Crais (1995). The numbers in Table V referring to the relative strengths and weaknesses reflect the seven points outlined above.

Cognitive Evaluation

Although the *Level 1* professional may have obtained a rough estimate of the child's cognitive status (mental age) by using screening tools or problem-solving milestone charts from preprinted well-child forms and textbooks, knowing the child's cognitive status is important in determining his overall level of functioning. This is, in turn, important when trying to establish a discrepancy between the child's level of social function and the overall cognitive and adaptive function, a key criterion in the diagnosis of autism.

As is true of language pathologists, clinical psychologists and developmental pediatricians are independent health care providers who have responsibilities at both levels of screening and diagnosis, which may or may not be accomplished in a single session rather than as discrete segments. Additional visits may be necessary for the child to adapt to change as well as to the newness of the procedures in order to optimize the chances that the results accurately represent the child's abilities. While the diagnosis of autism is based ultimately on clinical symptoms and early history, the results of cognitive assessment may assist in differential diagnosis, as well as provide important information for planning intervention and evaluating its effects. Research has demonstrated specific profiles on cognitive batteries, with spared performance on tasks that rely on rote, mechanical, or perceptual processes, and deficient performance on tasks requiring higher-order conceptual processes, reasoning, interpretation, integration or abstraction (Minshew & Goldstein, 1998). This pattern is present across multiple cognitive domains, with dissociations between simple and complex processing demonstrated in areas of language, memory, executive function, motor function, reading, mathematics, and

Table V. Strengths and Weaknesses of Specific Language Instruments[a]

Instrument	Strengths	Weaknesses
Evaluation of only receptive language		
Peabody Picture Vocabulary Test-Revised (PPVT-R; Dunn & Dunn, 1981)	5	1–4, 6–7
Receptive One-Word Picture Vocabulary Test-Revised (ROWPVT-R; Gardner, 1990b)	5	1–4, 6–7
Evaluation of only expressive language		
Expressive One-Word Picture Vocabulary Test-Revised (EOWPVT-R; Gardner, 1990a)	5	1–4, 6–7
Evaluation of both receptive and expressive language		
Birth to Three Developmental Scales (Bangs & Dodson, 1986)	2, 4 1, 3, 5 limited	6, 7
Clinical Evaluation of Language Fundamentals-3 (CELF-3; Semel, Wiig, & Secord, 1995)	5	1–4, 6–7
Communication and Symbolic Behavior Scales (CSBS; Wetherby & Prizant, 1993)	1–6	7 limited
MacArthur Communcative Development Inventories (MCDI; Fenson *et al.*, 1993)	1–3, 5–7	4
Preschool Language Scale-3 (PLS; Zimmerman, Steiner, & Pond, 1992)	1, 5	2–4, 6–7
Receptive-Expressive-Emergent-Language Scale-Revised (REEL-R; Bzoch & League, 1991)	1, 2 limited 5	3, 4, 6, 7
Rosetti Infant-Toddler Language Scale (1990)	1–6	7 limited
Sequenced Inventory of Communication Development (SICD; Hedrick, Prather, & Tobin, 1984)	1, 2 & 6 limited 5	3, 4, 7

[a] The numbers referring to the strengths and weaknesses are based on the seven points outlined in the text. This table was adapted from Wetherby and Prizant (1992) and Crais (1995).

perspective-taking (Klinger & Dawson, 1995; Minshew, Goldstein, Taylor, & Siegel, 1994; Ozonoff, personal communication; Reed & Peterson, 1990; Rumsey & Hamburger, 1988). However, few direct comparison studies between autism and other disorders have been conducted and it is possible that other disorders may share some aspects of this information-processing profile, which accounts for the differences in behavioral profile.

In terms of intellectual assessment, the Wechsler Intelligence Scale for Children/WISC-III (1991), and the Wechsler Adult Intelligence Scale/WAIS-III (1997) are the tests of choice for higher functioning and older individuals with relatively good verbal language. Numerous studies have demonstrated a particular pattern characteristic of autism: performance IQ (PIQ) higher than verbal IQ (VIQ) and specific inter-subtest scatter, with Block Design typically the highest subtest and Comprehension usually the lowest (see Lincoln, Allen, & Kilmasian, 1995; cited in Lincoln, Allen, & Kilman, 1995a. However, the PIQ–VIQ split is severity dependent. When Full-scale (FSIQ) and VIQ are both above 70, 80% of autistic individuals will have no sig-

nificant VIQ–PIQ disparity, and the remainder are evenly divided between those with PIQ>VIQ and those with PIQ<VIQ (Siegel, Minshew, & Goldstein, 1996). Thus, there is substantial variability in the intellectual profiles of people with autism. However, although these patterns may be typical, they are by no means universal and cannot be used for diagnostic or differential diagnostic purposes. No cognitive pattern confirms or excludes a diagnosis of autism.

Intellectual testing is essential for educational planning and, for some children, assists in projecting the long-term level of disability. It is usually beneficial to conduct these evaluations prior to entry into kindergarten, and to collaborate with educational professionals, including school psychologists, in order to address issues related to curriculum planning and school performance issues often addressed by school psychologists. In autism, however, it should be recognized that the predictive validity of such testing is not necessarily high.

There are particular concerns about the validity of testing younger, lower functioning, and nonverbal children. It is critical that care be taken in choosing which intellectual test to administer to lower functioning or nonverbal individual with autism (Groden & Mann, 1988; Johnson-Martin, 1988; Klin *et al.*, 1997; Watson & Marcus, 1988). It is recommended that tests be used which (1) are appropriate for both mental age and chronological age; (2) provide a full range (in the lower direction) of standard scores; (3) sample both verbal and nonverbal intellectual skills; (4) measure and score separately verbal and nonverbal skills; (5) provide an overall index of ability; and (6) have norms which are current and relatively independent of social function. With these principles in mind, the most appropriate and widely used intellectual tests for younger, low- or nonverbal individuals with autism are listed in Table VI.

Clinical judgment is required to properly interpret the findings of these measures for the purpose of differential diagnosis. Additional information regarding assessment and interpretation of psychological measures is provided in other resources (Jacobson & Mulick, 1996; Marcus, Lansing, & Schopler, 1993; Marcus & Stone, 1993).

Adaptive Behavior Evaluation

It is essential that a measure of adaptive function (the capability for self-sufficiency in acticities of daily living) be collected by the psychologist for any child evaluated for an associated mental handicap. Diagnosis of mental retardation relies upon both subaverage

intellectual functioning (IQ < 70) and concurrent deficits in adaptive functioning (APA, 1994).

The Vineland Adaptive Behavior Scales (VABS; Sparrow, Balla, & Cicchetti, 1984b) are considered to be the most widely used instrument to assess adaptive behavior (Klin *et al.*, 1997). The scales offer an estimate of adaptive development in the domains of Socialization (interpersonal relationships, play and leisure time, and coping skills); Daily Living Skills (personal, domestic, and community skills); Motor Skills (gross and fine motor); and Communication (receptive, expressive, and written communication), with developmentally ordered skills for each area. There are three available versions of the Vineland: (a) a survey form used as a diagnostic and classification tool for children and adults (Sparrow *et al.*, 1984b); (b) an expanded form for use in developing educational or rehabilitation plans (Sparrow, Balla, & Cicchetti, 1984a); and (c) a classroom edition to be used by teachers (Sparrow, Balla, & Cicchetti, 1985). Standard scores, percentile ranks, adaptive levels, and age equivalents are available. The expanded edition is the most useful for autistic children, whose adaptive function is usually lower than their cognitive level (Volkmar, Carter, Sparrow, & Cicchetti, 1993a). Recent supplementary norms have been published for individuals with autism (Carter *et al.*, 1998).

The Scales of Independent Behavior-Revised (SIB-R; Bruininks, Woodcock, Weatherman, & Hill, 1996) is a comprehensive norm-referenced assessment of adap-

Table VI. Strengths and Weaknesses of Specific Cognitive Instruments[a]

Instrument	Strengths	Weaknesses
Bayley Scales of Infant Development II (1993)	1: ≤42 months 3,5,6	1: not normed for >42 months 2: standard score (SS) ≥ 50 4: also mixes in social cannot always establish basal score
Mullen Scales of Early Learning (1997)	1: ≤60 months 3,4,5,6	
Leiter-Revised (Roid & Miller, 1997)	6 highlights visual strengths of autistic individuals	1: basal score = 24 months 3: nonverbal only 4,5
Merrill-Palmer (Stutsman, 1948)	3: verbal section is limited 5	1: basal score = 18 months 4 6: outdated
Differential Abilities Scales (DAS; Elliott, 1990)	1: extends from preschool through schoolage	2: SS to 45 only 3,4,5,6
Stanford-Binet IV (Thorndike, Hagen, & Sattler, 1986)	3,4,5,6	1: basal score = 24 months 2: SS to 70 only—highly verbal, long administration

[a] The numbers referring to the strengths and weaknesses are based on the six points outlined in the text.

tive and maladaptive behavior, for ages ranging from infancy through elderly adulthood. Fourteen Adaptive Behavior Clusters are offered in three forms: Early Development Form (15–20 minutes), Short Form (15–20 minutes), Full-scale Form (45–60 minutes). These cover motor skills, social interaction and communication skills, personal living, self-care, and community living skills. Age-equivalent scoring tables are included in the response booklets for each subscale, allowing examiners to get immediate developmental information.

Sensorimotor Assessment and Occupational Therapy Evaluation

Sensorimotor Assessment: Diagnostic practice has conventionally placed little emphasis on the assessment of sensorimotor behaviors in autism, with the exception that stereotypies are part of a "restricted behavioral repertoire" (APA, 1994; Lord, 1995). The reasons for this include the facts that there is a dearth of systematic empirical research in this domain and that the existing literature is controversial with respect to the usefulness of these variables for the differential diagnosis of autism. Thus, it seems particularly important to document qualitative dimensions of early sensory processing and motor behaviors (through both observation and parent report) rather than simply assess motor milestones during infant screenings.

Evaluation of sensorimotor functions should focus on the detection and localization of underlying neurologic deficits, whereas occupational therapists have specific expertise in the evaluation of their impact on the individual's functional skills or daily activities. Evaluation of motor skills is particularly important in situations where there is a question of delay, dysfunction, or regression in such skills, to document areas of strength as well as weakness for prognostic and intervention planning. Assessment of gross and fine motor skills may be completed by qualified professionals (e.g., occupational therapists or physical therapists) with a variety of standardized tools appropriate to the developmental level of the individual with autism; however, adaptations may be needed if the person with autism has difficulty understanding the tasks or is uncooperative. More important, qualitative observations of praxis (e.g., planning or sequencing of novel complex movement patterns; imitation of movements or pantomime; organization of goal-directed actions with materials in the environment) are a critical part of the sensorimotor evaluation for individuals with autism because these abilities are often deficient (Rogers, Bennetto, McEvoy, & Pennington, 1996; Stone & Lemanek, 1990), and require specific

interventions. Repetitive motor stereotypies, unusual posturing, object stereotypies, and self-injurious behaviors (SIBs) should be routinely documented through parental report or observation. Hand or finger mannerisms, body rocking, and other motor disturbances such as unusual posturing, are commonly reported in 37–95% of subjects studied (Adrien, Ornitz, Barthelemy, Sauvage, & Lelord, 1987; Elliott, 1990; Le Couteur et al., 1989; Ornitz, Guthrie, & Farley, 1977), and often manifest during the preschool years (Lord, 1995). The development of stereotypies, particularly in severe forms (e.g., SIB), may profoundly influence individual outcomes and prognosis for treatment in children with autism.

Sensory processing abilities are also prominently aberrant in autism. Preoccupations with sensory features of objects, sensory modulation difficulties reflected in over- and underresponsiveness to environmental stimuli, and paradoxical responses to sensory stimuli, among others, have been reported in 42–88% of persons with autism studied (Elliott, 1990; Kientz & Dunn, 1997; Le Couteur et al., 1989). Sensory processing requires assessment by expert clinical observations in tandem with parent reports or questionnaires because these disruptions may impact strongly on performance in daily activities.

The Sensory Integration and Praxis Tests (Ayres, 1989) are not routinely warranted as part of diagnostic evaluations of children with autism. However, this battery of tests may be prescribed on an individual basis to detect specific patterns of sensory integrative dysfunction in children between the ages of 4 and 9 years with average cognitive functioning.

Occupational Therapy Evaluation. The occupational therapist, as part of the evaluation team, should make a determination about the necessity to screen and fully evaluate an individual with autism about whom there are concerns regarding functional skills or occupational performance (i.e., goal-directed everyday routines). It is important that the occupational therapist have a comprehensive understanding of autism and be experienced in assessing persons in the age range of the clients being seen (e.g., child vs. adult). The occupational therapist first and foremost evaluates performance specifically in the areas of play or leisure, self-maintenance through activities of daily living, and productive school or work activities. Play is often disrupted in young children with autism (Restall & Magill-Evans, 1994; Stone & Lemanek, 1990) and particularly warrants assessment in a naturalistic context. Second, the occupational therapist should consider any specific performance components or contexts that may be impacting on the individual's daily functioning because this information is critical to the team diagnostic process as well as to an appropriate individualized intervention plan. Among specific components noted to be problematic, but not necessarily specific, to persons with autism, are complex motor planning abilities (Mailloux, Parham, & Roley, 1998; Minshew *et al.*, 1997), sensory processing abilities (Adrien *et al.*, 1993; Baranek, 1999; Dahlgren & Gillberg, 1989; Kientz & Dunn, 1997; Ornitz *et al.*, 1977), imitation skills (Rogers *et al.*, 1996; Stone & Lemanek, 1990), social and interpersonal skills (Gillberg *et al.*, 1990; Stone & Hogan, 1993; Volkmar *et al.*, 1993a), and coping with behavioral rigidities or restricted interests (Baranek, Foster, & Berkson, 1997). Supplemental interviews and parental reports should be used to corroborate observational findings or standardized assessments, particularly if those assessments were performed outside of the individual's typical routines and environments.

Neuropsychological, Behavioral, and Academic Assessment

Psychologists trained in evaluating autistic individuals can play a critical role in intervention planning, outcome assessment, and the diagnosis and treatment of comorbid psychological conditions. Standardized measures are used to establish baseline function in many domains of learning, performance, and socialization. Behavioral assessment by direct observation is used to address specific learning and behavior problems, to establish the functional or controlling relations of inappropriate behavior, to track behavioral progress, and to document the effectiveness of intervention. These are specialized psychological services, requiring appropriate training and experience. Specific assessments may address a child's psychological profile, motivation or reinforcement preferences, learning style, sensory and motor characteristics (and associated abnormalities), specific social skills deficits, academic skills, ritualistic or stereotyped patterns of behavior, and life-style and family relationships.

Recent research suggests that specific neuropsychological impairments can be identified in children in early childhood and that such impairments are correlated with the severity of autistic symptoms (Dawson, 1996; Dawson, Meltzoff, Osterling, & Rinaldi, 1998). Among the diverse types of neuropsychological impairments that may be exhibited by children with autism are deficits in explicit memory, in establishing rules governing reward contingencies, and in working memory, planning, and response inhibition (Dawson, 1996). Thus, it can be useful to assess a range of neuropsychological functions, including attention, memory, praxis, language and visual-spatial processing, so that educational strategies can address each child's specific strengths and weaknesses.

Assessment of Family Functioning and Resources

The family is a child's best resource. Parental intervention and behavior management strategies provided by a psychologist have a strong impact on the child's developmental status and autistic symptoms. Parental stress and exhaustion can adversely affect the child's well-being. Thus evaluation of the child must take place within the context of his or her family. One must determine the parents' level of understanding of their child's condition and offer appropriate counseling and education. One must determine if the family has informal supports, such as extended family, neighbors, or friends to assist them in their child-rearing responsibilities. The family's readiness to meet other families of children with similar conditions must also be assessed. Often families learn more and communicate more with other families than they do with professionals. Finally, based on the family's socioeconomic status and the status of the child, one must evaluate the need for and availability of various social services to provide respite and other supports.

Social workers, psychologists, or other professionals who specialize in families of autistic individuals may be best able to assess the family dynamics in relation to parenting and behavior management strategies as they specifically relate to the autistic child. These professionals may also know additional resources specifically tailored to families of autistic individuals. Finally, they themselves may facilitate parent support groups and plan parent seminars. This assessment will focus on the specific issues relating to the type of developmental profile identified during the *Level 2* evaluation. It cannot be overemphasized that *the family is the child's best resource.* Although there may be several confounding variables affecting a child's overall adult outcome, most autism specialists would agree that the family does play a very important role. This expanded assessment can also help determine the quality and quantity of community resources, educational programs and networking that a particular family needs. Each family is unique in its search for support and knowledge.

Level 2 Laboratory Investigation

Metabolic Testing

A wide range of biochemical determinations have been performed in urine, blood, and cerebrospinal fluid in an attempt to identify a specific metabolic abnormality in individuals with autism. Included are studies of inborn errors in amino acid, carbohydrate, purine, peptide, and mitochondrial metabolism, as well as toxicological studies. The reported co-occurrence of autistic-like symptoms in individuals with inborn errors of metabolism has led to consideration of screening tests as part of the routine assessment of patients with severe developmental impairment (Steffenburg, 1991). However, the percentage of children with autism who prove to have an identifiable metabolic disorder is probably less than 5% (Dykens & Volkmar, 1997; Rutter, Bailey, Bolton, & Le Couteur, 1994; Rutter *et al.*, 1994). Most of the biochemical analyses are useful at present *only as research tools* in the ongoing effort to understand the biology of autism.

Metabolic testing or consultation is indicated by a history of lethargy, cyclic vomiting, early seizures, dysmorphic or coarse features, mental retardation or if mental retardation cannot be excluded, questionable newborn screening, or birth out of the US because of the potential absence of newborn screening and maternal public health measures. As recommended by the American College of Medical Genetics, selective metabolic testing should be initiated only in the presence of suggestive clinical and physical findings (Curry *et al.*, 1997).

Genetic Testing

Of the chromosomal disorders found in association with autism, the most common abnormality described in recent studies is that involving the proximal long arm of chromosome 15 (15q11–q13), occurring in 1 to 4% of consecutive cases meeting criteria for Autistic Disorder (Cook *et al.*, 1998; Gillberg, 1998). These are usually maternally inherited duplications, either pseudodicentric 15 (inverted duplication 15) or other atypical marker chromosomes, with one or two extra copies of the area roughly corresponding to the typical Angelman syndrome (AS)/Prader Willi syndrome (PWS) deletion region of approximately 4 million base pairs. The 15q patients typically have moderate to profound mental retardation. In samples of patients with autistic disorder whose IQ was greater than 35, interstitial duplications of 15q11–13 have been found in more than 1% of patients and at a greater frequency than fragile X or other currently identifiable chromosomal disorders (Cook *et al.*, 1998; Gillberg, 1998; Pericak-Vance *et al.*, 1997; Schroer *et al.*, 1998; Weidmer-Mikhail, Sheldon, & Ghaziuddin, 1998).

Angelman syndrome, usually due to an absence (deletion) of maternally inherited 15q11–q13 material, has been found in patients with autism and profound mental retardation (Gillberg, 1998; Schroer *et al.*, 1998; Steffenburg, Gillberg, Steffenburg, & Kyllerman, 1996). Autism has also been found in patients with PWS (Demb

& Papola, 1995), although at a decreased rate relative to the frequency of autism in Angelman syndrome or duplications of 15q11–13. Confirmation by FISH probes for the PWS/AS region is necessary to confirm cytogenetic evidence of 15q11–13 abnormalities.

DNA analysis for fragile X and high resolution chromosome studies (karyotype) are indicated for a diagnosis of autism, mental retardation (or if mental retardation cannot be ruled out), if there is a family history of fragile X or undiagnosed mental retardation, or if dysmorphic features are present (American College of Medical Genetics: Policy Statement, 1994). It should be understood, however, that there is little likelihood of positive karyotype or fragile X testing in the presence of high-functioning autism. The absence of a positive genetic test does not exclude a genetic basis for autism. If the indications for DNA analysis for fragile X and high resolution chromosome studies are present but the family declines genetic testing, the family should be counseled to inform extended family members of the potential genetic risks of this disorder so they may seek appropriate genetic counseling.

In addition, the recurrence risk of autism is estimated to be between 3 and 7% across several studies (Bolton *et al.*, 1994; Jorde *et al.*, 1990; Piven *et al.*, 1990; Szatmari *et al.*, 1993).Therefore, although there is no current method to detect autism prenatally, parents should be counseled about the almost 50-fold increased risk of having a second child on the autistic spectrum (1 in 20 to 1 in 10, as compared with 1 in 1,000 to 1 in 500 for the general population).

Electrophysiologic Testing

The prevalence of epilepsy in a large cohort of preschool children with autism has been estimated as 7% (Rapin, 1996a), in another cohort, 14% (Tuchman *et al.*, 1991b), and the cumulative prevalence by adulthood is estimated at 20 to 35% (Minshew *et al.*, 1997). The peaks of seizure onset occurred in early childhood and again in adolescence (Gillberg & Steffenburg, 1987; Lockyer & Rutter, 1970; Minshew *et al.*, 1997; Rossi, Parmeggiani, Bach, Santucci, & Visconti, 1995; Volkmar & Nelson, 1990; Wong, 1993). Mental retardation, with or without motor abnormalities and family history of epilepsy, was a significant risk factor for the development of seizures in autistic individuals. The relationship between autism with an early regressive course (before 36 months), CDD (after 36 months), Landau-Kleffner syndrome (Landau & Kleffner, 1957, 1998), and electrical status epilepticus during slow wave sleep (ESES) is currently poorly understood, as are their underlying etiologies and pathophysiologies (Bristol *et al.*, 1996; Tuchman & Rapin, 1997). Regression in adolescence associated with seizure onset has also been reported, with further loss of language and cognitive skills (Lockyer & Rutter, 1970), but little is known about its cause or prevalence (Minshew *et al.*, 1997).

Seizures may be of all types, but partial complex seizures seem to be more prevalent, with EEG abnormalities occurring most often over the temporal lobes (Olsson *et al.*, 1988). The recognition of complex partial seizures in autistic individuals is complicated by the tendency to blame unusual behaviors on autism, and by the lack of direct correlation between clinical seizures and EEG paroxysmal activity (Minshew *et al.*, 1997). In addition, a recent study suggests that there may be a casual relationship between a subgroup of children with autistic regression and EEG-defined "benign focal epilepsies" (Nass, Gross, & Devinsky, 1998). Any behaviors such as staring, cessation of activity, or aggressive escalations associated with confusion should trigger a high index of suspicion of complex partial seizures in autistic individuals.

Indications for a prolonged sleep-deprived EEG with adequate sampling of slow wave sleep include evidence of clinical seizures, history of regression (clinically significant loss of social and communicative function) at any age but especially in toddlers and preschoolers, and in situations where there is a high index of clinical suspicion that epilepsy, clinical or subclinical, may be present. There is inadequate evidence at the present time to recommend EEG studies in all individuals with autism (Rapin, 1995, 1997; Rossi *et al.*, 1995; Tuchman, Jayakar, Yaylali, & Villalobos, 1997; Tuchman, 1994, 1995; Tuchman & Rapin, 1997; Tuchman *et al.*, 1991b.)

Except for the specific tests noted earlier, event-related potentials (Ciesielski, Knight, Prince, Harris, & Handmaker, 1995; Kemner, Verbaten, Cuperus, Cammferman, & Van Engeland, 1994; Kemner, Verbaten, Cuperus, Cammfferman, & van Engeland, 1995; Lincoln, Courchesne, Harms, & Allen, 1995b; Rapin & Dunn, 1997; Verbaten, Roelofs, van Engeland, Kenemans, & Slangen, 1991) and magnetoencephalography (Chuang, Otsubo, Hwang, Orrison, & Lewine, 1995; Morrell *et al.*, 1995; Salmelin, Service, Kiesila, Uutela, & Salonen, 1996) are considered to be research tools in the evaluation of autism, without evidence of routine clinical utility at present.

Neuroimaging

Computed tomographic (CT) studies during the 1970s and 1980s reported a wide range of brain imaging abnormalities, which contributed to the then prevalent view that most cases of autism would ultimately be found to be attributable to an underlying structural disorder. This perspective of autism, together with the general clinical practice in child neurology of including CT scanning in the search for etiologies of unexplained developmental delay in young children, led to the standardization of CT as part of the assessment of children diagnosed with autism during the 1970s and 1980s. This perspective changed substantially as a result of the landmark study of Damasio *et al.* (1980) demonstrating that CT abnormalities of the brain in autistic individuals were associated only with the presence of coexisting disorders rather than with autism itself. In a review of over 400 imaging studies in autistic subjects, a very low prevalence of focal lesions or other abnormalities was reported, and their inconsistent localization marked them as coincidental (Filipek *et al.*, 1992a). In a subsequent study, the prevalence of lesions on MRI in the children with autism was equal to that in the normal control volunteers (Filipek *et al.*, 1992b). A series of CT and magnetic resonance imaging (MRI) studies of autistic subjects screened to exclude those with identifiable disorders other than autism (see reviews by Minshew *et al.*, 1994, 1996b, Filipek *et al.*, 1992a, 1996, 1999) have confirmed the absence of significant detectable brain abnormalities characteristic of autism. The clinical perception that structural brain imaging should be routinely included in the assessment to identify gross brain abnormalities causing autism is, therefore, no longer viewed as valid (Filipek, 1999).

Functional imaging studies are a research endeavor in autism and do not have a role in clinical diagnosis at the present time. With the advent of functional imaging methods, such as functional MRI (fMRI), single photon emission tomography (SPECT), and positron emission tomography (PET), such studies are expected to play a major role in defining the brain basis for the behavioral impairments in autism, but as research tools only. The value of such studies will depend heavily on the design of activation paradigms, the documentation of the task demands of the paradigms for the individual, and the interpretation of the findings within the broader context of what is known about neurobehavioral function in autism. One construct of growing value in this regard is the cognitive model of autism as a selective disorder of complex information-processing abilities and as a disorder of multiple primary deficits (Minshew & Goldstein, 1998).

The presence of neurologic features not explained simply by the diagnosis of autism (e.g., asymmetric motor examination, cranial nerve dysfunction, severe headache) may be an indication for imaging, in which case the usual standards of practice apply (Filipek, 1999).

Autism *per se* is not considered an indication for neuro-imaging, even in the presence of megalencephaly.

Tests of Unproven Value

There is inadequate evidence to support routine clinical testing of individuals with autism for hair analysis for trace elements (Gentile, Trentalange, Zamichek, & Coleman, 1983; Shearer, Larson, Neuschwander, & Gedney, 1982; Wecker, Miller, Cochran, Dugger, & Johnson, 1985), celiac antibodies (Pavone, Fiumara, Bottaro, Mazzone, & Coleman, 1997), allergy testing (in particular food allergies for gluten, casein, candida and other molds) (Lucarelli *et al.*, 1995), immunological or neurochemical abnormalities (Cook, Perry, Dawson, Wainwright, & Leventhal, 1993; Singh, Warren, Averett, & Ghaziuddin, 1997; Yuwiler *et al.*, 1992), micronutrients such as vitamin levels (Findling *et al.*, 1997; LaPerchia, 1987; Tolbert, Haigler, Waits, & Dennis, 1993), intestinal permeability studies (D'Eufemia *et al.*, 1996), stool analysis, urinary peptides (Le Couteur, Trygstad, Evered, Gillberg, & Rutter, 1998), mitochondrial disorders (including lactate and pyruvate) (Lombard, 1998), thyroid function tests (D. J. Cohen, Young, Lowe, & Harcherik, 1980; Hashimoto *et al.*, 1991), or erythrocyte glutathione peroxidase studies (Michelson, 1998).

Referral to Early Intervention

Again, the Level 2 clinicians should refer to an appropriate early intervention or school team if the Level 1 clinicians did not do so. If the child is, indeed, enrolled in a program, the results of Level 2 evaluations by the psychologist, speech and occupational therapists should be communicated to the staff in an effort to better tailor their intervention strategies to the particular needs of the child.

RECOMMENDATIONS

Level 1: Routine Developmental Screening

1. All professionals involved in early child care (pediatricians, neurologists, psychiatrists, psychologists, audiologists, language pathologists, physical therapists, and occupational therapists) should be sufficiently familiar with the signs and symptoms of autism to recognize possible social, communicative, and behavioral indicators of the need for further diagnostic evaluation.

2. Developmental screening should be performed at each and every well-child visit throughout infancy, toddlerhood, the preschool years, and at any age thereafter if concerns are raised about social acceptance, learn-

ing and behavior. Recommended screening tools include *The Ages and Stages Questionnaire (ASQ), The BRIGANCE® Screens, The Child Development Inventories (CDIs)*, and the *Parents' Evaluation of Developmental Status (PEDS)*. Also recommended is the use of Specific Developmental Probes, as outlined in the text, to specifically identify any parental concerns about development. The *Denver-II* (formerly the *Denver Developmental Screening Test-Revised*) is *not* recommended as an appropriate developmental screen in this capacity.

3. The following developmental milestones are nearly universally present by the age indicated. Failure to meet any of these milestones is an absolute indication to proceed with further evaluations. Delay in referral for such testing may delay early diagnosis and treatment and affect the long-term outcome.

No babbling by 12 months.

No gesturing (pointing, waving bye-bye, etc) by 12 months.

No single words by 16 months.

No 2-word spontaneous (*not just echolalic*) phrases by 24 months.

Any loss of *any* language or social skills *at any age.*

4. Level 1 Laboratory Investigations. Concern regarding a speech, language, or hearing problem by parent or practitioner should prompt an immediate referral for a formal audiologic assessment, regardless of whether the child "passed" a neonatal hearing screen.

Audiological assessment should be performed at centers with qualified and experienced pediatric audiologists, with current audiological testing methods and technologies. Facilities without these qualifications should enter consortial arrangements with centers that are able to provide this type of comprehensive assessment of children with autism.

Periodic lead screens should be performed in any autistic child with pica.

5. Professionals involved in early child care should also become familiar with and use one of the screening instruments for children with autism (e.g., the *Checklist for Autism in Toddlers* (CHAT), the *Pervasive Developmental Disorders Screening Test* (PDDST), or, for older verbal children, the *Australian Scale for Asperger's Syndrome*).

6. The social, communication and play development and behavior of siblings of children with autism needs to be monitored very carefully not only for autism-related symptoms but also for language delays, learning difficulties, and anxiety or depressive symptoms.

7. As mandated by Public Law 99-457, and reauthorized as Public Law 105-17: Individuals with Disabilities Education Act- IDEA (1997), a referral for

early intervention should be initiated by the primary care practitioner. Children less than 36 months of age should be referred to the zero-to-three service system in their community; children ages 36 months and older should be referred to the local school district.

8. Health care providers and others need to increase their comfort level in talking with families about autism, which is a treatable disorder with a wide range of outcomes. Thus, information about the benefits of early intervention for children with autism needs to be widely disseminated to health care professionals and others working with young children and families.

9. Screening tools for older children with milder symptoms of autism need to be made widely available in educational and recreational settings, where these children's difficulties are often most visible, as well as in health and allied health settings. Pediatricians can and should play an important role in raising a suspicion of autism, paving the way to appropriate referral to professionals knowledgeable about autism in verbal individuals.

Level 2: Diagnosis and Evaluation of Autism

1. It is the consensus of this Panel that Level 2 Diagnosis and Evaluation should be performed by professionals who specialize in the treatment of children with autism.

2. The diagnosis of autism should be accurately made based on clinical and DSM-IV criteria, and should include the use of a diagnostic instrument with at least moderate sensitivity and good specificity for autism.

Sufficient time must be planned for both a standardized parent interview regarding current concerns and behavioral history related to autism, and direct, structured observation of social and communicative behavior and play.

Such interview instruments include the *Gilliam Autism Rating Scale* (GARS), *The Parent Interview for Autism* (PIA), *The Pervasive Developmental Disorders Screening Test- Stage 2* (PDDST), or the *Autism Diagnostic Interview-Revised* (ADI-R).

Direct, structured observation instruments include the *Screening Tool for Autism in Two-Year-Olds* (STAT), the *Childhood Autism Rating Scale (CARS)*, and the *Autism Diagnostic Observation Schedule-Generic* (ADOS-G).

3. Individuals with even mild autism must also receive adequate assessments and appropriate diagnoses, using practice standards similar to those outlined above.

4. Diagnostic evaluations must also address those factors that are not specific to autism, including degree

of language impairment, mental handicap, and presence of nonspecific behavioral disorders such as overactivity, aggression, anxiety, depression, or specific learning disabilities, which can significantly affect outcome and treatment of autistic individuals.

5. An expanded medical and neurological evaluation whose focus is on the search for acquired brain injury, comorbid condition, or difficulties common in autism: pregnancy, delivery, perinatal history, developmental history including milestones, regression in early childhood or later in life, encephalopathic events, attention deficit disorder, seizure disorder (absence or generalized), depression or mania, troublesome behaviors such as irritability, self-injury, sleep and eating disturbances, and pica for possible lead exposure.

Family History should specifically probe in nuclear and extended family for autism, mental retardation, fragile X syndrome, and tuberous sclerosis complex, because of their implications regarding the need for chromosomal or genetic evaluation. In addition, family members with affective or anxiety disorder should be identified, as these impact on the care of the child and family burden. The focus of the physical and neurological examination should include: longitudinal measurements of head circumference, unusual features (facial, limb, stature, etc.) suggesting the need for genetic evaluation, neurocutaneous abnormalities (requiring an ultraviolet Wood's-lamp examination), gait, tone, reflexes, cranial nerves, and mental status including verbal and nonverbal language and play.

6. A speech–language–communication evaluation should be performed on all children who fail language developmental screening procedures, by a language pathologist with training and expertise in evaluating children with autism.

A variety of strategies should be used in this assessment, including but not limited to direct standardized instruments, naturalistic observation, parental interviews, and procedures focusing on social-pragmatic abilities.

Results of a speech–language–communication assessment should always be interpreted relative to a child's cognitive, motor and socioemotional abilities.

7. A cognitive evaluation should be performed in all children with autism by a psychologist or developmental pediatrician experienced in autism testing, and should include assessment of family (parent and sibling) strengths, talents, stressors. and adaptation, as well as resources and supports. Psychologists working with children with autism should be familiar with a range of theories and approaches specific to this population.

Psychological instruments should be appropriate for the mental and chronological age, should provide a full range (in the lower direction) of standard scores, including independently scored measures of verbal and nonverbal abilities, should provide an overall index of ability, and should have current norms which are independent of social ability.

8. A measure of adaptive functioning should be collected by the psychologist for any child evaluated for an associated mental handicap. Recommended instruments include the *Vineland Adaptive Behavior Scales* and the *Scales of Independent Behavior-Revised* (SIB-R).

9. Screening and full evaluation for sensorimotor skills by qualified professionals (occupational therapists or physical therapists) with expertise in testing persons with autism should be considered, including an assessment of gross and fine motor skills, praxis, sensory processing abilities, unusual or stereotyped mannerisms, and the impact of these components on the autistic person's life.

10. An occupational therapy evaluation is indicated when an autistic individual is experiencing disruptions in functional skills or occupational performance in the areas of play or leisure, self-maintenance through activities of daily living, or productive school and work tasks. The occupational therapist may evaluate these performance areas in the context of different environments, and through activity analysis, the contributions of performance component abilities (e.g., sensory processing, fine motor skills, social skills) in goal-directed everyday routines.

11. A neuropsychological, behavioral, and academic assessment should be performed, in addition to the cognitive assessment, to include communication skills, social skills and relationships, educational functioning, problematic behaviors, learning style, motivation and reinforcement, sensory functioning, and self-regulation.

12. Assessment of family functioning should be performed to determine the parents' level of understanding of their child's condition and offer appropriate counseling and education. Based on the family's socioeconomic status and the status of the child, one must evaluate the need for and availability of various social services to provide respite and other supports.

13. Assessment of family resources should be performed by social workers, psychologists, or other professionals who specialize in families of autistic individuals, who may be better able to assess the family dynamics in relation to parenting and behavior management strategies as they specifically relate to the autistic child.

14. Level 2 Laboratory Evaluation may include the following, as indicated:

(a). Metabolic testing or consultation is indicated by a history of lethargy, cyclic vomiting, early seizures; dysmorphic or coarse features; mental retardation or if mental retardation cannot be excluded; if there is any question concerning the occurrence or adequacy of newborn screening for a birth within the US; or birth out of the U.S. indicating the potential absence of newborn screening and maternal public health measures.

As recommended by the American College of Medical Genetics, selective metabolic testing should be initiated by the presence of suggestive clinical and physical findings.

(b). Genetic testing, specifically DNA analysis for fragile X and high resolution chromosome studies (karyotype), are indicated for a diagnosis of autism, mental retardation (or if mental retardation cannot be excluded), if there is a family history of fragile X or undiagnosed mental retardation, or if dysmorphic features are present. It should be understood, however, that there is little likelihood of positive karyotype or fragile X testing is the presence of high-functioning autism.

If a family declines genetic testing, they should be counseled to inform extended family members of the potential genetic risks of this disorder so they may seek appropriate genetic counseling.

Although there is no current method to detect autism prenatally, parents of children with autism should be counseled to inform them of the 50-fold increased risk of having another autistic child (1 in 10 to 1 in 20, as compared with 1 in 500 in the general population).

(c). Indications for a prolonged sleep-deprived EEG with adequate sampling of slow wave sleep include evidence of clinical seizures, history of regression (clinically significant loss of social and communicative function) at any age but especially in toddlers and preschoolers, and in situations where there is a high index of clinical suspicion that epilepsy, clinical or subclinical, may be present. There is inadequate evidence at the present time to recommend EEG studies in all individuals with autism.

Other event-related potentials and magnetoencephalography are considered research tools in the evaluation of autism at the present time, without evidence of routine clinical utility.

(d). Neuroimaging may be indicated by the presence of neurologic features *not explained by the diagnosis of autism* (e.g., asymmetric motor examination, cranial nerve dysfunction, severe headache), in which case the usual standards of practice apply. Routine clinical neuroimaging does not have any role in the diagnostic evaluation of autism at the present time, even in the presence of autistic megalencephaly.

Functional imaging modalities (fMRI, SPECT, and PET) at present are considered solely as research tools in the evaluation of autism.

(e). Tests of unproven value: There is inadequate evidence to support routine clinical testing of individuals with autism for hair analysis for trace elements, celiac antibodies, allergy testing (in particular food allergies for gluten, casein, candida and other molds), immunological or neurochemical abnormalities, micronutrients such as vitamin levels, intestinal permeability studies, stool analysis, urinary peptides, mitochondrial disorders (including lactate and pyruvate), thyroid function tests, or erythrocyte glutathione peroxidase studies.

15. Reevaluation at least within a year of initial diagnosis and continued monitoring is an expected aspect of clinical practice, because relatively small changes in developmental level affect the impact of autism in the preschool years.

16. It is the consensus of this Panel that the role of medical professionals can no longer be limited to simply the diagnosis of autism. Professionals must expand their knowledge and involvement to be better able to counsel families concerning available and appropriate treatment modalities, whether educational, empirical, or "just off the web." In addition, professionals must be familiar with federal law which mandates a free and appropriate education for all children from the age of 36 months, and in some states, from zero to three as well.

Other Recommendations

1. Existing managed-care policy must change as follows:

Extremely brief well-child visits must increase in duration, with appropriate compensation, to permit the implementation of routine developmental screening as recommended above.

Short specialty visits must also increase in duration, with appropriate compensation, to permit the use of appropriate diagnostic instruments, as recommended above.

Autism must be recognized as a medical disorder, and managed care policy must cease to deny appropriate medical or other therapeutic care under the rubric of "developmental delay" or "mental health condition."

2. Existing governmental agencies that provide services for individuals with developmental disabilities must also change their eligibility criteria to include all individuals on the autistic spectrum, whether or not the relatively narrow criteria for Autistic Disorder are met, who nonetheless must also receive the same adequate

assessments, appropriate diagnoses, and treatment options as do those with the formal diagnosis of Autistic Disorder.

3. Public awareness and dissemination activities regarding the signs and symptoms of autism must occur throughout communities, to provide information to parents, child-care workers, health-care settings, and community centers. Small, attractive fliers targeting symptoms, needs, and outcomes of very young children and also older children should be developed and disseminated widely, in collaboration with the national autism societies and associations, schools, health, and allied health agencies which need to join in this concerted effort.

4. Increased education of health-related and education-related professionals about autism must occur at the preservice level. Professionals must learn to provide more than a diagnosis and a telephone number for governmental services to parents. Trainees in general and developmental pediatrics, psychiatry, neurology, early childhood education, speech and language pathology, occupational therapy, physical therapy, psychology, nursing, child-care providers, public health, education, and other disciplines need markedly increased knowledge about the range of symptoms of autism both early and later in life, about the educational and community needs of autistic individuals, and the potential outcomes of autism. They must also learn how to discuss potential risks of autism with families.

AN ANALYSIS OF DIFFERENCES RELATIVE TO OTHER PRACTICE PARAMETERS

This consensus recommendation parallels and expands upon many of the major points of the Cure Autism Now (CAN) Consensus Statement (CCS; Geschwind, Cummings, & the CAN Consensus Group, 1998), especially its recognition of the effectiveness of appropriate early intervention programs, the urgency of early identification and diagnosis of autistic spectrum disorders that follows, and the necessity for a careful neurologic and medical examination in all children with autism. Specific recommendations regarding imaging, electrophysiology, metabolic and genetic testing in this document are similar to those from the CCS (Geschwind *et al.*, 1998). The purpose of the CCS was to provide guidelines for first tier autism screening and diagnostic referral for primary care practitioners (primarily pediatricians). The major difference between the current recommendations and the CCS is that the CCS recommended only the CHAT (Baron-Cohen *et al.*, 1992) as a rapid and effective screening tool to screen all 18-month-old children for autism, whereas in this current consensus, the CHAT is grouped along with other screening instruments, and is felt not to be entirely sufficient for primary care screening purposes. Given the importance of early identification, and the currently unacceptable delays that occur between initial parental suspicion and diagnosis, the importance of widespread developmental screening beginning at 18 months cannot be overemphasized.

The American Academy of Child and Adolescent Psychiatry (AACAP) Practice Parameters (Volkmar *et al.*, in press) were consulted in the development of this document. The documents are similar with two main differences due to the difference in scope of the two documents. The AACAP practice parameters are concerned with aspects of diagnosis and treatment of particular relevance to psychiatrists in their care for children, adolescents, and adults with autism and related conditions. The present document is concerned primarily with aspects of assessment, including diagnostic screening, and does not address aspects of treatment. The AACAP looks forward to continued participation in the effort to provide consensus practice parameters for autism.

The American Academy of Pediatrics (AAP) Committee on Children with Disabilities was consulted regarding its own development of a Policy Statement regarding the role of the primary care pediatrician in the diagnosis and management of children with autism, which is in progress (American Academy of Pediatrics Committee on Children with Disabilities, 1994). The documents are also similar with main differences due to differences in scope of the target audience. The AAP document is concerned chiefly with the role of the primary care pediatrician and addresses management strategies as well as early diagnosis.

RECOMMENDATION FOR PARAMETER REVIEW

The Panel recommends review of these parameters in 2 to 3 years.

RECOMMENDATIONS FOR FUTURE RESEARCH

1. Develop and validate appropriate screening tools with adequate sensitivity and specificity for autism in children prior to age 1 year, which could be feasibly used by a wide range of practitioners. Current evidence suggests that it is likely that many children with autism can be identified by 12 to 18 months of age. It is the consensus of this Panel that early recognition can lead to early access to intervention, which would promote more positive long range outcomes for individuals with autism.

2. Continue to study the usefulness of electrophysiological techniques to clarify the role of epilepsy in autism, especially in children with a history of regression.

3. Continue efforts to identify contributing genes to determine whether the behavioral syndromes which constitute the basis of DSM-IV and ICD-10 have actual biologic validity.

4. Continue efforts to identify the harbingers, causes, and outcome of autistic regression.

5. Attempt to identify environmental factors, such as nonspecific infections or other immunologically mediated events, that might contribute to triggering the expression of autistic symptoms or regression.

6. Further research must focus on the development and validation of appropriate tools to accurately assess the cognitive and neuropsychological profile of individuals with autism, as it is clear that any of the current available tools has, despite the benefits listed in Table VI, significant limitations for use with autistic individuals.

7. A well-designed study of the prevalence of EEG abnormalities and seizures, of MRI abnormalities, and of genetic and metabolic abnormalities directly associated with autism.

8. Studies of the audiological characteristics of autistic individuals and development of appropriate clinical electrophysiological and behavioral procedures to assess peripheral hearing sensitivity and suprathreshold responses.

9. Further basic research on the development of complex auditory processing in children, to provide insight into the emergence of early auditory behaviors considered atypical.

10. Field trials on the results of implementing these guidelines to determine who is identified diagnostically by screening and the efficacy of the various screening instruments in detecting autism at different ages.

APPENDIX

Contact Information for Recommended Instruments

Ages and Stages Questionnaire (ASQ), Second Edition	Paul H. Brookes Publishing Company PO Box 10624, Baltimore, Maryland 21285 Telephone: 800-638-3775; Fax: 410-337-8539
Australian Scale for Asperger's Syndrome	Garnett, M. S., & Attwood, A. J. (1998). The Australian Scale for Asperger's Syndrome (pp. 17–19). In Attwood, T. (Ed.),

	Asperger's Syndrome. A Guide for Parents and Professionals. London; Jessica Kingsley Publisher, ISBN 1853025771.
Autism Diagnostic Interview-Revised Autism Diagnostic Observation Schedule-Generic	Catherine Lord Department of Psychiatry, MC3077, University of Chicago 5841 S. Maryland Ave, Chicago, IL 60637 Telephone: 773-702-9707; Fax: 773-834-2742
BRIGANCE® Screens	Curriculum Associates, Inc. P.O. Box 2001, North Billerica, MA 01862-0901 Telephone: 800-225-0248; Fax: 800-366-1158 E-mail: cainfo@curricassoc.com
Checklist for Autism in Toddlers (CHAT)	Baron-Cohen, S. *et al.* (1992). Can autism be detected at 18 months? The needle, the haystack, and the CHAT. *British Journal of Psychiatry, 161,* 839–843. Baron-Cohen, S. *et al.* (1996). Psychological markers in the detection of autism in infancy in a large population. *British Journal of Psychiatry, 168,* 158–163.
Child Development Inventories (CDIs)	Behavior Science Systems Box 580274, Minneapolis, MN 55458 Telephone: 612-929-6220
Childhood Autism Rating Scale (CARS)	Western Psychological Services 12031 Wilshire Boulevard Los Angeles, CA 90025-1251 Telephone: 800-648-8857; Fax: 310-478-7838
Parents' Evaluation of Developmental Status (PEDS)	Ellsworth and Vandermeer Press, Ltd. 4405 Scenic Drive, Nashville, TN 37204 Telephone: 615-386-0061; Fax: 615-386-0346
The Parent Interview for Autism (PIA) The Screening Tool for Autism in Two-Year-Olds (STAT)	Wendy Stone Vanderbilt Child Development Center Medical Center South, Room 426 2100 Pierce Avenue, Nashville, TN 37232-3573 Telephone: 615-936-0249 E-mail: wendy.stone@mcmail.vanderbilt.edu
Pervasive Developmental Disorders Screening Test (PDDST)	Bryna Siegel Langley Porter Psychiatric Institute, Box CAS University of California, San Francisco, CA 94143-0984 Telephone: 415-476-7385; Fax: 415-476-7160.

ACKNOWLEDGMENTS

The authors express their gratitude to the following people who contributed to this endeavor by their participation in the NIH State of the Science in Autism: Screening and Diagnosis Working Conference, June 15–17, 1998: George Anderson, Anthony Bailey, W. Ted Brown, Susan E. Bryson, Rebecca Landa, Jeffrey Lewine, Catherine Lord, William McIlvane, Sally Ozonoff, Joseph Piven, Ricki Robinson, Bryna Siegel, Vijendra K. Singh, Frank Symons, and Max Wiznitzer. The current authors, participants and NIH Liaisons also participated in this working conference.

The Panel acknowledges with gratitude the assistance of Stephen Ashwal as the AAN-QSS Facilitator for this project, the helpful consultations of Frances P. Glascoe, and Donald J. Siegel, and the assistance of Cheryl Jess, Kerry E. Shea, and Jody Sallah in this endeavor.

This project was supported in part by HD28202/HD27802/HD35458 (Filipek), HD35482 (Cook and Volkmar), HD34565 (Dawson), HD36080 (Gravel), HD3546a (Minshew), HD35468 (Rogers) and HD03008 (Volkmar) from the National Institute of Child Health and Human Development; DC00223 (Gravel) from the National Institute of Deafness and Communication Disorders; MH01389/MH52223 (Cook), MH47117 (Dawson), and MH50620 (Stone) from the National Institute of Mental Health; NS35896 (Filipek), NS33355 (Minshew), NS20489 (Rapin), from the National Institute of Neurologic Disorders and Stroke, National Institutes of Health, Bethesda, MD. This project was also supported by MCJ-369029 (Accardo) from the Maternal and Child Health Bureau, Health Resources and Services Administration, Department of Health and Human Resources.

REFERENCES

Accardo, P., Whitman, B., Caul, J., & Rolfe, U. (1988). Autism and plumbism. A possible association. *Clinical Pediatrics, 27,* 41–44.

Adkins, P. G., & Ainsa, T. A. (1979). The misdiagnosis of Matthew. *Academic Therapy, 14,* 335–339.

Adrien, J. L., Lenoir, P., Martineau, J., Perrot, A., Hameury, L., Larmande, C., & Sauvage, D. (1993). Blind ratings of early symptoms of autism based upon family home movies. *Journal of the American Academy of Child and Adolescent Psychiatry, 32,* 617–626.

Adrien, J. L., Ornitz, E., Barthelemy, C., Sauvage, D., & Lelord, G. (1987). The presence or absence of certain behaviors associated with infantile autism in severely retarded autistic and nonautistic retarded children and very young normal children. *Journal of Autism and Developmental Disorders, 17,* 407–416.

Adrien, J. L., Perrot, A., Sauvage, D., Leddet, I., Larmande, C., Hameury, L., & Barthelemy, C. (1992). Early symptoms in autism from family home movies. Evaluation and comparison between 1st and 2nd year of life using I.B.S.E. scale. *Acta Paedopsychiatrica, 55,* 71–75.

Allen, D. A. (1988). Autistic spectrum disorders: clinical presentation in preschool children. *Journal of Child Neurology, 3 (Suppl.),* S48–56.

Allen, D. A. (1989). Developmental language disorders in preschool children: Clinical subtypes and syndromes. *School Psychology Review, 18,* 442–451.

Allen, D. A. (1991). Variability in the clinical presentation of autism: Issues of diagnosis and treatment in the preschool years. In N. Amir, I. Rapin, & D. Branski (Eds.), *Pediatric neurology: Behavior and cognition of the child with brain dysfunction* (Pediatric and Adolescent Medicine, Vol. 1, pp. 36–49). Basel: Karger.

Allen, D. A., & Rapin, I. (1992). Autistic children are also dysphasic. In H. Naruse & E. M. Ornitz (Eds.), *Neurobiology of infantile autism* (pp. 157–163). Amsterdam: Elsevier.

American Academy of Pediatrics Committee on Children with Disabilities. (1994). Screening infants and young children for developmental disabilities. *Pediatrics, 93,* 863–865.

American College of Medical Genetics: Policy Statement. (1994). Fragile X Syndrome: Diagnostic and carrier testing. *American Journal of Medical Genetics, 53,* 380–381.

American Psychiatric Association. (1952). *Diagnostic and statistical manual of mental disorders.* Washington, DC: American Psychiatric Association.

American Psychiatric Association. (1968). *Diagnostic and statistical manual of mental disorders (2nd ed.).* Washington, DC: American Psychiatric Association.

American Psychiatric Association. (1980). *Diagnostic and statistical manual of mental disorders (3rd ed.).* Washington, DC: American Psychiatric Association.

American Psychiatric Association. (1987). *Diagnostic and statistical manual of mental disorders (3rd ed. Rev.).* Washington, DC: American Psychiatric Association.

American Psychiatric Association. (1994). *Diagnostic and statistical manual of mental disorders (4th ed.).* Washington, DC: American Psychiatric Association.

American Speech-Language-Hearing Association. (1991). Guidelines for the audiologic assessment of children from birth through 36 months of age. Committee on Infant Hearing. *American Speech-Language-Hearing Association (ASHA), 33(Suppl. 5),* 37–43.

Anderson, S. R., Avery, D. L., Dipietro, E. K., Edwards, G. L., & Christian, W. P. (1987). Intensive home-based early intervention with autistic children. *Education and Treatment of Children, 10,* 352–366.

Anderson, S. R., Campbell, S., & Cannon, B. O. (1994). The May Center for early childhood education. In S. Harris & J. Handleman (Eds.), *Preschool education programs for children with autism* (pp. 15–36). Austin, TX: Pro-Ed.

Armstrong, D. D. (1997). Review of Rett syndrome. *Journal of Neuropathology and Experimental Neurology, 56,* 843–849.

Asperger, H. (1991/1944). "Autistic psychopathy" in childhood. Translated and annotated by U. Frith. In U. Frith (Ed.), *Autism and Asperger syndrome* (pp. 37–92). New York: Cambridge University Press.

Attwood, A. J. (1998). *Asperger's syndrome. A guide for parents and professionals.* London: Kingsley.

Ayres, A. J. (1989). *Sensory integration and praxis tests.* Los Angeles: Western Psychological Services.

Bailey, A., Bolton, P., Butler, L., Le Couteur, A., Murphy, M., Scott, S., Webb, T., & Rutter, M. (1993a). Prevalence of the fragile X anomaly amongst autistic twins and singletons. *Journal of Child Psychology and Psychiatry, 34,* 673–688.

Bailey, A., Le Couteur, A., Gottesman, I., Bolton, P., Simonoff, E., Yuzda, E., & Rutter, M. (1995). Autism as a strongly genetic disorder: evidence from a British twin study. *Psychological Medicine, 25,* 63–77.

Bailey, A., Luthert, P., Bolton, P., Le Couteur, A., Rutter, M., & Harding, B. (1993b). Autism and megalencephaly. *Lancet, 341,* 1225–1226.

Bailey, A., Luthert, P., Dean, A., Harding, B., Janota, I., Montgomery, M., Rutter, M., & Lantos, P. (1998a). A clinicopathological study of autism. *Brain, 121,* 899–905.

Bailey, A., Palferman, S., Heavey, L., & Le Couteur, A. (1998b). Autism: The phenotype in relatives. *Journal of Autism and Developmental Disorders, 28,* 369–392.

Bailey, A., Phillips, W., & Rutter, M. (1996). Autism: towards an integration of clinical, genetic, neuropsychological, and neurobiological perspectives. *Journal of Child Psychology and Psychiatry, 37,* 89–126.

Baird, G., Charman, T., Baron-Cohen, S., Cox, A., Swettenham, J., Wheelwright, S., Drew, A., & Kernal, L. (1999). *Screening a large population of 18 month olds with the CHAT.* Paper presented at the Proceedings of the Society for Research in Child Development, Albuquerque, NM.

Bangs, T., & Dodson, S. (1986). *Birth to Three Developmental Scales.* Allen, TX: DLM Teaching Resources.

Baranek, G. T. (1999). Autism during infancy: A retrospective video analysis of sensory-motor and social behaviors at 9–12 months of age. *Journal of Autism and Developmental Disorders, 29,* 213–224.

Baranek, G. T., Foster, L. G., & Berkson, G. (1997). Tactile defensiveness and stereotyped behaviors. *American Journal of Occupational Therapy, 51,* 91–95.

Baron-Cohen, S., Allen, J., & Gillberg, C. (1992). Can autism be detected at 18 months? The needle, the haystack, and the CHAT. *British Journal of Psychiatry, 161,* 839–843.

Baron-Cohen, S., Cox, A., Baird, G., Swettenham, J., Nightingale, N., Morgan, K., Drew, A., & Charman, T. (1996). Psychological markers in the detection of autism in infancy in a large population. *British Journal of Psychiatry, 168,* 158–163.

Bauer, S. (1995a). Autism and the pervasive developmental disorders: Part 1. *Pediatrics in Review, 16,* 130–136.

Bauer, S. (1995b). Autism and the pervasive developmental disorders: Part 2. *Pediatrics in Review, 16,* 168–176.

Bauman, M. L. (1992a). Motor dysfunction in autism. In A. B. Joseph & R. R. Young (Eds.), *Movement disorders in neurology and psychiatry* (pp. 660–663). Boston: Blackwell.

Bauman, M. L. (1992b). Neuropathology of autism. In A. B. Joseph & R. R. Young (Eds.), *Movement disorders in neurology and psychiatry* (pp. 664–668). Boston: Blackwell.

Bauman, M. L. (1996). Brief report. Neuroanatomic observations of the brain in pervasive developmental disorders. *Journal of Autism and Developmental Disorders, 26,* 199–203.

Bauman, M. L., Filipek, P. A., & Kemper, T. L. (1997). Early infantile autism. In J. D. Schmahmann (Ed.), *The cerebellum and cognition* (pp. 367–386). San Diego: Academic Press.

Bauman, M. L., & Kemper, T. L. (1994). Neuroanatomic observations of the brain in autism. In M. L. Bauman & T. L. Kemper (Eds.), *The neurobiology of autism* (pp. 119–145). Baltimore: Johns Hopkins University Press.

Bauman, M. L., & Kemper, T. L. (1997). Is autism a progressive process? *Neurology, 48(Suppl.),* A285.

Bayley, N. (1993). *Bayley Scale of Infant Development (2nd ed.).* San Antonio, TX: Psychological Corp.

Bhaumik, S., Branford, D., McGrother, C., & Thorp, C. (1997). Autistic traits in adults with learning disabilities. *British Journal of Psychiatry, 170,* 502–506.

Bishop, D., Hartley, J., & Weir, F. (1994). Why and when do some language-impaired children seem talkative? A study of initiation in conversations of children with semantic-pragmatic disorder. *Journal of Autism and Developmental Disorders, 24,* 177–97.

Bishop, D. V. M. (1989). Autism, Asperger's syndrome and semantic-pragmatic disorder: Where are the boundaries? *British Journal of Disorders of Communication, 24,* 107–121.

Blomquist, H. K., Bohman, M., Edvinsson, S. O., Gillberg, C., Gustavson, K. H., Holmgren, G., & Wahlstrom, J. (1985). Frequency of the fragile X syndrome in infantile autism. A Swedish multicenter study. *Clinical Genetics, 27,* 113–117.

Bolton, P., Macdonald, H., Pickles, A., Rios, P., Goode, S., Crowson, M., Bailey, A., & Rutter, M. (1994). A case-control family history study of autism. *Journal of Child Psychology and Psychiatry, 35,* 877–900.

Bolton, P., & Rutter, M. (1990). Genetic influences in autism. *International Review of Psychiatry, 2,* 67–80.

Bolton, P. F., & Griffiths, P. D. (1997). Association of tuberous sclerosis of temporal lobes with autism and atypical autism. *Lancet, 349,* 392–395.

Bolton, P. F., Murphy, M., Macdonald, H., Whitlock, B., Pickles, A., & Rutter, M. (1997). Obstetric complications in autism: consequences or causes of the condition? *Journal of the American Academy of Child and Adolescent Psychiatry, 36,* 272–281.

Bonnet, K. A., & Gao, X. K. (1996). Asperger syndrome in neurologic perspective. *Journal of Child Neurology, 11,* 483–489.

Borowitz, K. C., & Glascoe, F. P. (1986). Sensitivity of the Denver Developmental Screening Test in speech and language screening. *Pediatrics, 78,* 1075–1078.

Braffman, B., & Naidich, T. P. (1994). The phakomatoses: Part I. Neurofibromatosis and tuberous sclerosis. *Neuroimaging Clinics of North America, 4,* 299–324.

Bricker, D., & Squires, J. (1994). *Ages and Stages Questionnaire.* Baltimore, MD: Paul H. Brookes.

Bricker, D., & Squires, J. (1999). *The Ages and Stages Questionnaires (2nd ed.).* Baltimore, MD: Paul H. Brookes.

Brigance, A. (1986). *The BRIGANCE® Screens.* North Billerica, MA: Curriculum Associates.

Bristol, M. M., Cohen, D. J., Costello, E. J., Denckla, M., Eckberg, T. J., Kallen, R., Kraemer, H. C., Lord, C., Maurer, R., Mcllvane, W. J., Minshew, N., Sigman, M., & Spence, M. A. (1996). State of the science in autism—Report to the National Institutes of Health. *Journal of Autism and Developmental Disorders, 26,* 121–154.

Brown, E., Dawson, G., Osterling, J., & Dinno, J. (1998). *Early identification of 8–10 month old infants with autism based on observations from home videotapes.* Paper presented at the International Society for Infant Studies, Atlanta, GA.

Brown, W. T., Jenkins, E. C., Cohen, I. L., Fisch, G. S., Wolf-Schein, E. G., Gross, A., Waterhouse, L., Fein, D., Mason-Brothers, A., Ritvo, E., & *et al.* (1986). Fragile X and autism: A multicenter survey. *American Journal of Medical Genetics, 23,* 341–352.

Bruininks, R. H., Woodcock, R. W., Weatherman, R. E., & Hill, B. K. (1996). *Scales of Independent Behavior-Revised (SIB-R).* Chicago: Riverside.

Bryson, S. E. (1996). Brief report—Epidemiology of autism. *Journal of Autism and Developmental Disorders, 26,* 165–167.

Bryson, S. E. (1997). Epidemiology of autism: Overview and issues outstanding. In D. J. Cohen & F. R. Volkmar (Eds.), *Handbook of autism and pervasive developmental disorders (2nd ed.)* pp. 41–46). New York: Wiley.

Bryson, S. E., Clark, B. S., & Smith, I. M. (1988a). First report of a Canadian epidemiological study of autistic syndromes. *Journal of Child Psychology and Psychiatry, 29,* 433–446.

Bryson, S. E., Smith, I. M., & Eastwood, D. (1988b). Obstetrical suboptimality in autistic children. *Journal of the American Academy of Child and Adolescent Psychiatry, 27,* 418–422.

Burd, L., Fisher, W., & Kerbeshian, J. (1989). Pervasive disintegrative disorder: are Rett syndrome and Heller dementia infantilis subtypes? *Developmental Medicine and Child Neurology, 31,* 609–616.

Bzoch, K., & League, R. (1991). *Receptive-Expressive-Emergent-Language Scale-Revised.* Baltimore, MD: University Park Press.

Cadman, D., Chambers, L. W., Walter, S. D., Feldman, W., Smith, K., & Ferguson, R. (1984). The usefulness of the Denver Developmental Screening Test to predict kindergarten problems in a general community population. *American Journal of Public Health, 74,* 1093–1097.

Camp, B. W., van Doorninck, W., Frankenburg, W., & Lampe, J. (1977). Preschool developmental testing in prediction of school problems. *Clinical Pediatrics, 16,* 257–263.

Carr, E., & Durand, V. (1985). The social communicative basis of severe behavior problems in children. In S. Reiss & R. Bootzin (Eds.), *Theoretical issues in behavior therapy.* New York: Academic Press.

Carter, A. S., Volkmar, F. R., Sparrow, S. S., Wang, J. J., Lord, C., Dawson, G., Fombonne, E., Loveland, K., Mesibov, G., &

Schopler, E. (1998). The Vineland Adaptive Behavior Scales: Supplementary norms for individuals with autism. *Journal of Autism and Developmental Disorders, 28,* 287–302.

Catalano, R. A. (1998). *When autism strikes: Families cope with childhood disintegrative disorder.* New York: Plenum Press.

Centers for Disease Control and Prevention. 1997, November. *Screening young children for lead poisoning: Guidance for state and local public health officials.* Atlanta, GA: Centers for Disease Control and Prevention- National Center for Environmental Health.

Chaffee, C. A., Cunningham, C. E., Secord-Gilbat, M., Elbard, H., & Richards, J. (1990). Screening effectiveness of the Minnesota Child Development Inventory expressive and receptive language scales: Sensitivity, specificity, and predictive value. *Psychological Assessment, 2,* 80–85.

Charman, T., Swettenham, J., Baron-Cohen, S., Cox, A., Baird, G., & Drew, A. (1997). Infants with autism: An investigation of empathy, pretend play, joint attention, and imitation. *Developmental Psychology, 33,* 781–789.

Charman, T., Swettenham, J., Baron-Cohen, S., Cox, A., Baird, G., & Drew, A. (1998). An experimental investigation of social-cognitive abilities in infants with autism: Clinical implications. *Infant Mental Health Journal, 19,* 260–275.

Chuang, S. H., Otsubo, H., Hwang, P., Orrison, W. W., Jr., & Lewine, J. D. (1995). Pediatric magnetic source imaging. *Neuroimaging Clinics of North America, 5,* 289–303.

Ciesielski, K. T., Knight, J. E., Prince, R. J., Harris, R. J., & Handmaker, S. D. (1995). Event-related potentials in cross-modal divided attention in autism. *Neuropsychologia, 33,* 225–246.

Cohen, D. J., Johnson, W. T., & Caparulo, B. K. (1976). Pica and elevated blood lead level in autistic and atypical children. *American Journal of Diseases of Children, 130,* 47–48.

Cohen, D. J., & Volkmar, F. R. (1997). *Handbook of autism and pervasive developmental disorders* (2nd ed.). New York: Wiley.

Cohen, D. J., Young, J. G., Lowe, T. L., & Harcherik, D. (1980). Thyroid hormone in autistic children. *Journal of Autism and Developmental Disorders, 10,* 445–450.

Cohen, I. L., Sudhalter, V., Pfadt, A., Jenkins, E. C., Brown, W. T., & Vietze, P. M. (1991). Why are autism and the fragile-X syndrome associated? Conceptual and methodological issues. *American Journal of Human Genetics, 48,* 195–202.

Cook, E. H., Jr., Courchesne, R. Y., Cox, N. J., Lord, C., Gonen, D., Guter, S. J., Lincoln, A., Nix, K., Haas, R., Leventhal, B. L., & Courchesne, E. (1998). Linkage-disequilibrium mapping of autistic disorder with 15q11–13 markers. *American Journal of Human Genetics, 62,* 1077–1083.

Cook, E. H., Jr., Perry, B. D., Dawson, G., Wainwright, M. S., & Leventhal, B. L. (1993). Receptor inhibition by immunoglobulins: specific inhibition by autistic children, their relatives, and control subjects. *Journal of Autism and Developmental Disorders, 23,* 67–78.

Courchesne, E., Muller, R. A., & Saiton, O. (1999). Brain weight in autism: normal in the majority of cases, megalencephalic in rare cases. *Neurology, 52,* 1057–1059.

Cox, A., Klein, K., Charman, T., Baird, G., Baron-Cohen, S., Swettenham, J., Drew, A., Wheelwright, S., & Nightengale, N. (1999). The early diagnosis of autism spectrum disorders: Use of the Autism Diagnostic Interview- Revised at 20 months and 42 months of age. *Journal of Child Psychology and Psychiatry,* in press.

Crais, E. R. (1995). Expanding the repertoire of tools and techniques for assessing the communication skills of infants and toddlers. *American Journal of Speech-Language Disorders, 4,* 47–59.

Cryan, E., Byrne, M., O'Donovan, A., & O'Callaghan, E. (1996). A case-control study of obstetric complications and later autistic disorder. *Journal of Autism and Developmental Disorders, 26,* 453–460.

Curatolo, P., Cusmai, R., Cortesi, F., Chiron, C., Jambeque, I., & Dulac, O. (1991). Neuropsychiatric aspects of tuberous sclerosis. New York Academy of Sciences and the National Tuberous

Sclerosis Association Conference: Tuberous sclerosis and allied disorders (1990, Bethesda, Maryland). *Annals of the New York Academy of Science, 615*, 8–16.

Curry, C. J., Stevenson, R. E., Aughton, D., Byrne, J., Carey, J. C., Cassidy, S., Cunniff, C., Graham, J. M., Jr., Jones, M. C., Kaback, M. M., Moeschler, J., Schaefer, G. B., Schwartz, S., Tarleton, J., & Opitz, J. (1997). Evaluation of mental retardation: recommendations of a Consensus Conference: American College of Medical Genetics. *American Journal of Medical Genetics, 72*, 468–477.

Dahlgren, S. O., & Gillberg, C. (1989). Symptoms in the first two years of life: A preliminary population study of infantile autism. *European Archives of Psychiatry and Neurological Sciences, 238*, 169–174.

Damasio, H., Maurer, R., Damasio, A. R., & Chui, H. (1980). Computerized tomographic scan findings in patients with autistic behavior. *Archives of Neurology, 37*, 504–510.

Davidovitch, M., Patterson, B., & Gartside, P. (1996). Head circumference measurements in children with autism. *Journal of Child Neurology, 11*, 389–393.

Dawson, G. (1996). Brief report: Neuropsychology of autism - a report on the state of the science. *Journal of Autism and Developmental Disorders, 26*, 179–184.

Dawson, G., Meltzoff, A. N., Osterling, J., & Rinaldi, J. (1998). Neuropsychological correlates of early symptoms of autism. *Child Development, 69*, 1276–1285.

Dawson, G., & Osterling, J. (1997). Early intervention in autism: Effectiveness and common elements of current approaches. In M. J. Guralnick (Ed.), *The effectiveness of early intervention: Second generation research* (pp. 307–326). Baltimore, MD: Paul H. Brookes.

Deb, S., & Prasad, K. B. (1994). The prevalence of autistic disorder among children with a learning disability. *British Journal of Psychiatry, 165*, 395–399.

DeLong, R. (1994). Children with autistic spectrum disorder and a family history of affective disorder. *Developmental Medicine and Child Neurology, 36*, 674–687.

DeLong, R., & Nohria, C. (1994). Psychiatric family history and neurological disease in autistic spectrum disorders. *Developmental Medicine and Child Neurology, 36*, 441–448.

Demb, H. B., & Papola, P. (1995). PDD and Prader-Willi syndrome. *Journal of the American Academy of Child and Adolescent Psychiatry, 34*, 539–540.

D'Eufemia, P., Celli, M., Finocchiaro, R., Pacifico, L., Viozzi, L., Zaccagnini, M., Cardi, E., & Giardini, O. (1996). Abnormal intestinal permeability in children with autism. *Acta Paediatrica, 85*, 1076–1079.

Deykin, E. Y., & MacMahon, B. (1980). Pregnancy, delivery, and neonatal complications among autistic children. *American Journal of Diseases of Children, 134*, 860–864.

Diamond, K. E. (1987). Predicting school problems from preschool developmental screening: A four-year followup of the Revised Denver Developmental Screening test and the role of parent report. *Journal of the Division of Early Childhood, 11*, 247–253.

DiLavore, P. C., Lord, C., & Rutter, M. (1995). The pre-linguistic autism diagnostic observation schedule. *Journal of Autism and Developmental Disorders, 25*, 355–379.

Dunn, L. M., & Dunn, L. (1981). *Peabody Picture Vocabulary Test-Revised*. Circle Pines, MN: American Guidance Service.

Dworkin, P. H. (1989). Developmental screening—expecting the impossible? *Pediatrics, 83*, 619–622.

Dworkin, P. H. (1992). Developmental screening: (still) expecting the impossible? *Pediatrics, 89*, 1253–1255.

Dykens, E. M., & Volkmar, F. R. (1997). Medical conditions associated with autism. In D. J. Cohen & F. R. Volkmar (Eds.), *Handbook of autism and pervasive developmental disorders* (2nd ed., pp. 388–410). New York: Wiley.

Ehlers, S., & Gillberg, C. (1993). The epidemiology of Asperger syndrome. A total population study. *Journal of Child Psychology and Psychiatry, 34*, 1327–1350.

Elliott, C. D. (1990). *Differential Abilities Scale (DAS)*. New York: Psychological Corp.

Evans-Jones, L. G., & Rosenbloom, L. (1978). Disintegrative psychosis in childhood. *Developmental Medicine and Child Neurology, 20*, 462–470.

Fein, D., Allen, D., Dunn, M., Feinstein, C., Green, L., Morris, R., Rapin, I., & Waterhouse, L. (1997). Pitocin induction and autism. *American Journal of Psychiatry, 154*, 438–439.

Feinstein, C., & Reiss, A. L. (1998). Autism: The point of view from fragile X studies. *Journal of Autism and Developmental Disorders, 28*, 393–405.

Fenske, E. C., Zalenski, S., Krantz, P. J., & McClannahan, L. E. (1985). Age at intervention and treatment outcome for autistic children in a comprehensive intervention program. Special Issue: Early intervention. *Analysis & Intervention in Developmental Disabilities, 5*, 49–58.

Fenson, L., Dale, P., Reznick, S., Thal, D., Bates, E., Hartung, J., Pethick, S., & Reilly, J. (1993). *MacArthur Communicative Development Inventories*. San Diego, CA: Singular.

Filipek, P. A. (1996). Brief report: Neuroimaging in autism - the state of the science 1995. *Journal of Autism and Developmental Disorders, 26*, 211–215.

Filipek, P. A. (1999). Neuroimaging in the developmental disorders: The state of the science. *Journal of Child Psychology and Psychiatry, 40*, 113–128.

Filipek, P. A. (1999). The autistic spectrum disorders. In K. F. Swaiman & S. Ashwal (Eds.), *Pediatric neurology. Principles and practice* (3rd ed., pp. 606–628). St. Louis, MO: Mosby.

Filipek, P. A., Kennedy, D. N., & Caviness, V. S., Jr. (1992a). Neuroimaging in child neuropsychology. In I. Rapin & S. Segalowitz (Eds.), *Handbook of neuropsychology: Vol. 6. Child neuropsychology* (pp. 301–329). Amsterdam: Elsevier.

Filipek, P. A., Richelme, C., Kennedy, D. N., Rademacher, J., Pitcher, D. A., Zidel, S. Y., & Caviness, V. S. (1992b). Morphometric analysis of the brain in developmental language disorders and autism. *Annals of Neurology, 32*, 475.

Findling, R. L., Maxwell, K., Scotese-Wojtila, L., Huang, J., Yamashita, T., & Wiznitzer, M. (1997). High-dose pyridoxine and magnesium administration in children with autistic disorder: An absence of salutary effects in a double-blind, placebo-controlled study. *Journal of Autism and Developmental Disorders, 27*, 467–478.

Finegan, J.-A., & Quarrington, B. (1979). Pre-, peri- and neonatal factors and infantile autism. *Journal of Child Psychology and Psychiatry, 20*, 119–128.

Fitzpatrick, T. B. (1991). History and significance of white macules, earliest visible sign of tuberous sclerosis. *Annals of the New York Academy of Science, 615*, 26.

Folstein, S., & Rutter, M. (1977a). Genetic influences and infantile autism. *Nature, 265*, 726–728.

Folstein, S., & Rutter, M. (1977b). Infantile autism: a genetic study of 21 twin pairs. *Journal of Child Psychology and Psychiatry, 18*, 297–321.

Fombonne, E., Bolton, P., Prior, J., Jordan, H., & Rutter, M. (1997). A family study of autism: Cognitive patterns and levels in parents and siblings. *Journal of Child Psychology and Psychiatry, 38*, 667–683.

Frankenburg, W. K. (1986). *Revised Denver Pre-Screening Developmental Questionnaire*. Denver, CO: Denver Developmental Materials.

Frankenburg, W. K., Dodds, J., Archer, P., Shapiro, H., & Bresnick, B. (1992). The Denver II: A major revision and restandardization of the Denver Developmental Screening Test. *Pediatrics, 89*, 91–97.

Gagnon, L., Mottron, L., & Joanette, Y. (1997). Questioning the validity of the semantic-pragmatic syndrome diagnosis. *Autism, 1*, 37–55.

Gardner, M. F. (1990a). *Expressive One-Word Picture Vocabulary Test-Revised*. Noyato, CA: Academic Therapy Publications.

Gardner, M. F. (1990b). *Receptive One-Word Picture Vocabulary Test-Revised*. Novato, CA: Academic Therapy Publications.

Garnett, M. S., & Attwood, A. J. (1998). The Australian Scale for Asperger's syndrome. In T. Attwood (Ed.), *Asperger's syndrome. A guide for parents and professionals* (pp. 17–19). London: Kingsley.

Gentile, P. S., Trentalange, M. J., Zamichek, W., & Coleman, M. (1983). Brief report: Trace elements in the hair of autistic and control children. *Journal of Autism and Developmental Disorders, 13,* 205–206.

Geschwind, D. H., Cummings, J. L., & the CAN Consensus Group. (1998). Autism screening and diagnostic evaluation: CAN Consensus Statement. *CNS Spectrums, 3,* 40–49. URL: http://www.canfoundation.org/newcansite/aboutcan/consensus.html

Ghaziuddin, M., Butler, E., Tsai, L., & Ghaziuddin, N. (1994). Is clumsiness a marker for Asperger syndrome? *Journal of Intellectual Disability Research, 38,* 519–27.

Ghaziuddin, M., & Gerstein, L. (1996). Pedantic speaking style differentiates Asperger syndrome from high-functioning autism. *Journal of Autism and Developmental Disorders, 26,* 585–595.

Ghaziuddin, M., Shakal, J., & Tsai, L. (1995). Obstetric factors in Asperger syndrome: comparison with high-functioning autism. *Journal of Intellectual Disability Research, 39,* 538–543.

Gillberg, C. (1990). Infantile autism: diagnosis and treatment. *Acta Psychiatrica Scandinavica, 81,* 209–215.

Gillberg, C. (1991). The treatment of epilepsy in autism. *Journal of Autism and Developmental Disorders, 21,* 61–77.

Gillberg, C. (1994). Debate and argument: having Rett syndrome in the ICD-10 PDD category does not make sense. *Journal of Child Psychology and Psychiatry, 35,* 377–8.

Gillberg, C. (1998). Chromosomal disorders and autism. *Journal of Autism and Developmental Disorders, 28,* 415–425.

Gillberg, C., Ehlers, S., Schaumann, H., Jakobson, G., Dahlgren, S. O., Lindbolm, R., Bagenhold, A., Tjuus, T., & Blidner, E. (1990). Autism under age 3 years: A clinical study of 28 cases referred for autistic symptoms in infancy. *Journal of Child Psychology and Psychiatry, 31,* 921–934.

Gillberg, C., & Gillberg, I. C. (1983). Infantile autism: A total population study of reduced optimality in the pre-, peri-, and neonatal period. *Journal of Autism and Developmental Disorders, 13,* 153–166.

Gillberg, C., & Gillberg, I. C. (1989). Asperger syndrome—some epidemiological considerations. A research note. *Journal of Child Psychology and Psychiatry, 30.*

Gillberg, C., & Steffenburg, S. (1987). Outcome and prognostic factors in infantile autism and similar conditions: a population-based study of 46 cases followed through puberty. *Journal of Autism and Developmental Disorders, 17,* 273–287.

Gillberg, C., Steffenburg, S., & Schaumann, H. (1991). Is autism more common now than ten years ago? *British Journal of Psychiatry, 158,* 403–409.

Gillberg, C., & Wahlstrom, J. (1985). Chromosome abnormalities in infantile autism and other childhood psychoses: a population study of 66 cases. *Developmental Medicine and Child Neurology, 27,* 293–304.

Gillberg, I. C., Gillberg, C., & Ahlsen, G. (1994). Autistic behaviour and attention deficits in tuberous sclerosis: A population-based study. *Developmental Medicine and Child Neurology, 36,* 50–56.

Gilliam, J. E. (1995). *Gilliam Autism Rating Scale (GARS).* Austin, TX: Pro-Ed.

Glascoe, F. P. (1991). Can clinical judgment detect children with speech-language problems? *Pediatrics, 87,* 317–322.

Glascoe, F. P. (1994). It's not what it seems. The relationship between parents' concerns and children with global delays. *Clinical Pediatrics, 33,* 292–6.

Glascoe, F. P. (1996). *A validation study and the psychometric properties of the BRIGANCE® Screens.* North Billerica, MA: Curriculum Associate.

Glascoe, F. P. (1997). Parents' concerns about children's development: prescreening technique or screening test? *Pediatrics, 99,* 522–528.

Glascoe, F. P. (1998) *Collaborating with parents: Using parents' evaluation of developmental status to detect and address developmental and behavioral problems.* Nashville, TN: Ellsworth & Vandermeer.

Glascoe, F. P., Altemeier, W. A., & MacLean, W. E. (1989). The importance of parents' concerns about their child's development. *American Journal of Diseases of Children, 143,* 955–958.

Glascoe, F. P., Byrne, K. E., Ashford, L. G., Johnson, K. L., Chang, B., & Strickland, B. (1992). Accuracy of the Denver-II in developmental screening. *Pediatrics, 89,* 1221–1225.

Glascoe, F. P., & Dworkin, P. H. (1995). The role of parents in the detection of developmental and behavioral problems. *Pediatrics, 95,* 829–836.

Glascoe, F. P., Foster, E. M., & Wolraich, M. L. (1997). An economic analysis of developmental detection methods. *Pediatrics, 99,* 830–837.

Glascoe, F. P., MacLean, W. E., & Stone, W. L. (1991). The importance of parents' concerns about their child's behavior. *Clinical Pediatrics, 30,* 8–11.

Gorga, M. P., Kaminski, J. R., Beauchaine, K. L., Jesteadt, W., & Neely, S. T. (1989). Auditory brainstem responses from children three months to three years of age. *Journal of Speech and Hearing Research, 32,* 281–288.

Grant, J., & Gittelsohn, A. M. (1972). The Denver Developmental Screening Test compared with the Stanford-Binet test. *Health Service Reports, 87,* 473–476.

Gravel, J. S., Kurtzberg, D., Stapells, D., Vaughan, H., & Wallace, I. (1989). Case studies. *Seminars in Hearing, 10,* 272–287.

Greer, S., Bauchner, H., & Zuckerman, B. (1989). The Denver Developmental Screening Test: how good is its predictive validity? *Developmental Medicine and Child Neurology, 31,* 774–781.

Grewe, T. S., Danhauer, J. L., Danhauer, K. J., & Thornton, A. R. (1994). Clinical use of otoacoustic emissions in children with autism. *International Journal of Pediatric Otorhinolaryngology, 30,* 123–132.

Groden, G., & Mann, L. (1988). Intellectual functioning and assessment. In G. Groden & M. G. Baron (Eds.), *Autism: Strategies for change* (pp. 75–97). New York: Gardner.

Guerin, D., & Gottfried, A. W. (1987). Minnesota Child Development Inventories: Predictors of intelligence, achievement, and adaptability. *Journal of Pediatric Psychology, 12,* 595–609.

Hagberg, B., Aicardi, J., Dias, K., & Ramos, O. (1983). A progressive syndrome of autism, dementia, ataxia, and loss of purposeful hand use in girls: Rett's syndrome: Report of 35 cases. *Annals of Neurology, 14,* 471–479.

Harnadek, M. C., & Rourke, B. P. (1994). Principal identifying features of the syndrome of nonverbal learning disabilities in children. *Journal of Learning Disabilities, 27,* 144–154.

Harper, D. C., & Wacker, D. P. (1983). The efficiency of the Denver Developmental Screening Test for rural disadvantaged pre-school children. *Journal of Pediatric Psychology, 8,* 273–283.

Harrison, J. E., & Bolton, P. F. (1997). Annotation: Tuberous sclerosis. *Journal of Child Psychology and Psychiatry, 38,* 603–614.

Hashimoto, O., Shimizu, Y., & Kawasaki, Y. (1993). Brief report: Low frequency of the fragile X syndrome among Japanese autistic subjects. *Journal of Autism and Developmental Disorders, 23,* 201–9.

Hashimoto, T., Aihara, R., Tayama, M., Miyazaki, M., Shirakawa, Y., & Kuroda, Y. (1991). Reduced thyroid-stimulating hormone response to thyrotropin-releasing hormone in autistic boys. *Developmental Medicine and Child Neurology, 33,* 313–319.

Hedrick, D. L., Prather, E. M., & Tobin, A. R. (1984). *Sequenced Inventory of Communication Development- Revised Edition.* Seattle, WA: University of Washington Press.

Hoshino, Y., Kaneko, M., Yashima, Y., Kumashiro, H., Volkmar, F. R., & Cohen, D. J. (1987). Clinical features of autistic children with setback course in their infancy. *Japanese Journal of Psychiatry and Neurology, 41,* 237–245.

Howlin, P., & Moore, A. (1997). Diagnosis of autism. A survey of over 1200 patients in the UK. *Autism, 1,* 135–162.

Hoyson, M., Jamieson, B., & Strain, P. S. (1984). Individualized group instruction of normally developing and autistic-like children: The LEAP curriculum model. *Journal of the Division of Early Childhood, 8,* 157–172.

Hughes, C., Leboyer, M., & Bouvard, M. (1997). Executive function in parents of children with autism. *Psychological Medicine, 27,* 209–220.

Hunt, A., & Shepherd, C. (1993). A prevalence study of autism in tuberous sclerosis. *Journal of Autism and Developmental Disorders, 23,* 323–339.

Individuals with Disabilities Education Act- IDEA'97. (1997). *Public Law 105–17.*

Ireton, H. (1992). *Child Development Inventories.* Minneapolis, MN: Behavior Science Systems.

Ireton, H., & Glascoe, F. P. (1995). Assessing children's development using parents' reports. The Child Development Inventory. *Clinical Pediatrics, 34,* 248–255.

Ishii, T., & Takahasi, O. (1983). The epidemiology of autistic children in Toyota, Japan: Prevalence. *Japanese Journal of Child and Adolescent Psychiatry, 24,* 311–321.

Jacobson, J. W., & Mulick, J. A. (1996). *Manual of diagnosis and professional practice in mental retardation.* Washington, DC: APA Books.

Jensen, V. K., Larrieu, J. A., & Mack, K. K. (1997). Differential diagnosis between Attention-Deficit/Hyperactivity Disorder and Pervasive Developmental Disorder- Not Otherwise Specified. *Clinical Pediatrics, 36,* 555–561.

Johnson, C. P., & Blasco, P. A. (1997). Infant growth and development. *Pediatrics in Review, 18,* 224–242.

Johnson-Martin, N. M. (1988). Assessment of low-functioning children. In E. Schopler & G. B. Mesibov (Eds.), *Diagnosis and assessment in autism* (pp. 303–319). New York: Plenum Press.

Jones, A. C., Daniells, C. E., Snell, R. G., Tachataki, M., Idziaszczyk, S. A., Krawczak, M., Sampson, J. R., & Cheadle, J. (1997). Molecular genetic and phenotypic analysis reveals differences between TSC1 and TSC2 associated familial and sporadic tuberous sclerosis. *Human Molecular Genetics, 6,* 2155–2161.

Jorde, L. B., Mason-Brothers, A., Waldmann, R., Ritvo, E. R., Freeman, B. J., Pingree, C., McMahon, W. M., Petersen, B., Jenson, W. R., & Moll, A. (1990). The UCLA-University of Utah epidemiologic survey of autism: genealogical analysis of familial aggregation. *American Journal of Medical Genetics, 36,* 85–8.

Jure, R., Rapin, I., & Tuchman, R. F. (1991). Hearing-impaired autistic children. *Developmental Medicine and Child Neurology, 33,* 1062–1072.

Kanner, L. (1943). Autistic disturbances of affective contact. *Nervous Child, 2,* 217–250.

Kemner, C., Verbaten, M. N., Cuperus, J. M., Camfferman, G., & Van Engeland, H. (1994). Visual and somatosensory event-related brain potentials in autistic children and three different control groups. *Electroencephalography and Clinical Neurophysiology, 92,* 225–237.

Kemner, C., Verbaten, M. N., Cuperus, J. M., Camfferman, G., & van Engeland, H. (1995). Auditory event-related brain potentials in autistic children and three different control groups. *Biological Psychiatry, 38,* 150–165.

Kientz, M. A., & Dunn, W. (1997). A comparison of the performance of children with and without autism on the Sensory Profile. *American Journal of Occupational Therapy, 51,* 530–537.

Klauck, S. M., Munstermann, E., Bieber-Martig, B., Ruhl, D., Lisch, S., Schmotzer, G., Poustka, A., & Poustka, F. (1997). Molecular genetic analysis of the FMR-1 gene in a large collection of autistic patients. *Human Genetics, 100,* 224–229.

Klin, A. (1993). Auditory brainstem responses in autism: brainstem dysfunction or peripheral hearing loss? *Journal of Autism and Developmental Disorders, 23,* 15–35.

Klin, A., Carter, A., Volkmar, F. R., Cohen, D. J., Marans, W. D., & Sparrow, S. (1997). Developmentally based assessments. In D. J. Cohen & F. R. Volkmar (Eds.), *Handbook of autism and pervasive developmental disorders* (2nd ed., pp. 411–447). New York: Wiley.

Klin, A., Volkmar, F. R., Sparrow, S. S., Cicchetti, D. V., & Rourke, B. P. (1995). Validity and neuropsychological characterization of Asperger syndrome: convergence with nonverbal learning disabilities syndrome. *Journal of Child Psychology and Psychiatry, 36,* 1127–1140.

Klinger, L. G., & Dawson, G. (1995). A fresh look at categorization abilities in persons with autism. In E. Schopler & G. B. Mesibov (Eds.), *Learning and cognition in autism* (pp. 119–136). New York: Plenum Press.

Kurita, H. (1985). Infantile autism with speech loss before the age of thirty months. *Journal of the American Academy of Child Psychiatry, 24,* 191–196.

Kurita, H. (1996). Specificity and developmental consequences of speech loss in children with pervasive developmental disorders. *Psychiatry and Clinical Neurosciences, 50,* 181–184.

Kurita, H. (1997). A comparative study of Asperger syndrome with high-functioning atypical autism. *Psychiatry and Clinical Neurosciences, 51,* 67–70.

Kurita, H., Kita, M., & Miyake, Y. (1992). A comparative study of development and symptoms among disintegrative psychosis and infantile autism with and without speech loss. *Journal of Autism and Developmental Disorders, 22,* 175–188.

Lainhart, J. E., Piven, J., Wzorek, M., Landa, R., Santangelo, S. L., Coon, H., & Folstein, S. E. (1997). Macrocephaly in children and adults with autism. *Journal of the American Academy of Child and Adolescent Psychiatry, 36,* 282–290.

Landau, W. M., & Kleffner, F. R. (1957). Syndrome of acquired aphasia with convulsive disorder in children. *Neurology, 7,* 523–530.

Landau, W. M., & Kleffner, F. R. (1998). Syndrome of acquired aphasia with convulsive disorder in children. 1957. *Neurology, 51,* 1241–1249.

LaPerchia, P. (1987). Behavioral disorders, learning disabilities and megavitamin therapy. *Adolescence, 22,* 729–738.

Le Couteur, A., Bailey, A., Goode, S., Pickles, A., Robertson, S., Gottesman, I., & Rutter, M. (1996). A broader phenotype of autism: the clinical spectrum in twins. *Journal of Child Psychology and Psychiatry, 37,* 785–801.

Le Couteur, A., Rutter, M., Lord, C., Rios, P., Robertson, S., Holdgrafer, M., & McLennan, J. (1989). Autism diagnostic interview: A standardized investigator-based instrument. *Journal of Autism and Developmental Disorders, 19,* 363–387.

Le Couteur, A., Trygstad, O., Evered, C., Gillberg, C., & Rutter, M. (1988). Infantile autism and urinary excretion of peptides and protein-associated peptide complexes. *Journal of Autism and Developmental Disorders, 18,* 181–190.

Levy, S., Zoltak, B., & Saelens, T. (1988). A comparison of obstetrical records of autistic and nonautistic referrals for psychoeducational evaluations. *Journal of Autism and Developmental Disorders, 18,* 573–581.

Lincoln, A. J., Allen, M. H., & Kilman, A. (1995a). The assessment and interpretation of intellectual abilities in people with autism. In E. Schopler & G. B. Mesibov (Eds.), *Learning and cognition in autism* (pp. 89–118). New York: Plenum Press.

Lincoln, A. J., Courchesne, E., Harms, L., & Allen, M. (1995b). Sensory modulation of auditory stimuli in children with autism and receptive developmental language disorder: event-related brain potential evidence. *Journal of Autism and Developmental Disorders, 25,* 521–539.

Lindquist, G. T. (1982). Preschool screening as a means of predicting later reading achievement. *Journal of Learning Disabilities, 15,* 331–332.

Lockyer, L., & Rutter, M. (1970). A five- to fifteen-year follow-up study of infantile psychosis. IV. Patterns of cognitive ability. *British Journal of Social and Clinical Psychology, 9,* 152–163.

Lombard, J. (1998). Autism: a mitochondrial disorder? *Medical Hypotheses, 50,* 497–500.

Lord, C. (1995). Follow-up of two-year-olds referred for possible autism. *Journal of Child Psychology and Psychiatry, 36,* 1365–1382.

Lord, C. (1998). *The Autism Diagnostic Observation Schedule-Generic (ADOS-G).* Paper presented at the NIH State of the Science in Autism: Screening and Diagnosis Working Conference, Bethesda, MD.

Lord, C., Mulloy, C., Wendelboe, M., & Schopler, E. (1991). Pre- and perinatal factors in high-functioning females and males with autism. *Journal of Autism and Developmental Disorders, 21,* 197–209.

Lord, C., & Paul, R. (1997). Language and communication in autism. In D. J. Cohen & F. R. Volkmar (Eds.), *Handbook of autism and pervasive developmental disorders* (2nd ed., pp. 195–225). New York: Wiley.

Lord, C., Pickles, A., McLennan, J., Rutter, M., Bregman, J., Folstein, S., Fombonne, E., Leboyer, M., & Minshew, N. (1997). Diagnosing autism: analyses of data from the Autism Diagnostic Interview. *Journal of Autism and Developmental Disorders, 27,* 501–517.

Lord, C., Rutter, M., Goode, S., Heemsbergen, J., Jordan, H., Mawhood, L., & Schopler, E. (1989). Autism Diagnostic Observation Schedule: A standardized observation of communicative and social behavior. *Journal of Autism and Developmental Disorders, 19,* 185–212.

Lord, C., Rutter, M., & Le Couteur, A. (1994). Autism Diagnostic Interview- Revised: A revised version of a diagnostic interview for caregivers of individuals with possible pervasive developmental disorders. *Journal of Autism and Developmental Disorders, 24,* 659–685.

Lord, C., Storoschuk, S., Rutter, M., & Pickles, A. (1993). Using the ADI-R to diagnose autism in preschool children. *Infant Mental Health Journal, 14,* 234–252.

Lotter, V. (1966). Epidemiology of autistic conditions in youg children. I. Prevalence. *Social Psychiatry, 1,* 124–137.

Lotter, V. (1967). Epidemiology of autistic conditions in young children: Some characteristics of the children and their parents. *Social Psychiatry, 1,* 163–173.

Lovaas, O. I. (1987). Behavioral treatment and normal educational and intellectual functioning in young autistic children. *Journal of Consulting and Clinical Psychology, 55,* 3–9.

Lucarelli, S., Frediani, T., Zingoni, A. M., Ferruzzi, F., Giardini, O., Quintieri, F., Barbato, M., P, D. E., & Cardi, E. (1995). Food allergy and infantile autism. *Panminerva Medica, 37,* 137–141.

Lund, N., & Duchan, J. (1993). *Assessing children's language in naturalistic contexts of early intervention.* Baltimore, MD: Paul H. Brookes.

Mailloux, Z., Parham, D., & Roley, S. (1998). *Performance of children with autism on the Sensory Integration and Praxis tests.* Paper presented at the World Federation of Occupational Therapy Conference, Toronto, Canada.

Majnemer, A., & Rosenblatt, B. (1994). Reliability of parental recall of developmental milestones. *Pediatric Neurology, 10,* 304–308.

Manjiviona, J., & Prior. M. (1995). Comparison of Asperger syndrome and high-functioning autistic children on a test of motor impairment. *Journal of Autism and Developmental Disorders, 25,* 23–39.

Marcus, L., Lansing, M., & Schopler, E. (1993). Assessment of children with autism and pervasive developmental disorder. In J. L. Culbertson & D. J. Willis (Eds.), *Testing young children: A reference guide for developmental, psychoeducational and psychosocial assessments.* Austin, TX: Pro-Ed.

Marcus, L. M., & Stone, W. L. (1993). Assessment of the young autistic child. In E. Schopler & G. B. Mesibov (Eds.), *Preschool issues in autism?* New York: Plenum Press.

Mars, A. E., Mauk, J. E., & Dowrick, P. (1998). Symptoms of pervasive developmental disorders as observed in prediagnostic home videos of infants and toddlers. *Journal of Pediatrics, 132,* 500–504.

Mason-Brothers, A., Ritvo, E. R., Guze, B., Mo, A., Freeman, B. J., Funderburk, S. J., & Schroth, P. C. (1987). Pre-, peri-, and postnatal factors in 181 autistic patients from single and multiple incidence families. *Journal of the American Academy of Child and Adolescent Psychiatry, 26,* 39–42.

Mason-Brothers, A., Ritvo, E. R., Pingree, C., Petersen, P. B., Jenson, W. R., McMahon, W. M., Freeman, B. J., Jorde, L. B., Spencer, M. J., Mo, A., & Ritvo, A. (1990). The UCLA-University of Utah epidemiologic survey of autism: prenatal, perinatal, and postnatal factors. *Pediatrics, 86,* 514–9.

McEachin, J. J., Smith, T., & Lovaas, O. I. (1993). Long-term outcome for children with autism who received early intensive behavioral treatment. *American Journal on Mental Retardation, 97,* 359–372.

McLennan, J. D., Lord, C., & Schopler, E. (1993). Sex differences in higher functioning people with autism. *Journal of Autism and Developmental Disorders, 23,* 217–227.

Michelson, A. M. (1998). Selenium glutathione peroxidase: Some aspects in man. *Journal of Environmental Pathology, Toxicology, and Oncology, 17,* 233–239.

Miller, J., & Paul, R. (1995). *The clinical assessment of language comprehension.* Baltimore, MD: Paul H. Brookes.

Miller, J. N., & Ozonoff, S. (1997). Did Asperger's cases have Asperger Disorder? A research note. *Journal of Child Psychology and Psychiatry, 38,* 247–251.

Minshew, N. J. (1996a). Autism. In B. O. Berg (Ed.), *Principles of child neurology* (pp. 1713–1730). New York: McGraw-Hill.

Minshew, N. J. (1996b). Brief report. Brain mechanisms in autism—Functional and structural abnormalities. *Journal of Autism and Developmental Disorders, 26,* 205–209.

Minshew, N. J., & Dombrowski, S. M. (1994). *In vivo* neuroanatomy of autism: Imaging studies. In M. L. Bauman & T. L. Kemper (Eds.), *The neurobiology of autism* (pp. 66–85). Baltimore, MD: Johns Hopkins University Press.

Minshew, N. J., & Goldstein, G. (1998). Autism as a disorder of complex information processing. *Mental Retardation and Developmental Disabilities Research Reviews, 4,* 129–136.

Minshew, N. J., Goldstein, G., Taylor, H. G., & Siegel, D. J. (1994). Academic achievement in high functioning autistic individuals. *Journal of Clinical and Experimental Neuropsychology, 16,* 261–270.

Minshew, N. J., Sweeney, J. A., & Bauman, M. L. (1997). Neurologic aspects of autism. In D. J. Cohen & F. R. Volkmar (Eds.), *Handbook of autism and pervasive developmental disorders,* (2nd ed., pp. 344–369). New York: Wiley.

Morrell, F., Whisler, W. W., Smith, M. C., Hoeppner, T. J., de Toledo-Morrell, L., Pierre-Louis. S. J., Kanner, A. M., Buelow, J. M., Ristanovic, R., Bergen, D., & *et al.* (1995). Landau-Kleffner syndrome. Treatment with subpial intracortical transection. *Brain, 118,* 1529–46.

Mullen, E. M. (1997). *Mullen Scales of Early Learning.* Los Angeles: Western Psychological Services.

Mundy, P., Sigman, M., & Kasari, C. (1990). A longitudinal study of joint attention and language development in autistic children. *Journal of Autism and Developmental Disorders, 20,* 115–128.

Naidu, S. (1997). Rett syndrome: A disorder affecting early brain growth. *Annals of Neurology, 42,* 3–10.

Nass, R., Gross, A., & Devinsky, O. (1998). Autism and autistic epileptiform regression with occipital spikes. *Developmental Medicine and Child Neurology, 40,* 453–458.

Nelson, K. B. (1991). Prenatal and perinatal factors in the etiology of autism. *Pediatrics, 87,* 761–766.

Olsson, I., Steffenburg, S., & Gillberg, C. (1988). Epilepsy in autism and autisticlike conditions. A population-based study. *Archives of Neurology, 45,* 666–668.

OMIM™. (1997). *Online Mendelian inheritance in man.* Baltimore and Bethesda, MD: Center for Medical Genetics, Johns Hopkins University and National Center for Biotechnology Information, National Library of Medicine.

Ornitz, E. M., Guthrie, D., & Farley, A. H. (1977). The early development of autistic children. *Journal of Autism and Childhood Schizophrenia, 7,* 207–229.

Osterling, J., & Dawson, G. (1994). Early recognition of children with autism: A study of first birthday home videotapes. *Journal of Autism and Developmental Disorders, 24,* 247–257.

Osterling, J., & Dawson, G. (1999). *Early identification of 1-year-olds with autism versus mental retardation based on home videotapes of first birthday parties.* Paper presented at the Proceedings of the Society for Research in Child Development, Albuquerque, NM.

Ozonoff, S., & Cathcart, K. (1998). Effectiveness of a home program intervention for young children with autism. *Journal of Autism and Developmental Disorders, 28,* 25–32.

Pavone, L., Fiumara, A., Bottaro, G., Mazzone, D., & Coleman, M. (1997). Autism and celiac disease: Failure to validate the hypothesis that a link might exist. *Biological Psychiatry, 42,* 72–75.

Percy, A., Gillberg, C., Hagberg, B., & Witt-Engerstrom, I. (1990). Rett syndrome and the autistic disorders. *Neurology, Clinics of North America, 8,* 659–676.

Pericak-Vance, M. A., Wolpert, C. M., Menold, M. M., Bass, M. P., DeLong, G. R., Beaty, L. M., Zimmerman, A., Potter, N., Gilbert, J. R., Vance, J. M., Wright, H. H., Abramson, R. K., & Cuccaro, M. L. (1997). Linkage evidence supports the involvement of chromosome 15 in autistic disorder. *American Journal of Human Genetics, 61,* A40.

Piven, J., Chase, G. A., Landa, R., Wzorek, M., Gayle, J., Cloud, D., & Folstein, S. (1991a). Psychiatric disorders in the parents of autistic individuals. *Journal of the American Academy of Child and Adolescent Psychiatry, 30,* 471–478.

Piven, J., Gayle, J., Chase, G. A., Fink, B., Landa, R., Wzorek, M. M., & Folstein, S. E. (1990). A family history study of neuropsychiatric disorders in the adult siblings of autistic individuals. *Journal of the American Academy of Child and Adolescent Psychiatry, 29,* 177–183.

Piven, J., Gayle, J., Landa, R., Wzorek, M., & Folstein, S. (1991b). The prevalence of fragile X in a sample of autistic individuals diagnosed using a standardized interview. *Journal of the American Academy of Child and Adolescent Psychiatry, 30,* 825–830.

Piven, J., Palmer, P., Jacobi, D., Childress, D., & Arndt, S. (1997a). Broader autism phenotype: evidence from a family history study of multiple-incidence autism families. *American Journal of Psychiatry, 154,* 185–190.

Piven, J., Palmer, P., Landa, R., Santangelo, S., Jacobi, D., & Childress, D. (1997b). Personality and language characteristics in parents from multiple-incidence autism families. *American Journal of Medical Genetics, 74,* 398–411.

Piven, J., Simon, J., Chase, G. A., Wzorek, M., Landa, R., Gayle, J., & Folstein, S. (1993). The etiology of autism: Pre-, peri- and neonatal factors. *Journal of the American Academy of Child and Adolescent Psychiatry, 32,* 1256–1263.

Piven, J., Wzorek, M., Landa, R., Lainhart, J., Bolton, P., Chase, G. A., & Folstein, S. (1994). Personality characteristics of the parents of autistic individuals. *Psychological Medicine, 24,* 783–795.

Porter, R., Goldstein, E., Galil, A., & Carel, C. (1992). Diagnosing the 'strange' child. *Child Care, Health and Development, 18,* 57–63.

Prieve, B. A. (1992). Otoacoustic emission in infants and children: Basic characteristics and clinical application. *Seminars in Hearing, 13,* 37–52.

Prizant, B. M., & Rydell, P. J. (1993). Assessment and intervention for unconventional considerations for unconventional verbal behavior. In J. Reichle & D. Wacker (Eds.), *Communicative alternatives to challenging behavior* (pp. 263–297). Baltimore, MD: Paul H. Brookes.

Prizant, B. M., & Wetherby, A. M. (1993). Communication assessment of young children. *Infants and Young Children, 5,* 20–34.

Prizant, B. M., Wetherby, A. M., Schuler, A. L., & Rydell, P. J. (1997). Enhancing communication: Language approaches. In

D. J. Cohen & F. R. Volkmar (Eds.), *Handbook of autism and pervasive developmental disorders* (2nd ed., pp. 572–605). New York: Wiley.

Rapin, I. (1995). Physicians' testing of children with developmental disabilities. *Journal of Child Neurology, 10 (Suppl.),* S11–15.

Rapin, I. (1996a). Historical data. In I. Rapin (Ed.), *Preschool children with inadequate communication: Developmental language disorder, autism, low IQ* (pp. 58–97). London: MacKeith.

Rapin, I. (1996b): Neurological examination. In I. Rapin (Ed.), *Preschool children with inadequate communication: Developmental language disorder, autism, low IQ* (pp. 98–122). London: MacKeith.

Rapin, I. (Ed.). (1996c): *Preschool children with inadequate communication: Developmental language disorder, autism, low IQ.* London: MacKeith.

Rapin, I. (1997). Autism. *New England Journal of Medicine, 337,* 97–104.

Rapin, I., & Allen, D. A. (1987). Syndromes in developmental dysphasia and adult aphasia. *Research Publications - Association for Research in Nervous and Mental Disease, 66,* 57–75.

Rapin, I., Allen, D. A., Aram, D. M., Dunn, M. A., Fein, D., Morris, R., & Waterhouse, L. (1996). Classification issues. In I. Rapin (Ed.). *Preschool children with inadequate communication: Developmental language disorder, autism, low IQ* (pp. 190–213). London: MacKeith.

Rapin, I., & Dunn, M. (1997). Language disorders in children with autism. *Seminars in Pediatric Neurology, 4,* 86–92.

Reed, T., & Peterson, C. C. (1990). A comparative study of autistic subjects' performance at two levels of visual and cognitive perspective taking. *Journal of Autism and Developmental Disorders, 20,* 555–567.

Reich, M., Lenoir, P., Malvy, J., Perrot, A., & Sauvage, D. (1997). Bourneville's tuberous sclerosis and autism. *Archives of Pediatrics, 4,* 170–175.

Restall, G., & Magill-Evans, J. (1994). Play and preschool children with autism. *American Journal of Occupational Therapy, 48,* 113–120.

Rett, A. (1966). Euber eine eigenartiges hirnatrophisches Syndrome bei hyperammonamie iim Kindesalter. *Weiner Medizmische Wochenschrift, 116,* 723–728.

Riikonen, R., & Amnell, G. (1981). Psychiatric disorders in children with earlier infantile spasms. *Developmental Medicine and Child Neurology, 23,* 747–760.

Riikonen, R., & Simell, O. (1990). Tuberous sclerosis and infantile spasms. *Developmental Medicine and Child Neurology, 32,* 203–209.

Ritvo, E. R., & Freeman, B. J. (1978). National society for autistic children definition of the syndrome of autism. *Journal of Autism and Childhood Schizophrenia, 8,* 162–167.

Ritvo, E. R., Mason-Brothers, A., Freeman, B. J., Pingree, C., Jenson, W. R., McMahon, W. M., Petersen, P. B., Jorde, L. B., Mo, A., & Ritvo, A. (1990). The UCLA-University of Utah epidemiologic survey of autism: The etiologic role of rare diseases. *American Journal of Psychiatry, 147,* 1614–1621.

Robinette, M. S. (1992). Clinical observations with transient evoked otoacoustic emissions with adults. *Seminars in Hearing, 13,* 23–36.

Robins, D., Fein, D., Barton, M., & Liss, M. (1999). *The Autism Screening Project: How early can autism be detected?* Paper presented at the American Psychological Association Meeting, Boston.

Rogers, S. J. (1996). Brief report: Early intervention in autism. *Journal of Autism and Developmental Disorders, 26,* 243–247.

Rogers, S. J. (1998). Empirically supported comprehensive treatments for young children with autism. *Journal of Clinical Child Psychology, 27,* 168–179.

Rogers, S. J. (in press). Differential diagnosis of autism before age 3. *International Review of Research in Mental Retardation.*

Rogers, S. J., Bennetto, L., McEvoy, R., & Pennington, B. F. (1996). Imitation and pantomime in high-functioning adolescents with autism spectrum disorders. *Child Development, 67,* 2060–2073.

Rogers, S. J., & DiLalla, D. L. (1990). Age of symptom onset in young children with pervasive developmental disorders. *Journal of the American Academy of Child and Adolescent Psychiatry, 29,* 863–872.

Rogers, S. J., & Lewis, H. (1989). An effective day treatment model for young children with pervasive developmental disorders. *Journal of the American Academy of Child and Adolescent Psychiatry, 28,* 207–214.

Roid, G., & Miller, L. (1997). *Leiter International Performance Scale- Revised.* Wood Dale, IL: Stoelting.

Rossetti, L. (1990). *Infant-Toddler Language Scale.* East Moline, IL: LinguiSystems.

Rossi, P. G., Parmeggiani, A., Bach, V., Santucci, M., & Visconti. P. (1995). EEG features and epilepsy in patients with autism. *Brain and Development, 17,* 169–174.

Rourke, B. (1989a). *Nonverbal learning disabilities: The syndrome and the model.* New York: Guilford.

Rourke, B. P. (1989b). Nonverbal learning disabilities, socioemotional disturbance, and suicide: A reply to Fletcher, Kowalchuk and King, and Bigler. *Journal of Learning Disabilities, 22,* 186–7.

Rumsey, J. M., & Hamburger, S. D. (1988). Neuropsychological findings in high-functioning autistic men with infantile autism, residual state. *Journal of Clinical and Experimental Neuropsychology, 10,* 201–221.

Rutter, M. (1996). Autism research—Prospects and priorities. *Journal Of Autism and Developmental Disorders, 26,* 257–275.

Rutter, M., Bailey, A., Bolton, P., & Le Couteur, A. (1994). Autism and known medical conditions: myth and substance. *Journal of Child Psychology and Psychiatry, 35,* 311–322.

Rutter, M., Bailey, A., Simonoff, E., & Pickles, A. (1997). Genetic influences and autism. In D. J. Cohen & F. R. Volkmar (Eds.), *Handbook of autism and pervasive developmental disorders* (2nd ed., pp. 370–387). New York: Wiley.

Rutter, M., & Hersov, R. (1977). *Child psychiatry: Modern approaches.* Oxford: Blackwell.

Rutter, M., & Lord, C. (1987). Language disorders associated with psychiatric disturbance. In W. Rule & M. Rutter (Eds.), *Language development and disorders* (pp. 206–233). Philadelphia: J. B. Lippincott.

Salmelin, R., Service, E., Kiesila, P., Uutela, K., & Salonen, O. (1996). Impaired visual word processing in dyslexia revealed with magnetoencephalography. *Annals of Neurology, 40,* 157–162.

Schopler, E. (1996). Are autism and Asperger syndrome (AS) different labels or different disabilities? *Journal of Autism and Developmental Disorders, 26,* 109–10.

Schopler, E., Mesibov, G. B., & Kunce, L. (1998). *Asperger syndrome or high-functioning autism?* New York: Plenum Press.

Schopler, E., Reichler, R., & Rochen-Renner, B. (1988). *The Childhood Autism Rating Scale (CARS).* Los Angeles, CA: Western Psychological Services.

Schopler, E., Reichler, R. J., DeVellis, R. F., & Daly, K. (1980). Toward objective classification of childhood autism: Childhood Autism Rating Scale (CARS). *Journal of Autism and Developmental Disorders, 10,* 91–103.

Schroer, R. J., Phelan. M. C., Michaelis, R. C., Crawford, E. C., Skinner, S. A., Cuccaro, M., Simensen, R. J., Bishop, J., Skinner, C., Fender, D., & E. S. R. (1998). Autism and maternally derived aberrations of chromosome 15q. *American Journal of Medical Genetics, 76,* 327–336.

Schuler, A. L., Prizant, B. M., & Wetherby, A. M. (1997). Enhancing communication: Prelinguistic approaches. In D. J. Cohen & F. R. Volkmar (Eds.), *Handbook of autism and pervasive developmental disorders* (2nd ed., pp. 539–571). New York: Wiley.

Sciarillo, W. G., Brown, M. M., Robinson, N. M., Bennett, F. C., & Sells, C. J. (1986). Effectiveness of the Denver Developmental Screening Test with biologically vulnerable infants. *Journal of Developmental and Behavioral Pediatrics, 17,* 77–83.

Semel, E., Wiig, E. H., & Secord, W. A. (1995) *Clinical Evaluation of Language Fundamentals-3 Examiner's Manual.* New York: Psychological Corp.

Shannon, M., & Graef, J. W. (1997). Lead intoxication in children with pervasive developmental disorders. *Journal of Toxicology-Clinical Toxicology, 34,* 177–182.

Shearer, T. R., Larson, K., Neuschwander, J., & Gedney, B. (1982). Minerals in the hair and nutrient intake of autistic children. *Journal of Autism and Developmental Disorders, 12,* 25–34.

Sheinkopf, S. J., & Siegel, B. (1998). Home based behavioral treatment of young autistic children. *Journal of Autism and Developmental Disorders, 28,* 15–24.

Short, A. B., & Schopler, E. (1988). Factors relating to age of onset in autism. *Journal of Autism and Developmental Disorders, 18,* 207–216.

Siegel, B. (1998). *Early screening and diagnosis in autism spectrum disorders: The Pervasive Developmental Disorders Screening Test (PDDST).* Paper presented at the NIH State of the Science in Autism. Screening and Diagnosis Working Conference, Bethesda, MD, June 15–17.

Siegel, D. J., Minshew, N. J., & Goldstein, G. (1996). Wechsler IQ profiles in diagnosis of high-functioning autism. *Journal of Autism and Developmental Disorders, 26,* 389–406.

Sigman, M., & Ungerer, J. A. (1984). Attachment behaviors in autistic children. *Journal of Autism and Developmental Disorders, 14,* 231–244.

Simonoff, E. (1998). Genetic counseling in autism and pervasive developmental disorders. *Journal of Autism and Developmental Disorders, 28,* 447–456.

Singh, V. K., Warren, R., Averett, R., & Ghaziuddin, M. (1997). Circulating autoantibodies to neuronal and glial filament proteins in autism. *Pediatric Neurology, 17,* 88–90.

Smalley, S., Smith, M. & Tanguay, P. (1991). Autism and psychiatric disorders in tuberous sclerosis. *Annals of the New York Academy of Science, 615,* 382–383.

Smalley, S. L., Tanguay, P. E., Smith, M., & Gutierrez, G. (1992). Autism and tuberous sclerosis. *Journal of Autism and Developmental Disorders, 22,* 339–355.

Smith, D. E., Miller, S. D., Stewart, M., Walter, T. L., & McConnell, J. V. (1988). Conductive hearing loss in autistic, learning-disabled, and normal children. *Journal of Autism and Developmental Disorders, 18,* 53–65.

Sparrow, S. S., Balla, D. A., & Cicchetti, D. V. (1984a). *Vineland Adaptive Behavior Scales (Expanded Edition).* Circle Pines, MN: American Guidance Service.

Sparrow, S. S., Balla, D. A., & Cicchetti, D. V. (1984b). *Vineland Adaptive Behavior Scales (Survey Edition).* Circle Pines, MN: American Guidance Service.

Sparrow, S. S., Balla, D. A., & Cicchetti, D. V. (1985). *Vineland Adaptive Behavior Scales (Classroom Edition).* Circle Pines, MN: American Guidance Service.

Squires, J., Bricker, D., & Potter, L. (1997). Revision of a parent-completed developmental screening tool: Ages and Stages Questionnaires. *Journal of Pediatric Psychology, 22,* 313–328.

Stapells, D. R., Gravel, J. S., & Martin, B. A. (1995). Thresholds for auditory brain stem responses to tones in notched noise from infants and young children with normal hearing or sensorineural hearing loss. *Ear and Hearing, 16,* 361–371.

Steffenburg, S. (1991). Neuropsychiatric assessment of children with autism: a population-based study. *Developmental Medicine and Child Neurology, 33,* 495–511.

Steffenburg, S., Gillberg, C. L., Steffenburg, U., & Kyllerman, M. (1996). Autism in Angelman syndrome: a population-based study. *Pediatric Neurology, 14,* 131–136.

Stone, W. L. (1998a). *Descriptive information about the Screening Tool for Autism in Two-Year-Olds (STAT).* Paper presented at the NIH State of the Science in Autism: Screening and Diagnosis Working Conference. Bethesda, MD, June 15–17.

Stone. W. L. (1998b). *STAT manual: Screening Tool for Autism in Two-Year-Olds.* Paper presented at the *NIH State of the Science in Autism: Screening and Diagnosis Working Conference,* Bethesda, MD, June 15–17.

Stone. W. L., & Caro-Martinez, L. M. (1990). Naturalistic observations of spontaneous communication in autistic children. *Journal of Autism and Developmental Disorders, 20,* 437–453.

Stone, W. L., & Hogan, K. L. (1993). A structured parent interview for identifying young children with autism. *Journal of Autism and Developmental Disorders, 23,* 639–652.

Stone. W. L., Lee, E. B., Ashford, L., Brissie, J., Hepburn, S. L., Coonrod, E. E., & Weiss. B. H. (1999). Can autism be diagnosed accurately in children under three years? *Journal of Child Psychology and Psychiatry, 40,* 219–226.

Stone, W. L., & Lemanek, K. L. (1990). Parental report of social behaviors in autistic preschoolers. *Journal of Autism and Developmental Disorders, 20,* 513–522.

Stone, W. L., Lemanek, K. L., Fishel, P. T., Fernandez, M. C., & Altemeier, W. A. (1990). Play and imitation skills in the diagnosis of autism in young children. *Pediatrics, 86,* 267–272.

Stone, W. L., Ousley, O. Y., Yoder, P. J., Hogan, K. L., & Hepburn, S. L. (1997). Nonverbal communication in two- and three-year-old children with autism. *Journal of Autism and Developmental Disorders, 27,* 677–696.

Sturner, R. A., Funk, S. G., Thomas, P. D., & Green, J. A. (1982). An adaptation of the Minnesota Child Development Inventory for preschool developmental screening. *Journal of Pediatric Psychology, 7,* 295–306.

Sturner, R. A., Green, J. A., & Funk, S. G. (1985). Preschool Denver Developmental Screening Test as a predictor of later school problems. *Journal of Pediatrics, 107,* 615–621.

Stutsman, R. (1948). *The Merrill-Palmer Scale of Mental Tests.* Chicago, IL: Stoelting.

Sugiyama, T., & Abe, T. (1989). The prevalence of autism in Nagoya, Japan: a total population study. *Journal of Autism and Developmental Disorders, 19,* 87–96.

Szatmari, P., Archer, L., Fisman, S., Streiner, D. L., & Wilson, F. (1995). Asperger's syndrome and autism: differences in behavior, cognition, and adaptive functioning. *Journal of the American Academy of Child and Adolescent Psychiatry, 34,* 1662–1671.

Szatmari, P., Bremner, R., & Nagy, J. (1989). Asperger's syndrome: A review of clinical features. *Canadian Journal of Psychiatry, 34,* 554–560.

Szatmari, P., Jones, M. B., Tuff, L., Bartolucci, G., Fisman, S., & Mahoney, W. (1993). Lack of cognitive impairment in first-degree relatives of children with pervasive developmental disorders. *Journal of the American Academy of Child and Adolescent Psychiatry, 32,* 1264–1273.

Teitelbaum, P., Teitelbaum, O., Nye, J., Fryman, J., & Maurer, R. G. (1998). Movement analysis in infancy may be useful for early diagnosis of autism. *Proceedings of the National Academy of Science U.S., 95,* 13982–13987.

Thorndike, R. L., Hagen, E. P., & Sattler, J. M. (1986). *The Stanford-Binet Intelligence Scale: Fourth Edition. Guide for administering and scoring.* Chicago, IL: Riverside.

Tolbert, L., Haigler, T., Waits, M. M., & Dennis, T. (1993). Brief report: Lack of response in an autistic population to a low dose clinical trial of pyridoxine plus magnesium. *Journal of Autism and Developmental Disorders, 23,* 193–199.

Towbin, K. E. (1997). Pervasive developmental disorder not otherwise specified. In D. J. Cohen & F. R. Volkmar (Eds.), *Handbook of autism and pervasive developmental disorders (2nd ed.,* pp. 123–147). New York: Wiley.

Truhan, A. P., & Filipek, P. A. (1993). Magnetic resonance imaging. Its role in the neuroradiologic evaluation of neurofibromatosis, tuberous sclerosis, and Sturge-Weber syndrome. *Archives of Dermatology, 129,* 219–226.

Tsai, L. Y. (1987). Pre-, peri- and neonatal factors in autism. In E. Schopler & G. B. Mesibov (Eds.), *Neurobiological issues in autism. Current issues in autism* (pp. 179–189). New York: Plenum Press.

Tsai, L. Y. (1992): Is Rett syndrome a subtype of pervasive developmental disorders? *Journal of Autism and Developmental Disorders, 22,* 551–61.

Tuchman, R. (1996). Pervasive developmental disorder: Neurologic perspective. *Acta Neuropediatrica, 2,* 82–93.

Tuchman, R., Jayakar, P., Yaylali, I., & Villalobos, R. (1997). Seizures and EEG findings in chidlren with autism spectrum disorders. *CNS Spectrums. 3,* 61–70.

Tuchman, R. F. (1994). Epilepsy, language, and behavior: clinical models in childhood. *Journal of Child Neurology, 9,* 95–102.

Tuchman, R. F. (1995). Regression in pervasive developmental disorders: Is there a relationship with Landau-Kleffner Syndrome? *Annals of Neurology, 38,* 526.

Tuchman, R. F., & Rapin, I. (1997). Regression in pervasive developmental disorders: seizures and epileptiform electroencephalogram correlates. *Pediatrics, 99,* 560–566.

Tuchman, R. F., Rapin, I., & Shinnar, S. (1991a). Autistic and dysphasic children. I: Clinical characteristics. *Pediatrics, 88,* 1211–1218.

Tuchman, R. F., Rapin, I., & Shinnar, S. (1991b). Autistic and dysphasic children. II: Epilepsy. *Pediatrics, 88,* 1219–1225.

Verbaten, M. N., Roelofs, J. W., van Engeland, H., Kenemans, J. K., & Slangen, J. L. (1991). Abnormal visual event-related potentials of autistic children. *Journal of Autism and Developmental Disorders, 21,* 449–470.

Verpoorten, R. A., & Emmen, J. G. (1995). A tactile-auditory conditioning procedure for the hearing assessment of persons with autism and mental retardation. *Scandinavian Audiology, Supplementum, 41,* 49–50.

Voeller, K. K. (1986). Right-hemisphere deficit syndrome in children. *American Journal of Psychiatry, 143,* 1004–1009.

Volkmar, F. R. (1992). Childhood disintegrative disorder: Issues for DSM-IV. *Journal of Autism and Developmental Disorders, 22,* 625–642.

Volkmar, F. R. (1994). Childhood disintegrative disorder. *Child and Adolescent Psychiatric Clinics of North America, 3,* 119–128.

Volkmar, F. R., Carter, A., Sparrow, S. S., & Cicchetti, D. V. (1993a). Quantifying social development in autism. *Journal of the American Academy of Child and Adolescent Psychiatry, 32,* 627–632.

Volkmar, F. R., & Cohen, D. J. (1991). Nonautistic pervasive developmental disorders. In R. Michels (Ed.), *Psychiatry (Child Psychiatry 2: 1–6).* Philadelphia: J. B. Lippincott.

Volkmar, F. R., Cook, E. H. J., Pomeroy, J., Realmuto, G., & Tanguay, P. (1999). Practice parameters for autism and pervasive developmental disorders. *Journal of the American Academy of Child and Adolescent Psychiatry, 38,* 32s–54s.

Volkmar, F. R., Kiln, A., Marans, W., & Cohen, D. J. (1997). Childhood disintegrative disorder. In D. J. Cohen & F. R. Volkmar (Eds.), *Handbook of autism and pervasive developmental disorders* (2nd ed.). New York: Wiley.

Volkmar, F. R., Klin, A., Schultz, R., Bronen, R., Marans, W. D., Sparrow, S., & Cohen, D. J. (1996). Asperger's syndrome [clinical conference]. *Journal of the American Academy of Child and Adolescent Psychiatry. 35,* 118–123.

Volkmar, F. R., Klin, A., Siegel, B., Szatmari, P., Lord, C., Campbell, M., Freeman, B. J., Cicchetti, D. V., Rutter, M., Kline, W., *et al.* (1994). Field trial for autistic disorder in DSM-IV. *American Journal of Psychiatry, 151,* 1361–1367.

Volkmar, F. R., & Nelson, D. S. (1990). Seizure disorders in autism. *Journal of the American Academy of Child and Adolescent Psychiatry, 29,* 127–129.

Volkmar, F. R., & Rutter, M. (1995). Childhood disintegrative disorder: results of the DSM-IV autism field trial. *Journal of the American Academy of Child and Adolescent Psychiatry, 34,* 1092–1095.

Volkmar, F. R., Stier, D. M., & Cohen, D. J. (1985). Age of recognition of pervasive developmental disorder. *American Journal of Psychiatry, 142,* 1450–1452.

Volkmar, F. R., Szatmari, P., & Sparrow, S. S. (1993b). Sex differences in pervasive developmental disorders. *Journal of Autism and Developmental Disorders, 23*, 579–591.

Wahlstrom, J., Gillberg, C., Gustavson, K. H., & Holmgren, G. (1986). Infantile autism and the fragile X. A Swedish multicenter study. *American Journal of Medical Genetics, 23*, 403–408.

Watson, L. R., & Marcus, L. M. (1988). Diagnosis and assessment of preschool children. In E. Schopler & G. B. Mesibov (Eds.), *Diagnosis and assessment in autism* (pp. 271–301). New York: Plenum Press.

Webb, D. W., Clarke, A., Fryer, A., & Osborne, J. P. (1996). The cutaneous features of tuberous sclerosis: a population study. *British Journal of Dermatology, 135*, 1–5.

Wechsler, D. (1991). *Wechsler Intelligence Scale for Children (WISC-III).* San Antonio, TX: Psychological Corp.

Wechsler, D. (1997). *Wechsler Adult Intelligence Scale- III (WAIS-III).* San Antonio, TX: Psychological Corp.

Wecker, L., Miller, S. B., Cochran, S. R., Dugger, D. L., & Johnson, W. D. (1985). Trace element concentrations in hair from autistic children. *Journal of Mental Deficiency Research, 29*, 15–22.

Weidmer-Mikhail, E., Sheldon, S., & Ghaziuddin, M. (1998). Chromosomes in autism and related pervasive developmental disorders: a cytogenetic study. *Journal of Intellectual Disability Research, 42*, 8–12.

Wetherby, A. M., & Prizant, B. M. (1992). Profiling young children's communicative competence. In S. Warren & J. Reichle (Eds.), *Causes and effects in communication and language intervention.* Baltimore, MD: Paul H. Brookes.

Wetherby, A. M., & Prizant, B. M. (1993). *Communication and Symbolic Behavior Scales (CSBS)- Normed Edition.* Chicago, IL: Applied Symbolix.

Wetherby, A. M., Prizant, B. M., & Hutchinson, T. (1998). Communicative, social-affective, and symbolic profiles of young children with autism and pervasive developmental disorder. *American Journal of Speech and Language Pathology, 7*, 79–91.

Wetherby, A. M., Schuler, A. L., & Prizant, B. M. (1997). Enhancing communication: Theoretical foundations. In D. J. Cohen & F. R. Volkmar (Eds.), *Handbook of autism and pervasive developmental disorders* (2nd ed., pp. 513–538). New York: Wiley.

Wetherby, A. M., Yonclas, D. G., & Bryan, A. A. (1989). Communicative profiles of preschool children with handicaps: implications for early identification. *Journal of Speech and Hearing Disorders, 54*, 148–158.

Wing, L. (1981a). Asperger's syndrome: a clinical account. *Psychological Medicine, 11*, 115–129.

Wing, L. (1981b). Language, social and cognitive impairments in autism and severe mental retardation. *Journal of Autism and Developmental Disorders, 11*, 31–44.

Wing, L. (1988). The continuum of autistic disorders. In E. Schopler & G. M. Mesibov (Eds.), *Diagnosis and assessment in autism* (pp. 91–110). New York: Plenum Press.

Wing, L. (1996). Wing Autistic Disorder Interview Checklist (WADIC). In I. Rapin (Ed.), *Preschool children with inadequate communication: Developmental language disorder, autism low IQ* (pp. 247–251). London: MacKeith.

Wing, L. (1997). The autistic spectrum. *Lancet, 350*, 1761–1766.

Wing, L., & Gould, J. (1979). Severe impairments of social interaction and associated abnormalities in children: Epidemiology and classification. *Journal of Autism and Developmental Disorders, 9*, 11–29.

Wong, V. (1993). Epilepsy in children with autistic spectrum disorder. *Journal of Child Neurology, 8*, 316–322.

Woodhouse, W., Bailey, A., Rutter, M., Bolton, P., Baird, G., & Le Couteur, A. (1996). Head circumference in autism and other pervasive developmental disorders. *Journal of Child Psychology and Psychiatry, 37*, 665–671.

World Health Organization. (1992). *The ICD-10 Classification of mental and behavioral disorders: Clinical descriptors and diagnostic guidelines.* Geneva: Author.

World Health Organization. (1993). *The ICD-10 Classification of mental and behavioral disorders: Diagnostic criteria for research.* Geneva: Author.

Yuwiler, A., Shih, J. C., Chen, C. H., Ritvo, E. R., Hanna, G., Ellison, G. W., & King, B. H. (1992). Hyperserotoninemia and antiserotonin antibodies in autism and other disorders. *Journal of Autism and Developmental Disorders, 22*, 33–45.

Zimmerman, I. L., Steiner, V. G., & Pond, R. E. (1992). *The Preschool Language Scale-3.* San Antonio, TX: Psychological Corp.

MENTAL RETARDATION AND DEVELOPMENTAL DISABILITIES
RESEARCH REVIEWS 4: 97–103 (1998)

EPIDEMIOLOGY OF AUTISM:
PREVALENCE, ASSOCIATED CHARACTERISTICS, AND IMPLICATIONS FOR RESEARCH AND SERVICE DELIVERY

Susan E. Bryson[1]* and Isabel M. Smith[2]

[1]Departments of Psychology, York University and The Hospital for Sick Children, Toronto, Ontario, Canada

[2]Departments of Pediatrics and Psychology, Dalhousie University, and IWK Grace Health Centre, Halifax, Nova Scotia, Canada

We provide an overview of research on the epidemiology of autism and related pervasive developmental disorders (PDDs). First, we provide data on the prevalence of autism, which now is estimated to be considerably higher than previously documented. Next, we focus on characteristics associated with autism, including psychosocial correlates, as well as associated physical and medical/psychiatric conditions. In this context, special consideration is given to the coexistence of autism and mental retardation, and to associated conditions that might be the most informative in advancing our understanding of the neurobiology and neuropsychology of autism. Data on outcome are also discussed, with special reference to early intervention and to empirically supported methods. We end by identifying potentially fruitful directions for future epidemiological research on autism/PDD, and by outlining implications of what already is known for the planning and delivery of services for this unique population.   © 1998 Wiley-Liss, Inc.
MRDD Research Reviews 1998;4:97–103.

Key Words: autism; epidemiology; prevalence; mental retardation; associated medical conditions; co-morbid psychiatric disturbance

Among the most important advances in the field of mental retardation / developmental disability has been the identification of etiologically distinct syndromes, each with unique profiles of neuropathology and psychosocial development [e.g., Lubs, 1969]. As our understanding of the etiology of various disabilities increases, so, too, does our ability to prevent them and/or to provide support to affected individuals and their families. The etiology of autism, however, remains elusive. Many fundamental questions remain unanswered. For example, why is the disorder often but not exclusively associated with mental retardation? This question and related ones are of considerable interest to both researchers and practitioners. As it stands, autism remains a major public heath problem. It exacts an enormous burden of suffering on individual families and service systems worldwide are struggling with the scope of the need. A better understanding of autism not only holds promise for earlier intervention and prevention, but will also yield important insights about both pathological and normal development.

© **1998 Wiley-Liss, Inc.**

Determining the epidemiology of autism is likely to help in understanding this puzzling disorder. This article provides an overview of what has been established thus far [see Wing, 1993, and Fombonne, 1996, for additional information]. First, we give a brief description of autism and related pervasive developmental disorders. Next, we turn to the data on prevalence. In that context, special consideration is given to the relationship between autism and mental retardation and to associated characteristics, both psychosocial and medical. Discussion also focuses on the course and outcome of autism, including recent findings from early intervention programs. We end by highlighting the implications of existing data for service delivery, and by suggesting directions for future epidemiological research on what is now considered a spectrum of autistic disorders.

DEFINITION

Presently, there is no biological marker for autism, and thus it has historically been defined in terms of behavior. Leo Kanner [1943] was the first to identify a unique group of children with an apparent failure to establish "affective contact" with others. Kanner provided a rich description of the prototype of autism, often referred to as "classic" or nuclear autism. Children so defined are socially aloof, showing little interest in human contact of any kind. They are also distinguished by the rigidity with which they cling to "sameness" and routine. This categorical conceptualization of autism prevailed for close to four decades. More recently, however, the definition has been extended to incorporate the idea of a continuum of related disorders, now referred to as pervasive developmental disorders (PDDs), of which autism is the most extreme form.

Recognition of the heterogeneity in the expression and severity of autism is attributable largely to the innovative work of Lorna Wing and colleagues. Social variants on the aloof child include children who are either passive or "active-but-odd," but

*Correspondence to: Susan E. Bryson, Department of Psychology, York University, 4700 Keele Street, Toronto, Ontario, Canada M3J 1P3. E-mail: sbryson@yorku.ca

who nonetheless share the core features of autism, notably, a lack of social reciprocity and behavioral inflexibility [Wing and Attwood, 1987; Wing and Gould, 1979]. The social-communicative problem is evident early in life and involves such basic dysfunctions as a lack of mutual gazing, reciprocal smiling, or pointing and looking to share interest with others, any one of which may vary in severity [see Travis and Sigman, this volume, and Wilkinson, this volume, for further discussion of these core deficits]. Differences in the expression and severity of autism also coexist with wide differences in the children's cognitive and linguistic abilities. For example, all affected individuals are relatively lacking in the social aspects of communication. However, some individuals have no speech, others can speak but lack fluency, and still others are verbally fluent but pedantic. The main point is that the behavioral manifestation of autism varies not only with the child's developmental level, but also with the severity of autism and the degree of mental retardation, the latter two of which appear to be nonorthogonal [McLennan et al., 1993; Volkmar et al., 1993].

Current diagnostic systems [e.g., APA, 1994; WHO, 1993] attempt to capture the marked variation in the expression of autism by requiring evidence of impairment in domains of function (socialization, communication, and imagination). The particular behaviors that represent such impairments include, but are not limited to, the most extreme or prototypic manifestations (e.g., social aloofness, as in Kanner's autism). Not surprisingly, this shift toward a broader definition of autism and related pervasive developmental disorders (notably, atypical autism/PDD-NOS and Asperger's syndrome) has yielded higher estimates of prevalence.

PREVALENCE

Autism occurs in 3–4 times as many males as females [e.g., Lotter, 1966]. Until fairly recently, it was considered a rare disorder, thought to occur in 4–5 per 10,000. This estimate derived from prevalence studies conducted prior to 1985, which relied heavily on Kanner's description of the classical autistic prototype. More recent studies have yielded rates more than twice as high, which has led to considerable controversy about whether or not there has been a real increase in prevalence [see, e.g., Bryson, 1996; Fombonne, 1996].

Central to the controversy is whether the higher rates reflect a real

increase in prevalence and/or changes over time in diagnostic criteria for autism [see Lord, this issue], as well as a general heightened awareness of the variability in its expression. Unfortunately, existing data preclude firm conclusions. What is needed are comparative studies, conducted within the same regions, in which the same methods of ascertainment and the same diagnostic criteria are used at different points in time. The effects of increased awareness of the heterogeneity in the expression of autism must also be considered. Such studies would provide comparative data not only on prevalence, but also on demographic and other associated psychological and biological characteristics. Only when such data are available will it be possible to ascertain whether rates are actually increasing, and if so, to test hypotheses regarding possible mechanisms. In their absence, we turn to the studies conducted over the last decade or so that led to higher prevalence estimates than those previously reported.

…the majority of individuals within the autistic spectrum do not have mental retardation, as measured by standard tests of intelligence.

Very recently, a prevalence for autism of 10–12 per 10,000 was reported by Gillberg [1997], who computed a mean (weighted for sample size) of the numerous studies conducted worldwide since 1985. Specifically, he reports mean prevalences of 10.2/10,000 for studies conducted between 1985 and 1994 and 11.7/10,000 for those conducted beyond 1995; confidence intervals were 9.3–11.1 and 9.1–14.3, respectively. These studies all adopted a broader definition of autism (e.g., DSM III-R or ICD-10) than that used in earlier work. However, it is important to note that none of these investigations screened for all PDD variants. In these revised estimates, the ratio of males to females remains largely unchanged from that reported in the pre-1985 studies (i.e., 3–4:1). Also, the number of individuals with IQs in the 50–70 IQ range (the range most representative of Kanner's autism) is about the same as those identified in the earlier studies. These consistencies indicate that the recent higher prevalence estimates are not due to a fundamental redefinition of

autism. Rather, these higher figures reflect increased awareness of the heterogeneity of its expression. More individuals with IQs less than 50 and greater than 70 now meet the criteria for autistic disorder. The interested reader is invited to compare the differences between the DSM-III [APA, 1984] and the DSM-IV [APA, 1994], which reflect the evolution of thinking on this issue.

It bears emphasizing that the more recent estimate of 10–12 per 10,000 is for autism specifically. Excluding the most capable variants (usually diagnosed as Asperger's syndrome), the only estimate we have for both autism (defined using traditional criteria) *and* related conditions (defined by a lack of social reciprocity, invariably associated with behavioral inflexibility) is 22 per 10,000 [Wing and Gould, 1979]. Recent epidemiological data suggest that Asperger's syndrome may be even more prevalent [3–4/1,000; Ehlers and Gillberg, 1993] than the combined estimate for autism *and* other less capable variants (2/1,000). Extrapolating from all existing data, we concur with Gillberg's [1997] conclusion that "the prevalence of autism spectrum disorders—including childhood autism, Asperger syndrome, disintegrative disorder and atypical autism—is at least 4–5 in 1,000 children." We also emphasize Wing and Gould's point that the lines of behavioral demarcation between autism, defined narrowly or broadly, and other PDD variants remain arbitrary, the significance of which is underscored in studies showing that different variants co-occur within families [Pickles et al., 1995].

ASSOCIATED PSYCHOSOCIAL CHARACTERISTICS

Results from recent epidemiological studies indicate that about 75% of those with autism also have mental retardation [e.g., Bryson et al., 1988]. Note, however, that while most people with autism have retardation (as traditionally assumed), this is not the case for the entire spectrum of autistic disorders. As noted, the prevalence of Asperger's syndrome (defined, in part, by IQ >70) is close to twice that reported for autism and other less capable PDD variants. Thus, the majority of individuals within the autistic spectrum do not have mental retardation, as measured by standard tests of intelligence. Data on adaptive functioning alter the picture somewhat. People with autism measure as more intelligent than their repertoire of life skills would (and does) indicate, a matter to which we return below.

98

58

Another way of looking at the relationship between autism and mental retardation is to ask about the proportion of those with retardation who have autism as well. This and other questions are being addressed by Bradley and Bryson in an ongoing epidemiological survey of mental retardation in 14–20-year-olds (hereafter, the Niagara prevalence study). Preliminary findings indicate that about 25% of these individuals with mental retardation also have autism, as identified by the Autism Diagnostic Interview—Revised [ADI-R; Lord et al., 1994]. This finding compares favorably with data reported by Wing and colleagues [Shah et al., 1982; Wing and Gould, 1979], who estimate that 30–40% of those with mental retardation have either autism or a lesser variant thereof. Findings from the Niagara prevalence study indicate further that autism is distributed roughly equally among those with mild and moderate-to-severe/profound levels of mental retardation [but see Deb and Prasad, 1994], whose relatively high rate among low-functioning children may reflect less stringent diagnostic criteria for autism. One potentially important finding is that the male-to-female ratio approaches 2:1 in individuals with autism and severe/profound mental retardation. Recall that this differs from the 3–4:1 ratio typically reported for the population with autism in general [Bryson et al., 1988; Gillberg et al., 1991; Lotter, 1966; Wing, 1981]. Such findings suggest different etiological factors, genetic or otherwise, in lower- and higher-functioning individuals with autism [see Bailey et al., 1996, for a review; see also Szatmari et al., 1996, for recent data on this issue].

In addition, the discrepancy in autism between measured IQ and functional (adaptive) skills bears emphasizing. Relative to IQ-matched comparison groups (most of whom have mental retardation), people with autism have significantly lower scores on measures of adaptive or life skills (typically measured via the Vineland Adaptive Behavior Scales), a difference that tends to widen with age [Bryson et al., 1988; Freeman et al., 1988; Loveland and Kelley, 1988]. The main point here is that certain aspects of intelligence (e.g., memory for facts and events, pattern recognition or the apprehension of underlying structure, as in language, for example) exceed practical knowledge. While people with autism may possess certain skills or knowledge, they have difficulty "seeing" their application to the circumstances of everyday life.

Learning by individuals with autism seems highly context-specific. Skills acquired in one setting may not be displayed when the setting changes. These individuals seemingly have to re-learn what to do in every new situation (i.e., there is a failure to generalize across experience, as noted by Harris [1975]). Conversely, what is learned by individuals with autism is learned rigidly; it may be extremely difficult for such individuals to modify their behavior to accommodate varying situational demands. Coping with the complexities and unpredictability of the social world is especially demanding, even overwhelming, for the person with autism. The associated anxiety experienced by the person clearly exacerbates the problem.

Findings from epidemiological research indicate that at least 25–30% of individuals with autism have associated medical conditions....

ASSOCIATED PHYSICAL CHARACTERISTICS AND MEDICAL/PSYCHIATRIC CONDITIONS

Epidemiological research informs us not only about the prevalence and associated psychosocial characteristics of autism, but also about its associated physical characteristics and medical/psychiatric conditions. Indeed, early reports of an association between autism and epilepsy [Lotter, 1974; Rutter et al., 1967] helped to implicate biological rather than psychogenic factors in the etiology of autism. Such reports also helped to foster a more scientific approach to understanding the neurobiological and neuropsychological bases of this unique developmental disorder. The etiological and neuropsychopathological significance of such reports, of course, depends on whether the documented association(s) differ significantly from those seen in the general population and, if so, whether mental retardation in general or autism specifically accounts for the association in question. Estimates of co-morbid conditions may well underestimate their actual co-occurrence. Existing data are constrained by several factors, most notably by limited access to the

necessary health/mental health resources and by "diagnostic overshadowing" (attributing all symptoms to an established diagnosis, in this case, autism and/or mental retardation). For our present purposes, therefore, we will focus on those conditions for which there appears to be reasonably strong and potentially informative relationships to autism specifically. We consider data from epidemiological as well as other sources in order to develop a more complete overall picture.

Medical Conditions

Findings from epidemiological research indicate that at least 25–30% of individuals with autism have associated medical conditions [e.g., Bryson et al., 1988; Lotter, 1967] (the reader is referred to Coleman and Gillberg [1985] for a comprehensive discussion of this issue). Among the most prevalent are sensory impairment (blindness and/or deafness), tuberous sclerosis, neurofibromatosis, and epilepsy, all of which predominate among individuals with the most severe mental retardation. Peripheral hearing loss may be more prevalent than previously reported and evidence of abnormal brain stem auditory-evoked responses implicates basic impairments in the processing of sensory information in some individuals [Klin, 1993]. Epilepsy, which may occur in as many as 30% of individuals, has a peak onset during early adolescence, but also occurs in infancy [see Rapin, 1997, for further discussion].

Two seizure conditions that may be informative for understanding autism are Landau Kleffner syndrome and infantile spasms. Landau Kleffner syndrome is characterized most often by a rather abrupt and dramatic loss of language (receptive and/or expressive) associated with epileptiform activity and autistic symptomatology [Dennis, 1996]. Autistic features also have been reported in cases of infantile spasms, notably in those who are either untreated or nonresponsive to existing pharmacological interventions [Martien et al., 1997; Riikonen and Amnell, 1981; also see Myzaki et al., 1993, for evidence of brain stem involvement]. It may be significant that in autism epilepsy has been reported to be particularly common when preceded by a period of relatively normal development (occurring in approximately 20% of such individuals, as compared to 10% in whom early dysfunction was more evident [Rapin, 1997]). These findings, however, need to be confirmed within a larger, more complete population than has been studied thus far.

Epidemiological data on minor physical anomalies (MPAs) in autism converge, with several lines of evidence that implicate an early brain stem injury [Rodier et al., 1996; also see Ornitz, 1985, and Rimland, 1964]. Because features of the ear develop during the latter part of the first month of gestation, MPAs of this structure point to an early operating process. In the Niagara prevalence study, posterior rotation of the ear was found to be common in children with autism (45% of cases) and to reliably distinguish them from controls (both from a mixed developmentally disordered group and from their own siblings [Rodier et al., 1997]). Complementing these findings, Rodier and colleagues [1996] have drawn attention to the report that thalidomide exposure during early embryological development (20th–24th day; the time of neural tube closure) resulted in autism in 30% of cases in a Scandinavian sample [Stromland and Miller, 1993]. These individuals are reported to share, to varying degrees, anomalies of the ear (hearing loss included) as well as the physical features diagnostic of Moebius syndrome (facial paralysis and a lack of eye abduction; see Gillberg, 1992; Gillberg and Steffenburg, 1989; Ornitz et al., 1977, for additional evidence of the co-occurrence of autism and Moebius syndrome). As predicted by the thalidomide cases, Rodier and colleagues have demonstrated abnormalities of brain stem development in an autopsy case of autism, as well as parallel neuroanatomical abnormalities in an animal model in which development was interrupted during the period of neural tube closure. This timing of the injury is also consistent with the well-documented associations between autism and both tuberous sclerosis [Valente, 1971] and rubella [Chess et al., 1971]. Rodier and colleagues' compelling argument for an early brain stem injury in autism constitutes a truly developmental account that has direct implications for studies on the etiological role of genetics and teratogens, and on brain–behavior relationships in autism and in normal development.

Psychiatric Conditions

Considerable attention has been focused on reports of co-morbid psychiatric disturbance in individuals with autism [see Lainhart and Folstein, 1994, for a review; also see Smalley et al., 1995]. Affective disorders appear to predominate and to co-occur in the families of some PDD variants [DeLong, 1994]. However, to date there has been little systematic study of co-morbid psychiatric

disturbance using well-defined diagnostic criteria. Moreover, there are no estimates for the population with autism. Indeed, the available reports are derived almost exclusively from relatively high-functioning individuals. Little is known about whether psychiatric disturbance co-occurs with autism in lower-functioning individuals. This state of affairs is not surprising, however, given the difficulties of making psychiatric diagnoses in individuals who are unable to speak and/or share their mental experiences.

Bradley and Bryson currently are addressing these and related issues in the Niagara prevalence study [Bryson, 1997]. Preliminary findings indicate that there is an elevated risk in autism for psychiatric disturbance, as defined by the Schedule for Assessment of Psychiatric Problems Associated with Autism [and Other Developmental Disorders; Bolton and Rutter, 1994]. At least 40% of individuals with ADI-R-defined autism experienced psychiatric "episodes," with mood disorder being particularly common. By comparison, such episodes were experienced by only 20% of a control group with mental retardation but not autism (matched for age, gender, and nonverbal IQ). Moreover, psychiatric disturbance may be more intractable in individuals with autism. Relative to comparable individuals without autism, they may have more difficulty "letting go" of the thoughts and/or emotional pain associated with distressing events. Similar observations have been reported by parents of higher-functioning 12–14-year-olds with autism or Asperger's syndrome (P. Szatmari, personal communication). Thus, individuals with autism spectrum disorders are at considerable risk for psychiatric problems and clearly need access to appropriate psychiatric as well as other medical and psychoeducational services. As the Niagara prevalence study progresses, we expect to provide further information on the nature of psychiatric disturbance in autism/PDD and its relationship to outcome; Szatmari's follow-up of more capable individuals will explore possible mechanisms, genetic and psychological, through which individuals with autism/PDD might be predisposed to additional psychiatric disturbance.

OUTCOME

Data on outcome, including that derived from epidemiological studies, has been reviewed elsewhere [Gillberg, 1991; Lotter, 1978; Venter et al., 1992]. In overview, findings from studies prior to the last decade or so indicated that outcome was poor for most people with

autism. Few (10–15%) had gainful employment; most required some degree of ongoing care and supervision; as many as 50% required a substantial amount of assistance. While more recent data are scarce (and possibly biased toward relatively young, higher-functioning individuals), the present picture looks somewhat more promising. Measures of educational attainment, employment status, self-sufficiency and social adaptation suggest that outcome for individuals with autism has improved with upgrades in diagnostic, psychoeducational, and social services [Gillberg, 1991; Kobayashi et al., 1992; Szatmari et al., 1992; Venter et al., 1992]. One unequivocal finding is that children and adults with autism fare best in environments that are suited to their needs. In such environments, other people understand the impairments associated with autism and are well versed in "proven" autism-specific methods for enhancing the development of life skills and personal happiness [e.g., Bryson, 1991; Smith, 1992; Van Bourgondien and Reichle, 1997].

Better outcomes have been consistently associated with, and are predicted by, higher IQs and functional language prior to five years of age [e.g., Lotter, 1974; Rutter et al., 1967], although a significant proportion of the variance in outcome remains to be explained. Some cognitively and linguistically capable individuals experience great difficulty educationally, vocationally, and socially. Such individuals are often misunderstood by educational, health, and social service providers. Moreover, they may be denied access to support services on some technicality (e.g., having an average or above average IQ, despite manifest evidence of autism-related behavioral impairment). Another high-risk, underserved subgroup are those who show evidence of behavioral regression or aggravation during adolescence which may persist well into adulthood [see, e.g., Gillberg, 1984; Kanner et al., 1972; Kobayashi et al., 1992]. This regression/aggravation is evident in a sizable subgroup (approximately 30%) and has been associated with the onset of seizures; most individuals in this group have moderate or severe cognitive impairments. The presence of additional psychiatric disturbance within this and other subgroups—indeed, within the entire spectrum of those with autism— may explain at least some of the unaccounted variance in outcome. Limitations in existing data on outcome serve to underscore the need for longitudinal data aimed at elucidating the nature of, and possible differences in, the developmental trajectories or pathways characteristic of autism and related pervasive disorders.

In Szatmari and colleagues' ongoing longitudinal study of cognitively capable individuals with autism or Asperger's syndrome, evidence has been provided for parallel developmental trajectories that differ in rate or timing, rather than kind [Szatmari et al., 1992]. Specifically, while there was a discrepancy in development at age 4–6 years between high-functioning children with autism and those with Asperger's syndrome, that discrepancy subsequently decreased considerably in a subgroup of autistic children who developed better language skills. Indeed, the later developmental trajectories of this subgroup paralleled those of younger children with Asperger's syndrome. These findings are consistent with and extend Wing's [1988] claim of a continuum of autistic conditions. Not yet known, however, is whether the developmental trajectories of lower-functioning children with autism differ from or are similar to those of their more capable counterparts. Also unknown is whether phenotypic differences in development serve as markers for differences in etiology. Research designed to address these issues also might consider the role of treatment in outcome. Recent reports suggest that early, intensive behavioral intervention is associated with better outcomes in autism [see Dawson and Osterling, 1997; Rogers, 1996, and this issue]. Among the questions that need to be asked are whether differences in method, intensity, and/or duration of treatment, or age of initiating treatment, contribute to the variability in outcome in autism/PDD.

SUMMARY

Autism is the most extreme form of a spectrum of related behaviorally defined, pervasive developmental disorders. These disorders share core impairments in socialization, communication, and imagination, but differ in specifics of their behavioral manifestation or severity. Recent prevalence estimates indicate that autism occurs with a frequency of about 10–12/10,000, and at least 2/1,000 have autism or a less severe variant thereof. In addition, about 3–4/1,000 meet diagnostic criteria for Asperger's syndrome. Thus, the prevalence of autism spectrum disorders is at least 5–6/1,000, and may be higher.

Of individuals with autism specifically, most (≈75%) also have mental retardation. Conversely, a significant proportion (≈25%) of people with mental

retardation also meet criteria for autism. Considering the entire spectrum of autistic disorders, fewer than 50% of individuals have mental retardation. However, all affected individuals are significantly impaired in the acquisition of adaptive skills. At least 25–30% of individuals with autism have associated medical conditions, which predominate among the most severely mentally retarded. Autism is further distinguished by the presence of minor physical anomalies and sensory impairments, the origin of which may be teratogenic and/or genetic. There is also evidence of elevated rates in autism of co-morbid psychiatric disturbance, notably mood disorder.

As to outcome, recent reports suggest that improvements in diagnostic, psychoeducational, and social services have begun to alter what was once a dismal picture for people with autism. Central to improving outcome is the use of empirically supported autism-specific behavioral interventions. Despite the well-documented relationship between better outcomes and higher IQs and functional language prior to age five, a good deal of the variability in outcome remains to be explained. Variables may include the onset of epilepsy, co-morbid psychiatric disturbance, and the nature of treatment (e.g., method and/or intensity, or age at which treatment commenced).

…autism is not only a severe developmental disorder associated with lifelong disability, it is also more prevalent than previously believed.

IMPLICATIONS FOR RESEARCH AND SERVICE DELIVERY

The research summarized here has important implications for planning and delivery of services, and for identifying potentially fruitful directions for research. Regarding research, little is known about borderline autistic conditions, including Asperger's syndrome. Also of interest is atypical autism/PDD-NOS, in which many affected individuals also have mental retardation. Even within the group with typical autism, we have only begun to explain the variability in outcome. Differences in developmental trajectories among those with autism/PDD may indicate different etiologies, but this

possibility has yet to be empirically established. Studies of developmental trajectories need to be extended to include the entire spectrum of autism, including those who are lower functioning. A question of particular concern is whether there has been a true increase in prevalence. Following Gillberg and colleagues [1991], we (Smith and Bryson) are positioned to conduct a second survey of autism in the same regions screened originally (one a relatively immobile rural region, the other a more transient urban-suburban region, both in the province of Nova Scotia; Bryson, 1996, 1997). Recent advances in the understanding of basic mechanisms, both biological and psychological, may render such a study particularly timely. We also need to understand better the contribution of treatment/intervention to outcome.

Future epidemiological studies need to be more theory-driven and conceptualized within a developmental framework. Such research has the potential to tell us much about the spectrum of autistic disorders, about differential outcomes, and about the role of treatment in outcome, while at the same time addressing basic questions about the etiology and neuropsychopathology of autism/PDD within an epidemiological context.

We end by emphasizing some of the implications of existing epidemiological research for the planning and delivery of services for individuals with autism/PDD. First and foremost, autism is not only a severe developmental disorder associated with lifelong disability, it is also more prevalent than previously believed. This fact must be recognized in order to provide appropriate services to the many individuals who are directly or indirectly affected. The true prevalence needs to be communicated to administrators, service providers, and funding agencies in order that sufficient resources are allocated to the problem. We add that a concerted effort is required to adequately train health, education, and social service providers about autism/PDD and its associated psychosocial and medical/psychiatric characteristics. Training needs to focus on state-of-the-science methods for identifying autism early in life, and for intervening and providing appropriate support then and throughout the life span. A sophisticated literature now exists on successful methods of intervention, as does considerable expertise in practical approaches to minimizing disability and developing the very real potential of those affected by autism. Children and adults with autism/PDD, with or without mental retardation, make remarkable progress when they are the beneficiaries of this knowledge and expertise. Greater accessibility by the many who actually need it is clearly a social, educational, and health care priority. ∎

REFERENCES

APA (American Psychiatric Association). Diagnostic and Statistical Manual of Mental Disorders (DSM-III). 2nd ed. Washington, DC: APA, 1984.

APA (American Psychiatric Association). Diagnostic and Statistical Manual of Mental Disorders (DSM-IV). 4th ed. Washington, DC: APA, 1994.

Bailey A, Phillips W, Rutter M. Autism: Towards an integration of clinical, genetic, neuropsychological and neurobiological perspectives. J Child Psychol Psychiatry 1996;37:89–126.

Bolton P, Rutter M. Schedule for Assessment of Psychiatric Problems Associated with Autism (and Other Developmental Disorders). Cambridge, UK: Developmental Psychiatry Section, University of Cambridge, London: Child Psychiatry Department, Institute of Psychiatry, 1994.

Bryson SE. Our Most Vulnerable Citizens: Needs of and Service Models for People with Autism. Toronto, ON: Autism Society Ontario, 1991.

Bryson SE. Epidemiology of autism. J Autism Dev Disord 1996;26:165–167.

Bryson SE. Epidemiology of autism: Overview and issues outstanding. In: Cohen DJ, Volkmar FR, eds. Handbook of Autism and Pervasive Developmental Disorders. 2nd ed. New York: John Wiley & Sons, 1997a:41–46.

Bryson SE. Epidemiology of Autism: Prevalence, Associated Characteristics and Implications for Service Delivery. Paper presented at the Autism Workshop of the U.S. Centers for Disease Control and Prevention and the National Alliance for Autism Research; Atlanta, GA, 1997b.

Bryson SE, Clark BS, Smith IM. First report of a Canadian epidemiological study of autistic syndromes. J Child Psychol Psychiatry 1988; 29:433–446.

Chess S, Korn SJ, Fernandez PB. Psychiatric Disorders of Children with Congenital Rubella. New York: Brunner/Mazel, 1971.

Coleman M, Gillberg C. The Biology of the Autistic Syndromes. New York: Praeger, 1985.

Dawson G, Osterling J. Early intervention in autism. In: Guralnick MJ, ed. The Effectiveness of Early Intervention. Baltimore: Paul H. Brookes, 1997:307–326.

Deb S, Prasad KB. The prevalence of autistic disorder among children with learning disabilities. Br J Psychiatry 1994;165:395–399.

DeLong R. Children with autism spectrum disorder and a family history of affective disorder. Dev Med Child Neurol 1994;36:674–687.

Dennis M. Acquired disorders of language in children. In: Feinberg TE, Farah MJ, eds. Behavioral Neurology and Neuropsychology. New York: McGraw-Hill, 1996:737–754.

Ehlers S, Gillberg C. The epidemiology of Asperger syndrome. A total population study. J Child Psychol Psychiatry 1993;34:1327–1350.

Fombonne E. Is the prevalence of autism increasing? J Autism Dev Disord 1996;26:673–676.

Freeman BJ, Yokota A, Childs J, et al. WISC-R and Vineland Adaptive Behavior scores in autistic children. J Am Acad Child Adolesc Psychiatry 1988;27:428–429.

Gillberg C. Autistic children growing up: Problems during puberty and adolescence. Dev Med Child Neurol 1984;26:122–129.

Gillberg C. Outcome in autism and autistic-like conditions. J Am Acad Child Adolesc Psychiatry 1991;30:375–382.

Gillberg C. Subgroups in autism: Are there behavioural phenotypes typical of underlying medical conditions? J Intellect Disabil Res 1992;36:201–214.

Gillberg C. Autism Is More Common Than Once Widely Held. Paper presented at the Autism Workshop of the U.S. Centers for Disease Control and Prevention and the National Alliance for Autism Research, Atlanta, GA, November, 1997.

Gillberg C, Steffenberg S. Autistic behaviour in Moebius syndrome. Acta Paediatr Scand 1989;78:314–317.

Gillberg C, Steffenburg S, Schaumann H. Is autism more common now than ten years ago? Br J Psychiatry 1991;158:403–409.

Harris SL. Teaching language to nonverbal children — With special emphasis on problems of generalization. Psychol Bull 1975;82:565–580.

Kanner L. Autistic disturbances of affective contact. Nervous Child 1943;2:217–250.

Kanner L, Rodriguez A, Ashenden B. How far can autistic children go in matters of social adaptation? J Autism Child Schizophr 1972;2: 9–33.

Klin A. Auditory brainstem responses in autism: Brainstem dysfunction or peripheral hearing loss? J Autism Dev Disord 1993;23:15–35.

Kobayashi R, Murata T, Yoshinaga K. A follow-up study of 201 children with autism in Kyushu and Yamaguchi areas, Japan. J Autism Dev Disord 1992;22:395–411.

Lainhart JE, Folstein SE. Affective disorders in people with autism: A review of published cases. J Autism Dev Disord 1994;24:587–601.

Lord C, Rutter M, Le Couteur A. Autism Diagnostic Interview—Revised: A revised version of a diagnostic interview for caregivers of individuals with possible pervasive developmental disorders. J Autism Dev Disord 1994;24:659–685.

Lotter V. Epidemiology of autistic conditions in young children. I. Prevalence. Soc Psychiatry 1966;1:124–137.

Lotter V. Epidemiology of autistic conditions in young children. II: Some characteristics of the parents and children. Soc Psychiatry 1967;1: 163–173.

Lotter V. Factors related to outcome in autistic children. J Autism Child Schizophr 1974;4: 263–277.

Lotter V. Follow-up studies. In: Rutter M, Schopler E, eds. Autism: A Reappraisal of Concepts and Treatment. New York: Plenum Press, 1978:475–495.

Loveland KA, Kelley MI. Development of adaptive behavior in adolescents and young adults with autism and Down syndrome. J Autism Dev Disord 1988;93:84–92.

Lubs HA. A marker X-chromosome. Am J Hum Genet 1969;2:231–244.

Martien KM, Banwell B, Hwang PA, et al. ACTH treatment in cryptogenic infantile spasms: Effects on later autistic features. Epilepsia 1997;38:184.

McLennan JD, Lord C, Schopler E. Sex differences in higher functioning people with autism. J Autism Dev Disord 1993;23:217–227.

Myazaki M, Hashimoto T, Tayama M, et al. Brainstem involvement in infantile spasms: A study employing brainstem evoked potentials and magnetic resonance imaging. Neuropediatrics 1993;24:126–130.

Ornitz EM. Neurophysiology of infantile autism. J Am Acad Child Psychiatry 1985;24:251–262.

Ornitz EM, Guthrie D, Farley AJ. The early development of autistic children. J Autism Schizophr 1977;7:207–229.

Pickles A, Bolton P, MacDonald H, et al. Latent-class analysis of recurrence risks for complex phenotypes with selection and measurement error: A twin and family history study of autism. Am J Hum Genet 1995;57: 717–726.

Rapin I. Autism. Curr Concepts 1997;337:97–103.

Riikonen R, Amnell G. Psychiatric disorders in children with earlier infantile spasms. Dev Med Child Neurol 1981;23:747–760.

Rimland B. Infantile Autism. New York: Appleton-Century-Crofts, 1964.

Rodier PM, Ingram JL, Tisdale B, et al. Embryological origin for autism: Developmental anomalies of the cranial nerve motor nuclei. J Comp Neurol 1996;370:247–261.

Rodier PM, Bryson SE, Welch P. Minor malformations and physical measurements in autism: Data from Nova Scotia. Teratology 1997;55: 319–325.

Rogers SJ. Early intervention in autism. J Autism Dev Disord 1996;26:243–246.

Rutter M, Greenfeld D, Lockyer L. A five-to-fifteen year follow-up study of infantile psychoses. II. Social and behavioral outcome. Br J Psychiatry 1967;113:1183–1199.

Shah A, Holmes N, Wing L. Appl Res Ment Handicap 1982;3:303–317.

Smalley SL, McCracken J, Tanguay P. Autism, affective disorders, and social phobia. Am J Med Genet 1995;60:19–26.

Smith M. Community integration and supported employment. In: Berkell DE, ed. Autism: Identification, Education, and Treatment. Hillsdale, NJ: Lawrence Erlbaum, 1992:253–271.

Stromland K, Miller MT. Thalidomide embryopathy: Revisited 27 years later. Acta Ophthalmol 1993;71:238–245.

Szatmari P, Archer L, Fisman S. A Two-Year Follow-up Study of High- Functioning Preschool Children with Pervasive Developmental Disorders. Annual Meeting of the American Academy of Child and Adolescent Psychiatry, Washington, DC, 1992.

Szatmari P, Jones MB, Holden J, et al. High phenotypic correlations among siblings with autism and pervasive developmental disorders. Am J Med Genet 1996;67:354–360.

Valente M. Autism: Symptomatic and idiopathic and mental retardation. Pediatrics 1971;48: 495–496.

Van Bourgondien ME, Reichle N. Residential treatment for individuals with autism. In: Cohen DJ, Volkmar FR, eds. Handbook of Autism and Pervasive Developmental Disorders. 2nd ed. New York: John Wiley & Sons, 1997:691–706.

Venter, A, Lord, C, Schopler, E. A follow-up study of high functioning autistic children. J Child Psychol Psychiatry 1992;33:489–507.

Volkmar FR, Szatmari P, Sparrow SS. Sex differences in pervasive developmental disorders. J Autism Dev Disord 1993;23:579–591.

Wing L. Sex ratios in early childhood autism and related conditions. Psychiatry Res 1981;5:129–137.

Wing L. The continuum of autistic disorders. In: Schopler E, Mesibov GM, Eds. Diagnosis and Assessment in Autism. New York: Plenum Press, 1988:91–110.

Wing L. The definition and prevalence of autism: A review. Eur Child Adolesc Psychiatry 1993;2:61–74.

Wing L, Attwood T. Syndromes of autism and atypical development. In: Cohen DJ, Donnel-lan AM, Eds. Handbook of Autism and Pervasive Developmental Disorders. New York: John Wiley & Sons, 1987:3–19.

Wing L, Gould J. Severe impairments of social interaction and associated abnormalities in children: Epidemiology and classification. J Autism Child Schizophr 1979;9:11–29.

WHO (World Health Organization) The ICD-10 Classification of Mental and Behavioural Disorders: Diagnostic Criteria for Research. Geneva: WHO, 1993.

Psychological Medicine, 1999, **29**, 769–786.   Printed in the United Kingdom
© 1999 Cambridge University Press

The epidemiology of autism: a review

ERIC FOMBONNE*

From the MRC Child Psychiatry Unit, Institute of Psychiatry, London

ABSTRACT

Background. There is some uncertainty about the rate and correlates of autism.

Method. Twenty-three epidemiological surveys of autism published in the English language between 1966 and 1998 were reviewed.

Results. Over 4 million subjects were surveyed; 1533 subjects with autism were identified. The methodological characteristics of each study are summarized, including case definition, case-finding procedures, participation rates and precision achieved. Across surveys, the median prevalence estimate was 5·2/10000. Half the surveys had 95% confidence intervals consistent with population estimates of 5·4–5·5/10000. Prevalence rates significantly increased with publication year, reflecting changes in case definition and improved recognition; the median rate was 7·2/10000 for 11 surveys conducted since 1989. The average male/female ratio was 3·8:1, varying according to the absence or presence of mental retardation. Intellectual functioning within the normal range was reported in about 20% of subjects. On average, medical conditions of potential causal significance were found in 6% of subjects with autism, with tuberous sclerosis having a consistently strong association with autism. Social class and immigrant status did not appear to be associated with autism. There was no evidence for a secular increase in the incidence of autism. In eight surveys, rates for other forms of pervasive developmental disorders were two to three times higher than the rate for autism.

Conclusion. Based on recent surveys, a minimum estimate of 18·7/10000 for all forms of pervasive developmental disorders was derived, which outlines the needs in special services for a large group of children.

INTRODUCTION

Epidemiology is the discipline that is concerned with patterns of disease occurrence in human populations and by the factors that influence them. Typical study designs are the prospective cohort study and the case–control study depending upon whether subjects are ascertained according to their exposure or disease status. Cross-sectional or prevalence studies are based on general population samples and characterized by the fact that both disease and exposure status are determined contemporaneously. Epidemiological investigations of psychiatric disorders have often started with cross-sectional surveys, which provide useful information on both the prevalence and the patterns of risk factors or correlates of the disorder among representative samples. In addition, these surveys are relevant to public health and services planning in portraying the needs that various professional groups have to meet.

Epidemiological surveys of autism started in the mid-1960s in England (Lotter, 1966, 1967) and have since then been conducted in many countries. All epidemiological surveys have focused on a psychiatric-diagnostic approach to autism that has relied over time on different sets of criteria. Thus, this review is concerned with autism defined as a severe developmental disorder and not with more subtle autistic features or symptoms that occur as part of other developmental disorders or as unusual personality traits. Most surveys have relied on operational definitions of autism, be they embodied by official classifications or not, and have

¹ Address for correspondence: Dr Eric Fombonne, MRC Child Psychiatry Unit, Institute of Psychiatry, De Crespigny Park, Denmark Hill, London SE5 8AF.

used the clinical judgement of experts to arrive at the final case groupings. It is worth emphasizing that the field trials of recent classifications such as DSM-III-R (Spitzer & Siegel, 1990) or DSM-IV/ICD-10 (Volkmar *et al*. 1994) have also relied upon the judgment of clinical experts as a gold standard to diagnose autism. Therefore, this review was conducted while recognizing the differences of particular diagnostic systems available in the last decades to define autism while making no *a priori* assumptions on their superiority relative to expert clinical judgement. The aims of this article are to provide an up-to-date review of the methodological features and substantive results of published studies. A key feature has been to rely on summary statistics throughout in order to derive quantitative conclusions for this review.

SELECTION OF STUDIES

The studies were identified through systematic searches from the major scientific literature databases and from prior reviews (Zahner & Pauls, 1987; Wing, 1993). Only studies published in the English language were included in this review. This led to the exclusion of several questionnaire-based studies and of small-scale investigations published in the national literature of the relevant countries (Haga & Miyamoya, 1971; Nakai, 1971; Ishii & Takahashi, 1983; Aussilloux *et al*. 1989; Herder, 1993) and, most certainly of other similar studies unknown to the author. Overall, 23 studies published between 1966 and 1998 were selected that surveyed autism in clearly demarcated, non-overlapping samples. They are listed in Table 1 by order of their appearance in the literature. Studies are numbered from 1 to 23, and these numbers are subsequently used in Tables 2–6, as well as in the text, to index each study. For several studies, the publication listed in Table 1 is the most detailed account or the earliest one; however, other published articles were used to extract relevant information from the same study, when appropriate. In the particular case of studies conducted in Göteborg by Gillberg and colleagues (Gillberg, 1984; Steffenburg & Gillberg, 1986; Gillberg *et al*. 1991), the examination of the samples studied in each of these three reports showed that there was a partial sample overlap between the first and the second report, and that

the sample of the second report was included in the sample of the third report. Accordingly, only the last report (Gillberg *et al*. 1991) was taken into consideration for this review. It is worth noting that the prevalence estimate from this last report is both the highest and the most recent.

RESULTS

Survey descriptions

The surveys were conducted in 12 countries and over half of the results have been published during the last decade (Table 1). Details on the precise sociodemographic composition and economical activities of the area surveyed in each study were generally lacking; most studies were, however, conducted in predominantly urban (seven studies) or mixed (10 studies) areas, with only two surveys (studies 6 and 11) carried out in rural areas. The proportion of children from immigrant families was generally not available and very low in four surveyed populations (studies 11, 12, 19 and 22); only in study 4 was there a substantial minority of children with an immigrant West-Indian background living in the area. The age range of the population included in the surveys is spread from birth to early adult life although the median age of 21 samples was comprised between 5 and 12 years, with an overall median age of 8·5 across the 23 studies. Similarly, there is huge variation in the size of the population surveyed (range: 5120–899750), with a median population size of 73301 subjects (mean = 182143) and about half of the studies relying on targeted populations ranging in size from 32000 to 275000. The total number of children surveyed in just over 4 million ($N = 4189295$).

Study designs

The case finding techniques and case definition adopted in each study are presented in Table 2. Most investigations have relied on a two-stage or multi-stage approach to identify cases in underlying populations. The first screening stage of these studies often consisted of sending letters or brief screening scales requesting school and health professionals to identify possible cases of autism. Each investigation varied in several key aspects of this screening stage. First, the coverage of the populations varied enormously from one

Table 1. *Description of the studies*

Number	Year of publication	Authors	Country	Region/State/ Province	Area	Year of data collection	Age group	Size of target population
1	1966	Lotter	UK	Middlesex	Mainly urban	1964	8–10	78 000
2	1970	Brask	Denmark	Aarhus county	Mostly urban	1962	2–14	46 500
3	1970	Treffert	USA	Wisconsin	Rural (36%) + Urban (64%)	1962–67	3–12	899 750
4	1976	Wing et al.	UK	Camberwell	Urban	1970–72	5–14	25 000
5	1982	Hoshino et al.	Japan	Fukushima-Ken	Mixed	1977–79	0–18	609 848
6	1983	Bohman et al.	Sweden	County of Västerbotten	Rural	1979	0–20	69 000
7	1984	McCarthy et al.	Ireland	East	—	1978	8–10	65 000
8	1986	Steinhausen et al.	Germany	West Berlin	Urban	1982	0–14	279 616
9	1987	Burd et al.	USA	North Dakota	—	—	2–18	180 986
10	1987	Matsuishi et al.	Japan	Kurume City	—	1983	4–12	32 834
11	1988	Tanoue et al.	Japan	Southern Ibaraki	Rural	1977–85	7	95 394
12	1988	Bryson et al.	Canada	part of Nova-Scotia	Suburban and rural	1985	6–14	20 800
13	1989	Sugiyama & Abe	Japan	Nagoya	Urban	1979–84	3	12 263
14	1989	Cialdella & Mamelle	France	1 'département' (Rhône)	Urban	1986	3–9	135 180
15	1989	Ritvo et al.	USA	Utah	Mixed	1984–88	3–27	769 620
16	1991	Gillberg et al.	Sweden	South-west Gothenburg + Bohuslän county	Mixed	1984–88	4–13	78 106
17	1992	Fombonne & du Mazaubrun	France	4 régions, 14 départements	Mixed	1985	9- and 13- year-olds	274 816
18	1992	Wignyosumarto et al.	Indonesia	Yogyakarita (South east of Jakarta)		1991	4–7	5 120
19	1996	Honda et al.	Japan	Yokohama	Urban	1994	5	8 537
20	1997	Fombonne et al.	France	3 'départements'	Mixed	1992–93	8–16	325 347
21	1997	Webb et al.	UK	South Glamorgan, Wales	Mixed	1992	3–15	73 301
22	1998	Sponheim & Skjeldal	Norway	Akershus County	Suburban and rural	1990–92	3–14	65 688
23	1999	Magnússon & Sæmundsen	Iceland	Whole Island	Mixed	1997	4–13	38 589

study to another. In some (i.e. studies 3, 17 and 20), only cases already known from educational or medical authorities could be identified, whereas in other surveys an extensive coverage of the entire population, including children attending normal schools (study 1) or children undergoing systematic developmental checks (studies 13 and 19) was achieved. In addition, the surveyed areas varied in terms of service development as a function of the specific educational or health care systems of each country and of the year of the study. Secondly, the type of information sent out to professionals invited to identify children varied from simple letters including a few clinical descriptors of autism-related syndromes or diagnostic check-lists re-phrased in non-technical terms, to more systematic screening based on questionnaires or rating scales of known reliability and validity. Thirdly, participation rates in the first screening

stages provide another source of variation in the screening efficiency of surveys. Refusal rates were available for eight studies (studies 1, 5, 6, 9, 12, 14, 19 and 20); the rate of refusal ranged from $< 0.27\%$ (study 12) to 27.4% (study 5), with a median value of 10%. Fewer studies could examine the extent to which refusal to participate or non-cooperativeness in surveys is associated with the likelihood that the corresponding children have autism. Bryson et al. (1988), however, provided some evidence that those families who refused cooperation in the intensive assessment phase had children with ABC scores similar to other false positives in their study, thereby suggesting that these children were unlikely to have autism. By contrast, in a Japanese study (Sugiyama & Abe, 1989; study 13) were 17.3% of parents refused further investigations for their 18-month old children who had failed a developmental check, the

Table 2. *Case identification and case definition methods*

Study	Screening		Intensive assessment			
	Instrument	Informants	Number assessed	Informants	Instruments	Diagnostic criteria
1 Lotter, 1966	22 items behaviour questionnaire	All sources (teachers + child guidance clinics + systematic screening of records of handicapped children)	124	Prof, Ch, Rec, Par	Multi-stage (children interview + tests) + parent interview + records	Rating scale
2 Brask, 1970	Inspection of case notes	Psychiatric hospital, institutions, medical wards	60	Rec, Prof	Review of all records + interview of professionals	Clinical
3 Treffert, 1970	Computer search of clinic attenders with a DSM-III diagnosis of childhood schizophrenia	Administrative data from clinics and hospitals	69	Rec	Review of diagnostic notes	Kanner
4 Wing et al. 1976	15 items interview	Teachers, speech therapists, observations	108	Prof, Ch, Rec, Par	Interview of professionals or parents, psychological tests	24 items rating scale of Lotter
5 Hoshino et al. 1982	Questionnaire requesting behavioural descriptions	Normal and special schools, medical and welfare institutions	386	Par, Ch	Parent and child interview	Kanner's criteria
6 Bohman et al. 1983	Two-stage screening questionnaire + follow-up telephone interview	716 professionals	272	Par, Ch, Rec	Clinical	Rutter criteria*
7 McCarthy et al. 1984	Letter + follow-up telephone calls	Psychiatrists + special schools	28	Ch, Rec, Prof	Observation + review of all data	Kanner
8 Steinhausen et al. 1986	Direct identification of children already known to child psychiatry clinics or attending an Autistic Society educational programme	Local professionals	52	Rec	Review of available data	Rutter
9 Burd et al. 1987	Letter with behavioural descriptors derived from DSM-III + telephone calls	All school and health professionals and parent associations	> 200	Par, Ch, Rec	Structured parental interview + review of all data available	DSM-III
10 Matsuishi et al. 1987	Screening of records	All schools and medical institutions	51	Rec, Ch	Direct clinical examination	DSM-III
11 Tanoue et al. 1988	Children referred to local child guidance centre	—	132	Ch	?	DSM-III
12 Bryson et al. 1988	19 items questionnaire	Teachers/counsellors	35	Par, Prof, Ch, Rec	WISC-R M-PSMT PPVT-R RDLS VABS WRAT-R ABC	New RDC
13 Sugiyama & Abe, 1989	Routine development checks at 18 months, with repeat follow-up investigations up to the age of 3	Paediatricians + nurses + parents + children	139	Ch	Gesell test + direct assessment + review of records	DSM-III
14 Cialdella & Mamelle, 1989	Completion of open-ended questionnaire for children with 'infantile psychosis'	Mental health professionals + special schools	220	Prof	Psychiatric diagnosis based on analysis of questionnaire information	DSM-III like

Table 2. (Cont.)

	Screening		Intensive assessment			
Study	Instrument	Informants	Number assessed	Informants	Instruments	Diagnostic criteria
15 Ritvo et al. 1989	Screening through media campaigns and advertising to a range of professionals	Review and quantitative rating of records by 2 blind psychiatrists	423	Prof, Par, Ch, Rec	Parent and child assessment + record review	DSM-III
16 Gillberg et al. 1991	Mailed questionnaire + register search	Doctors + teachers in institutions + associated professions	74	Ch, Rec, Prof, Par	Psychiatric assessment + review of all records VABS Griffiths + WISC-R ABC interview schedule	DSM-III-R
17 Fombonne & du Mazaubrun, 1992	Systematic survey of special education local authorities + survey of psychiatric hospitals	Child psychiatrists + parents + records	154	Rec	Review of all relevant information	Clinical – ICD-10 like
18 Wignyosumarto et al. 1992	19-items Bryson's screening scale	Professionals trained to the screening instrument	66	Par, Ch	Psychiatric interview + WISC-R + Merrill-Palmer	CARS
19 Honda et al. 1996	Health check-ups at 18 months + other referrals to local psychiatric services	Medical teams + schools	38	Ch, Rec, Par, Prof	Direct observation + psychological assessments + review of all data	ICD-10
20 Fombonne et al. 1997	Systematic survey of special education local authorities + survey of psychiatric hospitals	Child psychiatrists + parents + records	174	Rec	Review of all information	Clinical – ICD-10 like
21 Webb et al. 1997	Mailed check-list based on DSM-III-R descriptions + ABC if screened positive	Health and educational professionals + principal carer on screened positive	72	Ch, Par, Rec	Neuropsychiatric Developmental Interview (NDI)	DSM-III-R
22 Sponheim & Skjeldal, 1998	10 items screening schedule	Paediatricians + maternal-child health clinics + child psychiatrists	65	Par, Ch	Parental interview + direct observation CARS, ABC	ICD-10
23 Magnússon & Sæmundsen, 1999	All cases referred to 2 diagnostic centres	Educational and health professionals	—	Ch, Par, Rec	ADI-R, CARS + psychological tests	Mostly ICD-10

* Relaxed for the age of onset criterion.

Abbreviations: Par, parents; Prof, professionals; Ch, children; Rec, records. DSM-III, Diagnostic Statistical Manual, 3rd edn.; DSM-III-R, Diagnostic Statistical Manual, 3rd edn. revised; ICD-10, International Classification of Diseases, 10th revision; RDC, Research Diagnostic Criteria; WISC, Wechsler Intelligence Scale for Children; M-PSMT, Merrill-Palmer Scale of Mental Tests; PPVT-R, Peabody Picture Vocabulary Test – Revised; RDLS, Reynell Developmental Language Scales; VABS, Vineland Adaptive Behavioural Scales; WRAT-R, Wide Range Achievement Test-Revised; ABC, Autism Behavior Checklist; CARS, Childhood Autism Rating Scale; ADI-R, Autism Diagnostic Interview-Revised.

authors obtained follow-up data at age 3 that suggested that half of these children still displayed developmental problems. Whether or not these problems were connected to autism is unknown, but this study points to the possibility of having higher rates of developmental disorders among non-participants to surveys. Similarly, in Lotter's study (1966; study 1), 58 questionnaires covering schools for handicapped children were returned out of the 76 forms sent out, and an independent review of the records showed that four of the 18 missing forms corresponded to autistic children. Therefore, it is difficult to draw firm conclusions from these different accounts. Although there is no consistent evidence that parental refusal to co-operate is associated with autism in their offspring, it appears that a small proportion of cases may be missed in some surveys as a consequence of non-cooperation at the screening stage. No survey included a weighting procedure to compensate for non-response.

Only one study (study 1) provided an estimate of the reliability of the screening procedure. The sensitivity of the screening methodology is also difficult to gauge in autism surveys. The usual epidemiological approach, which consists of sampling at random screened negative subjects in order to estimate the proportion of false negatives, has not been used in these surveys for the obvious reason that, due to the very low frequency of the disorder, it would be both imprecise and very costly to undertake such estimations. The consequence of these remarks is that prevalence estimates must be seen as underestimates of 'true' prevalence rates because cases are being missed due either to lack of cooperation or to imperfect sensitivity of the screening procedure. The magnitude of this underestimation is unknown in each survey but it is, however, unlikely to be substantial.

Similar considerations about the methodological variability across studies apply to the intensive assessment phases of published surveys (Table 2). Participation rates in these second-stage assessments were not always available, either because they had simply not been calculated, or because the design and/or method of data collection did not lead easily to their estimation. When they were available (studies 1, 5, 8, 12, 13, 15 and 22), the participation rates were generally high, ranging from 76·1 % (study 12) to 98 % (study 8), with a median value of 92·5 %. The number of subjects included in intensive assessments varied from 28 to 423 (mean = 130), with a median number of 91 subjects per investigation. The source of information used to determine caseness usually involved a combination of informants and data sources, with a direct assessment of the person with autism in 14 studies.

The assessments were conducted with various diagnostic instruments, ranging from a classical clinical examination to the use of batteries of standardized measures. The precise diagnostic criteria retained to define caseness vary according to the study and, to a large extent, reflect historical changes in classification systems. Thus, Kanner's criteria, Lotter's and Rutter's definitions were used in the first eight surveys (all conducted before 1982), whereas DSM-based definitions took over thereafter as well as ICD-10 since 1990. Some studies have relaxed partly some diagnostic criteria such as the requirement of an age of onset before 30 months (study 6) or that of the absence of schizophrenic-like symptoms (studies 13 and 14). It is, however, impossible to assess the impact of a specific diagnostic scheme or of a particular diagnostic criterion on the estimate of prevalence since other powerful method factors confound between-studies comparisons of rates. Surprisingly, few studies have built in a reliability assessment of the diagnostic procedure; reliability during the intensive assessment phase was high in four surveys (studies 4, 13, 16 and 22) and moderate in a fifth one (study 14). All the methodological differences summarized in Table 2 should be borne in mind for between-studies comparisons as method factors are likely to account for most of the variation in rates.

Characteristics of identified samples

A total number of 1533 subjects assessed in the second stage of the 23 surveys were considered to suffer from autism, this number ranging from six to 241 across studies (median: 51). As indicated in Table 3 (third column), the positive predictive value of the screening procedure, or proportion of screened positive children who, in the intensive assessment phase, were confirmed to have autism, exceeded the 50 % figure only occasionally, with a median value of 33 % in 15 surveys (range: 9·1–73·6 %). Thus, on average, two non-autistic children were screened positively and assessed intensively for each autistic child. These features outline the costs of conducting population surveys of autism and they also reflect the relative lack of specificity of the screening procedures used in epidemiological surveys of such a rare disorder.

An assessment of intellectual function was obtained in 13 studies (Table 3). These assessments were conducted with various tests and instruments; furthermore, results were pooled together in broad bands of intellectual level that did not share the same boundaries across studies. As a consequence, differences in rates of cog-

Table 3. *Surveys of autism: main characteristics of identified samples*

Study, Author, Year	Number with autism	Positive predictive value	IQ distribution (%)			Sex ratio (M/F)		
			Normal range	Mild/ moderate retardation	Severe/ profound retardation	Overall	Normal IQ range	Moderate/ profound retardation
1 Lotter, 1996	32	25·8	15·6	15·6	68·8	2·6 (23/9)	∞ (10/0)	1·3 (12/9)
2 Brask, 1970	20	33·3	—	—	—	1·4 (12/7)	Higher proportion of boys	
3 Treffert, 1970	69	24·6	—	—	—	3·06 (52/17)	—	—
4 Wing et al. 1976	17*	15·7	30	35·0	35·0	16 (16/1)		
5 Hoshino et al. 1982	142	36·8	—	—	—	9·9 (129/13)	—	—
6 Bohman et al. 1983	39	54	20·5	30·8	48·7	1·6 (24/15)	—	Higher proportion of girls
7 McCarthy et al. 1984	28	—	—	—	—	1·33 (16/12)	—	0·6 (3·5)
8 Steinhausen et al. 1986	52	—	55·8	44·2†	(See prior column)	2·25 (36/16)	2·22 (20/9)	—
9 Burd et al. 1987	59	< 29·5	—	—	—	2·7 (43/16)	—	—
10 Matsuishi et al. 1987	51	—	—	—	—	4·7 (42/9)	—	—
11 Tanoue et al. 1988	132	—	—	—	—	4·07 (106/26)	—	—
12 Bryson et al. 1988	21	60	23·8	33·3	42·8	2·5 (15/6)	∞ (5/0)	1·25 (5/4)
13 Sugiyama & Abe, 1989	16	11·5	—	—	—	—	—	—
14 Cialdella & Marmelle, 1989	61	27·7	—	—	—	2·3	—	—
15 Ritvo et al. 1989	241	49	34	25·1	40·9	3·73 (190/51)	6·3 (69/11)	2·7 (70/26)
16 Gillberg et al. 1991	74	—	18	28	54	2·7 (54/20)	2·2 (9/4)	1·9 (26/14)
17 Fombonne & du Mazaubrun, 1992	154	—	13·3	18·1	68·6	2·1 (105/49)	6·0 (12/2)	1·9 (47/25)
18 Wignyosumarto et al. 1992	6	9·1	0	100·0	0	2·0 (4/2)	—	—
19 Honda et al. 1996	18	47·4	50·0	11·1	38·9	2·6 (13/5)	3·5 (7/2)	2·5 (5/2)
20 Fombonne et al. 1997	174	—	12·1	6·6	81·3	1·81 (112/62)	—	—
21 Webb et al. 1997	53	73·6	—	—	—	6·57 (46/7)	—	—
22 Sponheim & Skjeldal, 1998	34	53·8	47·1‡	(See other columns)	52·9‡	2·09 (23/11)	7·0‡ (14/2)	1·0 (9/9)
23 Magnússon & Sæmundsen, 1999	40	—	15	50	35	5·7 (34/6)	—	—

* This number corresponds to the sample described in Wing & Gould (1979) and it has been used for Tables 3, 5 and 6.
† Rate for combined levels of mental retardation (IQ < 70).
‡ In this study, mild mental retardation was combined with normal IQ, whereas moderate and severe levels of mental retardation were pooled together.

nitive impairment between studies should be interpreted with caution. With these caveats in mind, some general conclusions can, nevertheless, be reached (excluding study 22 results that relied upon different IQ groupings). The median proportion of subjects without intellectual impairment is 19·3 % (range: 0–55·8 %).

The corresponding figures are 29·4 % (range: 6·6–100 %) for mild to moderate intellectual impairments and 41·9 % (range: 0–81·3 %) for severe to profound level of mental retardation. In order to control for differences in sample sizes, these proportions were weighted by each study sample size. The three weighted averages

Table 4. *Prevalence rates estimates (per 10000)*

Study	Overall	95% CI*	By age group (years)			By type	
			Pre-school	School age	Teenage	Typical	Atypical
1 Lotter, 1966	4·1	2·7; 5·5	—	—	—	1·9	2·2
2 Brask, 1970	4·3	2·4; 6·2	—	—	—	—	—
3 Treffert, 1970	0·7	0·6; 0·9	—	—	—	—	—
4 Wing et al. 1976	4·8†	2·1; 7·5	—	—	—	2·0	2·8
5 Hoshino et al. 1982	2·33	1·9; 2·7	—	4·96 (4–10)	1·1* (11–16)	—	—
6 Bohman et al. 1983	5·6	3·9; 7·4	1·7 (0–3)	12·6 (7–9)	4·6 (13–15)	3·04*	2·6*
7 McCarthy et al. 1984	4·3	2·7; 5·9	—	—	—	2·15	2·15
8 Steinhausen et al. 1986	1·9	1·4; 2·4	—	2·37* (3–14)	—	1·9	—
9 Burd et al. 1987	3·26	2·4; 4·1	—	4·04 (5–14)	—	1·16	2·10
10 Matsuishi et al. 1987	15·5	11·3; 19·8	17·1 (4–6)	14·7 (7–12)	—	—	—
11 Tanoue et al. 1988	13·8	11·5; 16·2	—	—	—	—	—
12 Bryson et al. 1988	10·1	5·8; 14·4	—	—	—	—	—
13 Sugiyama & Abe, 1989	13·0	6·7; 19·4	—	—	—	—	—
14 Cialdella & Mamelle, 1989	4·5	3·4; 5·6	—	5·1 (5–9)	—	—	—
15 Ritvo et al. 1989	2·47	2·1; 2·8	2·17 (3–7)	3·57 (8–12)	3–16 (13–17)	—	—
16 Gillberg et al. 1991	9·5	7·3; 11·6	7·8 (4–7)	10·8 (8–10)	10·0 (11–13)	7·0	2·4
17 Fombonne & du Mazaubrun, 1992	4·9	4·1; 5·7	—	4·7 (9)	5·1 (13)	—	—
18 Wignyosumarto et al. 1992	11·7	2·3; 21·1	—	—	—	—	—
19 Honda et al. 1996	21·08	11·4; 30·8	—	—	—	—	—
20 Fombonne et al. 1997	5·35	4·6; 6·1	—	5·02 (8–12)	5·68 (13–16)	—	—
21 Webb et al. 1997	7·2	5·3; 9·3	—	—	—	—	—
22 Sponheim & Skjeldal, 1998	5·2	3·4; 6·9	4·9 (3–5)	4·7 (6–11)	6·4 (12–14)	3·8	1·4
23 Magnússon & Sæmundsen, 1999	10·4	7·2; 13·6	—	—	—	7·0	3·4

* Computed by the author.
† This rate corresponds to the first report on this study and is based on 12 subjects among the 5–14-year-olds.

were in close correspondence with the aforementioned median values (respectively: 25·4%, 23·2% and 55·5%). Other severity indices were used by some authors, such as the proportion of children without speech (studies 1, 2, 7, 12 and 18) which ranged from 19% (study 12) to 59% (study 4), or the proportion of subjects living in residential schools or institutions (studies 6, 12, 17 and 20) that ranged from 8·1% (study 6) to 34·5% (study 20).

Gender repartition among subjects with autism was reported in 22 studies and the male/female sex ratio varied from 1·33 (study 7) to 16·0 (study 4), with a median sex ratio of 2·6 (mean = 3·8). Thus, no epidemiological study ever identified more girls than boys with autism, a finding which parallels the gender differences found in clinically referred samples (Wing, 1981;

Lord et al. 1982). Weighting each sex ratio by the sample size, an average weighted estimate of 3·82:1 could be derived for an overall sample of 1517 subjects. The association between gender and intellectual functioning was assessed within subgroups with either normal or severely impaired intellectual function in 11 studies. The overall pattern supported the notion that gender differences were more pronounced when autism was not associated with mental retardation. In nine studies (representing a total sample of 800 subjects) where the sex ratio was available within the normal band of intellectual functioning, the median sex ratio was 6·0:1. Conversely, in eight studies including a total number of 748 subjects, the median sex ratio was 1·7:1 in the group of persons with autism and moderate to severe retardation.

Prevalence estimations

The findings on prevalence estimates are presented in Table 4. Prevalence estimates range from 0·7/10000 to 21·1/10000, with a median value of 5·2/10000. Confidence intervals were computed for each estimate and the width of these intervals (range: 0·3–19·4; mean = 5·2) indicates the variation in the sample sizes and in the precision achieved in each study. Prevalence rates were negatively correlated with sample size (Spearman $r = 0·71$; $P < 0·01$; small-scale studies tended to report higher prevalence rates. The weighted average estimate for 22 studies (excluding study 3 which had both a poorly sensitive case finding method and a high sample size) yielded an estimate of 4·4/10000. We then computed how many studies had confidence intervals including each of 30 possible population values ranging from 4·0 to 6·9/10000. Values of 5·4 and 5·5/10000 fell within the confidence limits of 11 studies, whereas fewer studies included either lower or higher values.

When surveys were combined in two groups according to the median year of publication (1988), the median prevalence rate for 12 surveys conducted in the period 1966–88 was 4·3/10000, and the median rate for the 11 surveys conducted in the period 1989–98 was 7·2/10000. Indeed, the correlation between prevalence rate and year of. publication reached statistical significance (Spearman $r = 0·55$; $P < 0·01$). However, within the 1989–98 period too, the same population values of 5·4 and 5·5/10000 fell within the confidence limits of the majority (six out of 11) of surveys, whereas a fewer number of studies were consistent with any other value ranging from 4·0 to 11·0/10000. The results of the nine surveys with prevalence rates over 6/10000 were all published since 1987. However, the estimated prevalence rates of these nine surveys somewhat lack precision (average width of the 95% CI = 9·7) and these surveys account for less than 9% ($N = 364944$) of the target populations of the 23 surveys. These findings, nevertheless, point towards an increase in prevalence estimates in the last decade, probably reflecting an improved recognition and detection of autism together with a broadening of the diagnostic concept and definitions.

Age-specific rates were available in some studies for the pre-school period (five studies),

the school age period (11 studies) and the teenage years (seven studies) (Table 4). A ratio of each of these age-specific rates to the overall study prevalence rate was computed for these studies. The average values were 0·81, 1·30 and 0·99 for pre-school, school and teenage years respectively. Thus, within studies, comparisons suggest that rates for the school-age period were on average 30% higher than unadjusted prevalence rates; conversely, adolescent rates were lower than school age rates, and rates for the very young were typically much lower, probably reflecting more difficulties in identifying and diagnosing cases in these age groups, developmental changes in autistic symptomatology, and variations with age in patterns of medical care and educational services. For the 11 studies which provided separate estimates for the school age period, the median rate was 5·0/10000.

In eight studies, the sample was broken down according to typical or atypical forms of autism, the precise meaning and reliability of this differentiation being somewhat questionable. Thus, atypical autism has been defined as either presentations departing from Kanner's original descriptions or as autism associated with neurological features (as in study 14). For these eight studies (studies 1, 4, 6, 7, 9, 16, 22 and 23), the mean prevalence rate ratio of typical to atypical forms was 1·49 (median = 1·08) thereby suggesting about equal frequency of both presentations.

Associated medical conditions

Rates of medical conditions associated with autism were reported in 11 surveys. It will be appreciated that these medical conditions were investigated by very different means ranging from questionnaires to full medical work-ups. However, some consistent findings derive from epidemiological samples (Table 5). The median rates and range for each disorder were: 16·8% for epilepsy (nine studies, range: 4·8–26·4%) 2·75% for cerebral palsy (four studies, range: 1·4–4·8%), 0·75% for fragile X (six studies, range: 0–6%), 1·2% for tuberous sclerosis (TS) (eight studies range: 0–3·1%), 0% for phenylketonuria (PKU) (five studies, range: 0–0%), 0·3% for neurofibromatosis (four studies, range: 0–1·4%), 1·3% for Down's syndrome (seven studies, range: 0–5·9%), 0·75% for congenital rubella (eight studies, range: 0–5·9%), 3·1% for

Table 5.   *Rates of associated medical characteristics*

Study[1]	Epilepsy		Cerebral palsy		Associated syndromes	Fragile X anomaly		Tuberous sclerosis	
	N	%	N	%		N	%	N	%
1 Lotter, 1966	4	12·5	—	—	—	—	—	1[2]	3·1
2 Brask, 1970	2	16·6	—	—		—	—	—	—
4 Wing et al. 1976	3	16·8	—	—	2 Encephalopathies	—	—	0	0·0
10 Matsuishi et al. 1987	—	—	—	—	—	0	0·0	0	0·0
12 Bryson et al. 1988	1	4·8	1[3]	4·8	1 Coffin–Lowry[4]	—	—	—	—
15 Ritvo et al. 1989[6]	34	14·6	—	—	1 Muccopolysaccharidose[5] 3 Chromosomal abnormalities 6 Viral/bacterial infections 7 Metabolic disorders 4 Retts syndrome 2 Tourette's syndrome	2	0·9	1	0·4
16 Gillberg et al. 1991	17	23·0	1	1·4	3 Moebius syndrome 1 Laurence-Moon-Biedl syndrome 1 Hydrocephalus 1 Williams' syndrome 3 Chromosomal abnormalities	6	8·1	1	1·4
17 Fombonne & du Mazaubrun, 1992	34	22·0	4	2·6	—	1	0·6	2	1·3
19 Honda et al. 1996	—	—	—	—	—	—	—	—	—
20 Fombonne et al. 1997	46	26·4	5	2·9	2 Chromosomal abnormalities	3	1·7	2	1·1
22 Sponheim & Skjeldal, 1998	8	23·6	—	—	1 Encephalopathy 1 Marinesco-Sjogren syndrome 1 Hydrocephalus (treated)	0	0·0	1	2·9

Study[1]	PKU		Neurofibromatosis		Down's syndrome		Congenital rubella		Sensory impairments			
									Hearing		Visual	
	N	%	N	%	N	%	N	%	N	%	N	%
1 Lotter, 1966	—	—	—	—	—	—	1	3·1	1	3·1	—	—
2 Brask, 1970	—	—	—	—	—	—	—	—	—	—	—	—
4 Wing et al. 1976	0	0·0	0	0·0	0[7]	0·0	1	5·9	1	5·9	0	0·0
10 Matsuishi et al. 1987	0	0·0	—	—	0	0·0	0	0·0	—	—	—	—
12 Bryson et al. 1988	—	—	—	—	—	—	—	—	—	—	—	—
15 Ritvo et al. 1989[6]	—	—	—	—	6	2·6	2	0·9	2	0·9	3	1·3
16 Gillberg et al. 1991	—	—	1	1·4	0	0·0	0	0·0	3	4·1	0	0·0
17 Fombonne & du Mazaubrun, 1992	0	0·0	0	0·0	2	1·3	2	1·3	9[8]	5·8[8]	(see previous col.)	
19 Honda et al. 1996	—	—	—	—	—	—	0	0·0	—	—	—	—
20 Fombonne et al. 1997	0	0·0	1	0·6	3	1·7	1	0·6	3	1·7	5	2·9
22 Sponheim & Skjeldal, 1998	—	—	—	—	2	5·9	—	—	—	—	—	—

[1] Findings from study 11 were not included in this Table since they applied to a broad definition including DSM-III like autism and other pervasive developmental disorders (results for the subgroup of children meeting stricter DSM-III criteria were not available).
[2] Based on a post-mortem examination at follow-up (see Lotter, 1974).
[3] Acquired haemiplegia.
[4] Provisional diagnosis.
[5] Tentative diagnosis.
[6] Based on 233 subjects whose medical records were available.
[7] Children with Down's syndrome and autistic features were, however, excluded from this study (see Wing et al. 1976, p. 95).
[8] These figures apply for both hearing and visual impairments.

hearing impairments (five studies, range: 0·9–5·9%), 1·3% for visual impairments (three studies, range: 0–2·9%). The number of studies from which these summary statistics derived was sometimes small, and the findings should also be checked against the characteristics of the samples included in each survey (see Tables 1–3), particularly regarding the rate of mental retardation.

Nevertheless, the results consolidate scientific knowledge on the association between autism and known medical conditions. Thus, conditions such as congenital rubella, and PKU account for almost no cases of autism. Prior studies suggesting an association of congenital rubella (Chess, 1971) and PKU (Knobloch & Pasamanick, 1975; Lowe et al. 1980) with autism were conducted before implementation of systematic prevention measures. Even then, the proportion of cases of autism attributable to these disorders remained low. Furthermore, follow-up studies of children with rubella suggested that unexpected improvements could occur (Chess, 1977), pointing towards strong differences of these presentations from typical autism. Likewise, our low estimate of 0·3 % for autism and neurofibromatosis is identical to that found in a large series of 341 referred cases (Mouridsen et al. 1992) and, contrary to earlier claims (Gillberg & Forsell, 1984), it does not exceed the rate expected under the assumption of independence of the two disorders. Similarly, bearing in mind the high rate of mental retardation among samples of autistic subjects, the rates found for cerebral palsy and Down's syndrome equally suggest no particular association. The recognition that Down's syndrome and autism co-occur in some individuals has been the focus of attention in recent reports (Bregman & Volkmar, 1988; Ghazziudin et al. 1992; Howlin et al. 1995); the epidemiological findings give further support to the validity of these clinical descriptions, although they do not suggest that the rate of co-morbidity is higher than that expected by chance once the effects of mental retardation are taken into account. For fragile X, the low rate available in epidemiological studies is most certainly an underestimate due to the fact that fragile X was not recognized until relatively recently and that, in the most recent surveys, systematic screening for fragile X was very rarely undertaken. In line with prior reports (Smalley et al. 1992), tuberous sclerosis (TS) has a consistently high frequency among autistic samples. Assuming a population prevalence of 1/10000 for TS (Hunt & Lindenbaum, 1984; Shepherd et al. 1991; Ahlsen et al. 1994), it appears that the rate of TS is about 100 times higher than that expected under the hypothesis of no association. The rate of TS in autistic samples is, however, much lower in these epidemiological studies than the 9 % minimum rate claimed in a recent study (Gillberg et al. 1994). Whether or not the association between

TS and autism is mediated by epilepsy, localized brain lesions or direct genetic effects is a matter for future research.

The overall proportion of cases of autism that could be causally attributed to known medical disorders therefore remains low. From the 10 surveys where rates of one of seven clear-cut medical disorders (cerebral palsy, fragile X, TS, PKU, neurofibromatosis, congenital rubella and Down's syndrome) were available, we computed the proportion of subjects with at least one of these recognizable disorders. Because the overlap between these conditions is expected to be low and because the information about multiply-handicapped subjects was not available, this overall rate was obtained by summing directly the rates for each individual condition within each study; the resulting rate might, therefore, be slightly overestimated. The fraction of cases of autism with a known medical condition ranged from 0 % (studies 10 and 19) to 12·3 % (study 16), with a median and mean values of 6·0 % and 5·8 % respectively. Even if some adjustment was made to account for the underestimation of the rate of fragile X in epidemiological surveys of autism, the attributable proportion of cases of autism would not exceed the 10 % figure for any medical disorder (excluding epilepsy and sensory impairments). Although this figure does not incorporate other medical events of potential aetiological significance, such as encephalitis, congenital anomalies, and other rare medical syndromes, it is similar to that reported in a recent review of the question (Rutter et al. 1994). It is worth noting that epidemiological surveys of autism in very large samples (i.e. studies 15, 17 and 20) provided estimates in line with our conservative summary statistics. By contrast, claims of average rates of medical conditions as high as 24 % appear to apply to studies of smaller size and relying on a broadened definition of autism (Gillberg & Coleman, 1996).

Rates of epilepsy are high among autism samples. The proportion suffering from epilepsy tends also to be higher in those studies which have higher rates of severe mental retardation (as in studies 16, 17 and 20). Age-specific rates for the prevalence of epilepsy were not available. The samples where high rates of epilepsy were reported tended to have a higher median age, although these rates seemed mostly to apply to

Table 6. *Informative studies on rates of non-autism pervasive developmental disorders*

Number	Study	Rates of autism	Prevalence rate of other PDD	Combined rate autism + other PDDs	Prevalence rate ratio*	Case definition for other PDDs
1	Lotter, 1966	4·1	3·3	7·8	1·90	Children with some behaviour similar to autistic children
2	Brask, 1970	4·3	1·9	6·2	1·44	Children with 'other psychoses' or 'borderline psychotic'
4	Wing *et al.* 1976	4·9	16·3	21·2	4·33	Socially impaired (triad of impairments)
5	Hoshino *et al.* 1982	2·33	2·92	5·25	2·25	Autistic mental retardation
9	Burd *et al.* 1987	3·26	> 7·79†	> 11·05†	3·39	Children referred by professionals with 'autistic-like' symptoms, not meeting DSM-III criteria for IA, COPDD or atypical PDD
14	Cialdella & Mamelle, 1989	4·5	4·7	9·2	2·04	Children meeting criteria for other forms of 'infantile psychosis' than autism, or a broadened definition of DSM-III
17	Fombonne & du Mazaubrun, 1992‡	4·6	6·6	11·2	2·43	Children with mixed developmental disorders
20	Fombonne *et al.* 1997	5·3	10·94	16·3	3·05	Children with mixed developmental disorders

* Combined rate divided by autism rate.
† Computed by the author.
‡ These rates are derived from the complete results of the survey of three birth cohorts of French children (Rumeau-Rouquette *et al.* 1994).

school-aged children. Thus, in light of the increased incidence of seizures during adolescence among subjects with autism (Rutter, 1970; Deykin & MacMahon, 1979), the epidemiological rates should be regarded as underestimates of the lifetime risk of epilepsy in autism. These rates are, nonetheless, high and support the findings of a bimodal peak of incidence of epilepsy in autistic samples, with a first peak of incidence in the first years of life (Volkmar & Nelson, 1990).

Finally, in light of the recent UK controversy about the possible association of autism with both inflammatory bowel diseases and exposure to measles and mumps infections and the MMR immunization (Fombonne, 1998; Wakefield *et al.* 1998), it is worth noting than there was no report in the epidemiological surveys of an association of autism with Crohn's disease, inflammatory bowel disorder or with wild measles or mumps infections. Moreover, surveys of autism conducted recently in the USA (study 15) or in France (study 20) after the introduction of the combined MMR immunization did not yield particularly high prevalence estimates.

Rates of other pervasive developmental disorders (PDDs)

Unspecified PDDs (PDDNOS)

Several studies have provided useful information on rates of syndromes similar to autism but falling short of strict diagnostic criteria (see Table 6). Because the screening procedures and subsequent diagnostic assessments differed from one study to another (Table 2), these groups of disorders are not strictly comparable across studies. In addition, as they were not the group on which the attention was focused, details are often lacking on phenomenological features in the available reports. Different labels have been used to characterize them such as the triad of impairments, defined by Wing & Gould (1979) as involving impairments in reciprocal social interaction, communication and imagination. These groups would be overlapping with current diagnostic labels such as atypical autism and PDDNOS, which does little to understand their relationship with a narrower definition of autism. Eight of the 23 surveys yielded estimates of the prevalence of these developmental disorders, with six studies showing higher rates for the non-autism disorders than the rates for autism. The ratio of the combined rate of all developmental disorders to the rate of autism varied between from 1·44 to 4·33 (Table 6) with a mean value of 2·6. In other words, for two children with autism assessed in epidemiological surveys, approximately three children were found to have severe impairments of a similar nature but falling short of strict diagnostic criteria for autism. This group has been less studied but it should be clear from these figures that they represent a very substantial group of children whose treatment needs are likely to be as important as those of children with autism.

Asperger syndrome

Asperger syndrome is a condition that has received much attention during the last decade. Yet, epidemiological studies of its prevalence and characteristics are sparse, probably due to the fact that it was acknowledged as a separate diagnostic category only recently in both ICD-10 and DSM-IV. At least four different diagnostic schemes have been proposed to operationalize its definition and no definite consensus has been reached yet about the respective validity of these competing definitions. Only one epidemiological study has been conducted which specifically investigated its prevalence (Ehlers & Gillberg, 1993). These authors surveyed 1519 7–16-year-old children from five normal schools on the outskirts of Göteborg (Sweden). A questionnaire was used for screening and the intensive assessment relied on a combination of direct assessment, observation and parent/teacher interviews. The prevalence for definite cases was estimated to be 28·5/10 000 (95 % CI computed by us: 0·6–56·5) for ICD-10 criteria and 35·7/10 000 (95 % CI: 4·5–66·9) for the authors' own diagnostic criteria. These estimates are based on a handful of cases ($N = 4$ and $N = 5$, respectively) and, as suggested by the wide confidence intervals, they are very imprecise. Higher rates were computed by the authors when they included possible or suspected cases. Replication of these figures in other samples is clearly needed before some meaningful picture can be drawn (Fombonne, 1997). Indeed, other recent studies have only identified very small numbers ($N = 2$) of children with Asperger syndrome which, subsequently, were included (study 22) or not (study 21) in the case definition; however, the case finding methodology of these studies had not been devised to efficiently identify this subgroup.

Other correlates

Time trends

Anecdotal reports have suggested that more cases of autism were being referred to specialized centres in recent years, suggesting that the incidence might perhaps be increasing. However, studies of clinically referred samples are confounded by many factors such as referral patterns, availability of services, and changes over time in diagnostic practices, to name only a few. Therefore, epidemiological studies are crucial in order to assess secular changes in the incidence of a disorder. As shown before, epidemiological surveys of autism each possess unique design features that could account almost entirely for the between-studies variations in rates, and time trends in the incidence of autism are therefore difficult to gauge from published prevalence rates. The significant correlation previously mentioned between prevalence rate and year of publication could merely reflect increased efficiency over time in case identification methods used in surveys as well as changes in diagnostic practices. Thus, changes in diagnostic practices were reported in Magnusson & Sæmundsen's study (1999) where ICD-9 based rates for the oldest cohorts born in the years 1964–83 were lower than the ICD-10 rates of the most recent 1984–92 birth cohorts. Similarly, lower rates in the oldest birth cohorts were thought to reflect changes in diagnostic practices and boundaries in Webb *et al.*'s study (1997). Nevertheless, epidemiological studies could be used to assess time trends in two particular instances: (*a*) when repeated surveys, using the same methodology, have been conducted in the same geographical area at different points in time; and (*b*) when large studies have produced specific prevalence rates for successive birth cohorts. In the latter case, increasing rates among the most recent birth cohorts could be interpreted as indicating a secular increase in the incidence of the disorder, provided that alternative explanations can confidently be ruled out.

The surveys conducted in Sweden and in France shed some light on this issue. The Göteborg studies (Gillberg, 1984; Gillberg *et al.* 1991) provided three prevalence estimates that increased over a short period of time from 4·0 (1980) to 6·6 (1984) and 9·5/10 000 (1988), the gradient being even steeper if rates for the urban area alone are considered (4·0, 7·5 and 11·6/ 10 000) (Gillberg *et al.* 1991). However, comparisons of these rates is not straightforward as different age groups were included in each survey. For example, the rate in the first survey for the youngest age group (which resembles more closely the children included in the two other surveys) was 5·1/10 000. Secondly, the increased prevalence in the second survey was explained by improved detection among the mentally retarded, and that of the third survey by cases born to immigrant parents. That the majority of the latter group was born abroad suggests that migration into the area could be a key explanation. Taken in conjunction with a progressive broadening of the definition of autism over time acknowledged by the authors (Gillberg et al. 1991), these findings do not provide solid evidence for an increased incidence in the rate of autism.

The French surveys (studies 17 and 20) derived from much larger sample sizes. In the first study (study 17), prevalence estimates were available for the two birth cohorts of children born in 1972 and 1976 surveyed in 1985–6. The rates were similar (5·1 and 4·9/10000) and not statistically different (Fombonne & du Mazaubrun, 1992). Furthermore, in a subsequent investigation conducted in 1989–90 in exactly the same areas, the age-specific rate of autism for the 1981 birth cohort was slightly lower (3·1/10000) (Rumeau-Rouquette et al. 1994). In any instance, the findings were not suggestive of increasing rates in the most recent cohorts. These findings of a stable prevalence rate were independently replicated in two different ways. First, another survey conducted with the same methodology but in different French regions a few years later (study 20) led to a similar (see Table 4) overall prevalence estimate as compared to the first survey. The latter survey included consecutive birth cohorts from 1976 to 1985, and the age-specific rates showed no upward trend (Fombonne et al. 1997). Secondly, another French survey (study 14) conducted at a different time, in a different area, with a different methodology, also yielded a similar prevalence estimate of 5·1/10000 for DSM-III defined autism among school aged children (Cialdella & Mamelle, 1989). The consistency of estimates from these various surveys and their stability across birth cohorts is impressive. Some weight should be given to these results as they derive from a total target population of 735000 children, 389 of whom had autism (Fombonne et al. 1997). The available epidemiological evidence does not therefore suggest that the incidence of autism has increased, and several other reasons could easily account for an artefactual impression of an increase (Fom-

bonne, 1996). As it stands now, the recent upward trend in rate of prevalence cannot be attributed to an increase in the incidence of the disorder.

Autism and immigrant status

Some investigators have mentioned the possibility that rates of autism might be higher among immigrants (Wing, 1980; Gillberg, 1987; Gillberg et al. 1991, 1995). Five of the 17 children with autism identified in the Camberwell study were from Caribbean origin (study 4; Wing, 1980) and the estimated rate of autism was 6·3/10000 for this group as compared to 4·4/10000 for the rest of the population (Wing, 1993). However, the wide confidence intervals associated with rates from this study (see Table 4) indicate no statistically significant difference. In addition, this area of London had received a large proportion of immigrants from the Caribbean region in the 1960s and, under circumstances where migration flux in and out of an area are happening, estimation of population rates should be viewed with much caution. Yet, Afro-Caribbean children referred from the same area were recently found to have higher rates of autism than referred controls (Goodman & Richards, 1995); however, the sample was again very small ($N = 18$) and differential referral patterns to a tertiary centre also providing services for the local area could not be ruled out. It is worth noting that only one child was born from British-born Afro-Caribbean parents in a recent UK survey (study 21; Webb et al. 1997), providing little support to this particular hypothesis. Similarly, the findings from the Göteborg studies paralleled an increased migration flux in the early 1980s in this area (Gillberg, 1987); they, too, were based on relatively small numbers (19 children from immigrant parents). Taken together, the combined results of these two studies (studies 4 and 16) should be interpreted in the specific methodological context of these investigations. Both studies had low numbers of identified cases, and both groups of authors have relied upon broadened definitions of autism. Unfortunately, other studies have not systematically reported the proportion of immigrant groups in the areas surveyed, with the exception of study 22 where a marginal, non-statistically significant, increase of parents from non-European immigrant origin was reported.

However, in five studies where the proportions of immigrant groups were low (studies 11, 12, 19, 21 and 23), rates of autism were in the upper range of rates. Conversely, in other populations where immigrants contributed substantially to the denominators (studies 14, 17 and 20), rates were in the rather low band. Finally, it is unclear what common mechanism could explain the putative association between immigrant status and autism, since the origins of the immigrant parents (especially in study 16) were very diverse and represented in fact all the continents. With this heterogeneity in mind, it is unclear what common biological features might be shared by these immigrant families and what would be a plausible mechanism explaining the putative association between autism and immigrant status. The hypothesis of an association between immigrant status and autism, therefore, remains largely unsupported by the empirical results.

Autism and social class

Twelve of the 23 studies provided information on the social class of the families of autistic children. Of these, four studies (1, 2, 3 and 5) suggested an association between autism and social class or parental education. The year of data collection for these four investigations was before 1980 (see Table 1), and all eight studies conducted thereafter provided no evidence for the association. Thus, the epidemiological results suggest that the earlier findings were probably due to artefacts in the availability of services and in the case-finding methods, as already shown in other samples (Schopler *et al.* 1979; Wing, 1980; Tsai *et al.* 1982).

DISCUSSION

Epidemiological surveys of autism have been extremely useful in establishing a baseline on the prevalence of this severe developmental disorder and in providing a relatively unbiased picture of its main correlates. Despite the methodological differences across surveys, survey results showed a fair amount of consistency, both for rates and correlates. Rates for the school-age period tended to be higher, reflecting more effective case identification methods at that age, and the median rate in 11 surveys with available estimates for this age group was 5·0/10000. We also

found that about half the surveys were consistent with population values of 5·4–5/10000. Based on these two highly convergent findings, the figure of 5·5/10000 appears to be the most robust estimate for the prevalence of autism currently available. The methodology of epidemiological surveys mentioned in this review is now well established and relies on a multi-stage case finding method. Epidemiological surveys can provide an invaluable starting point for the investigation of developmental disorders in countries where such investigations have not yet been conducted. Their planning and conduct can help to raise the awareness of health professionals and educational authorities about autism and other severe developmental disorders of development. Epidemiological samples may be used in various ways, i.e. to estimate the needs for specialized services or to provide a sampling base to select unbiased samples for case–control studies.

The main features of autism in the surveys included in this review lie in its consistent association with mental retardation in about 80% of the cases, in a clear preponderance of males (with a male/female ratio of 3·8:1), and in its association with some rare and genetically determined medical conditions, such as tuberous sclerosis. No evidence was found, in epidemiologically derived samples, for an association of autism with other disorders such as neurofibromatosis, Down's syndrome, or cerebral palsy. Congenital rubella and phenylketonuria, which were associated with a raised frequency of autistic syndromes 30 years ago, no longer account for more than a handful of cases, since prevention and screening programmes for these disorders have become systematic. The strength of the association between autism and fragile X is not exactly known since molecular biology techniques were not yet available when most of the surveys included in this review were conducted. Recent downward revisions of the actual incidence of fragile X in human populations (Turner *et al.* 1996) leave this issue open to further investigation. Overall, the median value of about 6% for combined rate of medical disorders in autism derived from this review is consistent with the 5% (Tuchman *et al.* 1991) to 10% (Rutter *et al.* 1994) figures available from other investigations and rules out claims of much higher rates deriving from studies relying on a rather different definition (Gillberg & Coleman, 1996).

A majority of surveys has ruled out social class as a risk factor for autism, a result once supported by studies of clinical, i.e. less representative, samples. The putative association of autism with immigrant status is, so far, not borne out by epidemiological studies. Such an association has been reported in studies based on small sample sizes and in which biases due to migration flux were not adequately controlled. Insofar as this question was examined in other surveys, the findings have been negative. The same considerations apply to the issue of secular changes in the incidence of autism. The little evidence that exists does not support this hypothesis but power to detect time trends is seriously limited in the existing datasets.

All surveys identified a larger group of children whose impairments have strong commonalities with those of autism and whose service needs are most certainly not different from those of autistic subjects. On average, we found that the rate ratio for autism and other non-autistic pervasive developmental disorders to that of narrowly defined autism was 2·6. Taking 5·5/10000 as the base-rate for autism, this means that a 8·8/10000 rate for non-autistic pervasive developmental disorders and, consequently, a 14·3/10000 rate for the combination of these disorders with autism, is likely to apply. If the median rate (7·2/10000) of surveys conducted since 1989 is taken as a reference, the corresponding figures would be 11·5/10000 and 18·7/10000. It could well be that, because these surveys were not focusing primarily on the non-autistic group, the actual rate of combined pervasive developmental disorders could be even higher. In addition, these figures do not include Asperger syndrome, which is typically not reflected in current epidemiological estimates for autism. In any instance, these figures carry strong implications for the planning of services, which cannot be overlooked. Future research should focus on this group of other pervasive developmental disorders on which basic descriptive clinical and developmental data are lacking, as well as on some more specific variants of autistic-spectrum disorders such as Asperger syndrome. In planning such epidemiological studies, reliance on current diagnostic methods of interview and observation (such as the Autism Diagnostic Interview (LeCouteur *et al.* 1989) and companion instruments), which have now become standards in clinical practice and research, would enhance comparability across epidemiological surveys and between epidemiological and clinical samples, and would allow for more meaningful differentiation within the group of pervasive developmental disorders.

A review by the author based on a smaller number of studies has also appeared as a chapter, entitled 'Epidemiological surveys of infantile autism', in *Autism and Pervasive Developmental Disorders* (ed. F. Volkmar), pp. 32–62, published by Cambridge University Press (1998) and it is used here with the permission of the publisher.

REFERENCES

Ahlsen, G., Gillberg, C., Lindblom, R., & Gillberg, C. (1994). Tuberous sclerosis in Western Sweden: a population study of cases with early childhood onset. *Archives of Neurology* 51, 76–81.

Aussilloux, C., Collery, F. & Roy, J. (1989). Epidémiologie de l'autisme infantile dans le département de l'Hérault. *Revue Française de Psychiatrie* 7, 24–28.

Bohman, M., Bohman, I. L., Björck, P. O. & Sjöholm, E. (1983). Childhood psychosis in a northern Swedish county: some preliminary findings from an epidemiological survey. In *Epidemiological Approaches in Child Psychiatry* (ed. M. H. Schmidt and H. Remschmidt), pp. 164–173. Georg Thieme Verlag: Stuttgart.

Brask, B. H. (1970). A prevalence investigation of childhood psychoses. In *Nordic Symposium on the Care of Psychotic Children*, pp. 145–153. Barnepsychiatrist Forening, Universitetsforlagets Trykningssentral: Oslo.

Bregman, J. D. & Volkmar, F. R. (1988). Autistic social dysfunction and Down's syndrome. *Journal of the American Academy of Child and Adolescent Psychiatry* 27, 440–441.

Bryson, S. E., Clark, B. S. & Smith, I. M. (1988). First report of a Canadian epidemiological study of autistic syndromes. *Journal of Child Psychology and Psychiatry* 4, 433–445.

Burd, L., Fisher, W. & Kerbeshan, J. (1987). A prevalence study of pervasive developmental disorders in North Dakota. *Journal of the American Academy of Child and Adolescent Psychiatry* 26, 700–703.

Chess, S. (1971). Autism in children with congenital rubella. *Journal of Autism and Childhood Schizophrenia* 1, 33–47.

Chess, S. (1977). Follow-up report on autism in congenital rubella. *Journal of Autism and Childhood Schizophrenia* 7, 69–81.

Cialdella, Ph. & Mamelle, N. (1989). An epidemiological study of infantile autism in a French department. *Journal of Child Psychology and Psychiatry* 30, 165–175.

Deykin, E. Y. & MacMahon, B. (1979). The incidence of seizures among children with autistic symptoms. *American Journal of Psychiatry* 136, 1310–1312.

Ehlers, S. & Gillberg, C. (1993). The epidemiology of Asperger syndrome. A total population study. *Journal of Child Psychology and Psychiatry* 34, 1327–1350.

Fombonne, E. (1996). Is the prevalence of autism increasing? *Journal of Autism and Developmental Disorders* 6, 673–676.

Fombonne, E. (1997). The prevalence of autism and other pervasive developmental disorders in the UK. *Autism* 1, 227–229.

Fombonne, E. (1998). Inflammatory bowel disease and autism. *Lancet* 351, 955.

Fombonne, E. & du Mazaubrun, C. (1992). Prevalence of infantile autism in four French regions. *Social Psychiatry and Psychiatric Epidemiology* 27, 203–210.

Fombonne, E., du Mazaubrun, C., Cans, C. & Grandjean, H. (1997). Autism and associated medical disorders in a large French epidemiological sample. *Journal of the American Academy of Child and Adolescent Psychiatry* **36**, 1561–1569.

Ghaziuddin, M., Tsai, L. & Ghaziuddin, N. (1992). Autism in Downs' syndrome: presentation and diagnosis. *Journal of Intellectual Disability Research* **35**, 449–456.

Gillberg, C. (1984). Infantile autism and other childhood psychoses in a Swedish region: epidemiological aspects. *Journal of Child Psychology and Psychiatry* **25**, 35–43.

Gillberg, C. (1987). Infantile autism in children of immigrant parents. A population-based study from Göteborg, Sweden. *British Journal of Psychiatry* **150**, 856–858.

Gillberg, C. & Coleman, M. (1996). Autism and medical disorders: a review of the literature. *Developmental ˜Medicine and Child Neurology* **38**, 191–202.

Gillberg, C. & Forsell, C. (1984). Childhood psychosis and neurofibromatosis – more than a coincidence. *Journal of Autism and Developmental Disorders* **13**, 1–8.

Gillberg, C., Steffenburg, S. & Schaumann, H. (1991). Is autism more common than ten years ago? *British Journal of Psychiatry* **158**, 403–409.

Gillberg, C., Gillberg, I. C. & Ahlsén, G. (1994). Autistic behaviour and attention deficits in tuberous sclerosis: a population-based study. *Developmental Medicine and Child Neurology* **36**, 50–56.

Gillberg, C., Schaumann, H. & Gillberg, I. C. (1995). Autism in immigrants: children born in Sweden to mothers born in Uganda. *Journal of Intellectual Disability Research* **39**, 141–144.

Goodman, R. & Richards, H. (1995). Child and adolescent psychiatric presentations of second-generation Afro-Caribbeans in Britain. *British Journal of Psychiatry* **167**, 362–369.

Haga, H. & Miyamoya, Y. (1971). A survey on the actual state of so-called autistic children in Kyoto prefecture. *Japanese Journal of Child Psychiatry* **12**, 160–167.

Herder, G. A. (1993). Infantile autism among children in the county of Nordland: prevalence and etiology. *Tidsskrift tarden Norske Laegeforening* **113**, 2247–2249.

Honda, W., Shimizu, Y., Misumi, K., Nimi, M. & Ohashi, Y. (1996). Cumulative incidence and prevalence of childhood autism in children in Japan. *British Journal of Psychiatry* **169**, 228–235.

Hoshino, Y., Yashima, Y., Ishige, K., Tachibana, R., Watanabe, M., Kancki, M., Kumashiro, H., Ueno, B., Takahashi, E. & Furukawa, H. (1982). The epidemiological study of autism in FukushimaKen. *Folia Psychiatrica et Neurologica Japonica* **36**, 115–124.

Howlin, P., Wing, L. & Gould, J. (1995). The recognition of autism in children with Down syndrome. Implications for intervention and some speculations about pathology. *Developmental Medicine and Child Neurology* **37**, 406–414.

Hunt, A. & Lindenmann, R. H. (1984). Tuberous sclerosis: a new estimate of prevalence within the Oxford region. *Journal of Medical Genetics* **21**, 272–277.

Ishii, T. & Takahashi, I. (1983). The epidemiology of autistic children in Toyota, Japan: prevalence. *Japanese Journal of Child and Adolescent Psychiatry* **24**, 311–321.

Knobloch, H. & Pasamanick, B. (1975). Some etiologic and prognostic factors in early infantile autism and psychosis. *Pediatrics* **55**, 182–191.

LeCouteur, A., Rutter, M., Lord, C., Rios, P., Robertson, S., Holdgrafer, M. & MacLennan, J. (1989). Autism Diagnostic Interview: a standardized investigator-based instrument. *Journal of Autism and Developmental Disorders* **19**, 363–387.

Lord, C., Schopler, E. & Revecki, D. (1982). Sex differences in autism. *Journal of Autism and Developmental Disorders* **12**, 317–330.

Lotter, V. (1966). Epidemiology of autistic conditions in young children: I. Prevalence. *Social Psychiatry* **1**, 124–137.

Lotter, V. (1967). Epidemiology of autistic conditions in young children: II. Some characteristics of the parents and children. *Social Psychiatry* **4**, 163–173.

Lotter, V. (1974). Social adjustment and placement of autistic children in Middlesex: a follow-up study. *Journal of Autism and Childhood Schizophrenia* **4**, 11–32.

Lowe, T. L., Tanaka, K., Seashore, M. R., Young, J. G. & Cohen, D. J. (1980). Detection of phenylketonuria in autistic and psychiatric children. *Journal of the American Medical Association* **243**, 126–128.

McCarthy, P., Fitzgerald, M. & Smith, M. A. (1984). Prevalence of childhood autism in Ireland. *Irish Medical Journal* **77**, 129–130.

Magnússon, P. & Sæmundsen, E. (1999). Prevalence of autism in Iceland. *Journal of Autism and Developmental Disorders* (in press).

Matsuishi, T., Shiotsuki, M., Yoshimura, K., Shoji, H., Imuta, F. & Yamashita, F. (1987). High prevalence of infantile autism in Kurume City, Japan. *Journal of Child Neurology* **2**, 268–271.

Mouridsen, S. E., Bachmann-Andersen, L., Sörensen, S. A., Rich, B. & Isager, T. (1992). Neurofibromatosis in infantile autism and other types of childhood psychoses. *Acta Paedopsychiatrica* **55**, 15–18.

Nakai, M. (1971). Epidemiology of autistic children in Gifu-Ken. *Japanese Journal of Child Psychiatry* **12**, 262–266.

Ritvo, E. R., Freeman, B. J., Pingree, C., Mason-Brothers, A., Jorde, L., Jenson, W. R., McMahon, W. M., Petersen, P. B., Mo, A. & Ritvo, A. (1989). The UCLA-University of Utah epidemiologic survey of autism: prevalence. *American Journal of Psychiatry* **146**, 194–199.

Rumeau-Rouquette, C., du Mazaubrun, C., Verrier, A., Mlika, A., Bréart, G., Goujard, J. & Fombonne, E. (1994). *Prévalence des Handicaps: Évolution dans Trois Générations d'enfants 1972, 1976, 1981*. Editions INSERM: Paris.

Rutter, M. (1970). Autistic children: infancy to adulthood. *Seminars in Psychiatry* **2**, 435–450.

Rutter, M., Bailey, A., Bolton, P. & Le Couteur, A. (1994). Autism and known medical conditions: myth and substance. *Journal of Child Psychology and Psychiatry* **35**, 311–322.

Schopler, E., Andrews, C. E. & Strupp, K. (1979). Do autistic children come from upper-middle-class parents? *Journal of Autism and Developmental Disorders* **9**, 139–151.

Shepherd, C. W., Beard, C. M., Gomez, M. R., Kurland, L. T. & Whisnant, J. P. (1991). Tuberous sclerosis complex in Olmsted County, Minnesota, 1950–1989. *Archives of Neurology* **48**, 400–401.

Smalley, S. L., Tanguay, P. E., Smith, M. & Gutierrez, G. (1992). Autism and tuberous sclerosis. *Journal of Autism and Developmental Disorders* **22**, 339–355.

Spitzer, R. L. & Siegel, B. (1990). The DSM-III-R field trial of pervasive developmental disorders. *Journal of the American Academy of Child and Adolescent Psychiatry* **6**, 855–862.

Sponheim, E. & Skjeldal, O. (1998). Autism and related disorders: epidemiological findings in a Norwegian study using ICD-10 diagnostic criteria. *Journal of Autism and Developmental Disorders* **28**, 217–227.

Steffenburg, S. & Gillberg, C. (1986). Autism and autistic-like conditions in Swedish rural and urban areas: a population study. *British Journal of Psychiatry* **149**, 81–87.

Steinhausen, H.-C., Göbel, D., Breinlinger, M. & Wohlloben, B. (1986). A community survey of infantile autism. *Journal of the American Academy of Child Psychiatry* **25**, 186–189.

Sugiyama, T. & Abe, T. (1989). The prevalence of autism in Nagoya, Japan: a total population study. *Journal of Autism and Developmental Disorders* **19**, 87–96.

Tanoue, Y., Oda, S., Asano, F. & Kawashima, K. (1988). Epidemiology of infantile autism in Southern Ibaraki, Japan: Differences in prevalence in birth cohorts. *Journal of Autism and Developmental Disorders* **18**, 155–166.

Treffert, D. A. (1970). Epidemiology of infantile autism. *Archives of General Psychiatry* **22**, 431–438.

Tsai, L., Stewart, M. A., Faust, M. & Shook, S. (1982). Social class distribution of fathers of children enrolled in the Iowa autism program. *Journal of Autism and Developmental Disorders* **12**, 211–221.

Tuchman, R. F., Rapin, I. & Shinnar, S. (1991). Autistic and dysphasic children. II. Epilepsy. *Pediatrics* **88**, 1219–1225.

Turner, G., Webb, T., Wake, S. & Robinson, H. (1996). Prevalence of the fragile X syndrome. *American Journal of Medical Genetics* **64**, 196–197.

Volkmar, F. R. & Nelson, D. S. (1990). Seizure disorders in autism. *Journal of the American Academy of Child and Adolescent Psychiatry* **1**, 127–129.

Volkmar, F. R., Klin, A., Siegel, B., Szatmark, I., Lord, C., Campbell, M., Freeman, B. J., Cicchetti, D. V., Rutter, M., Kline, W., Buitelaar, J., Hattab, Y., Fombonne, E., Fuentes, J., Werry, J., Stone, W., Kerbeshian, J., Hoshino, Y., Bergman, J., Loveland, K., Szymanski, L. & Towbin, X. (1994). Field trial for autistic disorder in DSM-IV. *American Journal of Psychiatry* **151**, 1361–1367.

Wakefield, A., Murch, S., Anthony, A., Linnell, J., Casson, D., Malik, M., Berelowitz, M., Dhillon, A., Thomson, M., Harvey, P., Valentine, A., Davies, S. & Walker-Smith, J. (1998). Ileal-lymphoid-nodular hyperplasia, non-specific colitis, and pervasive developmental disorder in children. *Lancet* **351**, 637–641.

Webb, E. V. J., Lobo, S., Hervas, A., Scourfield, J. & Fraser, W. I. (1997). The changing prevalence of autistic disorder in a Welsh health district. *Developmental Medicine and Child Neurology* **39**, 150–152.

Wignyosumarto, S., Mukhlas, M. & Shirataki, S. (1992). Epidemiological and clinical study of autistic children in Yogyakarta, Indonesia. *Kobe Journal of Medical Sciences* **38**, 1–19.

Wing, L. (1980). Childhood autism and social class: a question of selection? *British Journal of Psychiatry* **137**, 410–417.

Wing, L. (1981). Sex ratios in early childhood autism and related conditions. *Psychiatry Research* **5**, 129–137.

Wing, L. (1993). The definition and prevalence of autism: a review. *European Child and Adolescent Psychiatry* **2**, 61–74.

Wing, L. & Gould, J. (1979). Severe impairments of social interactions and associated abnormalities in children: epidemiology and classification. *Journal of Autism and Developmental Disorders* **9**, 11–29.

Wing, L., Yeates, S., Brierly, L. M. & Gould, J. (1976). The prevalence of early childhood autism: comparison of administrative and epidemiological studies. *Psychological Medicine* **6**, 89–100.

Zahner, G. E. P. & Pauls, D. L. (1987). Epidemiological surveys of infantile autism. In *Handbook of Autism and Pervasive and Developmental Disorders* (ed. D. J. Cohen, A. M. Donnellan and R. Paul), pp. 199–207. Wiley and Sons: New York.

Autistic and Dysphasic Children. II: Epilepsy

Roberto F. Tuchman, MD*; Isabelle Rapin, MD* ‡; and Shlomo Shinnar, MD, PhD* ‡

From the *Saul R. Korey Department of Neurology and the ‡Department of Pediatrics, the Albert Einstein College of Medicine and the Montefiore Medical Center, Bronx, New York

ABSTRACT. In a previously described population of 314 autistic and 237 dysphasic nonautistic children, after exclusion of 12 autistic girls with Rett syndrome, 14% (42 of 302) of autistic children and 8% (19 of 237) of dysphasic children had epilepsy ($P = .03$). The major risk factors for epilepsy were severe mental deficiency and the combination of severe mental deficiency with a motor deficit. In autistic children without severe mental deficiency, motor deficit, associated perinatal or medical disorder, or a positive family history of epilepsy, epilepsy occurred in 6% (10 of 160) which was analogous to the 8% (14 of 168) found in similar dysphasic nonautistic children. The language subtype of verbal auditory agnosia is associated with the highest risk of epilepsy in autistic (41%, 7 of 17) and dysphasic (58%, 7 of 12) children. The higher percentage of epilepsy in autistic girls, 24% (18 of 74) compared with boys 11% (25 of 228) ($P = .003$), is attributed to the increased prevalence of cognitive and motor deficit in girls. Once the risk attributable to associated cognitive and motor disabilities is taken into account, there is no difference in the risk of epilepsy between autistic and nonautistic dysphasic children. *Pediatrics* 1991;88:1219–1225; *autism, dysphasia, epilepsy, seizure, epidemiology.*

Epilepsy is a neurological disorder that is common in autistic children. Since 1960, rates of seizures in autistic children ranging from 11% to 42% have been reported in several publications.[1-11] Autism is a heterogeneous disorder, and the patients in these studies have differed in terms of sex ratio, cognitive deficit, motor deficit, and number and type of other associated medical disorders. These differences may account for the wide range of reported seizure rates.

Recent studies have attempted to address the types of seizures and the risk factors associated with epilepsy in autistic children.[7,11] In a study of 52 autistic children, Olson et al[7] found that all types of epilepsy occurred but "psychomotor epilepsy" and infantile spasms were the most common. They also stated that epilepsy could occur in the absence of mental deficiency, although they felt their numbers were too small for general conclusions. Volkmar and Nelson[11] observed 192 autistic children and found generalized motor seizures to be the most common seizure type. They found that the children without seizures had significantly higher IQ scores than the children with seizures and that only two of the children with seizures had IQ scores of 70 or greater.

The complex relationships between autistic behaviors, language dysfunction, cognitive deficits, associated motor disabilities, and epilepsy are not well understood. The purpose of this study was to determine risk factors associated with epilepsy in autistic and nonautistic dysphasic children and to describe the types of seizures and clinical characteristics of epileptic children within this population.

MATERIALS AND METHODS

All patients in this study were evaluated and diagnosed by one child neurologist whose diagnostic criteria for both autism and dysphasia have been published.[12,13] The diagnostic criteria applied for inclusion in the study were uniform and are described in the companion report.[16] Using this database, we identified and reviewed the records of 551 patients with the diagnosis of autism (n = 314) and dysphasia (n = 237) evaluated from May 1966 through May 1988 (2 patients, one autistic and the other dysphasic, were evaluated in 1960 and 1959, respectively). Children with language disorders

Received for publication Oct 26, 1990; accepted Feb 26, 1991.
Presented in part at the American Epilepsy Society Meeting, Boston, Massachusetts, December 1989.
Reprint requests to (I. R.) Rose F. Kennedy Center for Research in Mental Retardation and Human Development, Room 807, 1410 Pelham Parkway South, Bronx, NY 10461.

without severe mental deficiency who did not meet the criteria for autism were classified as dysphasic. In the autistic group, there were 12 girls who, in addition to meeting the criteria for autism, also met the criteria for Rett syndrome. As seizures are a supportive diagnostic criterion for Rett syndrome and are present in a high percentage of children with this syndrome,[14,15] we have analyzed this group of 12 girls separately. Unless otherwise stated, the data presented in this study exclude the children with Rett syndrome. The remaining 302 autistic and 237 dysphasic nonautistic children form the basis of this study.

Data regarding perinatal history, past medical history, language deficits, social deficits, diagnostic studies, and seizure history were extracted from the medical records and entered into a computer database. A detailed description of the methods and results are presented in the companion report.[16] When analyzing children by language subtypes, all children with severe cognitive deficit or hearing impairment were excluded.

The diagnosis of seizures was made on a clinical basis. Patients were divided into four groups: afebrile unprovoked seizures (epilepsy), febrile seizures only, neonatal seizures only, and questionable seizures. Epilepsy was defined as two or more unprovoked seizures occurring more than 24 hours apart.[17] These four groups were mutually exclusive, and a child with neonatal seizures who continued to have seizures past the neonatal period was categorized as having epilepsy. If a child had episodes of what may or may not have been seizures, he/she was classified as having only questionable seizures.

One of the authors (S. S.), a child neurologist and epileptologist who was blinded to the nonseizure aspects of the patients' history, independently reviewed the charts of all children with unprovoked seizures and assigned them a seizure type based on the International Classification of Seizures.[18] For the purpose of this study, all children with simple partial seizures, complex partial seizures, or partial seizures with secondary generalization were classified as having partial seizures. Children with a history of epileptic myoclonic jerks not characteristic of infantile spasms were classified as having myoclonic seizures. Children with a history of seizures typical for infantile spasms were classified as having infantile spasms.

Data regarding electroencephalographic (EEG) results were obtained from reports available in the medical records. There was considerable variability in the type of EEG (sleep vs no sleep), the number of EEGs performed on an individual child, and the age at which the EEG was performed. Patients who had EEG data were divided into three groups: 1)

normal EEG, 2) abnormal nonepileptiform EEG, and 3) epileptiform EEG (spikes, sharp waves, spike and wave, or hypsarrhythmia).

A statistical package, StatView SE+ Graphics was used for calculation of all P values given.[19] Total χ^2 and significance levels were calculated using 2×2 contingency tables. Kaplan-Meier methodology, which takes into account the variable length of follow-up, was used to determine the cumulative probability of developing epilepsy with age.[20]

RESULTS

Seizures and Epilepsy

There were a total of 47 autistic and 22 dysphasic children with afebrile seizures. Five autistic and 3 dysphasic patients had only one afebrile seizure. After exclusion of these 8 patients, 42 (14%) autistic and 19 (8%) dysphasic children met the criteria for epilepsy ($P = .03$). There were 8 (3%) autistic and 11 (5%) dysphasic children who only had febrile seizures. A history of exclusively neonatal seizures was present in 2 (1%) autistic and 5 (2%) dysphasic children. There were also 24 (8%) autistic and 14 (6%) dysphasic children in whom a seizure disorder was suspected but not confirmed. The results presented below pertain to children with epilepsy (autistic n = 42, dysphasic n = 19).

Cumulative Risk of Developing Epilepsy

The cumulative risk of developing epilepsy by age in the autistic and dysphasic population is shown in Fig 1. The cumulative probability of developing epilepsy by ages 1, 5, and 10 years was .06, .12, and .17, respectively, in the autistic group and .02, .08, and .12, respectively, in the dysphasic group. The risk of developing epilepsy in both groups is higher than one would expect in the general population

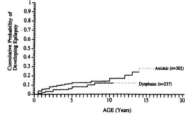

Fig 1. Cumulative risk of epilepsy in autistic and dysphasic children. Kaplan-Meier curves. Dotted line indicates less than 20 patients at risk being followed up at that age.

TABLE 1. Epilepsy and Intelligence

Cognitive Ability	Autistic		Dysphasic	
	n*	Epilepsy, %	n*	Epilepsy, %
Severe mental retardation	77 (16)	30 (19)	‡	‡
Mild/moderate mental retardation	145 (43)	8 (12)	116 (24)	9 (17)
Normal/near normal intelligence	68 (50)	9 (10)	115 (61)	8 (13)

* The numbers in parentheses are patients in whom formal intelligence data are available.
‡ Not applicable.

and remains high at least through the first decade of life.[17]

Risk Factors for Epilepsy

Table 1 shows the percent of children with epilepsy grouped by estimate of intelligence. Within each comparable intelligence subgroup, the rate of epilepsy in the autistic and dysphasic groups was very similar. The cumulative rate of epilepsy in children without severe mental deficiency or significant motor deficit was also very similar (Fig 2). In these subgroups the cumulative probability of developing epilepsy by age 1, 5, and 10 years was .02, .08, and .08 in the autistic population and .02, .08, and .13 in the dysphasic population.

The two major risk factors for epilepsy in the these populations were severe mental deficiency and motor handicap as shown in Fig 3. In the autistic subgroup with severe mental deficiency and motor deficit, the cumulative probability of developing epilepsy at 1, 5, and 10 years was .29, .35, and .67, respectively. In the subgroup with severe mental deficiency but no motor deficit the cumulative probability of developing epilepsy by age 1, 5, and 10 years was .07, .16, and .27, respectively. In the subgroup of autistic children with motor deficit who were not severely retarded the cumulative probability of developing epilepsy by age 1, 5, and 10 years was 0, .12, and .12, respectively. Within comparable subgroups, the rates of epilepsy in the autistic and dysphasic population was very similar (Table 2).

Once severe mental deficiency and motor deficit were taken into account, other risk factors such as a difficult perinatal course, presence of other medical conditions, or a family history of epilepsy did not materially affect the risk of epilepsy in this population. In the group of 188 autistic and 207 dysphasic children without severe mental deficiency or motor handicap, epilepsy occurred in 14 (7%) of the 188 autistic children with one or more of the other risk factors compared with 10 (6%) of the 160 autistic children with no other risk factors. Among the dysphasic children, epilepsy occurred in 17 (8%) of the 207 children with additional risk factors and 14 (8%) of the 168 children with no other risk factors.

Gender

Epilepsy occurred in 24% (18 of 74) of autistic girls as compared with 11% (25 of 228) of autistic boys ($P = .003$). However, in the group of autistic children without severe mental deficiency or motor deficit (150 boys and 38 girls), the percent with epilepsy was similar, 7% in boys and 8% in girls, respectively. There was no correlation between seizures and gender in the dysphasic population in

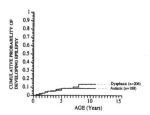

Fig 2. Cumulative risk of epilepsy in autistic and dysphasic children without motor deficit or severe mental deficiency. Kaplan-Meier curves. Dotted line indicates less than 20 patients at risk being followed up at that age.

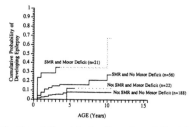

Fig 3. Cumulative risk of epilepsy in autistic children as a function of associated cognitive and motor deficits. Kaplan-Meier curves. Dotted line indicates less than 15 patients being followed up at that age. All groups are mutually exclusive. SMR = severe mental retardation.

TABLE 2. Risk Factors for Epilepsy*

Risk Factors	Autistic		Dysphasic	
	n	Epilepsy, %	n	Epilepsy, %
No motor deficit and not severe MR	188	7	207	8
Motor deficit and not severe MR	21	10	24	8
Severe MR and no motor deficit	56	25	0	‡
Motor deficit and severe MR	21	42	0	‡

* All groups are mutually exclusive. MR = mental retardation.
‡ Not applicable.

which 8% (13 of 168) of boys and 9% (6 of 69) of girls had epilepsy.

Types of Seizures

Figure 4 shows the different types of seizures in autistic and dysphasic children with epilepsy. All types of seizures occurred in both groups, except for myoclonic seizures which did not occur in dysphasic nonautistic children. The seizure types depicted in Figure 4 are not mutually exclusive, and some children had more than one seizure type. In the autistic group 45% (19 of 42) had more than one seizure type compared with 16% (3 of 19) of dysphasic children with epilepsy ($P = .03$).

Autistic children were significantly more likely than dysphasic children to have generalized seizures (74% vs 37%), whereas partial seizures were more common in the dysphasic group (63% vs 26%) ($P = .006$). A history of infantile spasms was present in 12% (5 of 42) autistic patients with epilepsy and in 16% (3 of 19) dysphasic patients with epilepsy. None of the dysphasic patients had myoclonic seizures not related to infantile spasms. A history of myoclonic seizures was present in 26% (11 of 42) epileptic autistic patients. All but two of the autistic patients with myoclonic seizures had other seizure types (generalized tonic-clonic, atypical absence, and atonic).

Electroencephalographic Data

EEG data were available on 60% (181 of 302) of autistic and 36% (85 of 237) of dysphasic children. EEG data were available on 95% (40 of 42) of autistic children with epilepsy and 54% (141 of 260) of autistic children without epilepsy. In the dysphasic group EEG data were available on 100% (19 of 19) of children with epilepsy and 30% (66 of 218) of children without epilepsy. Not surprisingly, patients in whom seizures were suspected were more likely to have had an EEG.

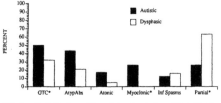

Fig 4. Autistic (n = 42) and dysphasic (n = 19) epileptic children grouped by seizure type. *$P \le .01$. GTC = generalized tonic-clonic; AtypAbs = atypical absence; Inf = infantile.

Of the 40 autistic children with epilepsy who had EEGs 33 (83%) had an abnormal EEG including 30 (75%) with epileptiform and 3 (8%) with nonepileptiform EEG abnormalities. The number of children with specific abnormalities on the EEG is shown in Table 3. In the autistic group with EEG data and without epilepsy (n = 139), 25 (20%) had an abnormal EEG including 11 children (8%) with epileptiform and 14 children (10%) with nonepileptiform EEG abnormalities.

In the dysphasic group with epilepsy with available EEG data (n = 19), 12 children (63%) had an abnormal EEG including 11 (58%) with epileptiform and 1 (5%) with nonepileptiform EEG abnormalities. In the dysphasic group with EEG data who did not have seizures (n = 66), 20% (13 of 66) had an abnormal EEG, including 6 children (9%) with epileptiform and 7 children (11%) with nonepileptiform EEG abnormalities. The proportion of EEG abnormalities and the type of abnormality in children with and without epilepsy were very similar in the autistic and dysphasic groups.

Regression of Language and Behavior and Epilepsy

There were 100 autistic and 11 dysphasic children whose parents reported regression of language and behavior. Epilepsy was present in 24% (20 of 100) of autistic and 36% (4 of 11) of dysphasic patients with regression.

Among autistic children, regression was not a significant risk factor for epilepsy. Epilepsy occurred in 33% of autistic children with severe mental deficiency and regression compared with 30% of children with severe mental deficiency and no history of regression. In the not severely retarded group of autistic children, epilepsy was present in 13% of children with a history of regression versus 6% without a history of regression.

In the dysphasic population there were only 11 children with a history of regression. By definition none of these children was severely retarded. In this group with regression, despite the small sample size, the rate of epilepsy of 38% (4 of 11) was significantly higher than the rate of epilepsy of 6% (14 of 218) in the dysphasic children without regression ($P = .0003$).

Language Subtypes, Regression, Epileptiform EEG, and Epilepsy

Figure 5 illustrates the percentage of autistic and dysphasic children with epilepsy within each language subtype.[21-23] As stated under "Materials and Methods," all children with severe mental deficiency or hearing impairment were excluded from this analysis. The highest rate of epilepsy occurred in children with verbal auditory agnosia. Epilepsy or a history of epilepsy was present in 48% (14 of 29) of 29 children with verbal auditory agnosia (7 of 17 autistic and 7 of 12 dysphasic).

An epileptiform EEG was present in 34% (10 of 29) of children with verbal auditory agnosia (5 of 17 autistic and 5 of 12 dysphasic children). Two children with verbal auditory agnosia (one autistic and one dysphasic) had an epileptiform EEG and regression without seizures. A temporal relationship between the onset of seizures and regression

TABLE 3. Electroencephalographic (EEG) Data in Autistic and Dysphasic Children with Epilepsy*

EEG Findings	Autistic	Dysphasic
Multifocal spikes, generalized spikes, or spike and wave	17	4
Hypsarrhythmia	3	3
Focal spikes	10	4
Total number of epileptiform EEGs	**30**	**11**
Total number of nonepileptiform abnormal EEGs	**3**	**1**
Normal EEGs	7	7
No EEG available	2	0
Total	42	19

* Data were available on 95% (40 of 42) autistic and 100% (19 of 19) dysphasic children with epilepsy.

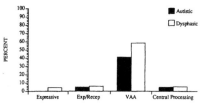

Fig 5. Percentage of children with epilepsy within language subtypes in autistic (n = 197) and dysphasic children (n = 215) whose language subtype could be classified. Exp/Recep = expressive/receptive; VAA, verbal auditory agnosia.

of language occurred in 36% (5 of 14) of children with verbal auditory agnosia and epilepsy (3 of 7 autistic and 2 of 7 dysphasic).

DISCUSSION

In this study, 14% of the autistic and 8% of dysphasic children had epilepsy. Recent studies have reported seizures in 16% to 35% of autistic children studied.[7,8,11,24,25] The major risk factors for epilepsy in this study were severe mental deficiency and the combination of severe mental deficiency with a motor deficit. The combination of severe mental deficiency and motor deficit in autistic patients was associated with epilepsy in 42% of autistic children. A higher rate of epilepsy in retarded autistic children is not unexpected, because these factors are known to be associated with an increased risk of seizures. The rates of epilepsy in autistic children with these handicaps are very similar to the rates of epilepsy found in other studies of children with developmental disabilities selected for the presence of mental deficiency or motor handicap.[26-28] The percentage of autistic children with epilepsy without severe mental deficiency and motor deficit (7%) is also essentially identical with the percentage found in similar dysphasic nonautistic children (8%). This suggests that, in this population, autism in and of itself is not an additional risk factor for developing epilepsy. However, both in autistic and dysphasic children, epilepsy occurs more commonly than one would expect in the general population.[17] This finding is most likely a reflection of the underlying brain dysfunction present in all autistic and dysphasic children.

The rate of epilepsy in autistic girls, even after exclusion of those meeting the diagnostic criteria for Rett syndrome, was significantly higher than in autistic boys. This difference was not found in the dysphasic population. The higher rate of epilepsy in autistic girls is attributed to the increased prevalence of cognitive and motor deficit in girls. Furthermore, epilepsy was present in 58% of autistic girls with severe mental deficiency and motor deficit, which is the same percentage found among the 12 autistic girls with Rett syndrome who were excluded from analysis in this paper. Since, as a group, autistic girls have a higher prevalence of associated disabilities than autistic boys, sex ratios must be taken into account when interpreting studies of epilepsy in autistic children. For example, in Schain and Yannett's study,[1] which found a rate of seizures of 42%, the sex ratio is 1.6:1; it is possible that the high percentage of girls accounts for the unusually high rate of seizures in that study. The importance of knowing the sex ratio applies to neurophysiological studies as well, as shown in a study by Tsai et al[29] in which the only difference found among autistic children with abnormal EEGs was the higher percentage of girls.

Another factor which will affect the observed rates of epilepsy is the length of follow-up. In this study, 79% of autistic and 68% of dysphasic children with epilepsy had their first seizure prior to age 5 years. Several authors have suggested that the risk of epilepsy in autistic children has two peaks, one in infancy and one in adolescence.[5,8,9] Our data do not include a sufficient number of children followed up through adolescence to address this issue fully. Although longer follow-up will provide valuable information on the cumulative rates of epilepsy in this population and may alter the fraction with onset at different ages, it will not affect the major findings of this study regarding the risk factors for epilepsy in autistic children and the comparison with dysphasic youngsters.

A variety of seizure types occurred in both autistic and dysphasic patients. A history of myoclonic seizures or infantile spasms was found in one third of autistic patients with epilepsy. Previous studies also have reported an association between infantile spasms and autism.[7,30,31] Similarly, a high percentage of children with infantile spasms are autistic.[32] What has not been reported previously is the high percentage (16%) of infantile spasms in nonautistic dysphasic children with epilepsy. We also found that autistic children were more likely to have generalized seizures, whereas partial seizures were more common in the dysphasic group. Because the International Classification of Seizures[18] is based on clinical observation, seizures whose partial onset is not witnessed may be classified mistakenly as generalized. Although this is an inherent bias of any classification scheme based on clinical history, it should not affect observed differences between groups. Multiple seizure types were more common in autistic than dysphasic children, and 43% of all autistic children with epilepsy had more than one seizure type.

Reviews of the literature on clinical EEG studies have found that abnormal EEGs have been reported in 13% to 83% of the cases studied.[33,34] In the present study, a very high rate of epileptiform abnormalities in patients with epilepsy was found (71% of autistic and 58% of dysphasic children with EEG data). Furthermore a high rate of epilepsy occurred in children with epileptiform EEG abnormalities (73% of autistic and 65% of dysphasic children). This latter finding was biased by the fact that children with seizures were more likely to get an EEG. Nevertheless, it suggests that in this population an EEG may be helpful in evaluating whether unusual stereotyped behaviors such as staring, eye blinking, or other unusual movements represent seizures or not.

Epilepsy occurred in 48% of children with verbal auditory agnosia. Furthermore, 34% of children with verbal auditory agnosia had an epileptiform EEG, and 36% of children with verbal auditory agnosia had a temporal association between onset of epilepsy and regression of language. The Landau-Kleffner syndrome is a disorder of childhood associated with an epileptiform EEG and an acquired aphasia.[35] Not all children with verbal auditory agnosia have the Landau-Kleffner syndrome; however, the most common type of language disorder in the Landau-Kleffner syndrome is verbal auditory agnosia.[36-38] The question of whether epilepsy causes the dysphasia or whether the epileptiform activity and the dysphasia are consequences of underlying abnormalities of cortical language areas remains in dispute.[39] There is no firm information about the localization of the brain dysfunction responsible for various clinically defined language disorder subtypes. The assumption is that differing clinical subtypes denote the dysfunction of different linguistic operations that engage anatomically distinct brain systems. Direct evidence on localization of brain dysfunction in the language subtypes encountered in autistic and nonautistic dysphasic children is not provided by our data; nonetheless, it is reasonable to hypothesize that the comprehension disorders engage the activity of the temporal cortex, a common source for epileptic activity.[37,40] The highest reported epilepsy occurs in children with the most severe deficit in the comprehension of oral language, those with verbal auditory agnosia.

The large reported variability in the number of autistic children with epilepsy is likely due to differences in associated disabilities among the populations studied.[6-8,11,24,41,42] Once cognitive and motor deficits are taken into account, no other risk factor except language type is associated with an increased risk of epilepsy in autistic children. Furthermore, once the risk attributable to associated cognitive and motor disabilities is taken into account, there is no difference in the risk of epilepsy between autistic and nonautistic dysphasic children.

ACKNOWLEDGMENTS

This work was supported in part by Program Project 20489 (to I. R.) and by a Teacher Investigator Development Award 1 K07 NS00930 and Grant 1RO1 NS26151 (to S. S.) from the National Institute of Neurological Disorders and Stroke.

The authors thank Dr Alfred Spiro for his initial suggestions, Dr Solomon Moshé for reviewing the manuscript and Dr Anne Berg for statistical consultation.

REFERENCES

1. Schain R, Yannet H. Infantile autism. *J Pediatr.* 1960;57:560–567
2. Creak ME. Childhood psychosis. *Br J Psychiatry.* 1963;109:84–89
3. Kolvin I, Ounsted C, Roth M. V. Cerebral dysfunction and childhood psychoses. *Br J Psychiatry.* 1971 ;1 18:407–414
4. Hauser SL, DeLong DR, Rosman NP. Pneumographic findings in infantile autism syndrome. *Brain.* 1975;98:667–688
5. Deykin EY, MacMahon B. The incidence of seizures among children with autistic symptoms. *Am J Psychiatry.* 1979;136:1310–1312
6. Golden GS. Neurological functioning. In: Cohen DJ, Donellan A, eds. *Handbook of Autism and Pervasive Developmental Disorders.* New York: John Wiley; 1987:133–147
7. Olson I, Steffenburg S, Gillberg C. Epilepsy in autism and autisticlike conditions. *Arch Neurol.* 1988;45:666–668
8. Rutter M. Autistic children: infancy to adulthood. *Semin Psychiatry.* 1970;2:435–450
9. Gillberg C, Steffenburg S. Outcome and prognostic factors in infantile autism and similar conditions: a population based study of 46 cases followed through puberty. *J Autism Dev Disord.* 1987:17:273–287
10. White PT, DeMyer W, DeMyer M. EEG abnormalities in early childhood schizophrenia: a double-blind study of psychiatrically disturbed and normal children during promazine sedation. *Am J Psychiatry.* 1964;120:950–958
11. Volkmar FR, Nelson DS. Seizure disorders in autism. *J Am Acad Child Adolesc Psychiatry.* 1990;29:127–129
12. Rapin I. Disorders of higher cerebral function in preschool children: part I. *AJDC.* 1988;142:1119–1124
13. Rapin I. Disorders of higher cerebral function in preschool children: part II. *AJDC.* 1988;142:1178–1182
14. The Rett Syndrome Diagnostic Criteria Work Group. Diagnostic criteria for Rett. *Ann Neurol.* 1988;23:425–428
15. Trevathan E, Naidu S. The clinical recognition and differential diagnosis of Rett syndrome. *J Child Neurol.* 1988;3:S6-S16
16. Tuchman R, Rapin I, Shinnar S. Autistic and dysphasic children, I: clinical characteristics. *Pediatrics.* 1991;88:1211–1218
17. Hauser W, Kurland L. The epidemiology of epilepsy in Rochester, Minnesota, 1935 through 1967. *Epilepsia.* 1975:1–66
18. Commission on Classification and Terminology of the International League Against Epilepsy. Proposal for revised clinical and electroencephalographic classification of epileptic seizures. *Epilepsia.* 1981;22:489–501
19. Feldman SD, Hofmann R, Gagnon J, Simpson J. StatView SE+ Graphics. Berkeley: Abacus Concepts; 1988
20. Kaplan EL, Meier P. Nonparametric estimation from incomplete observations. *J Am Stat Assoc.* 1958;53:457–481
21. Allen DA, Rapin I, Wiznitzer M. Communication disorders of preschool children: the physician's responsibility. *J Dev Behav Pediatr.* 1988;9:164–170
22. Allen D. Developmental language disorders in preschool children: clinical subtypes and syndromes. *Sch Psychol Rev.* 1989;18:442–451
23. Rapin I, Allen DA. Syndromes in developmental dysphasia and adult aphasia. In: Plum F, ed. *Language, Communication, and the Brain.* New York: Raven Press; 1988:57–75
24. Payton JB, Steele MW, Wenger SL, Minshew NJ. The fragile X marker and autism in perspective. *J Am Acad Child Adolesc Psychiatry.* 1989;28:417–421
25. Gillberg C. Infantile autism and other childhood psychoses in a swedish urban region. *J Child Psychol Psychiatry.* 1984;25:35–43
26. Benedetti MD, Shinnar S, Cohen H, et al. Risk factors for epilepsy in children with cerebral palsy and/or mental retardation. *Epilepsia.* 1986;27:614
27. Hauser W, Shinnar S, Cohen H, et al. Clinical predictors of epilepsy among children with cerebral palsy and/or mental retardation. *Neurology.* 1987;37:S150
28. Goulden KJ, Shinnar S, Koller H, et al. Incidence of seizures in the mentally retarded: a cohort study. *Epilepsia.* 1987;28:S623
29. Tsai LY, Tsai MC, August GJ. Brief report: implications of EEG diagnoses in the subclassification of infantile autism. *J Autism Dev Disord.* 1985;15:339–344
30. Taft LT, Cohen HJ. Hypsarrhythmia and infantile autism. *J Autism Child Schizophr.* 1971;1:327–336
31. Gillberg C, Schaumann H. Epilepsy presenting as infantile autism? Two case studies. *Neuropediatrics.* 1983;14:206–212
32. Riikonen R, Amnell G. Psychiatric disorders in children with earlier infantile spasms. *Dev Med Child Neurol.* 1981;23:747–760
33. James AL, Barry RJ. A review of psychophysiology in early onset psychosis. *Schizophr Bull.* 1980;6:506–525
34. DeMyer M, Hingtgen LN, Jackson RK. Infantile autism reviewed: a decade of research. *Schizophr Bull.* 1981;7:388–451
35. Landau WM, Kleffner FR. Syndrome of acquired aphasia with convulsive disorder in children. *Neurology.* 1957;7:523–530
36. Aicardi J. *Epilepsy in Children.* New York: Raven Press; 1986:176–182
37. Rapin I, Mattis S, Rowan JA, Golden G. Verbal auditory agnosia in children. *Dev Med Child Neurol.* 1977;19:192–207
38. Beaumanoir A. The Landau-Kleffner syndrome. In: Roger J, Dravet C, Bureau M, Dreifuss FE, Wolf P, eds. *Epileptic Syndromes in Infancy, Childhood, and Adolescence.* John Libbey Eurotext Ltd: Montrouge, France; 1985:181–191
39. Holmes GL, McKeever M, Saunders Z. Epileptiform activity in aphasia of childhood: An epiphenomenon? *Epilepsia.* 1981;22:631–639
40. Niedermeyer E. Epileptic seizure disorders. In: Niedermeyer E, Lopes da Silva F, eds. *Electroencephalography: Basic Principles, Clinical Applications and Related Fields.* Baltimore, MD: Urban & Schwarzenberg; 1987:405–510
41. Gillberg C, Steffenburg S. Outcome and prognostic factors in infantile autism and similar conditions: a population-based study of 46 cases followed through puberty. *J Autism Dev Disord.* 1987:17:273–287
42. Volkmar F, Cohen DJ. Neurobiologic aspects of autism. *N Engl J Med.* 1988;318:1390–1392

Psychological Medicine, 1995, **25**, 63–77. Copyright © 1995 Cambridge University Press

Autism as a strongly genetic disorder: evidence from a British twin study

A. BAILEY,[1] A. LE COUTEUR, I. GOTTESMAN, P. BOLTON, E. SIMONOFF, E. YUZDA
AND M. RUTTER

From the MRC Child Psychiatry Unit, Institute of Psychiatry, London; and Department of Psychology, University of Virginia, Charlottesville, VA, USA

SYNOPSIS   Two previous epidemiological studies of autistic twins suggested that autism was predominantly genetically determined, although the findings with regard to a broader phenotype of cognitive, and possibly social, abnormalities were contradictory. Obstetric and perinatal hazards were also invoked as environmentally determined aetiological factors. The first British twin sample has been re-examined and a second total population sample of autistic twins recruited. In the combined sample 60% of monozygotic (MZ) pairs were concordant for autism *versus* no dizygotic (DZ) pairs; 92% of MZ pairs were concordant for a broader spectrum of related cognitive or social abnormalities *versus* 10% of DZ pairs. The findings indicate that autism is under a high degree of genetic control and suggest the involvement of multiple genetic loci. Obstetric hazards usually appear to be consequences of genetically influenced abnormal development, rather than independent aetiological factors. Few new cases had possible medical aetiologies, refuting claims that recognized disorders are common aetiological influences.

INTRODUCTION

Autism is a severe neuropsychiatric disorder of children that results in characteristic and persistent social and language abnormalities and repetitive and stereotyped behaviours. The observation of an elevated recurrence risk in siblings (reviewed by Smalley *et al.* 1988) pointed to familial influences and sporadic reports of concordance for autism in monozygotic (MZ) twins suggested these might be genetically mediated. Doubts were expressed about this suggestion, however, and attention was drawn to the need to consider the biological peculiarities of twinning (Hanson & Gottesman, 1976).

The first epidemiological study of same-sex autistic twins (Folstein & Rutter, 1977*a, b*), found a pair-wise concordance rate for autism of 36% among the 11 MZ pairs, whereas none of the 10 dizygotic (DZ) pairs was concordant. Most of the non-autistic MZ cotwins had some form of cognitive impairment, usually involving

[1] Address for correspondence: Dr A. Bailey, MRC Child Psychiatry Unit, Institute of Psychiatry, De Crespigny Park, Denmark Hill, London SE5 8AF.

a speech or language deficit; pair-wise concordance rates for these impairments were 82% in the MZ pairs and 10% in the DZ pairs. Several non-autistic cotwins also showed some kind of emotional or social disability, but it was unclear whether these behaviours were inherited, or temporary reactions to cognitive and communication difficulties. The very different concordance rates for autism in the MZ and DZ twins, taken together with the rarity of the disorder suggested that the liability to autism was predominantly genetically determined (Folstein & Rutter, 1977*a*). It was also hypothesized that the identified cognitive impairments were part of an inherited broader phenotype that could include autism.

In the subsequent Scandinavian twin study (Steffenburg *et al.* 1989), 10 of the 11 MZ pairs (and a set of MZ triplets with Fragile X) were concordant for autism, but the one non-autistic MZ twin had neither cognitive nor social abnormalities. The concordance rate of 91% for both autism and cognitive disorder in MZ twins contrasted with zero concordance for autism and 30% concordance for cognitive disorder in the 10 DZ pairs. Among the three affected DZ

Table 1. *Three areas of dysfunction*

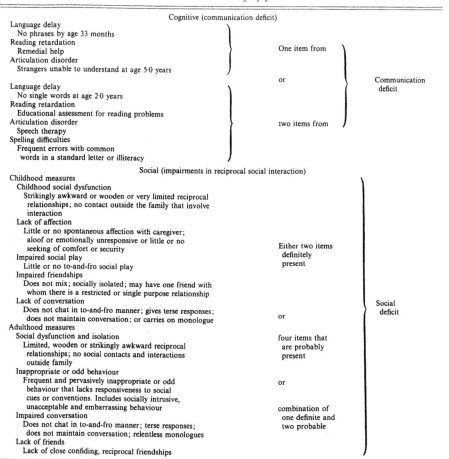

Cognitive (communication deficit)

Language delay
  No phrases by age 33 months
Reading retardation
  Remedial help
Articulation disorder
  Strangers unable to understand at age 5·0 years

One item from

or

Language delay
  No single words at age 2·0 years
Reading retardation
  Educational assessment for reading problems
Articulation disorder
  Speech therapy
Spelling difficulties
  Frequent errors with common
  words in a standard letter or illiteracy

two items from

Communication deficit

Social (impairments in reciprocal social interaction)

Childhood measures
  Childhood social dysfunction
    Strikingly awkward or wooden or very limited reciprocal
    relationships; no contact outside the family that involve
    interaction
  Lack of affection
    Little or no spontaneous affection with caregiver;
    aloof or emotionally unresponsive or little or no
    seeking of comfort or security
  Impaired social play
    Little or no to-and-fro social play
  Impaired friendships
    Does not mix; socially isolated; may have one friend with
    whom there is a restricted or single purpose relationship
  Lack of conversation
    Does not chat in to-and-fro manner; gives terse responses;
    does not maintain conversation; or carries on monologue
Adulthood measures
  Social dysfunction and isolation
    Limited, wooden or strikingly awkward reciprocal
    relationships; no social contacts and interactions
    outside family
  Inappropriate or odd behaviour
    Frequent and pervasively inappropriate or odd
    behaviour that lacks responsiveness to social
    cues or conventions. Includes socially intrusive,
    unacceptable and embarrassing behaviour
  Impaired conversation
    Does not chat in to-and-fro manner; terse responses;
    does not maintain conversation; relentless monologues
  Lack of friends
    Lack of close confiding, reciprocal friendships

Either two items
definitely
present

or

four items that
are probably
present

or

combination of
one definite and
two probable

Social deficit

cotwins, one individual had delayed speech development and two had difficulties in reading and writing; none of the non-autistic twins had severe social difficulties. While these results also pointed to strong genetic effects, the findings in MZ pairs suggested that these may be limited to autism.

In both studies concordance for autism was not attributable to obstetric hazards, but in discordant pairs it was usually the autistic twin who was affected by any obstetric hazards (Folstein & Rutter, 1977*a, b*; Steffenburg *et al.* 1989), or who was biologically disadvantaged compared to the non-autistic cotwin (Folstein & Rutter, 1977*a, b*). Consequently, despite the evidence for strong genetic influences, both groups implicated obstetric hazards as environmentally determined aetiological factors in some pairs; possibly leading to a small excess of autistic twins in the Scandinavian series (Gillberg *et al.* 1990). Moreover, Gillberg (1992) has suggested that only the minority of cases with a

Table 1—*cont.*

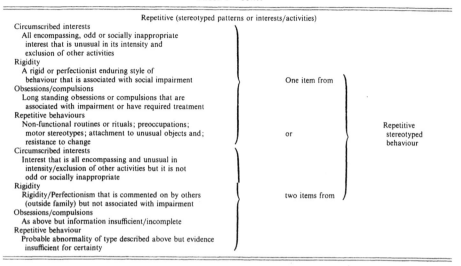

Repetitive (stereotyped patterns or interests/activities)

Circumscribed interests
 All encompassing, odd or socially inappropriate
  interest that is unusual in its intensity and
  exclusion of other activities
Rigidity
 A rigid or perfectionist enduring style of
  behaviour that is associated with social impairment
Obsessions/compulsions
 Long standing obsessions or compulsions that are
  associated with impairment or have required treatment
Repetitive behaviours
 Non-functional routines or rituals; preoccupations;
  motor stereotypes; attachment to unusual objects and;
  resistance to change
Circumscribed interests
 Interest that is all encompassing and unusual in
  intensity/exclusion of other activities but it is not
  odd or socially inappropriate
Rigidity
 Rigidity/Perfectionism that is commented on by others
  (outside family) but not associated with impairment
Obsessions/compulsions
 As above but information insufficient/incomplete
Repetitive behaviour
 Probable abnormality of type described above but evidence
  insufficient for certainty

One item from

or

two items from

Repetitive
stereotyped
behaviour

family history of autism of Asperger's syndrome represent a genetic form of the disorder, the majority being a consequence of obstetric hazards or medical disorders.

The findings from studies of autistic singletons provide support for the hypothesis of a genetically influenced broader phenotype and cast some doubt upon the pathogenicity of obstetric hazards. In the majority of family studies (for reviews see: Bolton & Rutter, 1990; Rutter *et al.* 1993a; Bolton *et al.* 1994) cognitive disorders extending well beyond any current diagnostic concepts of autism were more frequent among the siblings of autistic probands than controls. Bartak *et al.* (1975) also found an elevated rate of speech and language disorders among the parents of autistic probands. With respect to social deficits, three out of 67 siblings in Piven *et al.*'s uncontrolled study (1990) had a severe social disorder, and one out of 33 siblings in Gillberg *et al.*'s (1992) study had Asperger's syndrome; no studies have reported the incidence of less severe disorders. Wolff *et al.* (1988) and Landa *et al.* (1992) both found increased rates of social communication abnormalities in the parents of autistic individuals compared to controls. In summary, studies by several different research groups have found an elevated rate of cognitive and social abnormalities in the first-degree relatives of autistic individuals.

The hypothesis that autism is often a consequence of environmentally determined brain damage secondary to severe obstetric or perinatal hazards is at odds with a number of findings. First, studies of autistic singletons have not found an association with severe obstetric hazards that might cause brain damage. Statistical associations with minor hazards have also varied across studies (Torrey *et al.* 1975; Deykin & MacMahon, 1980). Secondly, the recent post mortem studies of autism have not detected lesions typical of perinatal brain damage (Williams *et al.* 1980; Ritvo *et al.* 1986; Bauman, 1991; Bailey *et al.* 1993a). Because twins are more frequently affected by obstetric hazards than singletons, it is possible that the apparent importance of such hazards may have been overestimated in the two previous twin studies. Finally, at least five studies of autistic singletons have found a higher number of minor congenital anomalies in probands than either siblings or normal controls (reviewed by Smalley *et al.* 1988), this suggests that the early in-utero development of autistic individuals may be suboptimal. These findings raise the possibility that late obstetric hazards may only be consequences of earlier abnormal development.

To resolve these contradictory findings, twin and family studies have been conducted using comparable diagnostic instruments and methods. The original British sample of autistic twins has been followed up and a new sample of twins examined. The outcome at follow-up of the original twin sample, and individual case vignettes are detailed elsewhere (Le Couteur et al. 1995). A companion paper describes the findings of the family genetic study (Bolton et al. 1994).

METHOD

The families included in the twin study of Folstein & Rutter (1977a, b) were recontacted and, when possible, reassessed; otherwise information from the original study was used. A new British twin sample was ascertained in a manner similar to the first. Information was requested from all consultant child psychiatrists; paediatricians interested in developmental and neurological disorders; community paediatricians; heads of district handicap teams; all special schools and units for autistic individuals; the National Autistic Society and two twin registers. Advertisements were also placed in the relevant professional journals. Details were requested on all same-sex pairs, identical and non-identical, in which one or both twins had autism; medical disorders were not exclusion criteria for referral. Case-note review then excluded opposite sex pairs and pairs in which neither twin had autism. Because this was a study of genetic influences upon idiopathic autism, pairs were also excluded in which the proband had a recognizable medical aetiology for a neurological disorder.

Diagnostic information upon participating pairs was obtained by administering the Autism Diagnostic Interview (ADI) (Le Couteur et al. 1989) to parents and/or the current caretaker. This standardized investigator-based interview, of demonstrated validity and reliability, gathers information on behaviours considered central to autism in ICD-10 (World Health Organization, 1992); a diagnostic algorithm allows the diagnosis of autism to be made according to ICD-10 criteria. Twins were also assessed using the Autism Diagnostic Observational Schedule (Lord et al. 1989). Additional information was

obtained from medical and educational authorities' notes. Extensive psychometry was conducted using the following instruments as appropriate: the Wechsler scales (Wechsler, 1974, 1981); Raven's Matrices (Raven & Court, 1982); the Reynell scales (Huntley, 1987); the British Picture Vocabulary Scale (Dunn et al. 1982) and the Merrill-Palmer test (Stutsman, 1931).

All relevant information on each twin was included in a randomly numbered case vignette from which names, exact ages and details of zygosity was removed. Psychiatric and educational diagnoses were made by three researchers using a coding booklet. The diagnosis of autism used in this report was based upon an overall summary coding using ICD-10 guidelines (World Health Organization, 1992). To identify abnormalities outside the ICD-10 diagnosis of autism, individuals were separately rated for impairments in each of the three behavioural domains that together characterize the autistic syndrome: impairments in reciprocal social interaction (social); communication impairments (cognitive); and restrictive, repetitive and stereotyped patterns of interests and activities (repetitive). The coding criteria (Table 1) required behaviour or development to be clearly deviant or markedly delayed and the definitions of impairment were constructed to identify disorders that were pervasive, persistent and/or severe. The communication domain was based on the specific cognitive deficits identified by Folstein & Rutter (1977a, b), the evidence from longitudinal studies for heterotypic continuities between language delay, articulation disorders and reading and spelling difficulties. The social domain tapped functioning in childhood and adulthood including affective reciprocity, social play and friendships. A measure of conversational ability was also included to tap pragmatic abnormalities. The restricted and repetitive interests and activities domain included measures of circumscribed interests, rigidity or perfectionism and obsessions or compulsions. When both childhood and adult functioning could be assessed, the more abnormal item was included in the relevant summary score for the three areas of abnormal functioning, giving a score of two for a severe abnormality and a score of one for a definite abnormality below the severe threshold. The social domain threshold was higher than that used for relatives in the family study (Bolton *et al.* 1994), as more data for coding the broader phenotype in the twins were available from the ADI.

Standardized obstetric and perinatal histories were taken from parents and collated with details from the birth records. If relevant an epilepsy diagnostic interview was administered. A neurodevelopmental examination included: a neurological examination; a search for the stigmata of tuberous sclerosis, neurofibromatosis and the Fragile X syndrome; and the minor congenital anomalies examination of Waldrop & Halverson (1971). Zygosity was determined by typing of nine blood groups. Cytogenetic examination (including Fragile X) and plasma and urine aminoacid chromatography were also performed.

RESULTS

The sample

Two probands from the original study did not meet ICD-10 criteria for autism and are not included in the present analysis. One proband in a discordant DZ pair had atypical autism: a disorder within the pervasive developmental disorder (PDD) grouping but not meeting ICD-10 criteria for autism. The other, in an MZ pair discordant for autism but concordant for cognitive and social disorder, had an onset just after 3 years of age. Both pairs are described elsewhere (Le Couteur *et al.* 1995). One DZ proband had died but the parents and cotwin agreed to take part in the diagnostic reassessment.

Eighteen newly referred pairs were excluded who, on review of case notes, or following discussion with medical staff, or at diagnostic assessment were not considered autistic. Three newly referred pairs with a recognized medical cause of a neurological disorder (trisomy 21, congenital rubella and William's syndrome) were not assessed and were not included in this genetic study.

The pairs from the original study and those subsequently ascertained are shown in Table 2. A female MZ pair from the original sample, concordant for social and cognitive disorder, had Fragile X (Le Couteur *et al.* 1988; Bailey *et al.* 1993*b*). In the new sample one pair of MZ twins had bilateral retinoblastomas; they were concordant for social and cognitive disorder and the non-autistic twin had an IQ in the normal range. Another newly referred MZ pair had infantile spasms without tuberous sclerosis; they were also concordant for social and cognitive disorder but the non-autistic cotwin had mild mental handicap. These two new pairs were assessed because the nature of the relationship between their medical disorders and autism is uncertain. All three assessed pairs with medical disorders have been conservatively excluded from the analysis that follows. Except in these three pairs, no clinical, chromosomal or biochemical evidence of abnormalities of aetiological significance were detected (both members of a discordant DZ pair had heterozygous cystinuria). Forty-four sets of twins and triplets were available for genetic analysis and these contained 59 autistic individuals.

The ratio of females to males in the sample was 1 to 3·4, 31% of tested autistic individuals had a non-verbal IQ within the normal range, while 36·4% had a non-verbal IQ less than 50. Verbal IQ was in the normal range in 19% of individuals and less than 30 in 65·5%. Performance and verbal IQ were both in the normal range in 17·9% of individuals. None of the non-autistic cotwins on whom psychometric data were available had a performance IQ outside the normal range. Nineteen autistic individuals (32·2%) in 15 pairs (34%) had epilepsy, but no non-autistic cotwin was affected. With one exception, affected individuals had a verbal IQ less than 30 and a performance IQ less than 70.

Follow-up of the original pairs

All 7 of the non-autistic DZ cotwins from the original sample on whom complete information was available had confiding social relationships, lived independently and were in education or stable employment. Only 1 of the 5 non-autistic MZ cotwins lived independently (his marriage was the only instance of a confiding relationship in an MZ cotwin), and only 2 were in stable employment (Le Couteur *et al.* 1995). None of the 5 MZ cotwins had been diagnosed as autistic in childhood and only 1 had an autistic-like disorder. Their social difficulties were similar to those seen in autism but of lesser degree and these had sometimes become more obvious with development. Their childhood cognitive difficulties were predominantly with language, and these were clinically less apparent in adulthood.

Table 2. *Pairs included in the study*

	Male		Female	
	MZ	DZ	MZ	DZ
Original sample	8	6*	2*†	3
New sample	13	7	4‡§	4¶

* Two probands from the original study do not meet ICD-10 criteria for autism and have been excluded.

† A pair concordant for social and cognitive disorder had the Fragile X anomaly.

‡ Includes two sets of triplets (concordant for autism); one triplet died in the neonatal period.

§ Includes a pair concordant for bilateral retinoblastomas and a pair concordant for hypsarrythmia; both pairs were concordant for social and cognitive disorder.

¶ One discordant pair was never seen; information from the referrer and telephone interview with the mother confirmed zygosity, the probands diagnosis, and, lack of social and cognitive difficulties in the co-twin.

Table 3. *Pair-wise concordance by zygosity*

Concordance	MZ pairs N = 25*† %	DZ pairs N = 20 %
Autism	60‡	0
Social or cognitive disorder	92	10
Social and cognitive disorder	76	0
Social disorder only	12	0
Cognitive disorder only	4	10
Neither social or cognitive disorder	8	90

* The three pairs affected by Fragile X, retinoblastoma and hypsarrhythmia are excluded from this and subsequent analyses.

† The surviving set of concordant triplets are conservatively treated as two rather than three concordant pairs.

‡ Proband-wise concordance rate = 73 %. Both twins were probands in 12 MZ pairs.

Concordance rates

The pair-wise concordance rates for autism in the new sample were 69 % in MZ pairs and 0 % in DZ pairs (as compared with 36 % and 0 % respectively in the original sample); while concordance for cognitive deficits was 88 % in MZ pairs and 9 % in DZ pairs (as compared with 82 % and 10 % in the original sample). Because the findings for the original and new samples were broadly similar, the data have been combined (Table 3). A broader phenotype of specific cognitive and social abnormalities, alone or in combination, was again identified in the new sample. Repetitive behaviours were only found in combination with social or cognitive difficulties. Three non-autistic MZ cotwins met ICD-10 (World Health Organization, 1992) diagnostic criteria for PDD. None of the non-

Table 4. *Summary of biological hazards and differences in discordant pairs*

Autistic twin	Non-autistic twin
MZ pairs	
*Multiple congenital anomalies	—
*Neonatal convulsions	—
†RDS + cardiac arrest	RDS
†Delay second birth	—
†540 grams lighter	—
DZ pairs	
*Severe haemolytic disease + apnoea	Delay second birth
*Severe haemolytic disease + apnoea	Mild haemolytic disease
*Delay second birth	—
*Delay second birth	—
*Delay second birth	—
†Multiple congenital anomalies	—
†RDS	—
—	†RDS
*840 grams lighter	—
*820 grams lighter	—
*800 grams lighter	—
*530 grams lighter	—
—	†800 grams lighter

* Old sample. † New sample. RDS = Respiratory distress syndrome.

autistic MZ cotwins had isolated mental handicap, and most cognitively affected MZ cotwins had substantial social difficulties (Table 3). These findings suggest that the genetic liability is for the development of specific cognitive and social abnormalities, with autism as the most severe phenotype.

Heritability

The heritability of the liability to autism can be estimated using a multifactorial threshold model (Falconer, 1965). The proband-wise concordance rate for autism in MZ pairs was 73 %. Because no concordant DZ pairs were ascertained during the time course of the study, the 2·9 % rate of autism among the siblings of autistic singletons in the accompanying family genetic study was used (Bolton et al. 1994); equivalent to a proband-wise rate of 5·8 % (assuming all affected individuals are probands). Prevalence estimates of autism vary widely depending upon the method and stringency of ascertainment. For this reason the calculations were performed using both the Department of Education's administrative prevalence rate of

1·75 in 10000 (cited in Wing *et al.* 1976) and the figure of 10 in 10000 suggested by Gillberg *et al.* (1991). Tetrachoric correlations were calculated from the proband-wise concordance rates using the Reich correction to the Falconer formula (Reich *et al.* 1972). The tetrachoric correlations for the MZ twins were 0·983 (S.E. 0·08) and 0·978 (S.E. 0·09) using the base rates of 1·75 and 10 in 10000 respectively. The tetrachoric correlations for the DZ pairs were 0·512 and 0·545 for the 1·75 and 10 in 10000 base rates. Standard errors for DZ correlations could not be calculated as no concordant pairs were ascertained. Cases continued to be collected, however, after the new sample was closed and the next DZ pair seen was concordant for autism. If this one concordant pair was included the standard errors would be 0·14 and 0·13 respectively. Structural equation modelling (Bentler, 1989) was used to calculate the heritability of the liability to autism using the twin correlations. The estimates of broad heritability were 93% and 91% for the base rates of 1·75 and 10 in 10000.

Obstetric and developmental data

In the combined sample there were no very low birthweight infants (< 1500 grams) and the average gestational age of both MZ and DZ pairs was 36 weeks. The mean age of mothers of both MZ (30·6 years) and DZ (30·6 years) twins born in England or Wales on whom data were available (39 pairs) was elevated: 39% were less than 30; 33% were between 30 and 34; and 28% were 35 or above. These rates show a significant and progressive increase with age (test of trend: *P* < 0·001) when compared with the corresponding figures of 65%, 22% and 13%[1]† for the mothers of all twins born over the same time period. The social class distribution of the fathers of the English families (41 pairs) was not significantly different from that of the general population.[2]

The role of obstetric and perinatal factors has been examined in a similar manner to that in the original study. Folstein & Rutter (1977*a*, *b*) identified pairs in which individuals experienced a biological hazard that might be associated with brain injury. In pairs in which severe hazards did not differentiate between the twins, any substantial biological differences between the twins were noted. When both twins were

† The notes will be found on p. 75.

affected by a severe hazard, biological differences were based upon evidence that one twin was more severely affected. In twins unaffected by hazards, biological differences were conceptualized as indexing possible biological disadvantage in one twin.

In the combined sample, twins with any of the following biological hazards were identified: severe haemolytic disease; multiple congenital anomalies; Respiratory Distress Syndrome (RDS); neonatal convulsions; second birth delayed by at least 30 min; and perinatal apnoea greater than 6 min. In only two MZ pairs concordant for autism were both individuals affected by a severe hazard (RDS in both pairs). The sister of one pair was also autistic but she was unaffected by RDS, suggesting that RDS was probably not an aetiological factor in this pair. As in the previous studies, concordance for autism was not attributable to the possible environmental causes of brain damage that were examined.

Turning to the 29 discordant pairs on whom systematic data were available, only the autistic twin was affected by a biological hazard in 8 pairs; both twins were affected in 3 pairs; and only the non-autistic twin was affected in one pair (Table 4). In discordant pairs not differentiated by possible biological hazards, biological differences between the twins were identified: more severe haemolytic disease with apnoea; more severe RDS with cardiac arrest; a birth weight difference of at least 500 grams. The autistic twin was disadvantaged in 8 pairs and the non-autistic twin in 1 pair (Table 4). In summary, in pairs discordant for autism any hazards usually affected the autistic individual, who was also usually disadvantaged when within-pair biological differences were examined. These data replicate those reported by Folstein & Rutter (1977*a*, *b*) and Steffenburg *et al.* (1989) and by themselves appear to suggest that some cases of autism might have been environmentally determined. A number of findings suggest, however, that biological hazards and differences might have been consequences of the processes leading to autism.

First, Gillberg *et al.* (1990) have argued that if obstetric complications were merely consequences of foetal abnormality, then they should be associated with autism *per se* and not just with autism in discordant pairs. Although obstetric

Table 5. *Within pairs comparison of minor congenital anomaly scores in pairs discordant for autism affected by biological hazards or differences*

	Autistic twin higher	Non-autistic twin higher	Identical scores	Missing data
Number of pairs	12*	0	2	4

* Also includes the two discordant pairs in which only the non-autistic twin was affected by a hazard or difference (RDS and birth weight difference).

hazards were found in both members of only two pairs concordant for autism, a hazard in one twin or a biological difference between the twins was found in a further 5 of the remaining 12 concordant sets (RDS; neonatal convulsion; two delays in second birth; weight difference). This compares with a hazard or difference affecting the autistic twin in 5 of 10 discordant MZ pairs and 11 of the 19 DZ pairs on whom information was available (Table 4). It appears that hazards and differences affected a similar proportion of both concordant and discordant pairs. Moreover, hazards that affected only one member of a concordant pair are unlikely to be aetiological factors for autism. Secondly, although both previous twin studies suggested that biological impairments were usually peri-natal events, in the combined sample many individuals were affected by adversities occurring earlier in gestation, such as congenital anomalies and substantial weight differences within pairs (Table 4).

Finally, if obstetric hazards affect develop-mentally abnormal foetuses, then minor con-genital anomalies might differentiate between autistic and non-autistic cotwins. The calculated minor congenital anomaly score was based upon the scale of Waldrop & Halverson (1971). Adult norms are not available for head circumference or interpupillary and intercanthal distances, so these data were excluded from the total score. The neurodevelopmental examination did, how-ever, include assessment of congenital ptosis, malocclusion and joint hyperextensibility, and these ratings were included in the scoring scheme. In the discordant pairs affected by a hazard or difference (Table 4), most examined autistic individuals had a higher minor congenital

anomaly score than their non-autistic cotwin (Table 5); no non-autistic twin had a higher score (binomial test $P = 0.0005$). As such anoma-lies arise relatively early in gestation (Smith & Jones, 1988), it appears that perinatal or neonatal hazards and differences did not occur randomly, but usually affected the individual whose development was apparently less optimal. Considering all the discordant pairs on whom data were available, the autistic twin had the higher score in 17 pairs; the non-autistic twin in 5 pairs (binomial test $P = 0.017$); and the scores were equal in 5 pairs. Four of the 5 non-autistic twins with higher scores were affected by the broader phenotype. In all pairs for whom systematic data were available, the highest anomaly score within each pair correlated -0.29 with gestational age ($P = 0.039$). Taken together, the concordance, obstetric and minor congenital anomaly data indicate that autism is unlikely to have been the consequence of perinatal or neonatal hazards, but that events that occur relatively early in gestation might influence phenotypic outcome.

The congenital anomaly score provided a relatively strong means of differentiating indi-viduals within discordant pairs; however, within pairs concordant for autism, the minor con-genital anomaly scores were more often dis-similar than identical. There were also differences between the two types of twin: the mean score of MZ autistic individuals was 1·7 compared to a score of 3·5 in DZ autistic individuals (t test on square roots of scores: $P = 0.003$). The mean score of MZ autistic individuals in discordant pairs was 1·1 *versus* 2·0 in concordant pairs ($P = 0.066$). The mean score of non-autistic individu-als was 1·5 in both types of twin.

The head circumference data were examined separately for individuals under 16 years of age. Nine of the 21 (42%) autistic individuals under 16 years of age had a head circumference greater than the 97th centile; eight of these individuals were male. None of the 11 non-autistic subjects had a head circumference of this magnitude. Although three of the individuals with macro-cephaly also had a height equal to or greater than the 97th centile, the finding of macro-cephaly was investigated further because of postmortem evidence of an association between megalencephaly and autism (Bailey *et al.* 1993*a*). Head circumferences appear to have increased since the normative data were collected, raising the possibility that the findings were the consequence of a secular trend. The male autistic twins were compared with a Caucasian sample of normal volunteer twins examined by Dr J. Buckler 5–7 years ago. Only 9% of the 120 normal male individuals under the age of 16 had a head circumference greater than the 97th centile compared to 38·9% of the male Caucasian autistic twins (exact test $P = 0·003$). It was also possible that the 9 individuals with enlarged heads had hydrocephalus. CT or MRI scans had been performed on 6 of these individuals, only one of whom was found to have moderately dilated ventricles.

As the number of individuals under 16 was small, the head circumference measurements of individuals age 16 and over were converted to percentiles using recent data taking account of adult height (Bushby *et al.* 1992). Among the 45 Caucasian autistic individuals of all ages on whom data were available, 12 (26·6%) had a head circumference above the 97th centile (none of the affected older subjects had a height greater than the 97th percentile); no non-autistic twin was similarly affected.

During the study some autistic individuals were observed to have an unusually broad nasal bridge or root. Photographs of the majority of twins were reviewed to ascertain the frequency of dysmorphic facial features not included in the Waldrop & Halverson scale (1971); this was done without reference to the other neurodevelopmental data. Broad nasal bridges or roots were observed in autistic individuals from 12 pairs, sometimes in association with increased interpupillary distance. A number of other dysmorphic facial features were also observed; the most frequent were synophrys (meeting of the eyebrows in the midline) and medial flare of the eyebrows (Smith & Jones, 1988), one or both were observed in autistic individuals from 10 pairs.

DISCUSSION

Nature of the sample

Before discussing the implications of these findings it is necessary to consider whether the probands in the twin sample were representative of autistic individuals in general. The sex ratio and psychometric findings are closely compar-

able with those in singletons (Smalley *et al.* 1988) as is the rate of epilepsy (Rutter, 1970; Gillberg & Steffenburg, 1987). The 0% rate of autism in DZ cotwins is also comparable with the rates of 2·9% (Bolton *et al.* 1994) and 3% (Smalley *et al.* 1988) reported in the siblings of autistic singletons. If the subsequently ascertained DZ pair concordant for autism is included, the rate of autism amongst DZ cotwins is 4·8%. In summary, the sample appears similar to singleton samples in terms of sex ratio, IQ distribution, the rate of epilepsy and the rate of autism in siblings.

A possible excess of autistic twin pairs was found in Sweden (Gillberg *et al.* 1990) and the expected number of pairs has been calculated for England and Wales. As probands had to be recognized as autistic by clinics and schools, the administrative prevalence figure of 1·75 per 10000 obtained by the Department of Education (Wing *et al.* 1976) is probably most appropriate (although the true prevalence rate may be higher; see: Wing *et al.* 1976). The total number of individuals in same sex DZ and MZ pairs was estimated assuming that the number of same sex DZ pairs equalled the number of opposite sex DZ pairs (the twins were born between 1952 and 1984 and the ratio of same sex MZ to DZ twins born during the time was approximately one, i.e. $1:1·03^3$). The number of autistic individuals surviving the first year can be estimated from the population data for live twin births[3] and infant mortality. When recorded, the infant death rate for liveborn twins was approximately 4 times the singleton rate,[4] and this factor was applied for years in which infant deaths in live multiple births were not recorded. The expected number of affected DZ individuals born in England and Wales (the prevalence rate × total number of surviving individuals in same sex DZ pairs) was 25. Assuming a concordance rate for autism of 3%, these individuals should occur in 25 pairs (Rutter *et al.* 1993*b*), whereas 20 DZ pairs were ascertained. The expected number of autistic individuals in MZ pairs was 24. Assuming a 60% concordance rate for autism, these 24 individuals should have been identified in 17 pairs (7 concordant and 10 discordant); 23 MZ pairs were in fact ascertained. The sample also contained two sets of female triplets concordant for autism (an individual in one set had died in the neonatal period). From 1952 to 1984 only

1315 same sex triplets were born, including stillbirths,[3] this suggests that no triplets with autism should have been identified.

If the finding of a possible small excess of MZ sets is not the result of ascertainment bias, would it affect the interpretation of the con- cordance rates? Any possible excess of MZ pairs is small, and because of the very low concordance rate for autism in DZ pairs, even a substantial reduction in the MZ rates would not alter the conclusion of strong genetic influences. Although MZ twinning is associated with an increased rate of congenital malformations (Little & Bryan, 1988), twins are usually dis- cordant for such abnormalities, which suggests that concordance for autism is unlikely to be attributable to MZ twinning.

Genetic factors

The findings from this study replicate the previous observations of substantial differences between the concordance rates for autism in MZ and DZ twins. In none of the three studies has concordance for autism been attributable to obstetric hazards, which suggests that the find- ings are a consequence of genetic influences. Although the magnitude of the difference be- tween the concordance rates in the two types of twin suggests that autism is unlikely to be a Mendelian disorder, the liability to autism appears to be largely genetically determined. This conclusion is unaffected by either the exclusion from the genetic analysis of the three pairs with medical disorders, or the rather different concordance rates for autism in MZ twins in the different studies. This is because autism is a rare disorder and the concordance rate in·DZ twins has always been very low. Consequently even modest concordance rates in MZ twins indicate the action of substantial genetic influences.

The findings from the Scandinavian study (Steffenburg et al. 1989) suggested that the genetic liability was usually manifest as autism; whereas variable expression was observed among the MZ cotwins in the British study (Folstein & Rutter 1977a, b). The findings from this study confirm that phenotypic expression is not confined to autism. At follow-up the MZ cotwins from the original sample had con- siderable social difficulties, and both cognitive and social difficulties were identified in the new

non-autistic cotwins. The finding that over 90% of MZ pairs were concordant for a broader phenotype of social and/or cognitive difficulties supports the conclusion of substantial genetic influences and suggests that these apply to most cases.

How may the differences between the twin studies have arisen? Diagnostic practice in the British study may have been unusual; others may have considered that the probands in discordant pairs were not affected by autism, or, they may have concluded that the non-autistic cotwins were in fact autistic. While differences in diagnostic practice do exist, they seem unlikely to account for the findings reported here. Probands were all referred with a diagnosis of autism, and the majority received specialist services for autistic individuals. The diagnosis was confirmed using both blindly coded interviews and the diagnostic algorithm for the ADI (Le Couteur et al. 1995). By contrast, the non- autistic cotwins were a heterogenous group. The three most severely affected individuals had PDD; they fulfilled ADI algorithm criteria in some but not all areas of functioning (Le Couteur et al. 1995). The more mildly affected individuals had a variety of difficulties, but in no case had the diagnosis of autism ever been raised. With the exception of cases with PDD, it is unlikely that any clinician would diagnose autism as defined by either ICD-10 or DSM-III-R criteria.

An alternative explanation for the difference in findings between the studies is referral bias. The tendency for the referral of concordant pairs may have been exacerbated by the Scandi- navian group accepting cases from five countries. Referral bias seems a more plausible explanation for the differences between the studies as the Scandinavian group did identify cognitive ab- normalities in 30% of non-autistic DZ cotwins, and Bolton et al. (1994) identified social and cognitive abnormalities among the siblings of singleton autistic probands. Social and cognitive abnormalities have also been found among the parents of the twin and singleton probands (Bailey et al. 1993c; Bolton et al. 1994). Taken together, the findings from the current and previous studies suggest that genetic influences may give rise to a phenotype considerably broader than autism as traditionally diagnosed. Of course the notion of an autistic spectrum has been frequently advocated (Wing & Attwood,

1987) and many of the non-autistic MZ cotwins would fall within such a grouping. The degree of aetiological and pathological heterogeneity within such a spectrum is unknown, however, and it remains to be determined whether all affected individuals have a disorder genetically related to autism.

The possibility that the genetic influences in autism apply to mental handicap, rather than to autism *per se* (Baird & August, 1985), is not supported by this study. Mental handicap only occurred in association with autism, and none of the non-autistic cotwins affected by the broader phenotype had a performance IQ outside the normal range, although some of their autistic cotwins were profoundly retarded.

The concordance findings from the various twin studies suggest that autism is a very strongly genetic neuropsychiatric disorder. Whether autism unassociated with medical conditions is a single or heterogeneous genetic disorder is unknown, although the findings for other medical disorders suggest that heterogeneity is likely. Consequently any conclusions about the nature of the genetic mechanisms are tentative. The large difference between the concordance rates for autism in MZ and DZ twins suggests that autism is probably a complex genetic trait involving more than one genetic locus (Risch, 1990). Furthermore, the relative risk for autism in either DZ cotwins or siblings is much larger than expected under any Mendelian model, but similar to that predicted by a multifactorial model (Emery, 1986). Support for a multilocus model comes from the accompanying family genetic study (Bolton *et al.* 1994), in which the rate of disorder in relatives was related to the severity of disorder in the probands.

If the genetic liability to autism is influenced by multiple genes, are these multiple genes of equal effect (an additive multilocus model characterized by no interlocus interaction), or are a specific combination of genes required (a multiplicative multilocus model representing epistasis)? The large difference between the relative risks for autism in MZ and DZ cotwins supports an epistatic model (Risch, 1990). Although the multifactorial model assumes a substantial number of genes, each of small effect, autism may be determined by a relatively small number of genes; an oligogenic mode of inheritance.

Gillberg (1992) has argued that genetic factors only operate in a minority of cases and that various medical disorders are frequent causes of autism. In the Scandinavian epidemiological twin study, the Fragile X anomaly was the only medical aetiology detected. This anomaly was detected in only one pair in this study (Le Couteur *et al.* 1988; Bailey *et al.* 1993*b*) and only two other pairs were excluded from the genetic analysis: one with bilateral retinoblastomas, the other with infantile spasms. Even if the three referred pairs with neurological disorders had also met ICD-10 diagnostic criteria for autism, possible medical aetiologies would account for only a small proportion of ascertained pairs. Of course some twins with autism may not have been recognized because they were only classified under the diagnosis of a medical disorder. The association between autism and medical disorders appears strongest in the most profoundly handicapped (Rutter *et al.* 1994) – the group in which diagnosis is most difficult – and in those with atypical autism. Nevertheless, a literature review (Rutter *et al.* 1994) does not support claims of a frequent association between autism and specific disorders. On balance it seems that genetic influences apply to the vast majority of cases; a conclusion supported by the lack of clustering of affected relatives in the accompanying family genetic study (Bolton *et al.* 1994).

Obstetric and developmental factors

The previous twin studies suggested that severe perinatal hazards may be environmental factors that convert an inherited broader phenotype into autism. Several findings suggest this conclusion should be reconsidered. First, although the concordance rates for autism in MZ pairs have varied, the findings in DZ pairs have been consistent. No concordant DZ pairs were ascertained in the previous studies, and only one pair was ascertained immediately after the close of the current study. Combining the DZ pairs in the Scandinavian and British studies, and including the recently ascertained concordant pair, the concordance rate in DZ pairs is 3·2%; virtually identical to the rate of autism in the siblings of autistic singletons (Bolton *et al.* 1994; Smalley *et al.* 1988). As twins suffer more obstetric difficulties than singletons, such factors seem unlikely to be aetiological factors. Furthermore, obstetric hazards did not account for concordance for autism, and possible hazards and differences affected autistic individuals in both concordant and discordant pairs. It seems that hazards and differences may be consequences of the processes leading to autism, rather than their cause.

This interpretation is supported by an examination of the nature of the obstetric hazards and differences and the minor congenital anomaly data. Although some potential causes of brain damages, such as RDS and delay in the second birth, are perinatal events, the minor congenital anomaly data suggested these hazards had been preceded by earlier suboptimal development. Consequently such hazards may be the result of foetal abnormalities that either precipitate premature labour or result in poor orientation in the birth canal; a conclusion supported by the correlation between the anomaly score and gestational age. Other hazards and differences, such as multiple congenital anomalies and substantial weight differences between cotwins, directly index early suboptimal development. Of course late hazards may not be consequences of early suboptimal development, but either manifestations of the continuing action of early adverse environmental factors, or de novo environmental aetiological factors. Such an argument is not supported by the findings from the family genetic study (Bolton et al. 1994), in which family loading for autism and the broader phenotype was related to a measure of obstetric suboptimality in the proband.

The minor congenital anomaly score discriminated best in pairs affected by hazards or differences, perhaps partially reflecting the fact that some hazards and differences probably arose early in gestation. The less adequate differentiation between autistic and non-autistic individuals within MZ than DZ pairs might be a consequence of the lower average score in MZ twins and a possible genetic contribution to some minor anomalies. While the difference between the mean minor congenital anomaly scores in MZ and DZ twins could reflect different intrauterine events in the two types of twin, the magnitude of the difference was small and a more extensive study of anomalies is needed before firm conclusions can be drawn.

Minor anomalies are most common in areas of complex and variable features, such as the face, auricles, hands and feet. Facial development is largely complete by 14 weeks gestation – although features such as mid-eyebrow patterning are influenced by the growth and form of underlying facial structures up to 16 weeks (Smith & Jones, 1988) – suggesting that some aspects of the abnormal development culminating in autism are manifest by this time. The observation of specific subtle mid-facial anomalies in some probands may, if replicated by others, provide clues as to the nature of some of the abnormal processes.

If phenotypic expression is possibly partly determined early in gestation, by what mechanisms does this arise? Variable phenotypic expression may simply be a consequence of the many non-deterministic processes occurring during the development of the nervous system (Goodman, 1991), sometimes called 'intangible variation' (Falconer, 1981). Phenotypic variability could also be the consequence of environmental factors that by themselves do not cause brain damage or autism, but which adversely affect brain development in combination with specific genetic influences. There may be many such environmental factors and some may be difficult to identify; elevated maternal age and MZ twinning are possible relevant factors.

Maternal age was significantly higher in the autistic twin sample than in the comparable total twin population. In the Scandinavian study, 9 of the 20 pairs were also born to mothers outside the age range 20–30, although it is not clear whether these were old or young mothers (Steffenburg et al. 1989). As the nature of the British sample resembles that of singleton samples, elevated maternal age is probably not a consequence of referral bias. Maternal age was similarly elevated in both MZ and DZ pairs, this suggests that the underlying mechanisms are more powerful than those that normally determine that the mothers of DZ twins are on average older than those of MZ twins (see for instance MacGillivray et al. 1988). Elevated maternal age has been reported in some (Finegan & Quarrington, 1979; Gillberg, 1980) but not all singleton samples. Links et al. (1980) also reported a correlation between maternal age and the minor congenital anomaly score, but there was no relationship in this study.

Elevated maternal age does not appear to be

a consequence of a social class bias in the twin sample, neither did mothers usually delay starting their families while gaining higher educational qualifications. In some cases marriage appeared delayed as a consequence of the mother's social behaviour (details upon first-degree relatives will be provided in a subsequent paper). Consequently, elevated maternal age may only reflect delayed reproduction secondary to mild social difficulties in parents. It is also possible, however, that delay was associated with a suboptimal intrauterine environment and led to more severe phenotypic expression in affected offspring.

If the possible small excess of MZ twins and triplets was not the result of ascertainment bias, what might be the nature of the link with autism? One possibility is the adverse sequelae of shared placental circulation, which can also expose twins to very different intrauterine environments. Systematic data on placentation, however, were not available in this study. Some processes associated with MZ twinning, such as the necessary doubling of cell replication, might place equally severe stresses on all progeny; whereas others, such as chance asymmetrical splitting might be a risk factor for one twin. Of course MZ twinning could be a consequence of autism rather than a contributory aetiological factor; a situation that could arise if the genes predisposing to autism were expressed very early in development and predisposed to division of the early cell mass.

This is the first epidemiological study of autistic individuals to report an association with increased head circumference. This association has also been observed in the family study (Bailey *et al.* 1993*c*, Bolton *et al.* 1994) and in a series of consecutive cases at the Maudsley Hospital (Woodhouse *et al.* 1995). There is some evidence that increased brain size contributes to the macrocephaly. Piven *et al.* (1992) reported an increase in mid-sagittal brain area using MRI. Three of the four post mortem cases examined in Great Britain had brain weights greater than 2·5 standard deviations above the population means for the relevant age cohorts (Bailey *et al.* 1993*c*); one of the two idiopathic cases reported by Williams *et al.* (1980) had an enlarged brain; and the brains examined by Bauman and colleagues are considerably heavier than age matched controls (Bauman, M., per-

sonal communication). While the pathology underlying megalencephaly may not be directly responsible for autistic behaviour, it does appear that this strongly genetic developmental disorder is sometimes associated with abnormal brain development.

NOTES

[1] Extracted from: The Registrar General's Statistical Review of England and Wales, 1952–1973, Table CC; Office of Population Census and Statistics publication, Birth Statistic series, FM1–11: Table 6.3 (FM1–7) and Table 6.2 (FM9–11) (data not collected in 1981).

[2] Extracted from Table 17 (usually resident population economically active: social class and socio-economic group by sex), 1981 census, Office of Population Censuses and Surveys.

[3] Extracted from: The Registrar General's statistical review of England and Wales, 1952–1973, Table DD; Office of Population Census and Statistics publication, Birth Statistic Series, FM1–11: Table 6.4 (FM1–7) and Table 6.3 (FM9–11) – data not collected in 1981.

[4] Extracted from: Office of Population Census and Statistics publications, Series DH3, 1–17 (multiple and singleton births); and The Registrar Generals Statistical Review of England and Wales 1952–1973 (singleton births).

We are grateful to: Susan Goode for psychometric testing; Les Butler and Doreen Summers at Queen Elizabeth's Hospital, Hackney, for cytogenetic analysis; Malcolm Carruthers and colleagues for metabolic analysis; Len Dobson at Lewisham Hospital for blood group analysis; John Buckler for data on normal twins; Andrew Pickles for statistical advice; Douglas Schmidt for data entry; and Linda Wilkinson and Elaine Hunt for secretarial support. We are also grateful to the many clinical colleagues who allowed access to their patients. This study would not have been possible without the generous cooperation of all the subjects and their families. Supported by grants to Michael Rutter from The MacArthur Foundation, The Mental Health Foundation and The Medical Research Council, UK.

REFERENCES

Bailey, A., Luthert, P., Bolton, P., Le Couteur, A., Rutter, M. & Harding, B. (1993*a*). Autism is associated with megalencephaly (letter). *Lancet* **341**, 1225–1226.

Bailey, A., Bolton, P., Butler, L., Le Couteur, A., Murphy, M., Scott, S., Webb, T. & Rutter, M. (1993*b*). Prevalence of the Fragile X anomaly amongst autistic twins and singletons. *Journal of Child Psychology and Psychiatry* **34**, 673–688.

Bailey, A., Le Couteur, A., Pickles, A. & Rutter, M. (1993c). British twin study of autism. Paper presented at Second World Congress on Psychiatric Genetics, New Orleans.

Baird, T. D. & August, G. J. (1985). Familial heterogeneity in infantile autism. *Journal of Autism and Developmental Disorders* **15**, 315–321.

Bartak, L., Rutter, M. & Cox, A. (1975). A comparative study of infantile autism and specific developmental language disorder: 1. The children. *British Journal of Psychiatry* **126**, 127–145.

Bauman, M. (1991). Microscopic neuroanatomic abnormalities in autism. *Pediatrics* **87**, (*suppl.*), 791–796.

Bentler, P. M. (1989). *EQS Structural Equations Program Manual.* BMDP Statistical Software: Los Angeles.

Bolton, P. & Rutter, M. (1990). Genetic influences in autism. *International Review of Psychiatry* **2**, 67–80.

Bolton, P., MacDonald, H., Pickles, A., Rios, P., Goode, S., Crowson, M., Bailey, A. & Rutter, M. (1994). A case–control family history study of autism. *Journal of Child Psychology and Psychiatry* **35**, 877–900.

Bushby, K. M. D., Cole, T., Matthews, J. N. S. & Goodship, J. A. (1992). Centiles for adult head circumference. *Archives of Disease in Childhood* **67**, 1286–1287.

Deykin, E. & MacMahon, B. (1980). Pregnancy, delivery and neonatal complications among autistic children. *American Journal of Disorders of Childhood* **134**, 860–864.

Dunn, L. M., Dunn, L. M., Whetton, C. & Pintillie, D. (1982). *British Picture Vocabulary Scale (Manual for long and short forms).* NFER Publishers: Windsor.

Emery, A. E. H. (1986). *Methodology in Medical Genetics.* Churchill Livingstone: Edinburgh.

Falconer, D. S. (1965). The inheritance of liability to certain diseases, estimated from the incidence among relatives. *Annals of Human Genetics* **29**, 51–77.

Falconer, D. S. (1981). *Introduction to Quantitative Genetics.* Longman: London.

Finegan, J. & Quarrington, B. (1979). Pre-, peri- and neonatal factors and infantile autism. *Journal of Child Psychology and Psychiatry* **20**, 119–128.

Folstein, S. & Rutter, M. (1977a). Genetic influences and infantile autism. *Nature* **265**, 726–728.

Folstein, S. & Rutter, M. (1977b). Infantile autism: a genetic study of 21 twin pairs. *Journal of Child Psychology and Psychiatry* **18**, 291–321.

Gillberg, C. (1980). Maternal age and infantile autism. *Journal of Autism and Developmental Disorders* **10**, 293–297.

Gillberg, C. (1992). Autism and autistic-like conditions. *Journal of Child Psychology and Psychiatry* **33**, 813–842.

Gillberg, C. & Steffenburg, S. (1987). Outcome and prognostic factors in infantile autism and similar conditions: a population-based study of 46 cases followed through puberty. *Journal of Autism and Developmental Disorders* **17**, 273–287.

Gillberg, C., Gillberg, I. & Steffenburg, S. (1990). Reduced optimality in the pre-, peri- and neonatal periods is not equivalent to severe peri- or neonatal risk: a rejoinder to Goodman's technical note. *Journal of Child Psychology and Psychiatry* **31**, 813–815.

Gillberg, C., Steffenburg, S. & Schaumann, H. (1991). Is autism more common now than ten years ago? *British Journal of Psychiatry* **158**, 403–409.

Gillberg, C., Gillberg, I. C. & Steffenburg, S. (1992). Siblings and parents of children with autism: a controlled population-based study. *Developmental Medicine and Child Neurology* **34**, 389–398.

Goodman, R. (1991). Growing together and growing apart: the non-genetic forces on children in the same family. In *The Genetics of Mental Illness* (ed. P. McGuffin and R. Murray), pp. 217–244. Butterworth-Heinemann: Oxford.

Hanson, D. R. & Gottesman, I. I. (1976). The genetics, if any, of infantile autism and childhood schizophrenia. *Journal of Autism and Childhood Schizophrenia* **6**, 209–234.

Huntley, M. (1987). *Reynell Developmental Language Scales* (2nd revision) NFER, Nelson Publishers: Windsor.

Landa, R., Piven, J., Wzorek, M. M., Gayle, J. O., Chase, G. A. & Folstein, S. E. (1992). Social language use in parents of autistic individuals. *Psychological Medicine* **22**, 245–254.

Le Couteur, A., Rutter, M., Summers, D. & Butler, L. (1988). Fragile X in female autistic twins. *Journal of Autism and Developmental Disorders* **18**, 458–460.

Le Couteur, A., Rutter, M., Lord, C., Rios, P., Robertson, S., Holdgrafer, M. & McLennan, J. (1989). Autism Diagnostic Interview: a standardized investigator-based instrument. *Journal of Autism and Developmental Disorders* **19**, 363–387.

Le Couteur, A., Bailey, A., Goode, S., Robertson, S., Gottesman, I. I., Schmidt, D. & Rutter, M. (1995). A broader phenotype of autism: the clinical spectrum in twins. (In preparation.)

Links, P., Stockwell, M., Abichandani, F. & Simeon, J. (1980). Minor physical anomalies in childhood autism. Part I. Their relationship to pre- and perinatal complications. *Journal of Autism and Developmental Disorders* **10**, 273–285.

Little, J. & Bryan, E. M. (1988). Congenital anomalies. In *Twinning and Twins* (ed. I. MacGillivray, D. M. Campbell and B. Thompson), pp. 207–240. John Wiley: Chichester.

Lord, C., Rutter, M., Goode, S., Heemsbergen, J., Jordan, H., Mawhood, L. & Schopler, E. (1989). Autism diagnostic observation schedule: a standardized observation of communicative and social behavior. *Journal of Autism and Developmental Disorders* **19**, 185–212.

MacGillivray, I., Samphier, M. & Little, J. (1988). Factors affecting twinning. In *Twinning and Twins* (ed. I. MacGillivray, D. M. Campbell and B. Thompson), pp. 67–97. John Wiley: Chichester.

Piven, J., Gayle, J., Chase, G. A., Fink, B., Landa, R., Wzorek, M. M. & Folstein, S. (1990). A family history study of neuropsychiatric disorders in the adult siblings of autistic individuals. *Journal of the American Academy of Child and Adolescent Psychiatry* **29**, 177–183.

Piven, J., Behme, E., Simon, J., Barta, P., Pearlson, G. & Folstein, S. (1992). Magnetic resonance imaging in autism: measurement of the cerebellum, pons and fourth ventricle. *Biological Psychiatry* **31**, 491–504.

Raven, J. C. & Court, J. H. (1982). *Manual for Raven's Progressive Matrices and Vocabulary Scales: Research and References.* H. K. Louis & Co. Ltd.: London.

Reich, T., James, J. W. & Morris, C. A. (1972). The use of multiple thresholds in determining the mode of transmission of semi continuous traits. *Annals of Human Genetics* **36**, 163–186.

Risch, N. (1990). Linkage strategies for genetically complex traits. 1. Multilocus models. *American Journal of Human Genetics* **46**, 222–228.

Rutter, M. (1970). Autistic children: infancy to adulthood. *Seminars in Psychiatry* **2**, 435–450.

Rutter, M., Bailey, A., Bolton, P. & Le Couteur, A. (1993a). Autism: syndrome definition and possible genetic mechanisms. In *Nature, Nurture and Psychology* (ed. R. Plomin and G. E. McClearn), pp. 269–284. American Psychological Association Press: Washington, DC.

Rutter, M., Simonoff, E. & Silberg, J. (1993b). How informative are twin studies of child psychopathology? In *Twins as A Tool of Behavioral Genetics.* (ed. T. J. Bouchard and P. Propping), pp. 180–194. John Wiley: Chichester.

Rutter, M., Bailey, A., Bolton, P. & Le Couteur, A. (1994) Autism and known medical conditions: myth and substance. *Journal of Child Psychology and Psychiatry* **35**, 311–322.

Smalley, S., Asarnow, R. & Spence, M. (1988). Autism and genetics: a decade of research. *Archives of General Psychiatry* **45**, 953–961.

Smith, D. W. & Jones, K. L. (1988). *Smith's Recognizable Patterns of Human Malformation* (ed. 4). W. B. Saunders: Philadelphia.

Steffenburg, S., Gillberg, C., Hellgren, L., Andersson, L., Gillberg, I., Jakobsson, G. & Bohman, M. (1989). A twin study of autism in Denmark, Finland, Iceland, Norway and Sweden. *Journal of Child Psychology and Psychiatry* **30**, 405–416.

Stutsman, R. (1931). *Mental Measurement of Preschool Children.* World Book: Yonkers-on-Hudson, N.Y.

104

Torrey, E., Hersh, S. & McCabe, K. (1975). Early childhood psychosis and bleeding during pregnancy: a prospective study of gravid women and their offspring. *Journal of Autism and Childhood Schizophrenia* 5, 287–297.

Waldrop, M. & Halverson, C., Jr. (1971). Minor physical anomalies and hyperactive behavior in young children. In *Exceptional Infant: Studies in Abnormalities*, Vol. 2 (ed. J. Hellmuth), pp. 343–381. Brunner/Mazel: New York.

Wechsler, D. (1974). *Manual for the Wechsler Intelligence Scale for Children – Revised*. The Psychological Corporation: New York.

Wechsler, D. (1981). *Manual for the Wechsler Adult Intelligence Scale – Revised*. The Psychological Corporation: New York.

Williams, R., Hauser, S., Purpura, D., Delong, G. & Swisher, C. (1980). Autism and mental retardation. *Archives of Neurology* 37, 749–753.

Wing, L. & Attwood, A. (1987). Syndromes of autism and atypical development. In *Handbook of Autism and Pervasive Developmental*

Disorders (ed. D. J. Cohen, A. Donellan and R. Paul), pp. 3–19. John Wiley: New York.

Wing, L., Yeates, S. R., Brierley, L. M. & Gould, J. (1976). The prevalence of early childhood autism: Comparison of administrative and epidemiological studies. *Psychological Medicine* 6, 89–100.

Wolff, S., Narayan, S. & Moyes, B. (1988). Personality characteristics of parents of autistic children. *Journal of Child Psychology and Psychiatry and Allied Disciplines* 29, 143–154.

Woodhouse, W., Bailey, A., Bolton, B., Baird, G., Le Couteur, A. & Rutter, M. (1995). Head circumference and pervasive developmental disorder. *Journal of Child Psychology and Psychiatry* (submitted).

World Health Organization (1992). *ICD-10 Classification of Mental and Behavioural Disorders: Clinical Descriptions and Diagnostic Guidelines*. World Health Organisation: Geneva.

American Journal of Medical Genetics (Neuropsychiatric Genetics) 54:27–35 (1994)

Genetics of Autism: Characteristics of Affected and Unaffected Children From 37 Multiplex Families

Donna Spiker, Linda Lotspeich, Helena C. Kraemer, Joachim Hallmayer, William McMahon, P. Brent Petersen, Peter Nicholas, Carmen Pingree, Susan Wiese-Slater, Carla Chiotti, Dona Lee Wong, Susan Dimicelli, Edward Ritvo, Luigi L. Cavalli-Sforza, and Roland D. Ciaranello

Autism Genetics Program (D.S., L.L., H.C.K., J.H., S.W.-S., C.C., D.L.W., S.D., L.L.C.-S., R.D.C.), Nancy Pritzker Laboratory of Developmental and Molecular Neurobiology, Department of Psychiatry and Behavioral Sciences (D.L.W., R.D.C.), and Department of Genetics (J.H., L.L.C.-S.), Stanford University School of Medicine, Stanford Department of Psychiatry (E.R.), UCLA School of Medicine, Los Angeles, California; and Department of Psychiatry (W.M., P.B.P., P.N., C.P.), University of Utah School of Medicine, Salt Lake City, Utah

Evidence from twin and family studies strongly suggests that genetic factors play a prominent role in the etiology of some cases of infantile autism. Genetic factors would be expected to be especially strong in families with multiple autistic members (multiplex families). This report describes the identification and evaluation of 44 families with two or more autistic children collected as part of a genetic linkage study in autism. Families were referred with a presumptive classification of multiplex autism. Children referred as autistic, as well as their presumptively normal siblings, were assessed using the Autism Diagnostic Interview (ADI) and the Autism Diagnostic Observation Scale (ADOS). Thirty-seven of the 44 families (87%) had at least two children who met diagnostic criteria for autism on the ADI. Of the total group of 117 children evaluated in these families, 83 (71%) met all ADI criteria and could be unambiguously classified as autistic (affected), 26 (22%) met none of the ADI criteria and were classified as not autistic (unaffected), and 8 (7%) were classified as uncertain because they met one or more but not all of the ADI cutpoints. Autistic siblings were not significantly concordant for most autism characteristics, for IQ, or for verbal ability. Significant concordances were found, however, for behaviors related to rituals and repetitive play, and for social impairments in the expression and understanding of facial expressions of emotion. The results of this study suggests two major points: first, there does not appear to be a highly variable autistic phenotype expressed in multiplex families; in the vast majority of cases, children are either clearly affected or clearly unaffected, so that linkage analysis should not be complicated by a large number of ambiguous or uncertain cases. Second, multiplex families do not appear to associate into subgroups defined by clustering of specific autism behaviors. © 1994 Wiley-Liss, Inc.

KEY WORDS: multiplex autism, genetic heterogeneity, etiology

INTRODUCTION

Accumulating evidence now strongly implicates genetic factors in the etiology of autism. Recently published reviews have summarized the empirical data leading to this conclusion. This includes data from twin and family studies, as well as data showing associations between autism and other known genetic disorders [Lotspeich and Ciaranello, 1993; Folstein and Piven, 1991; Smalley, 1991; Bolton and Rutter, 1990; Rutter, 1990; Rutter et al., 1990; Smalley et al., 1988]. The concordance rate reported for autism in monozygotic twins ranges from 36 to nearly 100%, while the concordance rate reported for dizygotic twins ranges from 0 to 24%; pooled estimates for these figures are 64% and 9%, respectively [Smalley et al., 1988]. The sibling recurrence risk rate pooled across several studies in 2.7% [Smalley et al., 1988]. Based on a prevalence rate for autism of 4 in 10,000 births, the recurrence risk in siblings is greater than 50 times the population risk, and may approach 100, making a linkage strategy aimed at finding a gene or genes in this disorder feasible [Risch, 1990].

While there is a growing consensus about the genetic etiology of some cases of autism, there is also widespread

Received for publication July 12, 1993; revision received October 5, 1993.

Address reprint requests to Donna Spiker, Ph.D., Autism Genetics Program, Department of Psychiatry and Behavioral Sciences, Stanford University School of Medicine, Stanford, CA 94305.

agreement that there are many importance obstacles to locating an autism gene or genes. Currently, linkage analysis using polymorphic DNA markers is the best available and most commonly used strategy for finding disease genes when the biology of a disorder is unknown [Cavalli-Sforza and King, 1986; Ott, 1991]. There are, however, several problems which can hinder or even invalidate a linkage analysis. These include genetic heterogeneity (several genes may cause a disorder, but only one or a few is responsible in any individual case), polygenic inheritance (the action of several genes is required to cause the disorder in each individual), and the presence of phenocopies, or nongenetic cases, which may appear identical to the genetic cases. Moreover, since linkage analysis requires dichotomization of cases into affected and unaffected categories, diagnostic accuracy and a correct definition of the affected phenotype are essential.

Genetic heterogeneity in autism has not been studied, and in the absence of any identified gene or linkage marker, is a problem of unknown magnitude. Genetic heterogeneity can arise by mutation at different points within a single gene locus (allelic heterogeneity), or by mutation in individual genes whose proteins subserve related functions. An example of the latter form of nonallelic heterogeneity is phenylketonuria, which can be caused by mutation in the phenylalanine hydroxylase gene, or in the gene for the enzyme tetrahydropteridine reductase, which is involved in formation of the cofactor essential to the phenylalanine hydroxylase reaction [Sugita et al., 1990; Takashima et al., 1991]. As the biochemical bases for more genetic diseases are uncovered, both types of genetic heterogeneity are increasingly likely to be observed.

The mode of inheritance of autism is unknown. The results to date indicate that autism does not follow classical Mendelian inheritance patterns, but several studies of the inheritance of autism have been contradictory. Smalley et al. [1988] proposed a polygenic model of inheritance, while Jorde et al. [1991], analyzing 185 nuclear families with autism, proposed a mixed model. If autism is indeed the product of the action of several genes, then the probability of finding any disease genes by linkage strategies rests on the number of genes involved and the fractional contribution each makes to the disorder.

The proportion of phenocopies to genetic cases of autism is unknown. However, several nongenetic causes, including prenatal viral infection, are associated with autism [reviewed in Lotspeich and Ciaranello, 1993], so phenocopies are likely to be an important potential confound in genetic analyses. In designing a linkage study attempting to identify disease genes in autism, we paid particular attention to diagnostic accuracy and the definition of the autistic phenotype. In the absence of genetic markers, elimination of phenocopies is extremely difficult. However, we expected that they would more likely occur in families with a single autistic offspring than in multiplex families. For this reason, we have collected only multiplex families for our linkage study.

This report describes the diagnostic procedures and the initial data accumulated for a group of 44 presump-

tively multiplex families. They are part of an ongoing genetic linkage study in which we are collecting behavioral data on all children using a standardized autism assessment instrument, the Autism Diagnostic Interview [ADI, LeCouteur et al., 1989] and carrying out DNA genotyping for linked markers [Hallmayer et al., 1993]. This report presents clinical and descriptive data on the autistic subjects and their siblings using the ADI. It addresses two questions important in autism genetic research. First, is there evidence for a partial or subclinical autism phenotype in the nonautistic siblings of autistic children in multiplex families? This question is relevant in determining the boundary of the autistic phenotype for linkage analysis. Second, are there specific signs and symptoms for which autistic siblings within a given family show significant concordance? If so, could they be used to identify diagnostically heterogeneous forms of autism which have implications for underlying genetic heterogeneity?

MATERIALS AND METHODS
Subject Recruitment

Forty-four families volunteered for this study. Fifteen are families who participated in the UCLA-University of Utah Epidemiologic Survey [Ritvo et al., 1989a,b]. The remainder are families seen for diagnostic evaluation in the Stanford Pervasive Developmental Disorders Clinic, families referred by professionals who conduct evaluations and/or research on autism, or families responding to recruitment notices placed in autism parent group newsletters. To be eligible for the study, a psychiatrist or psychologist had to have performed a clinical evaluation and determined that at least two children in the family were autistic, and those records had to be available for our review. The families we evaluated reside in California, Utah, Florida, Michigan, Illinois, Indiana, Maryland, and New Hampshire.

Data Collection Procedures

After referral to the study, a phone call was made to the family to explain the nature of the study, to obtain background information on the family members, to determine the presence of records to confirm a clinical diagnosis of autism in at least two children, and to determine availability for the diagnostic assessments. Previous diagnostic and medical records and written consents to participate were obtained prior to scheduling diagnostic appointments. Families were excluded if any presumed autistic member had a history of a neurologic disorder known to be associated with autism, such as Fragile X syndrome, Norrie syndrome, neurofibromatosis, phenylketonuria, or tuberous sclerosis. All referred families who gave informed consent and who met the eligibility criteria were seen for evaluations. All children in these families were assessed with the Autism Diagnostic Interview [ADI, LeCouteur et al., 1989]. Children under 17 years received the Autism Diagnostic Observation Schedule [ADOS, Lord et al., 1989].

One of us (D.K.S.) completed the ADI training course given by Dr. Catherine Lord, and subsequently trained four additional evaluators (L.L., W.Mc.M., P.B.P., and P.N.). At the completion of the training period, all interviewers scored 90% or better agreement on ADI practice tapes, which were scored by Dr. Lord or her staff at the University of North Carolina, Greensboro. Almost all the data collection took place in hospital or clinic settings, or schools; a few assessments were conducted in subjects' homes. Parents, usually the mothers, were interviewed with the ADI about each child in the family, and all interviews were videotaped. To achieve the greatest possible blinding of evaluators, different interviewers were used for each child in a family, when this was feasible. This was achieved 73% of the time in families with two children, while in larger families independent interviews for all children were achieved 21% of the time. The ADOS was administered after the ADI was completed, either by the ADI interviewer or by another trained person. The ADI interviewers did not have access to other clinical records or other family members' ADI data when administering or scoring a given ADI. Independent reliability checks (described below) served as a check for possible diagnostic bias associated with non-blindness.

Intelligence test scores were obtained from existing records for the autistic children in 30 of the 37 families. Nonverbal or performance IQ scores were used when available, otherwise full scale IQ scores were used to classify children as mentally retard (IQ<70) or non-retarded (IQ>70).

Testing for Fragile X

All children were tested for the fragile X mutation using polymerase chain reaction amplification of the (CGG)n trinucleotide repeat region of the fragile X locus. No occult cases of fragile X were detected in this sample [Hallmayer et al., 1993].

Scoring the ADI and Diagnostic Classifications

The ADI uses the ICD-10 criteria for autism [WHO, 1992]. To meet these, the child must have a score above a prespecified cutpoint in the three symptom areas of the ICD-10 diagnostic system, and also have an age of onset prior to 3 years of age. In this study, we classified a child as autistic or affected if s/he met all four cutpoints. The child was classified as not autistic or unaffected if s/he did not meet any of the cutpoints. A child was classified as uncertain if s/he met one or more but not all the ADI cutpoints.

Reliability Estimates

To assess the reliability of our ADI data, we selected 37 ADI videotapes at random, with oversampling for uncertain cases. These were sent to Dr. Catherine Lord at the University of North Carolina, Greensboro, for independent diagnosis. Dr. Lord was blinded to any information about the children.

Data Analysis: Sibling Concordance for Autism Signs and Symptoms

The ADI data from autistic siblings were analyzed using a one-way analysis of variance (ANOVA) model to estimate the within and between family variance. The ICD-10 criteria for autism are divided into three areas: social impairments, language impairments and re-stricted interests. For each area there are, respectively, 5, 5, and 6 criteria, and multiple ADI items (questions) are used to evaluate each criterion. Therefore scores may be obtained at the level of individual items, criteria or areas. For these analyses, the full range of item scores (0–3) were used to provide maximal information. We performed the analysis on the scores for the 49 ADI items, the 16 ICD-10 autism criteria, and on the total scores for the three major symptom areas covered by the ICD-10 diagnostic scheme. With a components of variance model, the proportion of total variance that was intrafamilial was estimated. The F-test comparing families was used to test the null hypothesis of random variation within families.

A high concordance could reflect nongenetic familial traits, in particular, maternal reporting bias. Mothers could be describing their autistic and non-autistic children in a similar way on a particular behavior. To test for this, we compared scores for the autistic and nonautistic siblings in the same family and using a matched pair t-test procedure. The standardized mean difference (d) between autistic and non-autistic siblings was used to describe the difference; the greater the d, the greater the difference between autistic and nonautistic siblings.

RESULTS
Reliability Measures

Table I compares the diagnoses obtained by our group with those obtained by the North Carolina evaluators. The kappa coefficient for autistic vs. non-autistic was 0.90 (95% confidence limit > 0.80). The sensitivity was 0.90 and the specificity was 1.00. The kappa coefficient for not-autistic vs. all others was 0.90 (95% confidence limit > 0.76). The sensitivity was 0.91 and the specificity was 1.00. These findings suggest that good interrater reliability can be obtained using blinded, trained evaluators.

Comparison of Referral and ADI Diagnoses

We recruited 44 families presumptive for multiplex autism with a total of 142 children into the study. We classified all children as autistic, not-autistic, or uncertain, and compared the results with the referring classifications (Table II). There was agreement in 123 of 142 cases between the referring diagnosis and our ADI as-

TABLE I. Reliability of Diagnoses*

| | | Diagnosis by North Carolina | | |
	N	Autistic	Not autistic	Uncertain
Diagnosis by Stanford				
Autistic	20	18	0	2
Not autistic	11	0	10	1
Uncertain	6	0	0	6
Total	37	18	10	9

* Thirty-seven videotapes of children from multiplex autistic families were randomly selected for reliability determination by Dr. Catherine Lord and her group at the University of North Carolina, Greensboro, as described in Materials and Methods. An oversampling of children classed as uncertain was done.

TABLE II. Comparison of Presumptive and ADI Diagnoses*

ADI Diagnoses	N	Presumptive diagnosis		
		Autistic	Not autistic	Uncertain

A. Relationship between presumptive (referral) diagnosis and ADI diagnosis for children in presumed autism multiplex families (N = 44 families)

Autistic	90	90	0	0
Not autistic	32	0	32	0
Uncertain	20	7	12	1
Total	142	97	44	1

B. Relationship between referral diagnosis and ADI diagnosis for children in strictly defined multiplex families (N = 37 families)

Autistic	83	83	0	0
Not autistic	26	0	26	0
Uncertain	8	0	7	1
Total	117	83	33	1

* A shows the relation between the referral diagnosis and ADI diagnosis for all 44 families. B provides the same information after 8 families who had one but not two autistic children were excluded ("strict" definition of multiplex).

sessments. The referral diagnosis of autism matched the ADI diagnosis in 90 of 97 cases (sensitivity = 0.93), and in 32 of 44 non-cases (specificity = 0.73). On the basis of the research diagnoses, seven presumptively multiplex families were excluded. In these seven families, one child of the presumed affected pair met all ADI cutpoints, but the other did not. This latter sib was classified as uncertain. In most cases s/he would have been given a clinical diagnosis of pervasive developmental disorder, (PDD-NOS) [American Psychiatric Association, 1987], a category many autism researchers believe is related to, if not part of, the autistic syndrome.

Thus 37 families could be strictly defined as multiplex for autism because they had two or more children who met ADI criteria for the disorder. In this group of 37 families, 83 of 117 children (70.9%) were autistic, 26 (22.2%) were not-autistic, and only 8 (6.8%) had an uncertain classification. Results for the 37 eligible families are shown in Figure 1.

Clinical Characteristics of Autism Multiplex Families

Table III shows the ages, sex, and family sizes of the 37 autism multiplex families. Thirty-three (89%) of the families had two autistic children, two had four and two had five. It should be noted that 15 families (40.5%) had no non-autistic children. Thirty-four of the families were Caucasian and 3 were African-American. Table IV shows the ADI area scores by diagnostic status. Note that the ranges and medians for the autistic versus other two groups are quite different. The implications of this for a linkage study are important. Children in the uncertain group met some but not all the ADI cutoffs. The observation that their ADI scores were much lower than the autistic group and not different from the unaffected group indicates that including the uncertain children in either the affected (autistic) or unaffected group in a linkage analysis would not be justified.

Characteristics of Unaffected Siblings in Autism Multiplex Families

We next examined further the clinical characteristics of the 26 individual unaffected siblings. The ADI area scores for this group are shown in Table V. Although this group was judged, both clinically and by the ADI area scores, as being non-autistic, there were a few slightly elevated but still subthreshold scores.

Characteristics of Uncertain Siblings in Autism Multiplex Families

Table VI shows the ADI area scores for the 8 children in 6 families who were classified as uncertain because they met one or more but not all of the ADI cutpoints. One of these (258-3) was referred to the study with an uncertain diagnosis; the remainder were considered unaffected by their referring source. We examined in more detail why children in the uncertain group received this classification. Five met the ADI cutpoint for age of onset only, meaning parents or professionals identified some developmental problem before 3 years of age. These were usually language delays or behavioral irritability. Two met only the ADI cutpoint for ritualistic behaviors. One (258-3) met the social, rituals, and age of onset cutpoints, and also had language deficits, but with a subthreshold score.

Concordance of Autistic Behaviors in Multiplex Families

As previously described, one of the important problems facing a linkage study is genetic heterogeneity. We attempted to address this question in a preliminary fashion by examining the concordance of autistic behaviors within multiplex families. Our hypothesis was that diagnostic heterogeneity might be revealed by a clustering of certain behaviors within families. We tested this by comparing the intrafamilial vs. interfamilial variation for each ADI item, criterion and area scores. The results are shown in Table VIIA–C. For all ADI items,

TABLE III. Ages, Sex, and Family Size in Autism Multiplex Sibling Families (N = 37)*

	Autistic N = 83	Not autistic N = 26	Uncertain N = 8
Age (yr)			
Mean (S.D.)	13.6 (9.2)	16.2 (9.9)	13.8 (6.9)
Median	11	14	13
Sex			
Male N	59	14	3
Female N	24	12	5
M/F	2.45	1.16	0.6

	Number of non-autistic children						
Autistic children	0	1	2	3	4	5	6
2 (33)	14	10	5	3	0	0	1
4 (2ᵃ)	1	1	0	0	0	0	0
5 (2)	0	1	1ᵇ	0	0	0	0

* The ages, sex ratios, and family sizes for the 37 strictly defined autism multiplex families are shown.
ᵃ Includes one family with four autistic children, two of whom are monozygotic twins.
ᵇ One child in this family died at 18 months of age.

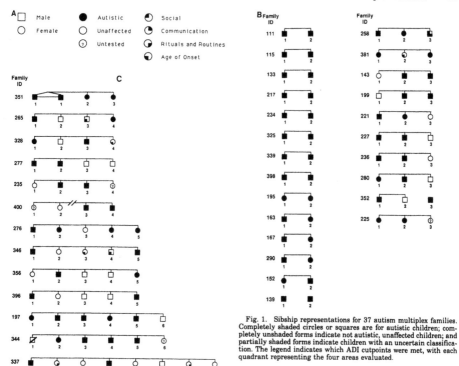

Fig. 1. Sibship representations for 37 autism multiplex families. Completely shaded circles or squares are for autistic children; completely unshaded forms indicate not autistic, unaffected children; and partially shaded forms indicate children with an uncertain classification. The legend indicates which ADI cutpoints were met, with each quadrant representing the four areas evaluated.

TABLE IV. ADI Area Scores for Children in Autism Multiplex Sibling Families
(N = 37 Families, 117 Children)*

	Autistic (N = 83) (In 37 families)	Not Autistic (N = 26) (In 22 families)	Uncertain (N = 8) (In 6 families)
Social total			
Range	17–44	0–9	0–14
Median	36	1	1.5
Language total (V)[a]			
No. of children	58	26	8
Range	11–29	0–8	0–7
Median	21	0.5	0
Language total (NV)[b]			
No. of children	25	0	0
Range	9–16	—	—
Median	15	—	—
Ritual total			
Range	3–12	0–2	0–4
Median	8	0	1.5
Onset present?[c]			
N (% Yes)	83 (100)	0 (0)	6 (75)

* Social cutpoint = 12, range = 0–42; language cutpoint = 10 for verbal subjects, range = 0–30, and cutpoint for nonverbal subjects is 8, range = 0–16; rituals cutpoint = 3, range = 0–12.
[a]V = verbal: having phrase speech by age 5 years.
[b]NV = non-verbal: not having phrase speech by age 5 years.
[c]Meets onset criteria; developmental delays or deviance < 3 years.

111

TABLE V. Distributions of ADI Area Scores for
Non-Autistic Children in Autism Multiplex Sibling
Families
(N = 22 Families, 26 Children)

	Total ADI scores[a]		
Area score[a]	Social N (%)	Language N (%)	Rituals N (%)
0	6 (23.1)	13 (50.0)	21 (80.8)
1	9 (34.6)	5 (19.2)	4 (15.4)
2	4 (15.4)	3 (11.5)	1 (3.8)
3	2 (7.7)	0 (0)	
4	1 (3.8)	2 (7.7)	
5	2 (7.7)	2 (7.7)	
6	1 (3.8)	0 (0)	
7	0 (0)	0 (0)	
8	0 (0)	1 (3.8)	
9	1 (3.8)		

[a]Social cutpoint = 12, range = 0–42; language cutpoint = 10 for verbal
subjects, range = 0–30, and cutpoint for nonverbal subjects = 8, range
= 0–16; rituals cutpoint = 3, range = 0–12.

criteria and area scores tested, the effect sizes (d) were
large (>0.8), indicating that mothers were describing
their autistic children differently than their unaffected
children, so reporting bias could be eliminated as a factor in these results. For the majority of ADI items and
criteria, and for the three area scores, concordance scores
were non-significant, indicating that intrafamilial variation among autistic siblings was similar to interfamilial variation among multiplex families.

For a few items and criteria, we observed significant
concordances between sibling scores ($R^2 = 0.16$–0.33). In
the area of social impairment (Table VIIA), there was
significant concordance for three individual items tap-
ping behaviors concerning the display and understanding of emotional expression: limited facial expressions,
seeking to share one's own enjoyment and showing inappropriate facial gestures.

In the language impairment area (Table VIIB), one
criterion, the use of gestures, showed a significant clustering within families, as did one item in this criterion,
pointing to express interest. Two items under the repeti-

tive speech criterion showed evidence of concordance
as well: use of stereotyped utterances and pronominal
reversals.

The greatest number of significant concordances was
in the area concerning restricted interests and rituals
(Table VIIC). Two criteria and four items scores were
significant. These included ritualistic behaviors and
play, and repetitive sensory behaviors. To illustrate this,
we plotted data for individual autistic children, ordered
by mean within each family for the item about compulsions and rituals and for the criterion about idiosyncratic
and repetitive play. While some families showed evidence
of clustering, in general the results are not impressive
(data not shown).

Concordance for IQ Scores Among Autistic Siblings

IQ scores were available for both autistic siblings in 30
of the 37 families. As an overall indicator of intellectual
functioning, autistic children in multiplex families may
show concordance for IQ. To examine this hypothesis, we
first examined the IQ data by classifying children as
retarded (IQ<70) or normal (IQ>70). In seven families,
all autistic sibs had IQ scores below 70. In eleven families, all autistic siblings had IQs in the normal range
(>70). In the remaining twelve families, some autistic
children had normal and some had retarded scores.
Overall, using a binomial test, families were not more
likely to be concordant than discordant (chi-square =
1.18, n.s.) Because the classification of normal vs. retarded might be too broad, we next examined the IQ
scores within a more restricted numerical range. In 15
families the autistic sibs had IQ scores within 15 points
(1 standard deviation) of each other. In the other 15
families, the IQ scores of autistic sibs differed by more
than 15 points. Again, families were no more likely to be
concordant when the data were examined in this fashion
(chi-square = 0.00, n.s.).

Since language ability correlates with IQ in autistic
children [Bartak and Rutter, 1976; Wing, 1981], we examined concordance for verbal ability in these multiplex
families. On the ADI, the child is classified as verbal if

TABLE VI. ADI Scores for Uncertain Cases*

Subject ID	Age (yr), Sex	Verbal type[b]	Total ADI Area Scores[a]			Onset (Y/N)[c]
			Social	Language	Rituals	
258-3	3,M	V	12	7	4	Yes
337-2	20,F	V	2	1	3	No
337-7	10,F	V	0	0	3	No
381-2	26,F	V	5	0	1	Yes
346-3	14,F	V	3	1	0	Yes
346-4	12,M	V	1	0	2	Yes
328-4	15,F	V	0	0	0	Yes
265-3	10,M	V	0	0	0	Yes

* Siblings of autistic subjects who were classed as uncertain are shown here; the
subject ID matches the pedigree drawings in Figure 1.
[a]Social cutpoint = 12, range 0–42; language cutpoint = 10 for verbal subjects, range
= 0–30, and cutpoint for nonverbal subjects is 8, range 0–16; rituals cutpoint = 3,
range 0–12.
[b]V = verbal, NV = nonverbal status on ADI: presence vs. absence of phrase speech by
age 5 years.
[c]Meets onset criteria: developmental delays or deviance <3 yr.

TABLE VII. Concordances for ADI Criteria, Items, Area Scores

Criteria/items	R^2	d	Criteria/items	R^2	d
A: Concordances for ADI criteria and items:			C5 Make-believe or imitative play	0.02	5.26
social behavior impairments			Spontaneous imitation	0.09	2.66
B1 Nonverbal communication	−0.03	3.23	Imaginative play	0.00	4.07
Direct gaze	0.07	3.24	Imitative social play	0.10	3.32
Social smiling	0.05	2.24	Verbal children		
Range of facial expressions	0.17*	2.35	C2V Conversational interchanges	0.11	3.36
Arms up to be lifted	0.05	1.51	Chat	0.01	3.26
B2 Peer friendships	−0.02	4.59	Reciprocal conversation	0.13	3.07
Imaginative play with peers	0.08	4.80	C3V Stereotyped or repetitive	0.16	2.16
Interest in children	−0.05	2.95	speech		
Response to other children	0.08	2.58	Stereotyped utterances	0.33**	2.00
Group play with peers (4–10 yrs)	0.05	3.59	Inappropriate questions	0.12	1.62
Friends (10–15 yrs)	0.05	3.59	Pronominal reversal	0.28*	1.26
B3 Comfort and affection	0.02	2.96	Neologisms/idiosyncratic language	0.04	0.68
Offers comfort	0.15	2.47	C4V Prosody	0.04	1.95
Coming for comfort	−0.03	2.10	Intonation/volume/rhythm/rate	0.12	1.74
Affection	0.14	1.87	Vocal expression	0.03	1.70
Secure base	0.02	1.83			
Separation anxiety	0.14	0.93	Total: All C criteria	0.12	1.87
B4 Shared enjoyment	0.08	3.93	C: Concordances for ADI criteria and items:		
Showing and directing attention	0.10	2.82	restricted interests and unusual repetitive behaviors		
Offering to share	0.02	2.45	R1 Restricted interests	−0.01	1.61
Seeking to share own enjoyment	0.24**	2.81	Circumscribed interested	−0.04	0.79
Sharing others' pleasure	0.02	2.82	Unusual preoccupations	0.05	1.57
B5 Integration of social behaviors	0.07	4.39	R2 Idiosyncratic play	0.21*	2.54
Greeting	0.04	2.60	Repetitive use of objects	0.07	2.53
Quality of social overtures	−0.02	2.63	Unusual sensory interests	0.19*	1.39
Inappropriate facial expressions	0.30**	2.22	Abnormal idiosyncratic neg response	0.18*	0.87
Appropriateness of social response	0.03	3.28	R3 Attachment to unusual objects	0.09	1.09
Use of others' body			Unusual attachments	0.08	1.20
			R4 Distress over trivial changes	0.12	2.01
Total: All B criteria	0.07	5.42	Minor changes in routines	0.09	2.50
			Minor changes in environment	0.18*	1.21
			R5 Stereotyped hand or body	0.10	1.87
B. Concordances for ADI criteria and items:			movements		
language and communication impairments			Hand and finger mannerisms	0.09	1.38
All children			Complex mannerisms	0.11	1.65
C1 Gestures	0.16*	3.51	R6 Compulsive routines and rituals	0.03	1.13
Pointing to express interest	0.19	2.32	Verbal rituals	−0.05	0.84
Conventional gestures	0.04	3.38	Compulsions/rituals	0.25**	1.18
Nod head to mean 'yes'	0.04	2.40	Total: All R criteria	0.03	2.64
Shake head to mean 'no'	0.12	2.20			

* p < .05.
** p < .001.

s/he has phrase speech by 5 years of age, and as nonverbal if s/he does not. In 19 families the autistic siblings were all verbal, in three they were nonverbal and in 15 families the autistic siblings had discrepant verbal status. Once again, no significant concordance was observed using a one-sample chi-square test (chi-square = 1.31, n.s.). Taken together, the results from these three analyses do not support the hypothesis that there are strong concordance of IQs and verbal ability within autism multiplex families.

DISCUSSION

Problems in a diagnostic accuracy and phenotypic definition have had an adverse impact on genetic studies of psychiatric disorders. Genetic linkage analyses have proven to be very sensitive to diagnostic errors resulting in subject misclassification, and to the presence of phenocopies or false positives [Ott, 1991]. For these reasons,

in designing our genetic study we employed several strategies aimed at minimizing diagnostic error. These included (1) the use of a standardized diagnostic instrument, the Autism Diagnostic Interview, (2) evaluation by multiple trained diagnosticians with blinding of evaluators, and (3) independent verification of our diagnoses by a separate, blinded diagnostic group. To minimize the problem of subject misclassification, we limited the definition of affected individuals to those meeting all of the ADI criteria for autism.

This study is the first to determine the presence of autistic behaviors in all children, both the presumed affected and unaffected, in a large sample of multiplex autism families, and the results of our analyses are of interest in several ways. First is the question of presumptive or referral diagnosis vs. research diagnoses. Second is the definition of affected status, and third is the question of genetic heterogeneity.

Referral vs. Research Diagnoses

In genetic studies, it may be difficult or costly for the research team to examine blindly every subject. To what extent can the evaluations done by professionals outside the study be used in linkage analyses? Our data suggest that there is good agreement between our referral sources and our own diagnoses in classifying children as autistic rather than not autistic and vice versa, but we classified some cases in both groups as uncertain (Table II). Of 20 children whom we classified as uncertain, outside clinicians classified 7 as autistic, 12 were presumed to be unaffected, and only one was referred with an uncertain diagnosis. One important consequence of the differences in classification seen in Table II is that we had to exclude seven presumptively multiplex families from the study because there were seven false positive presumptive diagnoses using the research diagnoses. For purposes of genetics studies, the research team must treat the referral diagnosis as presumptive and arrive at its own diagnostic conclusions. The practical implications of this conclusion are that classification by chart review or clinical records of individuals who are unavailable for assessment is probably unwise. Additionally, clinical information is unlikely to be obtained by individuals who are blinded to status of other family members, and for the presumably unaffected siblings, clinical records are especially likely to be sparse or unavailable.

In this study we used a standardized diagnostic instrument, the ADI/ADOS, for diagnostic purposes. There are several advantages to this approach. First, without such standardized procedures, it is unclear whether the children being classified as autistic are comparable from study to study, from cohort to cohort, or even within a single study where different diagnosticians have participated. Second, although affected status might be appropriately defined by the referral diagnosis (e.g., autism), a decision to define affected status by individual signs and symptoms or clusters of these might later be warranted for linkage analysis. Such data is only available when standardized instruments are used and information about individual behaviors is collected systematically for each subject.

Definition of Affected Status

A second important question addressed by these findings is the matter of the autistic phenotype. There is general consensus that an autistic spectrum exists, with variation both in severity and clinical expression [Rutter and Schopler, 1992; Szatmari, 1992]. If this is true, then who, in a linkage study, should be included as affected? There have been numerous studies attempting to define the boundaries of the autism phenotype. Classically autistic subjects, those meeting criteria for pervasive developmental disorder, as well as those with developmental language disorders have all been included in the definition of affected [Wing, 1988; Bolton and Rutter, 1990]. One of the goals of our study was to determine the proportion of children in multiplex families who could be unambiguously classified, so that we could arrive at a suitable definition of the affected phenotype for linkage analysis.

At the outset of this study we hypothesized that ADI analysis of all children in multiplex families would yield a broad distribution of phenotypes, spanning more or less a continuum from unaffected to affected, without clear breakpoints. We expected to find a large group of children falling into an ambiguous, or uncertain, phenotype. Such a phenotypic distribution would present a daunting challenge to a linkage analysis.

The data indicated otherwise: children were either unambiguously autistic (~71%), or unaffected (~22%), with only a small uncertain group. These proportions were not greatly affected by excluding the seven families who were not strictly multiplex; taking all 44 families, the autistic group was 63%, the unaffected group 22% and the uncertain group 14% of all children (Table II). Some important points emerge from this. First, a conservative or strict definition of autism can be used without undue concern for the presence of an ambiguous group. Linkage can then be performed by defining affected individuals as solely those meeting strict criteria for autism. The uncertain group can be treated as "unknown," and excluded from linkage analysis. Some information is lost this way, but the risk of false positive classification is avoided.

Second, the distinction between affected and unaffected is clear. A few children in the unaffected group had mildly elevated ADI scores in some areas. In the absence of additional data from ADI evaluations of children taken randomly from the general population, the significance of subthreshold scores is unclear, but there is no empirical reason to classify these children as other than unaffected. Third, because there is only a very small uncertain group, we may not need to collect a great number of families to accumulate sufficient numbers for linkage analysis. Power calculations to determine the needed sample size are dependent on estimates of genetic heterogeneity, which is unknown in autism. Therefore these calculations are tenuous at best, but we have estimated that 100–200 families should provide sufficient power to detect linkage, even in the presence of substantial genetic heterogeneity (Hallmayer, unpublished observations). Fourth, because of the problems of phenotypic spectrum, Pauls [1993] has advocated the use of multidimensional or continuous approaches to diagnosis in psychiatric genetics. While our results indicate this might not be necessary in autism, the data from the ADI, which includes information on the degree of severity, as well as the presence or absence of a large number of autism symptoms is ideally suited for such an approach.

Genetic Heterogeneity

A third point which we attempted to address was genetic heterogeneity. Our hypothesis was that there might be diagnostically distinct subgroups of autistic subjects that could be defined on the basis of high intrafamilial concordance for certain autistic behaviors. From the analyses of individual ADI items, criteria, and areas, we could find only limited evidence in support of this hypothesis. The familial concordances for specific autistic symptoms were generally not strong, and high intrafamilial variability was the rule. There were, however, significant intrafamilial concordances for autistic behaviors concerning ritualistic and repetitive behaviors that may yield clues for identifying behaviorally defined subgroups of multiplex families. This possibility should be pursued with a larger sample of multiplex families. Additionally, the possibility of stronger concordances among distinct subgroups exhibiting *patterns* of behaviors needs to be explored. While we will continue to examine these possibilities as we collect additional families, we think it likely that further attempts at identifying genetic heterogeneity in autism must await the finding of a linkage marker or an actual gene locus.

Such a marker will answer many questions left unresolved or raised by this study. Among the most important of these is the boundary of the autistic phenotype, which we have drawn tightly around the ADI definition, but which others have argued quite persuasively should be extended. But where should the line be drawn? Examining the "uncertain" and even the "unaffected" siblings of autistic subjects with a linked marker or gene probe will shed critical light on this question, as well as providing important independent biologic evidence for an autism classification.

ACKNOWLEDGMENTS

This work was supported by a program project grant from the National Institute of Mental Health (MH39437), and by grants from the Scottish Rite, the Spunk Fund, the Solomon and Rebecca Baker Fund, and the endowment fund of the Nancy Pritzker Laboratory. L.L. and J.H. are the recipients of Young Investigator Awards from the National Alliance for Research in Schizophrenia and Affective Disorders (NARSAD). R.D.C. is the recipient of a Career Scientist Award from the NIMH (MH 00219). We are grateful to the families who are participating in this research.

REFERENCES

American Psychiatric Association (1987): "Diagnostic and Statistical Manual of Mental Disorders III-R" (Third ed.). Washington, DC: American Psychiatric Association.

Bartak L, Rutter M (1976): Differences between mentally retarded and normally intelligent autistic children. J Autism Child Schizophr 4:109–120.

Bolton P, Rutter M (1990): Genetic influences in autism. Int Rev Psychiatry 2:67–80.

Cavalli-Sforza LL, King MC (1986): Detecting linkage for genetically heterogeneous diseases and detecting heterogeneity with linkage data. Am J Hum Genet 38:599–616.

Folstein SE, Piven J (1991): Etiology of autism: Genetic influences. Pediatrics 87:767–773.

Hallmayer J, Underhill P, Spiker D, Lotspeich L, Kraemer HC, McMahon WM, Peterson PB, Nicholas P, Pingree C, Wong DL, Ciaranello RD, Cavalli-Sforza LL (1993): A linkage study of autism. Biol Psychiatry 33:104a.

Hallmayer J, Pintado E, Lotspeich L, Spiker D, McMahon WM, Petersen PB, Nicholas P, Pingree C, Kraemer HC, Wong DL, Ritvo E, Cavalli-Sforza LL, Ciaranello RD (In preparation): Exclusion of linkage between the Fragile X gene and familial autism.

Jorde LB, Hasstedt SJ, Ritvo ER, Mason-Brothers A, Freeman BJ, Pingree C, McMahon WM, Peterson B, Jenson WR, Moll A (1991): Complex segregation analysis of autism. Am J Hum Genet 49: 932–938.

LeCouteur A, Rutter M, Lord C, Rios P, Robertson S, Holdgrafer M, McLennan J (1989): Autism Diagnostic Interview: A standardized investigator-based instrument. J Autism Dev Disord 19:363–387.

Lord C, Rutter M, Good S, Heemsbergen J, Jordan H, Mawhood L, Schopler E (1989): Autism Diagnostic Observation Scale: A standardized observation of communicative and social behavior. J Autism Dev Disord 19:185–212.

Lotspeich LJ, Ciaranello RD (1993): The neurobiology and genetics of infantile autism. Int Rev Neurobiol 35:87–129.

Ott J (1991): "Analysis of Human Genetic Linkage," Revised Edition. Baltimore: The Johns Hopkins University Press.

Pauls DL (1993): Behavioural disorders: lessons in linkage. Nature 3:4–5.

Risch N (1990): Genetic linkage and complex diseases, with special reference to psychiatric disorders. Genet Epidemiol 7:1–16.

Ritvo ER, Freeman BJ, Pingree C, Mason-Brothers A, Jorde L, Jenson WR, McMahon WM, Petersen PB, Mo A, Ritvo A (1989a): The UCLA-University of Utah epidemiologic survey of autism: Prevalence. Am J Psychiatry 146:194–199.

Ritvo ER, Jorde LB, Mason-Brothers A, Freeman BJ, Pingree C, Jones MB, McMahon WM, Petersen PB, Jenson WR, Mo A (1989b): The UCLA-University of Utah epidemiologic survey of autism: Recurrence risks estimates and genetic counseling. Am J Psychiatry 146:1032–1036.

Rutter M (1990): Autism as a genetic disorder. In McGuffin P, Murray R (eds): "The New Genetics of Mental Illness." Stoneham, MA: Butterworth-Heinemann, pp 225–244.

Rutter M, Schopler E (1992): Classification of pervasive developmental disorders: some concepts and practical considerations. J Autism Dev Disord 22:459–482.

Rutter M, MacDonald H, LeCouteur A, Harrington R, Bolton P, Bailey A (1990): Genetic factors in child psychiatric disorders - II: empirical findings. J Child Psychol Psychiatry 31:39–83.

Smalley SL (1991): Genetic influences in autism. Psychiatr Clin North Am 14:125–139.

Smalley SL, Asarnow RF, Spence MA (1988): Autism and genetics. Arch Gen Psychiatry 45:953–961.

Sugita R, Takahashi S, Ishii K, Matsumoto K, Ishibashi T, Sakamoto K, Narisawa K (1990): Brain CT and MR bindings in hyperphenylalaninemia due to dihydropteridine reductase deficiency (variant of phenylketonuria). J Comp Assist Tomogr 14(5):699–703.

Szatmari P (1992): The validity of autistic spectrum disorders: a literature review. J Autism Dev Disord 22:583–600.

Takashima S, Chan F, Becker LE (1991): Cortical dysgenesis in a variant of phenylketonuria (dihydropteridine reductase deficiency). Pediatr Pathol 11(5):771–779.

Wing L (1981): Language, social and cognitive impairments in autism and severe mental retardation. J Autism Dev Disord 11:31–44.

Wing L (1988): The continuum of autistic characteristics. In Schopler E, Mesibov GB (eds.): "Diagnosis and Assessment in Autism." New York: Plenum Press, pp 91–100.

World Health Organization (1992): "ICD-10. Classification of Mental and Behavioural Disorders. Clinical Description and Diagnostic Guidelines." Geneva: Author.

American Journal of Medical Genetics (Neuropsychiatric Genetics) 105:406–413 (2001)

Rapid Publication

Evidence Supporting WNT2 as an Autism Susceptibility Gene

Thomas H. Wassink,[1*] Joseph Piven,[2] Veronica J. Vieland,[1,3] Jian Huang,[4] Ruth E. Swiderski,[5] Jennifer Pietila,[5] Terry Braun,[5,6] Gretel Beck,[5] Susan E. Folstein,[7] Jonathon L. Haines,[8] and Val C. Sheffield[5]

[1]Department of Psychiatry, University of Iowa College of Medicine, Iowa City, Iowa
[2]Neurodevelopmental Disorders Research Center and Department of Psychiatry, University of North Carolina, North Carolina
[3]Department of Biostatistics, University of Iowa College of Public Health, Iowa City, Iowa
[4]Department of Statistics and Actuarial Science, University of Iowa, Iowa City, Iowa
[5]Department of Pediatrics and the Howard Hughes Medical Institute, University of Iowa College of Medicine, Iowa City, Iowa
[6]Interdepartmental Genetics Ph.D. Program, University of Iowa, Iowa City, Iowa
[7]Department of Psychiatry, Tufts University College of Medicine, Medford, Massachusetts
[8]Program in Human Genetics, Vanderbilt Medical Center Nashville, Tennessee

We examined WNT2 as a candidate disease gene for autism for the following reasons. First, the WNT family of genes influences the development of numerous organs and systems, including the central nervous system. Second, WNT2 is located in the region of chromosome 7q31–33 linked to autism and is adjacent to a chromosomal breakpoint in an individual with autism. Third, a mouse knockout of Dvl1, a member of a gene family essential for the function of the WNT pathway, exhibits a behavioral phenotype characterized primarily by diminished social interaction. We screened the WNT2 coding sequence for mutations in a large number of autistic probands and found two families containing nonconservative coding sequence variants that segregated with autism in those families. We also identified linkage disequilibrium (LD) between a WNT2 3'UTR SNP and our sample of autism-affected sibling pair (ASP) families and trios. The LD arose almost exclusively from a subgroup of our ASP families defined by the presence of severe language abnormalities and was also found to be associated with the

evidence for linkage to 7q from our previously published genomewide linkage screen. Furthermore, expression analysis demonstrated WNT2 expression in the human thalamus. Based on these findings, we hypothesize that rare mutations occur in the WNT2 gene that significantly increase susceptibility to autism even when present in single copies, while a more common WNT2 allele (or alleles) not yet identified may exist that contributes to the disorder to a lesser degree © 2001 Wiley-Liss, Inc.

KEY WORDS: autism; candidate gene; linkage disequilibrium; chromosome 7q

INTRODUCTION

Autism is a behavioral syndrome consisting of deficits in social interaction and communication, specific ritualistic-repetitive behaviors, and a characteristic course [Rutter et al., 1993]. Onset is typically first noted at the age when relevant behaviors such as speech and complex social interactions become observable, and symptoms generally continue throughout life [Gillberg, 1993]. Family and twin studies have demonstrated that the predisposition to develop autism is largely genetically determined with a sibling relative risk of between 50 and 100 and a heritability estimate of at least 90% [Szatmari et al., 1998]. These same studies also show that the mode of inheritance for

Val C. Sheffield is an associate investigator of the Howard Hughes Medical Institute.
*Correspondence to: Dr. Thomas H. Wassink, University of Iowa College of Medicine, Psychiatry Research/MEB, Iowa City, IA 52242. E-mail: thomas-wassink@uiowa.edu
Received 10 January 2001; Accepted 15 February 2001

116

autism is likely to be complex, due to multiple genes interacting in variable combinations in additive, multiplicative, epistatic, or as yet unknown fashions [Szatmari, 1999], with estimates of the number of genes involved ranging from 3 [Pickles et al., 1995] to more than 15 [Risch et al., 1999].

These heritability data have stimulated a concerted search to identify the specific genes conferring autism susceptibility, with chromosome 7q31–33 emerging as a primary region of interest. Suggestive evidence for linkage to broad regions of 7q was found in two of four genomewide screens of autism [International Molecular Genetic Study of Autism Consortium, 1998; Collaborative Linkage Study of Autism, 1999], while the others reported positive, though less significant, scores [Philippe et al., 1999; Risch et al., 1999]. A subsequent focused examination of 7q also produced suggestive evidence for linkage [Ashley-Koch et al., 1999], with the region most consistently implicated across studies being 7q31–33 [Wassink and Piven, 2000]. In addition, 7q abnormalities from six autistic individuals have now been reported, most of which are also in the 7q31–33 region [Ashley-Koch et al., 1999; Sultana et al., 1999; Vincent et al., 2000; Warburton et al., 2000]. Lastly, data from related phenotypes supports this locus and suggests that it may relate specifically to the language abnormalities characteristic of autism, as both specific language impairment (SLI) and a complicated speech phenotype from a single large pedigree have been linked or associated with genetic markers in 7q31–33 [Tomblin et al., 1998; Lai et al., 2000].

In light of this evidence, we began examining the 7q31–33 interval for autism candidate genes, and our attention was drawn to WNT2 (wingless-type MMTV integration site family member 2). WNT2 is in the linked region and is immediately adjacent to RAY1, a gene interrupted by a chromosomal breakpoint in an autistic patient but otherwise not shown to be involved in autism [Vincent et al., 2000]. WNT2 is one of more than a dozen WNT genes that are expressed during development in a variety of tissues [Cadigan and Nusse, 1997]. Knockout and expression studies in mice [Uusitalo et al., 1999], zebrafish [Hauptmann and Gerster, 2000], and Xenopus [Landesman and Sokol, 1997] have demonstrated specific and important contributions of WNT genes to the development and patterning of the vertebrate central nervous system. Further piquing our interest was a report describing the mouse knockout of disheveled 1 (Dvl1) [Lijam et al., 1997]. Transmission of the WNT signal is dependent on the disheveled (DVL) family of proteins, and the report of Lijam et al. [1997] described a phenotype consisting primarily of reduced social interaction, characterized by a lack of huddling during sleep, the absence of grooming of cage mates, and diminished mothering behaviors in mice deficient for Dvl1.

Our investigation of the potential contribution of WNT2 to the autism disease phenotype included the following elements. First, thoroughly screening the coding sequence for functional sequence variants in unrelated autistic individuals and in control subjects.

Second, testing for linkage disequilibrium (LD) using intragenic SNPs in our total sample of autism families and separately in a language-impaired subset of these families. Third, examining the relationship between LD in the SNPs and our prior evidence for linkage. Fourth, assessing WNT2 expression in the human central nervous system.

MATERIALS AND METHODS

Patient and Ascertainment Sample

All autistic probands and their families were ascertained and diagnosed through the Collaborative Linkage Study of Autism under a previously described protocol [Collaborative Linkage Study of Autism, 1999]. Briefly, families were recruited from three regions of the United States (Midwest, New England, and mid-Atlantic) through four clinical data collection sites: the University of Iowa, Tufts University–New England Medical Center, Johns Hopkins University, and the University of North Carolina. All probands were at least 3 years old and were assessed with the Autism Diagnostic Interview–Revised (ADI-R) and the Autism Diagnostic Observation Schedule (ADOS or the more recent ADOS-G). Affected sibling pair (ASP) and trio families were recruited. All probands were required to meet ADI algorithm criteria for autism. Probands were excluded if they had fragile X syndrome (based on fragile X DNA testing) or any other neurological or medical condition suspected to be associated with autism. All individuals (or, when appropriate, their guardians) provided written, informed consent for participation in this study.

In addition to examining our entire sample, analyses were also performed on phenotypically defined subgroups. Based on the evidence suggesting the potential language specificity of the 7q locus, and following the genomewide analysis reported by our group [Collaborative Linkage Study of Autism, 1999], we split our initial sample of 75 autism affected sibling pair (ASP) families into two groups defined by their speech and language characteristics. Families were classified as language-abnormal if neither proband had developed phrase speech by 36 months, and otherwise as language-normal [Folstein, 2000; Folstein and Mankoski, 2000]. The average normal onset of phrase speech is 18 months, and the vast majority of children in the general population begin to speak in phrases between 12 and 24 months of age. Fifty families were thus classified as language-abnormal and the remaining 25 as language-normal. Furthermore, in the initial genomewide screen, parental phenotypes were classified as unknown. For the language-related analyses, however, information regarding parental language phenotype was available, which had been gathered by direct questioning. Parents with probable or definite delayed onset of speech, trouble learning to read, or persistent trouble with spelling were classified as language-abnormal and otherwise as language-normal. There were similar proportions of language-abnormal and -normal parents in each of the two proband groups.

Linkage analyses of the two resultant subgroups revealed that virtually all of our 7q linkage signal arose from the language-abnormal families, while the signal from the normal group was negligible [Folstein, 2000; Folstein and Mankoski, 2000]. This supported the hypothesis that language impairment might be genetically related to autism and that it defined a more homogeneous subgroup of families for subsequent analyses.

Mutation Screening

DNA for exon screening was available from 135 unrelated autistic individuals and a comparison group of 160 unrelated individuals of similar ethnicity presumed not to have autism. DNA was extracted from whole blood using standard procedures. The 2,301 bp WNT2 cDNA contains 1,082 bp of coding sequence across five exons. Intron/exon boundaries were determined by BLASTing the cDNA against human genomic sequence. Exons, including flanking splice junction sequences, were screened with a total of eight amplicons (primers available upon request), none of which exceeded 250 bp, using single-strand conformational polymorphism (SSCP) analysis. PCR of amplicons was performed with 20 ng of genomic DNA amplified in a reaction mixture containing 1.0 µL of PCR buffer [100 mM Tris-HCl (pH 8.8), 500 mM KCl, 15 mM MgCl$_2$, 0.01% gelatin (w/v)], 200 µM each of dATP, dCTP, dGTP, and dTTP, 2.5 pM of each primer, and 0.05 units of Taq DNA polymerase, increased to a final volume of 10.0 µL with water. Samples were initially denatured at 94°C for 3 min, followed by 40 cycles of 94°C for 30 sec, 54°C or 58°C for 30 sec, and 72°C for 30 sec. PCR products were electrophoresed on 6% nondenaturing polyacrylamide gels at 20 W for approximately 3 hr at ambient temperature. The gels were then silver-stained using standard protocols [Bassam et al., 1991].

Amplicons containing SSCP shifts were forward- and reverse-sequenced on an Applied Biosystems (ABI, Foster City, CA) model 377 automated sequencer using dye terminator chemistry. Sequence data were compared with published sequence for WNT2 using the Sequencher 3.1 gene analysis computer program (Gene Codes, Ann Arbor, MI). Sequence variants detected in this manner were then sequenced with dye terminator chemistry in all available family members from the proband's family of origin.

In addition, because SSCP is not 100% sensitive, all coding sequence amplicons were also completely sequenced in 64 of these same autistic individuals. These 64 individuals included one proband from each of the 50 language-impaired ASP families and one proband from 14 other randomly selected ASP families.

Linkage Disequilibrium

Testing for linkage disequilibrium was carried out in 75 ASP families, 45 trios, and separately in the two language-based subgroups of the ASP families. 3' and 5' sequences were screened for polymorphisms using SSCP. Amplicons displaying shifts on SSCP gels were sequenced to confirm the polymorphism. A robust SSCP assay was developed for each SNP, and multiplex autism families and trios were then genotyped using the SSCP analysis. To test the SNPs for linkage disequilibrium, we constructed a likelihood ratio test assuming that WNT2 is an autism disease gene and allowing for locus heterogeneity. The likelihood has two parameters, λ and α, where λ is the probability of a heterozygous parent transmitting allele 1 to one child of a trio family or to both children of an ASP family, α is the proportion of families in which the recombination fraction $\theta \approx 0$, and $1 - \alpha$ is the proportion of families in which $\theta = 0.5$. The null hypothesis is $\lambda = 0.5$ and the alternative hypothesis is $\lambda \neq 0.5$. The likelihood ratio is $L(\hat{\lambda}\hat{\alpha})/L(0.5, \hat{\alpha})$, where $L(\hat{\lambda}\hat{\alpha})$ is the value that maximizes $L(\lambda, \alpha)$, and $\hat{\alpha}$ is the value that maximizes $L(0.5, \alpha)$. Note that the recombination fraction is not a parameter in this likelihood under the assumption that WNT2 is the susceptibility gene in some families $(\theta \approx 0)$.

Association of SNPs With Evidence for Linkage

Greenberg [1993] and Hodge [1993] have examined the relationship between LD and linkage [Horikawa et al., 2000]. They argue that if both are present, one can test whether an allele that is in disequilibrium is also a susceptibility allele by splitting the sample of families into two groups based on the presence of that allele, and then reassessing the evidence for linkage in the two resultant subgroups. If the allele confers susceptibility, this analysis should demonstrate an association between that allele and the evidence for linkage (i.e., the group defined by the presence of the allele should contain the preponderance of the linkage signal, whereas the other group should not). Conversely, if the associated allele does not directly confer susceptibility, such subsetting should simply split the linkage signal proportionally between the two resultant subgroups. We therefore tested this hypothesis with any marker(s) found to be in LD.

This analysis focused on the language-impaired ASP families, as these contained virtually all of our original evidence for linkage. These families were split into two groups based on the appropriate SNP genotype, and evidence for linkage was examined separately in each group. In keeping with findings from our previous work [Collaborative Linkage Study of Autism, 1999], we first performed all linkage analyses in these two groups under a simple recessive model with 50% penetrance and a disease allele frequency of 0.10. We then sought to identify the best heritability model [Clerget-Darpoux et al., 1986; Elston, 1989; Greenberg; Vieland and Hodge, 1996] for our data, using it to perform the same analyses. Lastly, though WNT2 is located on 7q at approximately 125 cM, we examined such subsetting effects on linkage at 104–109 cM, as this was the location of our strongest 7q linkage signal (maximum heterogeneity LOD = 2.2 at 104 cM), while our study actually found no evidence for linkage in the 7q31–33 region [Collaborative Linkage Study of Autism, 1999].

Northern Blot Analysis

Central nervous system expression of *WNT2* across vertebrates is not constant and had not previously been demonstrated in humans. To investigate this, we searched the NCBI Serial Analysis of Gene Expression (SAGE) database and found that *WNT2* contains a SAGE tag that is expressed at a high level in a human thalamus cDNA library (tag = CATCTGGTAT). To confirm this expression, we performed a Northern blot analysis using a Human Brain Blot IV Northern blot (Clontech, San Francisco, CA). This blot was hybridized with a human *WNT2* DNA probe corresponding to 450 bp of the 3'UTR prepared by PCR amplification of human genomic DNA using the forward primer 5'-GGAACAGTAAAGAAAGCAG-3' and the reverse primer 5'-GTATATCTGTACAGATCAAG-3'. The probe was labeled with ^{32}P-dCTP using an RTS RadPrime DNA Labeling System (Life Technologies, Gaithersburg, MD). Hybridization and autoradiography were performed as described previously [Swiderski et al., 1999]. The blot was stripped of radioactivity and rehybridized with a cDNA probe for β-actin (Clontech, Palo Alto, CA) to assess equal loading of RNA.

RESULTS

Mutation Screening

In the 135 autistic probands screened for mutations, a total of three shifts visualized on SSCP gels were confirmed by sequencing to involve nucleotide base pair substitutions. Of these, two were nonconservative missense mutations, while the third change was a synonymous codon change. Both missense variants were found in one parent and only the affected siblings from both ASP families.

Mutation 1. This mutation was a C-to-T transition at nucleotide 1189 that produced Arg299Trp, which is in exon 5 in the *WNT*-defining region. The mutation was found in the father and two affected siblings, but in neither the mother nor two unaffected siblings (Figs. 1 and 2). Phenotypically, though the father did not meet full criteria for autism, he had significant deficits in childhood conversation, adult conversation, and reading, and his speech, as mea-

sured by the Pragmatic Language Scale [Piven et al., 1997], was impaired. The mother, on the other hand, had no structural or pragmatic language abnormalities.

Mutation 2. This mutation was a T-to-G transversion at nucleotide 14 that produced Leu5Arg, which is a conserved amino acid in the signal domain of exon 1. The mutation occurred in the mother and two affected siblings, but not in the father (Figs. 1 and 2). Detailed phenotypic information was not available for these parents.

Both of these mutations alter the charges of evolutionarily conserved residues (Fig. 3). No sequence variations were found by an SSCP screen of the entire coding region in 160 control subjects. Direct sequencing of the 64 autism probands revealed no additional coding sequence variants.

Linkage Disequilibrium

Screening of noncoding regions revealed two SNPs, one in the 3'UTR and a second approximately 0.5 kb upstream from *WNT2*. The 3'UTR SNP was a C/T transition 783 bases downstream from the stop codon, while the 5' SNP was a C/T change 519 bp upstream from the start codon. These SNPs were genotyped in the sample of 75 ASPs and 45 trios using SSCP analysis.

Transmission of alleles for the 3' and 5'UTR SNPs are shown in Table I. Transmission of the 3'UTR SNP gives a likelihood ratio of 22. Asymptotically, this corresponds to a chi-square value of 6.2 ($P = 0.013$), with the data showing that the T-allele is transmitted to affected offspring more often than expected by chance. Analyzing the ASP and trio families separately shows that nearly all the evidence for LD is from the ASP families, as the likelihood ratio for this group is 21 (chi-square = 6.13; $P = 0.013$), while that for the trio families is about 1. Within the ASP families, when the language-abnormal and -normal families are analyzed separately, the likelihood ratio is 8.1 for the abnormal group and 2.8 for the normal group, demonstrating that most of the signal comes from the language-abnormal group.

In contrast, the 5'UTR SNP demonstrated no disequilibrium. Though the T-allele was transmitted more frequently than the C-allele, the difference was not significant. The likelihood ratio for the entire sample was 2.7 (chi-square = 2; $P = 0.16$) and for the ASPs alone was 1.6 (chi-square = 1; $P = 0.30$). Similarly, separate analysis of the language-impaired subgroup of the ASP families showed no evidence for LD.

We also tested for LD between the 3'UTR and 5'UTR SNPs. Our test hypothesized that LD between the two markers would manifest as differences between the conditional genotype frequencies of the 5'UTR SNP for each of the three genotypes at the 3'UTR SNP. A likelihood ratio test comparing these genotype frequencies (Table I) with four df based on the trinomial distributions provided no significant evidence for LD between the two markers (chi-square = 7.6; $P = 0.11$).

A   **B**

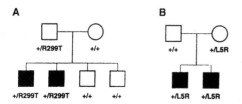

Fig. 1. Pedigrees for two autism-affected sibling pair families segregating mutations of *WNT2*. A: Mutation 1. B: Mutation 2.

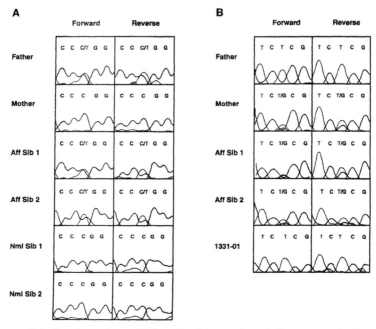

Fig. 2. Sequencing waveforms for *WNT2* mutations. **A:** Sequence showing C-to-T transition at nucleotide 1189 in family with mutation 1. **B:** Sequence showing T-to-G transversion at nucleotide 14 segregating with autism in family with mutation 2.

Association of 3'UTR SNP With Evidence for Linkage

The 3' SNP found to be in LD with autism was tested for association with our prior evidence for linkage to 7q. The language-impaired ASP families (n = 50) were split into two groups based on the presence (n = 24) or absence (n = 26) of a T/T 3'UTR SNP genotype in a randomly chosen affected sibling. Table II shows two-point homogeneity as well as heterogeneity LOD scores for the resultant groupings of families at our two most strongly linked 7q markers: D7S1813 (104 cM) and D7S821 (109 cM). For both markers, the LOD scores in the T/T subset are higher than in the total sample, and considerably higher than in the non-T/T subset.

Furthermore, the best heritability model for our sample was found to be a simple (no phenocopies) recessive model with full penetrance. Under this model,

```
                       5                          299
Human        ----MNAPLGGIWLW  . . .  LGTAGRVCNLTSRGM
Mouse        ----MNVPLGGIWLW  . . .  LGTAGRVCNLTSRGM
Rat          ----MNVPLGGIWLW  . . .  LGTAGRVCNLTSRGM
Xenopus      ---------MHFA    . . .  LGTAGRVCDKVSRGT
Danio Rerio  ---MNFLPNGICFY   . . .  VGTGGRVCNRTSRGT
Drosophila   ------------MW   . . .  QGTSGRTCQRTGHGP
C. Elegans   MIPRRSCWLILLLNL  . . .  LGTEGRVCKRGSGGA
```

Fig. 3. Protein alignment showing conservation of mutated *WNT2* amino acids across species.

TABLE I . Comparison of Data

Transmission of SNP alleles in autism-affected sibling pair
(ASP) Families

	3'UTR SNP	5'UTR SNP
Heterozygous parents	61	62
Heterozygous parents transmitting T-allele to both siblings	22	12
Heterozygous parents transmitting C-allele to both siblings	8	7
Heterozygous parents transmitting a different allele to each sibling	23	35
Ambiguous transmissions from heterozygous parents	8	8
Transmission of SNP alleles in autism trios		
Heterozygous parents	39	44
Heterozygous parents transmitting T-allele	13	21
Heterozygous parents transmitting C-allele	12	15
Ambiguous transmissions from heterozygous parents	14	8

5' SNP genotype frequencies given 3' SNP genotypes for parents of probands

	3' UTR SNP		Conditional 5'UTR SNP genotype frequencies		
Genotype		n	T/T	T/C	C/C
T/T		96	0.46	0.46	0.08
T/C		109	0.35	0.48	0.17
C/C		18	0.23	0.55	0.22

the maximum two-point homogeneity LOD was 3.7 in the T/T language-abnormal subset with no evidence of heterogeneity and an estimate of 0.06 recombination (at marker D7S1813). By comparison, the maximum LOD in the non-T/T language-abnormal families was 0.14.

WNT2 Expression in Human Brain

Our analysis of poly(A) mRNA isolated from selected regions of the adult human brain demonstrated WNT2 expression in the thalamus (Fig. 4). The blot showed two bands at ~2.2 and 2.4 kb, similar to the pattern previously reported in other tissues [McMahon and McMahon, 1989]; the two bands have been attributed to alternative polyadenylation [Wainwright et al., 1988]. Signal was undetectable in the poly(A) mRNA of the whole brain, indicating that WNT2 is expressed in low abundance in specific regions of the brain, such as the thalamus. WNT2 expression was also undetectable in the poly(A) mRNA of 16- to 32-week human whole brain fetal tissue as assessed by Northern blotting using a Clontech Human Fetal Multiple Tissue Northern blot (data not shown), and no blot was available

specifically for fetal thalamus. We also detected expression in fetal lung, adult lung, and placenta (data not shown).

DISCUSSION

Previous work describing the function and expression of WNT proteins, the location of WNT2 in the 7q31–33 linked region and its proximity to the RAY1 breakpoint, and the phenotype of the Dvl1 mouse knockout had suggested WNT2 as a strong candidate for an autism susceptibility gene. We add to this information a substantial array of data suggesting that rare coding sequence mutations in the WNT2 gene, even when present in single copies (heterozygous state), strongly increase susceptibility to autism, while a more common WNT2 allele (or alleles) may exist that contributes to the disorder to a lesser degree.

First, we have found two nonconservative missense mutations in functionally significant segments of WNT2 that occur in one parent, both affected siblings, and no unaffected siblings in the two families in which they are found. Both mutations (Arg299Trp and Leu5Arg) result in a change in the charge of an

TABLE II. Evidence for Linkage in Language Impairment Positive Families Across WNT2 3'UTR SNP Genotype Subgroups

Marker	cM	All families (n = 50)		T/T families (n = 24)		Non-T/T families (n = 26)	
		Z	Z_{HET}	Z	Z_{HET}	Z	Z_{HET}
D7S1813	104	1.8	2.7	2.5	2.9	0.2	0.3
D7S821	109	2.2	2.2	2.3	2.7	0.4	0.4

*Z = maximum two-point LOD scores: Z_{HET} = maximum two-point heterogeneity LOD scores. Subgroups were determined by the genotype of a randomly chosen affected sibling from each family.

This work was supported by the following grants: KO2-MH01568 and MH 55284 (to J. Piven), MH55135 (to S.E.F.), 5K21-MH01338, K02-MH01432, and MH 52841 (to V.J.V.), K08-MH01541 and K08-MH62123-01 (to T.H.W.).

REFERENCES

Ashley-Koch A, Wolpert CM, Menold MM, Zaeem L, Basu S, Donnelly SL, Ravan SA, Powell CM, Qumsiyeh MB, Aylsworth AS, Vance GR, Cuccaro ML, Pericak-Vance MA. 1999. Genetic studies of autistic disorder and chromosome 7. Genomics 61:227-236.

Bassam BJ, Caetano-Anolles G, Gresshoff PM. 1991. Fast and sensitive silver staining of DNA in polyacrylamide gels. Anal Biochem 196:80-83.

Cadigan KM, Nusse R. 1997. Wnt signaling: a common theme in animal development. Genes Dev 11:3286-3305.

Chugani DC, Muzik O, Rothermel R, Behen M, Chakraborty P, Mangner T, da Silva EA, Chugani HT. 1997. Altered serotonin synthesis in the dentatothalamocortical pathway in autistic boys. Ann Neurol 42:666-669.

Clerget-Darpoux F, Bonaiti-Pellie C, Hochez J. 1986. Effects of misspecifying genetic parameters in lod score analysis. Biometrics 42:393-399.

Collaborative Linkage Study of Autism. 1999. An autosomal genomic screen for autism. Am J Med Genet (Neuropsychiatr Genet) 88:609-615.

Ellsworth RE, Jamison DC, Touchman JW, Chissoe SL, Braden Maduro VV, Bouffard GG, Dietrich NL, Beckstrom-Sternberg SM, Iyer LM, Weintraub LA, Cotton M, Courtney L, Edwards J, Maupin R, Ozersky P, Rohlfing T, Wohldmann P, Miner T, Kemp K, Kramer J, Korf I, Pepin K, Antonacci-Fulton L, Fulton RS, Green D, et al. 2000. Comparative genomic sequence analysis of the human and mouse cystic fibrosis transmembrane conductance regulator genes. Proc Natl Acad Sci USA 97:1172-1177.

Elston RC. 1989. Man bites dog? the validity of maximizing lod scores to determine mode of inheritance. Am J Med Genet 34:487-488.

Folstein SE. 2000. Autism LOD on chromosome 7q was increased subsetting the sample on language acquisition. Am J Hum Genet 67:1944.

Folstein SE, Mankoski RE. 2000. Chromosome 7q: where autism meets language disorder? Am J Hum Genet 67:278-281.

Fougerousse F, Bullen P, Herasse M, Lindsay S, Richard I, Wilson D, Suel L, Durand M, Robson S, Abitbol M, Beckmann JS, Strachan T. 2000. Human-mouse differences in the embryonic expression patterns of developmental control genes and disease genes. Hum Mol Genet 9:165-173.

Gerhart J. 1999. 1998 Warkany lecture: signaling pathways in development. Teratology 60:226-239.

Gillberg C. 1993. Autism and related behaviours. J Intellect Disabil Res 37:343-372.

Greenberg DA. 1989. Inferring mode of inheritance by comparison of lod scores. Am J Med Genet 34:480-486.

Greenberg DA. 1993. Linkage analysis of "necessary" disease loci versus "susceptibility" loci. Am J Hum Genet 52:135-143.

Hauptmann G, Gerster T. 2000. Regulatory gene expression patterns reveal transverse and longitudinal subdivisions of the embryonic zebrafish forebrain. Mech Dev 91:105-118.

Hodge SE. 1993. Linkage analysis versus association analysis: distinguishing between two models that explain disease-marker associations. Am J Hum Genet 53:367-384.

Horikawa Y, Oda N, Cox NJ, Li X, Orho-Melander M, Hara M, Hinokio Y, Lindner TH, Mashima H, Schwarz PE, del Bosque-Plata L, Oda Y, Yoshiuchi I, Colilla S, Polonsky KS, Wei S, Concannon P, Iwasaki N, Schulze J, Baier LJ, Bogardus C, Groop L, Boerwinkle E, Hanis CL, Bell GI. 2000. Genetic variation in the gene encoding calpain-10 is associated with type 2 diabetes mellitus. Nat Genet 26:163-175.

International Molecular Genetic Study of Autism Consortium. 1998. A full genome screen for autism with evidence for linkage to a region on chromosome 7q. Hum Mol Genet 7:571-578.

Lai CS, Fisher SE, Hurst JA, Levy ER, Hodgson S, Fox M, Jeremiah S, Povey S, Jamison DC, Green ED, Vargha-Khadem F, Monaco AP. 2000. The SPCH1 region on human 7q31: genomic characterization of the

critical interval and localization of translocations associated with speech and language disorder. Am J Hum Genet 67:357-368.

Landesman Y, Sokol SY. 1997. Xwnt-2b is a novel axis-inducing Xenopus Wnt, which is expressed in embryonic brain. Mech Dev 63:199-209.

Lijam N, Paylor R, McDonald MP, Crawley JN, Deng CX, Herrup K, Stevens KE, Maccaferri G, McBain CJ, Sussman DJ, Wynshaw-Boris A. 1997. Social interaction and sensorimotor gating abnormalities in mice lacking Dvl1. Cell 90:895-905.

McMahon JA, McMahon AP. 1989. Nucleotide sequence, chromosomal localization and developmental expression of the mouse int-1-related gene. Development 107:643-650.

Muller RA, Chugani DC, Behen ME, Rothermel RD, Muzik O, Chakraborty PK, Chugani HT. 1998. Impairment of dentato-thalamo-cortical pathway in autistic men: language activation data from positron emission tomography. Neurosci Lett 245:1-4.

Philippe A, Martinez M, Guilloud-Bataille M, Gillberg C, Rastam M, Sponheim E, Coleman M, Zappella M, Aschauer H, van ML, Penet C, Feingold J, Brice A, Leboyer M. 1999. Genome-wide scan for autism susceptibility genes. Paris autism research international sibpair study. Hum Mol Genet 8:805-812.

Pickles A, Bolton P, Macdonald H, Bailey A, Le CA, Sim CH, Rutter M. 1995. Latent-class analysis of recurrence risks for complex phenotypes with selection and measurement error: a twin and family history study of autism. Am J Hum Genet 57:717-726.

Piven J, Palmer P, Landa R, Santangelo S, Jacobi D, Childress D. 1997. Personality and language characteristics in parents from multiple-incidence autism families. Am J Med Genet (Neuropsychiatr Genet) 74:398-411.

Risch N, Spiker D, Lotspeich L, Nouri N, Hinds D, Hallmayer J, Kalaydjieva L, McCague P, Dimiceli S, Pitts T, Nguyen L, Yang J, Harper C, Thorpe D, Vermeer S, Young H, Hebert J, Lin A, Ferguson J, Chiotti C, Wiese-Slater S, Rogers T, Salmon B, Nicholas P, Myers RM. 1999. A genomic screen of autism: evidence for a multilocus etiology. Am J Hum Genet 65:493-507.

Rutter M, Bailey A, Bolton P, Le Couteur A. 1993. Autism: syndrome definition and possible genetic mechanisms. In: Baron-Cohen S, H. T-F, D. C, editors. Nature, nurture, and psychology. Washington, DC: APA Books. p 269-284.

Sultana R, Yu J, Raskind W, Disteche C, de La Barra Monsalvo F, Villacres E. 1999. Cloning of a candidate gene (ARG1) from the breakpoint of t(7;20) in an autistic twin pair. Am J Hum Genet 65 (suppl):A44.

Swiderski RE, Ying L, Cassell MD, Alward WL, Stone EM, Sheffield VC. 1999. Expression pattern and in situ localization of the mouse homologue of the human MYOC (GLC1A) gene in adult brain. Brain Res Mol Brain Res 68:64-72.

Szatmari P, Jones MB, Zwaigenbaum L, MacLean JE. 1998. Genetics of autism: overview and new directions. J Autism Dev Disord 28:351-368.

Szatmari P. 1999. Heterogeneity and the genetics of autism. J Psychiatry Neurosci 24:159-165.

Tomblin JB, Nishimura C, Zhang X, Murray JC. 1998. Association of developmental language impariment with loci at 7q3. Am J Hum Genet 63 (suppl):A312. .

Uusitalo M, Heikkila M, Vainio S. 1999. Molecular genetic studies of Wnt signaling in the mouse. Exp Cell Res 253:336-348.

Vieland VJ, Hodge SE. 1996. The problem of ascertainment for linkage analysis. Am J Hum Genet 58:1072-1084.

Vincent JB, Herbrick JA, Gurling HM, Bolton PF, Roberts W, Scherer SW. 2000. Identification of a novel gene on chromosome 7q31 that is interrupted by a translocation breakpoint in an autistic individual. Am J Hum Genet 67:510-514.

Wainwright BJ, Scambler PJ, Stanier P, Watson EK, Bell G, Wicking C, Estivill X, Courtney M, Boue A, Pedersen PS, et al. 1988. Isolation of a human gene with protein sequence similarity to human and murine int-1 and the Drosophila segment polarity mutant wingless. EMBO J 7:1743-1748.

Warburton P, Baird G, Chen W, Morris K, Jacobs BW, Hodgson S, Docherty Z. 2000. Support for linkage of autism and specific language impairment to 7q3 from two chromosome rearrangements involving band 7q31. Am J Med Genet (Neuropsychiatr Genet) 96:228-234.

Wassink TH, Piven J. 2000. The Molecular Genetics of Autism. Curr Psychiatry Rep 2:170-175.

Wei J, Hemmings GP. 2000. The NOTCH4 locus is associated with susceptibility to schizophrenia. Nat Genet 25:376-377.

NeuroReport 10, 1647–1651 (1999)

The neuroanatomy of autism: a voxel-based whole brain analysis of structural scans

Frances Abell, Michael Krams,[1]
John Ashburner,[1]
Richard Passingham,[2] Karl Friston,[1]
Richard Frackowiak,[1]
Francesca Happé,[3] Chris Frith[1]
and Uta Frith[CA]

Institute of Cognitive Neuroscience and
Department of Psychology, UCL, 17 Queen
Square, London WC1B 3AR; [1]Wellcome
Department of Cognitive Neurology, Institute of
Neurology, UCL, 12 Queen Square, London WC1N
3BG; [2]Department of Experimental Psychology,
University of Oxford, South Parks Road, Oxford;
[3]SGDP Institute of Psychiatry, 111 Denmark Hill,
London SE5 8AF, UK

[CA]Corresponding Author

Introduction

Autism is a biologically based disorder with a behavioral definition, spanning a wide range of manifestations and showing characteristic impairments in social communication [1]. While the majority of patients suffer from intellectual retardation and often have little or no useful language, explorations of the cognitive impairments in autism have focused on high-functioning individuals, in whom general intellectual and linguistic impairment is not a contributory factor [2]. High-functioning individuals, often labeled as having Asperger syndrome, appear to suffer from the relatively subtle developmental consequences of a cognitive deficit in 'theory of mind', a deficit that accounts well for the more conspicuous social impairments of children with severe forms of autism.

Recently, a PET scan study contrasted tasks where reasoning about other minds and the attribution of mental states is essential with tasks where it is not [3]. A circumscribed region on the border of medial frontal cortex and anterior cingulate was found to be specifically active for theory of mind tasks in normal volunteers but was significantly less active in individuals with Asperger syndrome. However, little is known about the link between this functional deficit and the underlying neuroanatomy.

The evidence from histopathological studies suggests abnormalities in the limbic system and in the cerebellum, in both low- and high-functioning patients with autistic disorder [4,5]. Reduced numbers of Purkinje cells in the cerebellum, reduced neuronal cell size and increased cell packing density have been identified in the hippocampal complex, subiculum, entorhinal cortex, amygdala, mamillary body, medial septal nucleus and anterior cingulate gyrus. The limbic abnormalities have been related to lesion studies in primates where removal of the amygdala results in decreases in affiliative behavior, social communication and emotional response to other animals [6]. Neonatal lesions of amygdala and hippocampus in monkeys produce a pattern of social withdrawal that has led to an animal model for autism [7]. In humans, amygdala damage has been found to cause abnormal affect, impaired face recog-

123

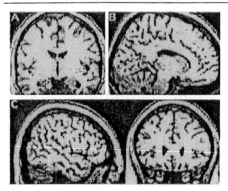

FIG. 2. Areas with significant differences of relative grey matter volume at *p* < 0.001, superimposed onto the standard template. (A) Left amygdala/peri-amygdaloid cortex (−14, −5, −28): increased relative grey matter volume in the autism group (coronal cut). (B) Right paracingulate sulcus (−14, +50, +22): decreased relative grey matter volume in the autism group (sagittal cut). (C) Left inferior frontal gyrus BA 45 (−49, +26, +5): decreased relative grey matter volume in the autism group (sagittal and coronal cut).

emotional significance, and the connections with the frontal lobe (ventral and orbital frontal cortex and anterior cingulate cortex) provide pathways through which mental states, such as emotions, can be monitored and modulated. The abnormalities in the cerebellum, which relate to previous anatomical studies of autism [5], may have to be accounted for separately, as they do not seem to be part of this amygdala-centered system.

The same areas that differentiated the present groups, whether in terms of increased or reduced relative volume, have shown increased cell packing density in post-mortem studies of seven autistic brains [4], including in particular, amygdala, anterior cingulate and cerebellum. The medial frontal focus in the anterior cingulate region was close to the focus found in the PET study of theory of mind by Happé *et al.* [3]. Thus the same areas have been highlighted in independent studies using entirely unrelated measurement techniques.

Since impairments of social communication, and specifically deficits in the ability to attribute mental states to self and others, can be seen as the common denominator across the spectrum of autistic disorders [2], we propose that the neural system identified in the present study is critical to self- and other-awareness. The anterior cingulate in particular is known to be implicated in the awareness of mental states and in the reportable experience of emotions [20]. The set of brain areas showing group differences in the present study fits well with the 'social brain' delineated on the basis of animal and human neuropsychological studies [6]. According to this model, the social behavior required in two-way

communication is critically dependent on a specialized circuit centered on the amygdala, involving orbital frontal cortex, anterior cingulate and temporal pole cortex.

We cannot of course interpret increases and decreases of relative volumes of grey matter as mapping onto absolute increases or decreases of brain tissue, since this was not measured directly. It is not clear what relationship should be expected between cell packing density and grey matter volume. A possible explanation of greater volume of grey matter would be a failure of programmed cell death (apoptosis) in certain regions [21]. Speculatively, we suggest that the anatomical abnormalities found correspond to functional abnormalities. The anterior (executive) components of the amygdala-centered system may underlie poor monitoring and control of mental states. The posterior (sensory) components of the system may underlie the often reported overwhelming sensory overload and high anxiety levels in autism. For example, abnormality in the amygdala/peri-amygdaloid cortex might lead fear conditioning to be more swiftly established and less amenable to extinction in autism. Abnormally fast classical eye-blink conditioning in autism has indeed been shown [22]. Further, as the system pinpointed is particularly rich in opioid receptors, and since abnormalities in opioid metabolism have been found in autism [23], it is possible that some further symptoms (e.g. self-injury, high pain threshold, self-reports of sensory overload) can also be illuminated.

Conclusion

Our results and those of previous studies converge on a distributed system which shows structural abnormalities in individuals with autism. This system, which appears to be centered on the amygdala, is strongly implicated in emotional and social learning and, more speculatively, self-awareness. One theoretical formulation of brain plasticity posits a central role for the amygdala that relates directly to the current findings [24]. According to this theory, the amygdala integrates highly processed perceptual inputs that have value or salience. This synthesis is then used to modulate or consolidate adaptive changes in synaptic efficacy throughout the brain via its vicarious projections to the ascending modulatory neurotransmitter systems. A critical component of this theory is that the amygdala is responsible for consolidating its own inputs. This model suggests that a neurodevelopmental abnormality involving the amygdala, or its targets, would be sufficient to explain the impairments in emotional and social learning in autism, and can account for morphological abnormalities at the sources of amygdala inputs.

Although highly speculative, there is compelling convergence among the neuropsychological deficits of autism, the functional anatomy of an amygdala centered system, and finally, the neuroanatomical correlates of self-awareness identified by this work.

References

1. *Diagnostic and Statistical Manual of Mental Disorders*, 4th edn (DSM-IV). Washington, DC: American Psychiatric Association, 1994.
2. Happé F and Frith U. *Brain* **119**, 1377–1400 (1996).
3. Happé F, Ehlers S, Fletcher P *et al*. *NeuroReport* **8**, 197–201 (1996).
4. Bauman ML and Kemper TL. Neuroanatomic observations of the brain in autism. In: Bauman ML and Kemper TL, eds. *The Neurobiology of Autism*. Baltimore: Johns Hopkins Press, 1994: 119–145.
5. Courchesne E, Townsend J and Saitoh O. *Neurology* **44**, 214–223 (1994).
6. Kling SL and Brothers L. The amygdala and social behaviour. In: Aggleton J, ed. *The Amygdala: Neurobiological Aspects of Emotion, Memory and Mental Dysfunction*. New York: Wiley-Liss, 1992: 353–377.
7. Bachevalier J. The contribution of medial temporal lobe structures in infantile autism: A neuro-behavioural study in primates. In: Bauman ML and Kemper TL, eds. *The Neurobiology of Autism*. Baltimore: Johns Hopkins Press, 1994: 146–169.
8. Cahill L, Babinsky R, Markowitsch HJ *et al*. *Nature* **377**, 295–296 (1995).
9. Hoon AH and Reiss AL. *Dev Med Child Neurol* **34**, 252–259 (1992).
10. Bolton P and Griffiths P. *Lancet* **349**, 392–395 (1997).
11. Ammons RB and Ammons CH. *The Quick test*. Missouri: Psychological Test Specialists, 1962.
12. Raven J. *Raven's Advanced Progressive Matrices*. Windsor: NFER-Nelson, 1994.
13. Vargha-Khadem F, Watkins KE, Price C *et al*. *Proc Natl Acad Sci USA* **95**, 12695–12700 (1998).
14. Ashburner J and Friston KJ. *NeuroImage* **6**, 209–217 (1997).
15. Friston KJ, Ashburner J, Frith CD *et al*. *Hum Brain Mapp* **3**, 165–189 (1995).
16. Talairach J and Tournoux P. *A Co-planar Stereotaxic Atlas of the Human Brain*. Stuttgart: Thieme, 1988.
17. Evans AC, Collins DL, Mills SR *et al*. *IEEE Nucl Sci Symp Med Imag Conf* 1813–1817 (1993).
18. Friston KJ, Holmes AP, Worsley KJ *et al*. *Hum Brain Mapp* **3**, 189–210 (1995). (http://www.fil.ion.ucl.ac.uk/spm).
19. Amaral D, Price JL, Pitkanen A *et al*. Anatomical organisation of the primate amygdaloid cortex. In: Aggleton J, ed. *The Amygdala: Neurobiological Aspects of Emotion, Memory and Mental Dysfunction*. New York: Wiley-Liss, 1992: 1–66.
20. Lane RD, Fink GR, Chua PML *et al*. *NeuroReport* **8**, 3969–3972 (1997).
21. Margolis RL, Chuang DM and Post RM. *Biol Psychiat* **35**, 946–56 (1994).
22. Sears LL, Finn PR and Steinmetz JE. *J Autism Dev Disord* **24**, 737–51 (1994).
23. Gillberg C. *Dev Med Child Neurol* **37**, 239–45 (1995).
24. Friston KJ, Tononi KG, Reeke GN Jr *et al*. *Neuroscience* **39**, 229–243 (1994).

ACKNOWLEDGEMENTS: This research was funded by the Wellcome Trust and the Medical Research Council.

**Received 17 March 1999;
accepted 30 March 1999**

125

Abnormal Processing of Social Information from Faces in Autism

Ralph Adolphs, Lonnie Sears, and Joseph Piven

Abstract

■ Autism has been thought to be characterized, in part, by dysfunction in emotional and social cognition, but the pathology of the underlying processes and their neural substrates remain poorly understood. Several studies have hypothesized that abnormal amygdala function may account for some of the impairments seen in autism, specifically, impaired recognition of socially relevant information from faces. We explored this issue in eight high-functioning subjects with autism in four experiments that assessed recognition of emotional and social information, primarily from faces. All tasks used were identical to those previously used in studies of subjects with bilateral amygdala damage, permitting direct comparisons. All subjects with autism made abnormal social judgments regarding the trustworthiness of faces; however, all were able to make normal social judgments from lexical stimuli, and all had a normal ability to perceptually discriminate the stimuli. Overall, these data from subjects with autism show some parallels to those from neurological subjects with focal amygdala damage. We suggest that amygdala dysfunction in autism might contribute to an impaired ability to link visual perception of socially relevant stimuli with retrieval of social knowledge and with elicitation of social behavior. ■

INTRODUCTION

Autism is a developmental neuropsychiatric syndrome defined by deficits in social behavior and communication, and by stereotyped, repetitive behaviors, which show a characteristic course. Although most autistic subjects show impairments in multiple cognitive domains, there is some evidence that high-functioning autism may be a disorder that disproportionately affects those aspects of cognition most relevant to social functioning. The theoretical support for this idea comes from the hypothesis that social cognition may be functionally modular, in the sense that it can be, in principle, dissociated from other aspects of cognition, and in the sense that relatively dedicated neural systems may have evolved to subserve some of its component processes (Karmiloff-Smith, Bellugi, Klima, Grant, & Baron-Cohen, 1995; see also for a review Adolphs, 1999). The empirical support for this idea comes from findings that suggest subjects with autism can be impaired relatively selectively on tasks that assess their knowledge of other people's mental states, with relative sparing of other perceptual and cognitive abilities (see for a review Baron-Cohen, 1995).

In regard to processing social information, high-functioning subjects with autism (we use the term "high-functioning autism" interchangeably with "Asperger Syndrome") show relatively selective impairments in recognizing higher-order mental states from faces. Baron-Cohen, Wheelwright, and Jolliffe (1997) found that higher-order social/mental states, which were signalled primarily by the eyes (e.g., states such as "flirtatiousness"), were not recognized normally by subjects with high-functioning autism. However, the subjects in that study were readily able to recognize the facial expression of other basic emotions such as happiness (cf. also Baron-Cohen, Spitz, & Cross, 1993). These findings from tasks involving recognition of social and emotional information from faces show some parallels to a variety of other tasks that have been used to assess the processes by which we normally attribute mental states to other individuals. In particular, Baron-Cohen (1995) and others (Leslie, 1987) have argued that the social impairments seen in autism result in large part from an impaired ability to use a "theory of mind" mechanism. The details of this latter hypothesis are contentious, and in the present paper, we do not wish to take any particular stance on that issue.

The neurobiological basis for autism is a topic of intense recent research investigations (Piven, 1997). It remains unclear to what extent the abnormal processing of social and emotional information in subjects with autism could be due, at least in part, to dysfunction in specific limbic neural structures, such as the amygdala. The proposal that amygdala pathology could contribute to some of the neuropsychological impairments in social and emotional processing seen in autism (Baron-Cohen et al., 2000) is supported by the finding that subjects

University of Iowa

Journal of Cognitive Neuroscience 13:2, pp. 232–240

with damage to the amygdala also show abnormal emotional and social processing. In particular, several studies using either subjects with amygdala lesions (Broks et al., 1998; Adolphs, Tranel, Damasio, & Damasio, 1994; Adolphs et al., 1999), or using functional imaging of the amygdala in normal individuals (Breiter et al., 1996; Morris et al., 1996), have demonstrated that the amygdala is important for recognition of certain emotions, such as fear, from facial expressions, and that it is also important for making more complex social judgments about faces, such as their perceived trustworthiness (Adolphs, Tranel, & Damasio, 1998). Further support for a possible link between amygdala dysfunction and autism is provided by a recent functional imaging study, which showed that the amygdala is activated in normal individuals, but not in subjects with autism, on a task in which autistic subjects are impaired (Baron-Cohen et al., 1999; see also Baron-Cohen et al., 2000).

In addition to these investigations of the functions of the human amygdala, Bauman and Kemper (1985) found morphological abnormalities in the amygdalas of autistic subjects, and structural MRI studies have also reported differences between amygdala volume in high-functioning autistic subjects compared to normal controls (Abell et al., 1999). A direct functional role for the amygdala has been proposed from animal studies: Experimental lesions of the amygdala in young monkeys (Bachevalier, 1991) result in social impairments that bear some resemblance to the abnormal behavior seen in human autism. All these disparate findings suggest the hypothesis that impaired emotional and social cognition in autism may be, in part, caused by amygdala dysfunction (Baron-Cohen et al., 2000; Damasio & Maurer, 1978). However, to date, no investigations have specifically compared subjects with amygdala lesions to subjects with autism on the same tasks.

The present study provides such a direct comparison. We used four experimental tasks to assess the recognition of emotional and social information from faces, as well as from lexical stimuli, in eight high-functioning subjects diagnosed with autism. All of the tasks were identical in both format and in stimuli to tasks previously published on subjects with amygdala lesions. Data from subjects with autism were compared to those from normal controls and from subjects with bilateral amygdala damage. All data from normal subjects and from subjects with bilateral amygdala damage have been published previously in several reports (Adolphs et al., 1994; Adolphs, Tranel, Damasio, & Damasio, 1995; Adolphs et al., 1998, 1999). We here provide summaries of the findings from these prior studies for the purpose of direct comparisons with autistic subjects.

Due to time and testing constraints, not all of the eight subjects participated on all tasks; details on all subjects are provided in Tables 1 and 2. Taken together, the data permit a detailed investigation of how emotional and social stimuli are processed by subjects with autism, and further allow direct comparisons with the performances on the same tasks given by neurological patients with focal brain damage, with a special emphasis on the amygdala.

RESULTS

Experiment 1: Discriminating the Intensity of Facial Emotion (Jansari, Tranel, & Adolphs, 2000; Adolphs et al., 1998)

Subjects with autism did not have any visuoperceptual impairments in processing faces. Their abilities to discriminate faces on the basis of identity were in the normal range on a standard neuropsychological test (the Benton Facial Recognition Task; Benton, Hamsher, Varney, & Spreen, 1983; Table 1). Similarly, their ability

Table 1. Demographic and Background Neuropsychological Information on Participants with Autism

					Autism Diagnostic Interview		
ID No.	Age	PIQ	VIQ	Benton	Social	Communication	Repetitive
1	21	130	108	71	18	8	5
2	17	120	90	71	27	21	8
4	28	115	90	90	38	24	9
5	24	117	88	90	25	13	4
6	21	109	127	71	24	12	7
7	21	91	119	22	21	13	9
8	19	93	84	85	15	15	5
10	18	91	96	22	12	14	4

Subscale scores are shown for the Autism Diagnostic Interview (LeCouteur et al., 1989); percentiles for the Benton Facial Recognition Task (Benton et al., 1983), a measure of the ability to discriminate face identity. IQ scores are from the WAIS-R or WISC-R.

Table 2. Summary of Sample Sizes, Ages, and IQs for the Different Subject Groups and Experiments

		Autistic	Normal	Amygdala
N	Experiment 1	6	28	3
	Experiment 2	7	18	8
	Experiment 3	8	47	3
	Experiment 4	5	20	3
Age	Experiment 1	22±3	43±16	47±18
	Experiment 2	21±4	56±16	53±17
	Experiment 3	21±4	19±1	47±18
	Experiment 4	23±3	19±1	47±18
IQ	Experiment 1	106±16	–	98±9
	Experiment 2	102±15	–	–
	Experiment 3	104±15	–	98±9
	Experiment 4	109±15	–	98±9

to discriminate faces on the basis of the intensity of emotional expression (Experiment 1; Figure 1) did not differ from normal controls. No autistic subject was more than two SD below the normal mean in the accuracy with which they discriminated very faint morphs of emotional facial expressions from neutral faces. These findings are particularly relevant, since they demonstrate normal discrimination for the same

class of stimuli that we used in further tasks reported below.

Experiment 2. Recognition of Basic Emotions from Facial Expressions (Adolphs et al., 1994, 1995, 1999)

Most autistic subjects tested gave normal ratings to facial expressions of happiness, surprise, anger, disgust, sadness, and fear (Figure 2). Their performances on this task were in general within the range given by normal subjects (Figure 2, gray bars). As a group, the performance of subjects with autism ($n = 7$) was better on all emotions than were the performances of subjects with bilateral amygdala damage ($n = 8$). A repeated-measures ANOVA with a within-subjects factor of emotion type (happy, surprised, afraid, angry, disgusted, or sad) and a between-subjects factor of subject group (autistic, amygdala damage, normal control) revealed significant effects of both emotion [$F(5) = 18$; $p < .0001$] and subject group [$F(2) = 5.1$; $p < .01$], but no interaction between the two.

There were some provocative individual performances. Notably, one of the autistic subjects (Subject

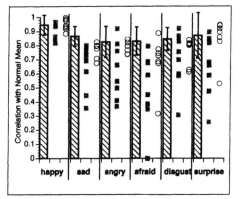

Figure 2. Recognition of basic emotions in facial expressions. Shown are correlations between ratings given by autistic subjects with mean normal ratings (circles), compared to the same correlation measures for eight subjects with bilateral amygdala damage (gray squares) and 18 normal controls (bars, means ± SD). Thus, correlations near 1 correspond to a normal rating profile given to that emotion, whereas low correlations correspond to an abnormal rating profile. Each emotion category consisted of six face stimuli depicting that emotion. While most autistic subjects performed normally, one subject gave a severely impaired performance when rating faces of fear, disgust, and surprise; and another subject gave an impaired performance when rating faces of disgust, a pattern of impairment similar to that seen in subjects with bilateral amygdala damage. Data for subjects with bilateral amygdala damage are from Adolphs et al. (1999), and details regarding the method of analysis can be found in Adolphs et al. (1995).

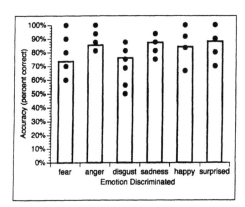

Figure 1. Discrimination of emotional facial expressions. Accuracy in discriminating morphs of the six basic emotions in facial expressions is shown as % correct on a two-alternative forced-choice task (50% is chance), for six autistic subjects (filled circles) compared to the mean of 28 normal controls (bars). Every autistic subject performed within two SD of the control mean.

7) gave very impaired performances when rating faces expressing fear, disgust, and surprise, a pattern of impairment that is similar to that seen in some subjects with bilateral amygdala damage. Another subject (Subject 2) also yielded abnormally low scores when rating disgust. The pattern of impaired recognition of fear, disgust, and surprise, with entirely normal recognition of happiness, is precisely what has been reported for subjects with bilateral amygdala damage (Adolphs, et al., 1999).

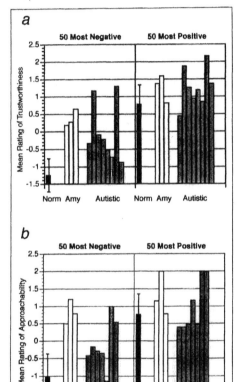

a

Figure 3. Ratings of (a) trustworthiness and (b) approachability from 100 unfamiliar faces. Shown are mean ratings of the 50 faces that normally receive the most negative ratings (left half of each split graph), and the 50 faces that normally receive the most positive ratings (right half of each split graph). Solid black bars are the means (±SD) data from 47 normal controls; three white bars are data from three individual subjects with bilateral amygdala damage; gray bars are individual data from autistic subjects. All data except for the data from autistic subjects are from Adolphs et al. (1998). Norm = Normal; Amy = Amygdala.

Experiment 3. Social Judgment of Faces (Bellugi, Adolphs, Cassady, & Chiles, 1999; Adolphs et al., 1998)

We analyzed data from these tasks separately in regard to those 50 stimuli that normally receive the most negative ratings, and those 50 stimuli that normally receive the most positive ratings. These are shown as the split graphs in Figure 3.

As a group, autistic subjects tended to give abnormally positive ratings to those 50 faces that normally receive the most negative ratings and there were some autistic subjects who gave highly abnormal ratings that were more positive than those given by any normal subject, as is also the case in subjects with bilateral amygdala damage. In particular, when rating that half of the stimuli that normally receive the most negative ratings with respect to trustworthiness (left half of Figure 3a), every autistic subject gave a mean rating that was more positive than the mean normal rating, and subjects 2 and 8 gave highly abnormally positive ratings of trustworthiness, a pattern previously reported for subjects with bilateral amygdala damage. Similarly, for ratings of approachability (Figure 3b), all but one of the autistic subjects gave ratings that were more positive than the mean control rating, and subjects 8 and 10 gave abnormally positive ratings to those half of the stimuli that normally receive the most negative ratings.

Despite the small sample sizes, some of these effects were statistically significant. When examining those 50 faces that normally receive the most negative trustworthiness ratings, Mann–Whitney U tests revealed that both autistic subjects (corrected $p < .005$) and subjects with bilateral amygdala damage (corrected $p < .01$; all ps are Bonferroni-corrected for multiple comparisons) gave higher ratings than did normal controls; but ratings given by autistic subjects did not differ significantly from those given by subjects with bilateral amygdala damage (corrected $p > .8$). For approachability ratings of the 50 faces that normally receive the most negative ratings, ratings given by autistic subjects did not differ significantly from either those given by subjects with bilateral amygdala damage (corrected $p > .3$) or those given by normal controls (corrected $p > .9$).

Experiment 4. Social Judgment from Lexical Stimuli (Adolphs et al., 1998)

When autistic subjects were given adjectives that describe personality attributes, they did not differ from normals in rating their likeability of those attributes (Mann–Whitney U test comparing autistic subjects to normal controls; $p > .6$). In fact, ratings given by autistic subjects were highly correlated with ratings given by normal control subjects (Spearman rank correlations: Spearman $\rho = 0.71$–0.90; all ps $< .0001$).

When given short biographies that described people, autistic subjects likewise gave normal ratings ($p > .8$; Mann–Whitney U test) that correlated significantly with those given by normal controls (Spearman ρ: 0.65–0.84; all $ps < .005$). Both these above findings are very similar to those previously reported for subjects with bilateral amygdala damage, who also perform entirely normally in their social judgments of adjectives and biographies (Adolphs et al., 1998).

DISCUSSION

The findings of the present study can be summarized as follows. First, subjects with autism did not have any visuoperceptual impairments in discriminating human faces, either on the basis of identity or on the basis of emotional expression. These data make it unlikely that the impairments discussed below could be attributable to a simple perceptual impairment in processing the stimuli. In this regard, the findings from subjects with autism parallel those from subjects with focal damage to limbic structures important to social cognition, such as the amygdala and the orbitofrontal cortices: Such lesion patients also show a normal visuoperception of faces, despite impairments in linking visual percepts to the social and emotional information that such stimuli might signal (Adolphs et al., 1995; Damasio, 1994).

Second, while the findings on the other tasks show a large variance, there is an overall pattern, of which some, but not all, components bear similarity to what has been reported in subjects with bilateral amygdala damage. (a) Unlike subjects with bilateral amygdala damage, subjects with autism generally performed normally in their recognition of basic emotions from facial expressions. However, one of the subjects with autism showed impaired recognition of certain negative emotions from human facial expressions, notably fear, disgust, and surprise, a pattern of impaired emotion recognition that is also seen in some subjects with bilateral amygdala damage. (b) Like subjects with bilateral amygdala damage, autistic subjects gave ratings of trustworthiness that were more positive than the mean normal ratings, when judging those faces that normally receive the most negative ratings. Several autistic subjects gave highly abnormally positive ratings of trustworthiness and of approachability to unfamiliar faces. These findings are the most striking in our paper, as three out of the three subjects with bilateral amygdala damage gave abnormally positive ratings of trustworthiness, as did eight out of the eight subjects with autism. (c) Autistic subjects gave normal social judgments when the stimuli were lexical, as did subjects with bilateral amygdala damage.

While our results must be taken as preliminary, given the small sample sizes, they nonetheless suggest a pattern that is consistent with the hypothesis of amygdala dysfunction in a subset of subjects with autism. Taken together,

the data suggest that some of the same processes that are impaired in subjects with bilateral amygdala damage may also be dysfunctional in some subjects with autism. The impairment we report appears to be most striking (and most similar to that reported in subjects with bilateral amygdala damage) for higher-level social judgments from faces (such as trustworthiness judgments), but not for recognizing basic emotions from faces.

It is worth reiterating that the performances given by subjects with autism were quite heterogeneous: Some subjects were impaired on some tasks, whereas other subjects were impaired on different tasks. An important future goal will be to investigate whether this heterogeneity reflects differences between subjects (e.g., some subjects had a particular brain pathology, and others not) or if it reflects heterogeneity in performances within a single subject. It is possible that autistic subjects, like subjects with bilateral amygdala damage (Adolphs et al., 1999) give variable performances, an issue that could be addressed with future retesting of the same subjects on the same tasks.

The overall pattern of results points towards a disproportionate impairment in those processes that subserve higher-level social cognition, with relative sparing of perceptual processing of faces, and of the recognition of basic emotions. The data are thus consistent with the idea that autistic subjects are able to form normal perceptual representations of faces (Experiment 1), and that they are able to retrieve knowledge regarding the basic emotion expressed (Experiment 2), but that they fail to link perception of the face to the social judgments called for in our task (Experiment 3)—possibly either because they cannot trigger normal retrieval of social knowledge, or because they have not acquired normal social knowledge to begin with. It is important to note that, like subjects with bilateral amygdala damage, the impaired social judgment disappears when the information is presented in a more explicit, lexical format (Experiment 4). This suggests that at least some basic social knowledge and some ability to form social judgments are intact in autism. It would appear that autism features dysfunction in those neural structures necessary to link percepts of visual, nonlexical stimuli with their social meaning, an interpretation we have previously put forth in regard to subjects with bilateral amygdala damage (Adolphs et al., 1995, 1998).

It is of interest also to compare the above findings with those from subjects with Williams Syndrome, a genetic disorder that, in some respects, presents the converse of the social impairments seen in autism (Bellugi, Lichtenberger, Mills, Galaburda, & Korenberg, 1999). Subjects with Williams Syndrome are often hypersocial, and appear unusually empathic and skilled in their social interactions, in the face of severe impairments in other cognitive domains. We recently assessed social judgment in subjects with Williams Syndrome, using identical stimuli and a similar task to the one used here (Bellugi, Adolphs, et al., 1999). In that study, subjects with Williams Syndrome showed an abnormal positive bias in their social judgments, consistent with their real-life prosocial behavior. Surprisingly, the present report also found a positive bias in subjects with autism, although from their real-life behavior one might have expected a negative bias. While entirely speculative, one possibility would thus be that subjects with Williams Syndrome and subjects with autism both share some social processing impairments in common, and, moreover, that this impairment may result in part from amygdala dysfunction.

As we pointed out above, it is quite possible that our sample of autistic subjects may have been heterogeneous with respect to underlying brain abnormalities, so that only a subset of our subjects had amygdala dysfunction, and others had autistic behavior resulting from dysfunction in structures other than the amygdala. Furthermore, we wish to stress that, while the present findings may implicate the amygdala in some of the social dysfunction seen in autism, our data say nothing about the amygdala's role in accounting for other aspects of the autistic phenotype, nor do they imply that the amygdala is the only contributor. Indeed, it seems most probable to us that the amygdala will be only one component of a distributed neural system that is dysfunctional in autism (Damasio & Maurer, 1978).

Comparisons between the present data and findings from other investigations of face processing in autism are made difficult by the differences in subject selection criteria, and differences in stimuli and procedures amongst studies. Furthermore, a limitation of the present study is the relatively small sample size. The literature on face processing in autism suggests a key abnormal component in regard to how individual features of faces are processed: While normal subjects tend to process faces holistically, there is some evidence that subjects with autism process them in a more analytical, feature-based fashion, and attend to different features than normals would (Hobson, Ouston, & Lee, 1988b; Langdell, 1978). Autistic subjects were impaired in a task of facial emotion matching, when the faces to be matched were presented at separate times rather than concurrently, thus making feature-based strategies of comparison difficult, suggesting that holistic processing of facial emotion is abnormal in autism (Celani, Battacchi, & Arcidiacono, 1999). Other studies have reported impairments in perceiving identity (Boucher, Lewis, & Collis, 1998) or emotion (Capps, Yirmiya, & Sigman, 1992; Hobson, Ouston, & Lee, 1988a, Hobson, Ouston, & Lee, 1989) from faces in autistic subjects, and a case study of Asperger Syndrome reported relatively impaired recognition of specific emotions (anger and disgust) in facial expressions (Ellis & Leafhead, 1996). No study to date has carried out such investigations using the same experimental tasks that were used in the present paper.

Faces, as a close second possibly only to language, convey critical social information and are a key channel for social communication. The ability to use the face as a channel for social communication develops early in infancy, and was already noted as an apparent defect in subjects with autism by Kanner (1943). Despite the general consensus that autistic subjects do not process social and emotional information from faces normally, it has been difficult to ascertain precisely the nature of the impairment. The present study provides an additional piece of evidence, and suggests a possible set of specific processes that might be impaired in autism. Given the intact visuoperceptual discrimination of autistic subjects on our tasks, it appears plausible that early perceptual processing is intact, but that autism features an impaired ability subsequently to trigger normal retrieval of knowledge, and normal social behaviors, on the basis of the visual representations of faces. Possibly, amygdala dysfunction is one neuroanatomical correlate of this impaired mechanism, a hypothesis that will need to be tested in additional experiments with larger sample sizes, and that could be explored also with functional imaging studies of amygdala activation in autism.

METHODS

Subjects

Eight male subjects who all met DSM-IV/ICD-10 diagnostic criteria for autism participated in our studies. All subjects met the cutoff scores for autism on the Autism Diagnostic Interview (LeCouteur, Rutter, & Lord, 1989), all had verbal and performance IQs in the normal range (from WAIS-R or WISC-R), and all had a normal ability to discriminate faces of different individuals, as determined by normal performances on the Benton Facial Recognition Task. Our sample, thus, comprised a group of high-functioning autistic subjects (Table 1). All subjects were tested individually by the same experimenters in the same room.

Experimental Tasks

We used tasks that ranged from simple perceptual discrimination of emotions (Experiment 1), to recognition of the intensity of basic emotions in facial expressions (Experiment 2), to more subtle social judgments (Experiments 3 and 4). Tasks were administered in randomized order. There was no time limit for any task, and breaks were taken between and, in some cases, in the middle of tasks, as suited to particular subjects.

Experiment 1: Discriminating the Intensity of Facial Emotion

To provide a sensitive measure of the visuoperceptual ability with respect to the same class of stimuli (Ekman

& Friesen, 1976) used in some of the experimental tasks below (facial expressions of emotion), we administered a standardized two-alternative forced-choice discrimination task. Subjects were shown 80 pairs of faces. Each pair of faces was shown side-by-side, and the two faces in the pair differed in the intensity of emotion expressed. Subjects were asked to identify the face that showed the more intense emotion. The stimuli were computer-generated morphs that showed only a very faint emotion, permitting us to calculate a threshold above which subjects were able to discriminate the stimuli, and below which their performances were equivalent to chance. Six of the autistic subjects (Subjects 1, 4, 5, 6, 7, 8) participated in this task, and their data were compared to those from 28 normal subjects (Jansari et al., 2000) and from three subjects with bilateral amygdala damage (Adolphs et al., 1998).

Experiment 2: Recognition of Basic Emotions

This task has been used in several prior published reports to investigate recognition of the intensity of facial emotion following focal brain damage; (e.g., to demonstrate impaired recognition of emotion in subjects with bilateral amygdala damage; Adolphs et al., 1994, 1995, 1999). Briefly, subjects were shown 39 facial expressions of basic emotions (six instances each of happiness, surprise, fear, anger, disgust, and sadness, as well as three neutral faces) from Ekman and Friesen (1976) and asked to rate each face with respect to the intensity of each of the six basic emotions. Thus, a subject would see, e.g., a facial expression of fear, and be asked to rate that face with respect to the intensity of fear, happiness, surprise, anger, disgust, and sadness that they thought the depicted person would feel. Ratings from subjects were correlated with mean normal ratings to obtain a correlation score (Adolphs et al., 1994). Fisher Z-transforms of the correlations were used in all averaging procedures and in all parametric statistical analyses. Seven autistic subjects participated in this task (Subjects 1, 2, 4, 5, 7, 8, 10). Their scores were compared with an identical measure obtained from 18 normal control subjects, and from 8 subjects with amygdala damage (Adolphs et al., 1999).

Experiment 3: Complex Social Judgments of Faces

(a) Judgments of trustworthiness. Subjects were shown 100 faces of unfamiliar people and asked to judge how much they would trust the person, by giving a rating on a seven-point scale. The 100 stimuli had been carefully chosen so as to uniformly span the range of ratings from minimum to maximum, and so as to minimize the variance in the ratings given by normal subjects (cf. Adolphs et al., 1998). All eight autistic subjects participated in this task. Data were compared to those obtained from 47 normal controls, and to those from 3

subjects with bilateral amygdala damage (Adolphs et al., 1998).

(b) Judgments of approachability. Subjects were shown the same 100 faces as for the judgments of trustworthiness, and asked to judge how much they would like to approach the person and initiate a conversation with them if they were to meet them on the street. Seven of the autistic subjects (Subjects 1, 4, 5, 6, 7, 8, 10) participated in this task. Data were again compared to those obtained from 47 normal controls and 3 subjects with bilateral amygdala damage (Adolphs et al., 1998).

Experiment 4: Complex Social Judgments of Lexical Stimuli

(a) Words. We chose 88 adjectives that described personality attributes from a large standardized set (Anderson, 1968). We chose the words to span the range from very likeable to very dislikeable, and to exhibit maximal reliability and common usage (cf. Adolphs et al., 1998). Subjects were asked to rate on a seven-point scale how much they would like a person who exhibited the given adjective. Five of the subjects with autism (Subjects 1, 4, 5, 6, 7) participated in the task. Data were compared to those given by 20 normal controls, and could also be compared to those from three subjects with bilateral amygdala damage (Adolphs et al., 1998).

(b) Biographies. We constructed 20 short stories, which described people, containing information about the person's lifestyle and activities. Subjects were asked to rate how much they liked the individuals described by the stimuli, on a seven-point scale. Five autistic subjects participated in this task (Subjects 1, 4, 5, 7, 10). Data were compared to those given by 20 normal controls, and could also be compared to those from three subjects with bilateral amygdala damage (Adolphs et al., 1998).

Note Added in Proof

Since acceptance of our manuscript, several additional relevant studies have appeared. Critchley et al. (2000) found that high-functioning autistic subjects failed to show normal amygdala activation in response to implicit processing of emotional facial expressions. In a study that bears some similarity to ours, Howard et al. (2000) found impaired recognition of emotion from facial expressions, as well as abnormalities on structural MR images of the amygdala, in subjects with autism. A study by Grossman, Klin, Carter and Volkmar (2000) found, as we did, that high-functioning subjects with autism may not be impaired in simple recognition of basic emotions from faces, but that they are impaired on more demanding social judgments from faces; the authors proposed that autism may feature impaired emotion recognition,[1] but that high-functioning subjects may be able to compensate in part for their impairment via strategies that use verbal mediation. Taken together, these recent reports corroborate our present findings that autism may result from an impaired ability to link perception of faces to the retrieval of social knowledge, and that this impairment may result, in part, from dysfunction involving the amygdala.

Acknowledgments

We thank Jeremy Nath and Ashok Jansari for help in testing subjects. Supported in part by grants from NIMH, the Sloan Foundation, and the EJLB Foundation to R.A.

Reprint requests should be sent to: Ralph Adolphs, Department of Neurology, University of Iowa Hospitals and Clinics, 200 Hawkins Drive, Iowa City, IA 52242, USA. E-mail: ralph-adolphs@uiowa.edu.

REFERENCES

Abell, F., Krams, M., Ashburner, J., Passingham, R., Friston, K., Frackowiak, R., Happe, F., Frith, C., & Frith, U. (1999). The neuroanatomy of autism: A voxel-based whole brain analysis of structural scans. NeuroReport, 10, 1647–1651.

Adolphs, R. (1999). Social cognition and the human brain. Trends in Cognitive Sciences, 3, 469–479.

Adolphs, R., Tranel, D., & Damasio, A. R. (1998). The Human amygdala in social judgment. Nature, 393, 470–474.

Adolphs, R., Tranel, D., Damasio, H., & Damasio, A. (1994). Impaired recognition of emotion in facial expressions following bilateral damage to the human amygdala. Nature, 372, 669–672.

Adolphs, R., Tranel, D., Damasio, H., & Damasio, A. R. (1995). Fear and the human amygdala. The Journal of Neuroscience, 15, 5879–5892.

Adolphs, R., Tranel, D., Hamann, S., Young, A., Calder, A., Anderson, A., Phelps, E., & Damasio, A. R. (1999). Recognition of facial emotion in nine subjects with bilateral amygdala damage. Neuropsychologia, 37, 1111–1117.

Anderson, N. H. (1968). Likableness ratings of 555 personality-trait words. Journal of Personality and Social Psychology, 9, 272–279.

Bachevalier, J. (1991). An animal model for childhood autism: Memory loss and socioemotional disturbances following neonatal damage to the limbic system in monkeys. In C. A. Tamminga & S. C. Schulz (Eds.), Advances in neuropsychiatry and psychopharmacology, vol. 1, Schizophrenia research (pp. 129–140). New York: Raven.

Baron-Cohen, S. (1995). Mindblindness: An essay on autism and theory of mind. Cambridge: MIT Press.

Baron-Cohen, S., Ring, H. A., Bullmore, E. T., Wheelwright, S., Ashwin, C., & Williams, S. C. R. (2000). The amygdala theory of autism. Neuroscience and Biobehavioral Reviews, 24, 355–364.

Baron-Cohen, S., Ring, H. A., Wheelwright, S., Bullmore, E. T., Brammer, M. J., Simmons, A., & Williams, S. C. R. (1999). Social intelligence in the normal and autistic brain: An fMRI study. European Journal of Neuroscience, 11, 1891–1898.

Baron-Cohen, S., Spitz, A., & Cross, P. (1993). Can children with autism recognize surprise? Cognition and Emotion, 7, 507–516.

Baron-Cohen, S., Wheelwright, S., & Jolliffe, T. (1997). Is there are a "language of the eyes"? Evidence from normal adults and adults with autism or Asperger Syndrome. Visual Cognition, 4, 311–332.

Bauman, M., & Kemper, T. L. (1985). Histoanatomic observations of the brain in early infantile autism. Neurology, 35, 866–874.

Bellugi, U., Adolphs, R., Cassady, C., & Chiles, M. (1999). Towards the neural basis for hypersociability in a genetic syndrome. NeuroReport, 10, 1653–1659.

Bellugi, U., Lichtenberger, L., Mills, D., Galaburda, A., & Korenberg, J. R. (1999). Bridging cognition, the brain, and molecular genetics: Evidence from Williams syndrome. Trends in Neurosciences, 22, 197–207.

Benton, A. L., Hamsher, K., Varney, N. R., & Spreen, O. (1983). Contributions to neuropsychological assessment. New York: Oxford University Press.

Boucher, J., Lewis, V., & Collis, G. (1998). Familiar face and voice matching and recognition in children with autism. Journal of Child Psychology and Psychiatry, 39, 171–181.

Breiter, H. C., Etcoff, N. L., Whalen, P. J., Kennedy, W. A., Rauch, S. L., Buckner, R. L., Strauss, M. M., Hyman, S. E., & Rosen, B. R. (1996). Response and habituation of the human amygdala during visual processing of facial expression. Neuron, 17, 875–887.

Broks, P., Young, A. W., Maratos, E. J., Coffey, P. J., Calder, A. J., Isaac, C., Mayes, A. R., Hodges, J. R., Montaldi, D., Cezayirli, E., Roberts, N., & Hadley, D. (1998). Face processing impairments after encephalitis: Amygdala damage and recognition of fear. Neuropsychologia, 36, 59–70.

Capps, L., Yirmiya, N., & Sigman, M. (1992). Understanding of simple and complex emotions in non-retarded children with autism. Journal of Child Psychology and Psychiatry, 33, 1169–1182.

Celani, G., Battacchi, M. W., & Arcidiacono, L. (1999). The understanding of the emotional meaning of facial expressions in people with autism. Journal of Autism and Developmental Disorders, 29, 57–66.

Critchley, H. D., Daly, E. M., Bullmore, E. T., Williams, S. C., van Amelsvoort, T., Robertson, D. M., Rowe, A. M. P., McAlonan, G., Howlin P., & Murphy, D. G. (2000). The functional neuroanatomy of social behavior: Changes in cerebral blood flow when people with autistic disorder process facial expressions. Brain, 123, 2203–2212.

Damasio, A. R. (1994). Descartes' error: Emotion, reason, and the human brain. New York: Grosset/Putnam.

Damasio, A. R., & Maurer, R. G. (1978). A neurological model for childhood autism. Archives of Neurology, 35, 777–786.

Ekman, P., & Friesen, W. (1976). Pictures of facial affect. Palo Alto, CA: Consulting Psychologists Press.

Ellis, H. D., & Leafhead, K. M. (1996). Raymond: A study of an adult with Asperger syndrome. In P. W. Halligan & J. C. Marshall (Eds.), Methods in madness: Case studies in cognitive neuropsychiatry (pp. 79–92). Hove, UK: Psychology Press.

Grossman, J. B., Klin, A., Carter, A. S., & Volkmar, F. R. (2000). Verbal bias in recognition of facial emotions in children with Asperger syndrome. Journal of Child Psychology and Psychiatry, 41, 369–379.

Hobson, R. P., Ouston, J., & Lee, A. (1988a). Emotion recognition in autism: Co-ordinating faces and voices. Psychological Medicine, 18, 911–923.

Hobson, R. P., Ouston, J., & Lee, A. (1988b). What's in a face? The case of autism. British Journal of Psychology, 79, 441–453.

Hobson, R. P., Ouston, J., & Lee, A. (1989). Naming emotion in faces and voices: Abilities and disabilities in autism and mental retardation. British Journal of Developmental Psychology, 7, 237–250.

Howard, M. A., Cowell, P. E., Boucher, J., Broks, P., Mayes, A., Farrant, A., & Roberts, N. (2000). Covergent neuroanatomical and behavior evidence of an amygdala hypothesis of autism. NeuroReport, 11, 2931–2935.

Jansari, A., Tranel, D., & Adolphs, R. (2000). A valence-specific lateral bias for discriminating emotional facial expressions in free-field. *Cognition and Emotion* (in press).

Kanner, L. (1943). Autistic disturbances of affective contact. *Nervous Child, 2,* 217–250.

Karmiloff-Smith, A., Bellugi, U., Klima, E., Grant, J., & Baron-Cohen, S. (1995). Is there a social module? Language, face processing, and theory of mind in individuals with Williams Syndrome. *Journal of Cognitive Neuroscience, 7,* 196–208.

Langdell, T. (1978). Recognition of faces: An approach to the study of autism. *Journal of Child Psychology and Psychiatry, 19,* 255–268.

LeCouteur, A., Rutter, M., & Lord, C. (1989). Autism diagnostic interview: A standardized investigator-based instrument. *Journal of Autism and Developmental Disorders, 19,* 363–387.

Leslie, A. (1987). Pretense and representation: The origins of "theory of mind". *Psychological Review, 94,* 412–426.

Morris, J. S., Frith, C. D., Perrett, D. I., Rowland, D., Young, A. W., Calder, A. J., & Dolan, R. J. (1996). A differential neural response in the human amygdala to fearful and happy facial expressions. *Nature, 383,* 812–815.

Piven, J. (1997). The biological basis of autism. *Current Opinion in Neurobiology, 7,* 708–712.

134

The human amygdala in social judgment

Ralph Adolphs*, Daniel Tranel* & Antonio R. Damasio*†

* Department of Neurology, Division of Cognitive Neuroscience, University of Iowa College of Medicine, 200 Hawkins Drive, Iowa City, Iowa 52242, USA
† The Salk Institute for Biological Studies, La Jolla, California 92037, USA

Studies in animals have implicated the amygdala in emotional[1-3] and social[4-6] behaviours, especially those related to fear and aggression. Although lesion[7-10] and functional imaging[11-13] studies in humans have demonstrated the amygdala's participation in recognizing emotional facial expressions, its role in human social behaviour has remained unclear. We report here our investigation into the hypothesis that the human amygdala is required for accurate social judgments of other individuals on the basis of their facial appearance. We asked three subjects with complete bilateral amygdala damage to judge faces of unfamiliar people with respect to two attributes important in real-life social encounters: approachability and trustworthiness. All three subjects judged unfamiliar individuals to be more approachable and more trustworthy than did control subjects. The impairment was most striking for faces to which normal subjects assign the most negative ratings: unapproachable and untrustworthy looking individuals. Additional investigations revealed that the impairment does not extend to judging verbal descriptions of people. The amygdala appears to be an important component of the neural systems that help retrieve socially relevant knowledge on the basis of facial appearance.

Data from three subjects with complete bilateral amygdala damage (subjects SM, JM and RH) and seven with unilateral amygdala damage were compared to those from normal and from brain-damaged control subjects (see Table 1 and Methods). Ratings of approachability and of trustworthiness were analysed separately for the 50 faces to which normal controls assigned the most negative ratings, and for the 50 most positive faces. Subjects with bilateral amygdala damage rated the 50 most negative faces more positively than did either normal controls ($P < 0.01$) or brain-damaged controls ($P < 0.05$; Mann–Whitney U-tests on subjects' mean ratings, Bonferroni corrected) (Fig. 1). Groups with unilateral amygdala lesions did not differ from controls on either rating. All subject groups gave similar ratings to the 50 most positive faces.

136

Subject SM spontaneously commented during the experiment that, in real life, she would not know how to judge if a person were trustworthy, consistent with her tendency to approach and engage in physical contact with other people rather indiscriminately[7,14]. All subjects with bilateral amygdala damage had normal ability to discriminate faces (Table 1), clear evidence that there were no visuoperceptual impairments that might account for the above findings.

Data from subjects with bilateral amygdala damage showed two effects: the subjects tended to rate all faces more positively than did controls, and they also showed the largest deviation from control ratings specifically when rating the most negative faces (Fig. 2). This suggests an overall positive bias, as well as a disproportionate impairment in rating the most negative faces. To establish the independence of these two effects, we carried out a detailed two-alternative forced-choice task with JM, RH and SM, using the same 100 face stimuli. We asked JM and RH to choose the more approachable face in pairwise comparisons between an anchor face that received a mean normal rating of 0.0 and each of the remaining 99 faces. We compared subjects' choices on this task to the choices that would be expected from the mean approachability ratings given to the faces in each pair by normal controls. JM and RH consistently made more incorrect choices when making comparisons to very negative faces, than when making comparisons to very positive faces (Fig. 3a). By contrast, the small number of errors made by normal controls occurred in the opposite direction, with positive rather than with negative faces (Fig. 3a), indicating that the impairments seen in amygdala subjects cannot be explained by stimulus difficulty.

In subject SM, we carried out forced-choice tasks with a total of five anchor faces, including faces normally rated very negatively and very positively. Each anchor face was paired with the remaining 99 faces, for a total of 5 × 99 = 495 pairwise comparisons. SM made the largest number of incorrect choices in comparisons involving those of the five anchor faces that normally receive the most negative

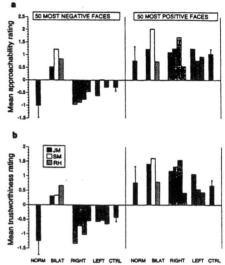

Figure 1 Mean judgments. **a**, Approachability; **b**, trustworthiness of the faces of 100 unfamiliar people, shown for the 50 faces that received the most negative (left) and most positive (right) mean ratings from normal controls. Data are shown from 46 normal controls (NORM; means and s.d.), 3 subjects with bilateral amygdala damage (BILAT; individual means), 4 subjects with unilateral right (RIGHT) and 3 with unilateral left (LEFT) amygdala damage, and 10 brain-damaged controls with no damage to amygdala (CTRL; means and s.e.m.).

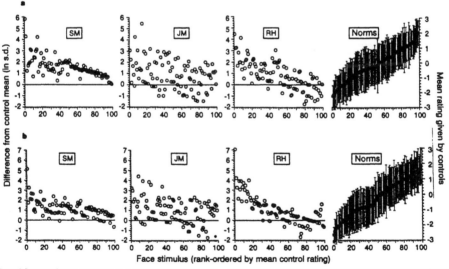

Figure 2 Deviations from normal judgments. **a**, Approachability; **b**, trustworthiness given by subjects with bilateral amygdala damage (circles; left y-axis). Units are standard deviations of the normal control ratings. Stimuli are rank-ordered on the x-axis according to the ratings normal controls gave them (squares; far right y-axis; means and s.d.).

137

ratings, a performance that was highly abnormal compared to control subjects' forced-choices in the same task (Fig. 3b). The findings from the forced-choice tasks cannot be explained solely on the basis of a general positive bias, and confirm that judgments given by subjects with bilateral amygdala damage are disproportionately impaired relative to individuals who are normally classified as unapproachable.

Might the impairment seen in subjects with bilateral amygdala damage extend to judging people from word descriptions rather than from faces? We asked subjects to rate the likeability of different individuals based on short verbal biographies or on single words (adjectives describing people). All three subjects with bilateral amygdala damage made entirely normal judgments when the stimuli were verbal (Fig. 4). This critical dissociation supports the

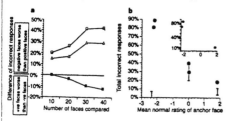

Figure 3 Disproportionate impairment in choosing the most unapproachable faces. **a**, JM's (empty squares), RH's (triangles) and normal controls' (filled squares) judgments of approachability from two-alternative forced-choice tasks. We calculated the per cent incorrect choices for pairings involving faces at either extreme of the normal rating scale (that is, faces that were normally rated as either very approachable or very unapproachable). The x-axis shows the number of faces at either extreme of the normal rating scale over which the per cent incorrect choices was calculated. The y-axis shows the difference in the errors made (unapproachable – approachable). **b**, SM's judgments of approachability from two-alternative forced-choice tasks. The mean normal rating of approachability given to each of 5 anchor faces is shown on the x-axis, and the proportion of incorrect forced choices (out of 99) made by SM (circles) and by normal controls (grey bars show range) are shown on the y-axis. Inset, analysis of SM's data from this task for only those pairs of faces whose mean control rating differed by more than 2 rating points. Data from comparisons involving the two faces with mean control ratings of 0 were not analysed, as very few faces with ratings <−2 or >2 could be paired with them. No normal control made any incorrect choices in this analysis.

following interpretation. The amygdala appears necessary to trigger the retrieval of information on the basis of prior social experience or innate bias in regard to certain classes of faces[15]. The retrieved information might be either covert or overt, or both (compare with ref. 16). The failure due to amygdala damage thus occurs after basic visual processing has taken place, by blocking the retrieval of information normally linked either to negative past experiences with similar stimuli, or to innately specified feature configurations. By contrast, sentences and words evoke a broad sweep of information directly, without the need for the amygdala's assistance, thus providing a sufficient basis for performing judgments normally.

A further question concerns the specific facial cues that would normally engage the amygdala in social judgment. Might amygdala lesions impair judgments based only on certain facial features? This does not seem to be the case, as subjects with bilateral amygdala lesions gave idiosyncratic ratings to specific negative faces (Fig. 2; intersubject Spearman rank correlations of ratings given by subjects with bilateral amygdala lesions for the 50 most negative faces: $-0.23 < r < 0.31$). We further explored this complex issue by choosing the 10 faces to which SM had given the most abnormal ratings of approachability (all rated very negatively by controls), and systematically manipulating individual features in each face. We showed subjects 109 pairs of faces in which each pair showed the same individual differing by only one single feature. We manipulated direction of gaze (45 stimuli), expression of the eyes (27 stimuli), expression of the mouth (14 stimuli), or visibility of the eyes (for example, with glasses of different tint; 23 stimuli), all features that might conceivably contribute to the subjects' judgments. In a two-alternative forced-choice task, SM and 16 normal controls were asked to choose the face they would prefer to approach. SM performed entirely normally on this task. Logistic linear analysis, with subjects' binary choices as the dependent variable and the manipulated features as factors, showed that SM did not differ from controls in her choices with respect to any of the above features that we had manipulated. Insensitivity to particular features, in isolation, is thus unlikely to account for the impairment in judging approachability or trustworthiness in faces.

The findings suggest that the human amygdala triggers socially and emotionally relevant information in response to visual stimuli. The amygdala's role appears to be of special importance for social judgment of faces that are normally classified as unapproachable and untrustworthy, consistent with the amygdala's demonstrated role in processing threatening and aversive stimuli. An intriguing question that remains to be addressed is the amygdala's relative participation in triggering information that is innate, versus infor-

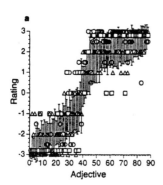

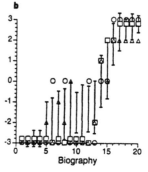

Figure 4 Likeability ratings of lexical stimuli. **a**, Ratings given by SM (2 experiments; circles), JM (squares), RH (triangles) and 20 normal controls (s.d. shown as bars) to 88 adjectives describing personality. **b**, Ratings given by SM, JM, RH and 20 normal controls to 20 biographical descriptions of people.

138

Table 1 Neuropsychology background data

Subject	SM	JM	RH	Left	Right	BD Ctrl	N Ctrl
N				3	4	10	46
Age	31	67	42	29 ± 5	31 ± 5	66 ± 10	19 ± 1
PIQ	90	95	108	104 ± 24	103 ± 24	98 ± 11	-
Benton (%ile)	71st	12th	20th	32nd	50th	48th	-
Expression discrimination	70 (40)	45 (20)	59 (15)	-	-	-	-
Gender discrimination	75th	65th	65th	-	-	-	-
Gaze discrimination	64th	86th	86th	-	-	-	-

SM, JM, RH, bilateral amygdala damage; Left, Right, unilateral amygdala damage; BD Ctrl and N Ctrl, brain-damaged and normal controls. PIQ, performance IQ from the Wechsler Adult Intelligence Scale-revised. Benton, percentile score on the Benton Facial Recognition Test, a measure of ability to discriminate among unfamiliar faces[4]. Expression, gender, gaze discrimination, percentile score on two-alternative forced-choice discrimination tasks of emotional facial expressions (average and minimum (in parentheses) for the 6 basic emotions), gender, and direction of gaze. See Methods for details.

mation that is acquired through individual experience in a cultural setting[17]. □

Methods

Subjects. All subjects had given informed consent to participate in these studies. Brain-damaged subjects were selected from the Patient Registry of the Department of Neurology at the University of Iowa, and had been fully characterized neuropsychologically[18] and neuroanatomically[19,20].

Amygdala damage. Subject SM has complete lesions of both amygdalae, as well as minimal damage to anterior entorhinal cortex, resulting from Urbach-Wiethe disease[7,14,21,22]. Subjects RH and JM had encephalitis at ages 28 and 62, respectively, resulting in complete bilateral destruction of the amygdala and substantial damage to surrounding structures. Both patients are severely amnesic. Seven subjects with unilateral amygdala lesions (4 right, 3 left) had surgical temporal lobectomy for the treatment of epilepsy, and also had damage to hippocampus and surrounding temporal cortices.

Control subjects. We examined 10 brain-damaged controls with lesions that did not include the amygdala. Four of the subjects had bilateral lesions. Three of the subjects were amnesic consequent to anoxia and hippocampal damage. We also examined 46 normal controls (16M/30F) who were undergraduates at the University of Iowa.

Stimuli and tasks. In all tasks, stimuli within each session were presented in randomized order, and without time limit.

Approachability and trustworthiness ratings of faces. We selected from a larger set of photographs 100 final stimuli whose ratings had low variance and were evenly distributed (Fig. 2). There was no effect of subject gender on rating the faces (P > 0.7, ANOVA on normal data). Stimuli were black-and-white photographs of unfamiliar male (N = 55) and female (N = 45) faces in natural poses.

Subjects were asked to rate the stimuli, shown one at a time on a slide projector, on a 7-point scale (−3 to +3) with respect to either approachability or trustworthiness. For approachability, subjects were asked to imagine meeting the person on the street, and to indicate how much they would want to walk up to that person and strike up a conversation. For trustworthiness, subjects imagined trusting that person with all their money, or with their life. Each of the two attributes was rated in two independent sessions in counterbalanced order; there were no order effects.

Approachability and trustworthiness were chosen because (1) they are clear measures of real-life social judgment; (2) they are easy to understand; and (3) pilot data indicated that ratings of these specific attributes had lower variance than those obtained with other words, such as 'nice' or 'good'. Although approachability and trustworthiness ratings in normals were somewhat correlated (mean r = 0.52), there were many stimuli that received discrepant ratings on the two attributes, indicating that they were non-redundant measures of social judgment.

Forced-choice tasks. Direct pairwise comparisons of approachability were made between an anchor face, and each of the remaining 99 faces, all drawn from the same 100 face stimuli used in other tasks. We calculated the proportion of subjects' choices that differed from the choices that would be expected on the basis of the mean normal control ratings given to each of the two faces in a pair.

In one experiment (Fig. 3a), each of two anchor faces with a mean normal approachability rating of 0.0 was compared to other faces that were either very

approachable or very unapproachable; data obtained with both anchor faces were very similar and were pooled. In a second experiment (Fig. 3b), each of 5 anchor faces (which included faces with a range of ratings) was compared to all other 99 faces (a total of 495 pairwise comparisons).

Lexical stimuli. We chose 88 adjectives that described personality attributes from a large standardized set[23] so as to span the range from very likeable to very dislikeable, and to exhibit maximal reliability and common usage. Twenty short biographies described people by giving information about the person's lifestyles and activities. Subjects rated how much they liked individuals described by the stimuli, on a scale of −3 to +3. Words were presented visually on a sheet of paper; biographical descriptions were read to subjects.

Control tasks. For each of the control tasks, we calculated thresholds at which subjects were just able to discriminate stimuli. Data were converted to percentiles compared to performances given by normal subjects (N = 28 for expression, 20 for gender, 28 for gaze).

Expression discrimination. Two-alternative forced-choice discriminations were made between 80 images of a neutral face, and 80 images that were linear morphs between the neutral face and facial expressions of emotion[24] (happiness, surprise, fear, anger, disgust, sadness). Subjects were asked to choose the image that showed more of a stated emotion.

Gender discrimination. Two-alternative forced-choice discriminations were made between 84 pairs of images that were morphs between an average composite of a neutral male face, and an average composite of a neutral female face, of equal age.

Gaze discrimination. Two-alternative forced-choice discriminations were made between 16 pairs of images showing the same, neutral, male face in which only direction of gaze had been varied by manipulating the digital image on a computer.

Received 7 January; accepted 30 March 1998.

1. Weiskrantz, L. Behavioral changes associated with ablation of the amygdaloid complex in monkeys. J. Comp. Physiol. Psychol. 49, 381–391 (1956).
2. Blanchard, D. C. & Blanchard, R. J. Innate and conditioned reactions to threat in rats with amygdaloid lesions. J. Comp. Physiol. Psychol. 81, 281–290 (1972).
3. Le Doux, J. The Emotional Brain (Simon and Schuster, New York, 1996).
4. Rosvold, H. E., Mirsky, A. F. & Pribram, K. Influence of amygdalectomy on social behavior in monkeys. J. Comp. Physiol. Psychol. 47, 173–178 (1954).
5. Kling, A. Steklis, H. D. & Deutsch, S. Radiotelemetered activity from the amygdala during social interactions in the monkey. Exp. Neurol. 66, 88–96 (1979).
6. Kling, A. S. & Brothers, L. A. in The Amygdala: Neurobiological Aspects of Emotion, Memory, and Mental Dysfunction (ed. Aggleton, J. P.) 353–378 (Wiley-Liss, New York, 1992).
7. Adolphs, R., Tranel, D., Damasio, H. & Damasio, A. Impaired recognition of emotion in facial expressions following bilateral damage to the human amygdala. Nature 372, 669–672 (1994).
8. Young, A. W. et al. Face processing impairments after amygdalotomy. Brain 118, 15–24 (1995).
9. Calder, A. J. et al. Facial emotion recognition after bilateral amygdala damage: differentially severe impairment of fear. Cogn. Neuropsychol. 13, 699–745 (1996).
10. Broks, P. et al. Face processing impairments after encephalitis: amygdala damage and recognition of fear. Neuropsychologia 39, 59–70 (1998).
11. Morris, J. S. et al. A differential neural response in the human amygdala to fearful and happy facial expressions. Nature 383, 812–815 (1996).
12. Breiter, H. C. et al. Response and habituation of the human amygdala during visual processing of facial expression. Neuron 17, 875–887 (1996).
13. Morris, J. S. et al. A neuromodulatory role for the human amygdala in processing emotional facial expressions. Brain 121, 47–57 (1998).
14. Tranel, D. & Hyman, B. T. Neuropsychological correlates of bilateral amygdala damage. Arch. Neurol. 47, 349–355 (1990).
15. Damasio, A. R. Toward a neurobiology of emotion and feeling: operational concepts and hypotheses. Neuroscientist 1, 19–25 (1995).
16. Lewicki, P., Hill, T. & Czyzewska, M. Nonconscious acquisition of information. Am. Psychol. 47, 796–801 (1992).
17. Saarni, C., Mumme, D. L. & Campos, J. J. in Handbook of Child Psychology, Vol. 3: Social, Emotional, and Personality Development (ed. Damon, W.) 237–309 (Wiley, New York, 1997).

139

letters to nature

18. Tranel, D. in *Neuropsychological Assessment of Neuropsychiatric Disorders* (eds Grant, I. & Adams, K. M.) 81–101 (Oxford Univ. Press, New York, 1996).
19. Damasio, H. & Frank, R. Three-dimensional *in vivo* mapping of brain lesions in humans. *Arch. Neurol.* 49, 137–143 (1992).
20. Frank, R. J., Damasio, H. & Grabowski, T. J. Brainvox: an interactive, multi-modal visualization and analysis system for neuroanatomical imaging. *NeuroImage* 5, 13–30 (1997).
21. Adolphs, R., Tranel, D., Damasio, H. & Damasio, A. R. Fear and the human amygdala. *J. Neurosci.* 15, 5879–5892 (1995).
22. Nahm, F. K. D., Tranel, D., Damasio, H. & Damasio, A. R. Cross-modal associations and the human amygdala. *Neuropsychologia* 31, 727–744 (1993).
23. Anderson, N. H. Likableness ratings of 555 personality-trait words. *J. Person. Social Psychol.* 9, 272–279 (1968).
24. Ekman, P. & Friesen, W. *Pictures of Facial Affect* (Consulting Psychologists, Palo Alto, CA, 1976).

Acknowledgements. We thank J. Suhr and J. Nath for technical assistance in testing subjects, D. Krutzfeldt for help in scheduling subjects and H. Damasio for comments on the manuscript. This study was supported by a grant from the National Institute for Neurological Diseases and Stroke.

Correspondence and requests for materials should be addressed to R.A. (e-mail: ralph-adolphs@uiowa.edu).

140

Brain (1998), **121**, 889–905

A clinicopathological study of autism

A. Bailey,[1] P. Luthert,[2,]* A. Dean,[2] B. Harding,[3] I. Janota,[2] M. Montgomery,[2,]* M. Rutter[1] and P. Lantos[2]

[1]*MRC Child Psychiatry Unit, and [2]Department of Neuropathology, The Institute of Psychiatry and [3]Department of Histopathology, Institute of Child Health, London, UK*

Correspondence to: A. Bailey, MRC Child Psychiatry Unit, The Institute of Psychiatry, De Crespigny Park, Denmark Hill, London SE5 8AF, UK

*Present address: The Department of Pathology, The Institute of Ophthalmology, University College, London, UK

Summary

A neuropathological study of autism was established and brain tissue examined from six mentally handicapped subjects with autism. Clinical and educational records were obtained and standardized diagnostic interviews conducted with the parents of cases not seen before death. Four of the six brains were megalencephalic, and areas of cortical abnormality were identified in four cases. There were also developmental abnormalities of the brainstem, particularly of the inferior olives. Purkinje cell number was reduced in all the adult cases, and this reduction was sometimes accompanied by gliosis. The findings do not support previous claims of localized neurodevelopmental abnormalities. They do point to the likely involvement of the cerebral cortex in autism.

Keywords: autism; neuropathology; megalencephaly; cortical dysgenesis

Abbreviations: ADI = Autism Diagnostic Interview; GFAP = glial fibrillary acidic protein

Introduction

Autism is a severe developmental disorder characterized by impairments in reciprocal social interaction and communication, restricted and stereotyped patterns of behaviour and interests, and an onset before 3 years of age (World Health Organization, 1992). The core disorder affects approximately four in 10 000 children, and is much commoner in males, in a ratio of ~4 : 1. The syndrome was first described by Leo Kanner (1943); he assumed that affected children were of normal intelligence and for several decades the disorder was thought to be psychogenic. An organic basis was first suggested by the finding that three-quarters of sufferers are mentally handicapped (Lockyer and Rutter, 1969) and that at least one-quarter develop epilepsy (Rutter, 1970; Gillberg and Steffenburg, 1987). Subsequently autism was often assumed to be an unusual consequence of brain damage, caused either by medical disorders or obstetric hazards. More recently it has been appreciated that only a minority of cases of autism are associated with medical causes of mental handicap, then most commonly with tuberous sclerosis or Fragile X (Rutter et al., 1994). The findings from twin and family studies suggest that the vast majority of idiopathic cases arise on the basis of strong specific genetic influences

(Bailey et al., 1996). Thus, autism usually appears to represent a severe expression of a specific disease process.

Many regions of the brain have been implicated in the genesis of autism, but the neurobiological basis of the disorder remains unknown. Autism is a rare disorder which was described relatively recently and there have been only a few post-mortem studies. Darby (1976) reviewed 33 diverse cases and found no consistent abnormalities. Two of the four cases reported by Williams et al. (1980) had associated disorders (phenylketonuria and probable Rett's syndrome); in one of the two idiopathic cases pyramidal cell dendritic spine density was reduced in the mid-frontal gyrus and the number of cerebellar Purkinje cells was also diminished. Coleman et al. (1985) undertook cell counts in several cortical regions from a single case and two control subjects. Consistent differences were not found, although the glia : neuron ratio was smaller in the autistic brain than in the two control subjects. Recent examination of the brainstem of this case (Rodier et al., 1996) revealed a hypoplastic facial nucleus and superior olive. Ritvo et al. (1986) measured Purkinje cell density in the brains of four autistic and four control subjects and reported significantly lower counts in the autistic brains (the

141

histopathological findings in the cerebral hemispheres and brainstem have not been reported). There have been two case reports of extremely retarded individuals who were also considered to have autism (Hof *et al.*, 1991; Guerin *et al.*, 1996).

Bauman and Kemper's study of six brains is the most comprehensive post-mortem study of autism to-date (Kemper and Bauman, 1993). In all cases there was a reduction in Purkinje cell density, but this varied in severity (Bauman, 1991). In four of the cases Purkinje cell density was decreased by 50–95% in some areas (Arin *et al.*, 1991); three of these individuals had a history of epilepsy (Kemper and Bauman, 1993) which could be relevant. In two brains there was also a qualitative decrease in cerebellar granule cell density (Kemper and Bauman, 1993). The neurons of the cerebellar nuclei were enlarged in the brains of two children and decreased in both size and number in those of three adults (Kemper and Bauman, 1993). The dentate nucleus was distorted in one brain (Bauman and Kemper, 1985). Inferior olivary neurons were preserved; they were enlarged in the younger individuals and unusually small in the adults. In five brains the inferior olivary neurons tended to cluster at the periphery of the convolutions.

In the forebrain, abnormally small, densely packed neurons were noted in all areas of the hippocampus, subiculum, mamillary body, septal nuclei and amygdala (Kemper and Bauman, 1993). Hippocampal neuronal counts have been published on only the first of these six cases (Bauman and Kemper, 1985). The size of hippocampal pyramidal cells has been measured in areas CA1 and CA4 of two cases; only the neurons in CA4 were significantly smaller than in the control brains (Raymond *et al.*, 1989). The only consistent cerebral cortical abnormalities were in the anterior cingulate region.

Because neuropathological abnormalities have been largely confined to the cerebellum and medial temporal structures, their possible involvement in autism has been the subject of much interest. Bauman and Kemper (1985) argued that decreased Purkinje cell density, in the absence of either glial cell hyperplasia or retrograde olivary cell loss, suggested that the cerebellar abnormality developed at or before 30 weeks gestation. An MRI study of autistic individuals and control subjects (Courchesne *et al.*, 1988) found hypoplasia of cerebellar vermal lobules VI–VII, but not of vermal lobules I–V. On the basis of the post-mortem and neuroimaging findings, Courchesne's group have argued that developmental cerebellar abnormalities are the most consistent neuroanatomical lesion in autism, and that such abnormalities can lead to the characteristic symptomatology by several different routes (Courchesne *et al.*, 1994). Nevertheless the cerebellar abnormality has not been replicated using similar imaging protocols (see Bailey and Cox, 1996). Temporal horn dilatation, visualized by pneumoencephalography (Hauser *et al.*, 1975), has been cited in support of the hypothesis that medial temporal abnormalities underlie the autistic syndrome (Bauman and Kemper, 1985; DeLong, 1992; Kemper and

Bauman, 1993; Bachevalier, 1994). The finding of temporal horn dilatation has not been replicated, and the only quantitative MRI study of the posterior hippocampus did not find any differences between autistic and control subjects (Saitoh *et al.*, 1995).

The focus upon the cerebellum and medial temporal lobe structures arose largely because of the limited post-mortem evidence of abnormalities in other areas. Nevertheless, because autism is associated with epilepsy, EEG abnormalities and mental handicap, the possibility of neocortical involvement in autism has been raised (Minshew, 1991). The main goals of the present study were to determine whether neuropathological abnormalities are more extensive than previously supposed, and to evaluate the previous observations. The brain weights of the first four cases in this study have been previously reported (Bailey *et al.*, 1993).

Methods

Case material

Post-mortem brain tissue was obtained from six individuals with autism. Contact was made with clinical colleagues specializing in the diagnosis and treatment of autism and advertisements were placed in the publications of several of the national and international autistic societies. UK pathologists were also informed of the study. By these means post-mortem brain tissue from two cases (1 and 3) and whole brains from four individuals who died since 1991 were obtained. In addition, post-mortem findings, but no tissue, were available from a further 14 cases.

Diagnostic assessment

The parents of five of the six cases included in the study were interviewed using the Autism Diagnostic Interview (ADI), an investigator based instrument of known reliability and validity (Le Couteur *et al.*, 1989). A diagnostic algorithm for autism, based upon ICD-10 criteria, was completed using the information gathered with the ADI. Case 3 was reviewed by one of the authors (M.R.) in adulthood; because he died in the 1970s the parents were not recontacted. The available clinical and educational notes of all cases were reviewed.

Clinical details

The six patients were all male and diagnosed as showing autism in life. Cases 1, 2, 4, 5 and 6 all met ADI algorithm criteria for autism. Relevant medical information and any psychometric findings are noted below. Case histories are provided in the Appendix. To maintain confidentiality details of the circumstances of death have been omitted.

Case 1, age 4 years

Born at 41 weeks gestation weighing 8 lb. No history of peri- or neonatal brain damage. Head circumference just above the 10th percentile at birth, above the 25th percentile by 9 months and above the 50th percentile by 22 months. Left convergent squint noticed from birth. Advice was sought for head lag and hypotonia at 9 months. He sat unaided at 9 months, cruised at 24 months and walked slowly by 29 months. Developmental ages (months) on the Griffiths scales at 24 months were: locomotor 11; personal–social 18.5; hearing and speech 11.5; eye–hand co-ordination 13.5 and performance 16. At 30.5 months the scores were: locomotor 16.5; personal–social 20.5; hearing and speech 16.5; eye–hand co-ordination 19 and performance 17.5. Extensive biochemical investigations, chromosomal analysis and skull X-ray were normal. He was seen a few weeks before death by his paediatrician; he could run well but flapped his arms and was socially aloof.

Case 2, age 23 years

Induced at 42 weeks gestation, weighed 7 lb 2 oz; no history of peri- or neonatal brain damage. Head circumference at 2 years 7 months was 51.5 cm (above 75th percentile). At 3 years 6 months, head circumference was 54 cm (above 97th percentile); a lumbar puncture and EEG were normal. Severe self-injury was a significant management problem and included autoamputation of part of a digit and anal gouging. Medication, used in an effort to control his over-active and difficult behaviour, included: flupenthixol, chlor-promazine, chlorpheniramine, amitriptyline, lithium, carbamazepine and benzodiazepines. There was no definite evidence of epilepsy but, ~6 months prior to death, the subject had two falls accompanied by diminished awareness.

Case 3, age 27 years

Born at 38 weeks gestation weighing 5 lb 12 oz; no history of peri- or neonatal brain damage. He sat at 11 months, stood at 18 months and did not walk until 25 months. At the age of 6 years he sustained a depressed right frontal fracture. He had two seizures at the age of 13 years which involved head deviation to the right, and at the age of 18 years developed generalized seizures which occurred approximately once a month. He had received phenytoin, phenobarbital and carbamazepine. He completed several performance IQ tests at the age of 16 years and performed best on spatial items; his estimated IQ was 43. Using the Vineland scale his social age was estimated as 1.35 years.

Case 4, age 24 years

Born at term weighing 8 lb 7 oz; no history of peri- or neonatal brain damage. His head circumference at 6 years and 10 months was 57 cm (above 97th percentile). An EEG at the age of 6 years was dysrhythmic and slow. His first grand mal seizure occurred at 19 years of age; an EEG showed only minor diffuse abnormalities. His seizures con-tinued, were difficult to control and were preceded by

aggressive behaviour. He had been treated with sodium valproate, primidone, lamotrigine and clobazam.

Case 5, age 20 years

Born at term weighing 7 lb 11 oz; mother took a progesterone drug during the first 16 weeks of pregnancy. No history of peri- or neonatal brain damage. The first grand mal seizure occurred at the age of 11 years. These seizures occurred approximately weekly, mainly at night or on waking. An EEG recording consisted mainly of slow wave activity; short bursts of generalized spike and wave activity were also seen. He was initially treated with sodium valproate. This was changed to carbamazepine and then vigabritin added. At the age of 10 years his mental age scores on the Griffiths Scales were (in months): locomotor 46, personal social 38, hearing and speech 22, eye–hand co-ordination 31.5 and perform-ance 52.

Case 6, age 24 years

Delivered by forceps at 39 weeks gestation because of a broad head (head circumference not recorded); he weighed 7 lb 15 oz. No history of peri- or neonatal brain damage. In childhood there were four febrile convulsions and sub-sequently four afebrile seizures. A convulsion at the age of 22 years may have been a drop attack. He was prescribed ritalin between the ages of 7 and 8 years but he never received anticonvulsants.

Control material

For the morphometric studies, identically processed, indi-vidual male control subjects for Cases 2, 4, 5 and 6 were chosen from the cases available at the Institute of Psychiatry. Potential control subjects were not included when intercurrent disease could have affected neuronal counts. An identically processed male control for Case 3 was obtained from the Institute of Neurology, but no cerebellum was available. No suitable, identically processed age-matched male control subjects were available at the Institute of Child Health for Case 1, and tissue from two age-matched females was used. The weight of the brain was not recorded for two control cases.

Tissue processing of whole brains (Cases 2, 4, 5 and 6)

Brains were weighed intact, and the brainstem and cerebellum was separated and weighed. A cerebral hemisphere (left or right, chosen at random) was fixed intact and has not yet been examined histologically. The other hemisphere was freshly sliced and blocks removed for short fixation, cryopro-tection and electron microscopy when tissue preservation was adequate. The remaining tissue was fixed in 10% buffered formol saline, and blocks were subsequently taken for paraffin

Table 1 *Brain weight of six mentally handicapped autistic males*

Case	Age (years)	Brain weight (kg)	Normal range* (kg)	Weight of brainstem and cerebellum (kg)	Ratio of total brain to brainstem and cerebellar weights
1	4	1.53	1.25–1.35	0.15	10.2 : 1
2	23	1.60	1.39–1.49	0.19	7.6 : 1
3	27	1.45	1.39–1.49	0.21	7.6 : 1
4	24	1.81	1.39–1.49	0.22	8.2 : 1
5	20	1.41	1.39–1.49	0.21	6.6 : 1
6	24	1.82	1.39–1.49	0.23	7.9 : 1

*Normal ranges given as mean ± 2.5 SD (from Dekaban and Sadowsky, 1978).

embedding, routine staining and examination. Where possible, the cerebral cortex, hippocampus and cerebellum were compared histologically with material from identically processed age- and sex-matched control subjects.

Immunohistochemistry for glial fibrillary acidic protein (GFAP; DAKO, 1 : 1600) and phosphorylated neurofilaments (RT97; Courtesy of BH Anderton, 1 : 100) was performed using the avidin–biotin complex method (DAKO) with diaminobenzidine as the chromogen.

Morphometric studies

As a supplement to subjective assessment, limited morphometry was undertaken. Neuronal counts were performed on sections from three areas: (i) the medial aspect of the superior frontal gyrus at the level of the corpus callosum; (ii) the CA1, CA3 and CA4 sub-fields of the hippocampus (as close as possible to the lateral geniculate body); and (iii) the Purkinje cell layer of the superior aspect of the cerebellar hemisphere.

Sections cut at ~14 μm thickness were stained with cresyl violet and examined with a ×40 objective (×10 eyepiece). Neurons were identified on the basis of classical morphological criteria. For neocortical counts, successive fields, as defined by a rectangular eyepiece graticule were counted from pia to white matter. Neurons whose nucleus lay on either of two adjacent borders of the field boundary (forbidden lines) were excluded. Neurons were considered to lie within the thickness of the section if the mid-point of the nucleus, as defined by a sharply focussed nuclear outline, was present (Everall *et al.*, 1991). All section thicknesses were measured by focusing from the top to the bottom of the section with a ×100 oil immersion objective and measuring the distance the microscope stage travelled with a microcator. The product of field size and section thickness provided the reference volume.

In the hippocampus, a single ×40 field of CA1, CA3 and CA4 was counted as described above. The number of nucleolated Purkinje cells was counted and the length of the counted Purkinje cell layer was measured using an IBAS 2000 Kontron image analyser. The product of this length and section thickness yielded a reference area. Purkinje cell

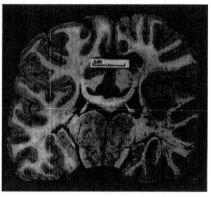

Fig. 1 Case 1. Coronal slice showing large, hyperconvoluted temporal lobes with upturned hippocampi and abnormal lateral ventricles (see text).

counts were therefore expressed as the number per unit area of Purkinje cell layer.

White matter neurons were counted deep to the superior frontal sulcus at the level of the head of the caudate nucleus and deep to the superior temporal sulcus at the level of the lateral geniculate nucleus. Sixteen non-overlapping ×400 magnification fields of 7-μm thick haematoxylin and eosin stained sections were counted. Again neurons were identified on the basis of classical morphological criteria.

Results

Post-mortem and histopathological findings in the nervous system of Cases 1–6

Case 1, age 4 years

The brain was large and weighed 1525 g (normal range 1250–1350 g). The weight of the brainstem and cerebellum was disproportionately low at 145 g (Table 1). The convolutional pattern of the cerebral cortex was abnormal, with overlarge hyperconvoluted temporal lobes and upwardly rotated hippocampi (Fig. 1). Anteriorly there was a cavum

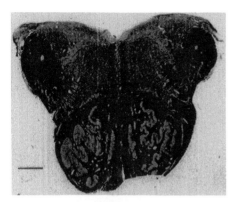

Fig. 2 Case 1. Medulla oblongata. The inferior olives show an abnormal outline; the band of neurons is irregular and broken up. (Luxol fast blue and cresyl violet; bar represents 2.5 mm.)

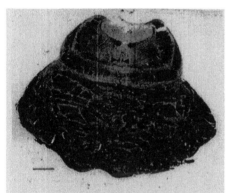

Fig. 3 Case 1. Pons. An aberrant tract, (arrow heads) is seen on both sides adjacent to the midline in the pontine tegmentum. (Luxol fast blue and cresyl violet; bar represents 3.0 mm.)

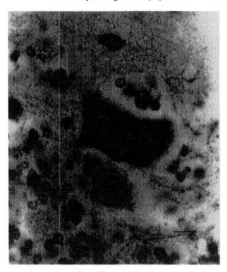

Fig. 4 Case 1. Cerebellum. The Purkinje cells contain round, darkly stained cytoplasmic inclusions (Luxol fast blue and cresyl violet; bar represents 10 μm.)

septi pellucidi but the septum was completely absent posteriorly. The outer angles of the lateral ventricles were abnormally acute. The medulla oblongata was large but the pyramids were relatively small. There was mild widening of the sulci of the superior cerebellar vermis. The inferior olives did not form a continuous ribbon (Fig. 2). There was apparent reduplication of the medial accessory olive, and multiple small bilateral groups of ectopic neurons lay lateral to the olives and in the inferior cerebellar peduncles. An aberrant tract was present in both sides of the pontine tegmentum (Fig. 3). The midbrain was unusually small and the periaqueductal grey matter and raphe nuclei appeared disproportionately large.

The perikaryon and proximal dendrites of 30–40% of Purkinje cells in the vermis contained well-defined, round or oval eosinophilic inclusions (mean number two but ranging up to six per cell) that stained homogeneously deep blue with Luxol fast blue and cresyl violet stain and measured up to 7 μm across (Fig. 4). The inclusions were less frequent in the cerebellar hemispheres and were not observed elsewhere. Electron microscopy confirmed that the inclusions were oval or circular and had a uniform intermediate electron density (Fig. 5). No limiting membrane was identified. The dentate ribbon was discontinuous and there were patches of subcortical ectopic grey matter consisting of large mature neurons.

The laminar pattern in the superior frontal gyrus was slightly irregular with clusters of abnormally orientated pyramidal cells, particularly in layer 5 (Fig. 6). There were no neurons that were unusual in size, configuration or neurofilament expression. In some areas in the frontal lobe there was blurred grey–white matter differentiation, and numerous patches of ectopic grey matter and many solitary mature neurons in the white matter. There was a little gliosis subpially and in the white matter of the temporal and frontal lobes. The hippocampal formation and the deep grey matter were unremarkable.

Case 2, age 23 years

The brain weighed 1600 g and was large and slightly swollen, but there was no herniation. There was no atrophy of the

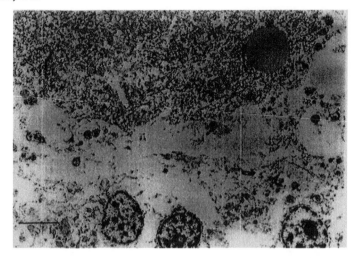

Fig. 5 Case 1. Cerebellum. The Purkinje cell at the top of the figure contains, on the right, a well-defined, homogeneous, moderately electron-lucent inclusion. Note three granule cell neurons at the bottom of the figure. (Electron micrograph; bar represents 5 μm.)

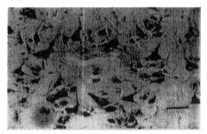

Fig. 6 Case 1. Lamina 5 of the superior frontal gyrus showing irregular orientation of pyramidal neurons. The top of the figure is closest to the pia. (Luxol fast blue and cresyl violet; bar represents 40 μm.)

cerebellar vermis or hemisphere. The inferior olivary ribbon was normally formed, but there were groups of ectopic neurons lateral to both olives. There was also a group of ectopic neurons in an inferior cerebellar peduncle adjacent to the brainstem. The cross-sectional area of the lower end of the aqueduct at the midbrain–pons junction was unusually small (0.2 mm²). In the cerebellum the number of Purkinje cells was reduced, more so in the hemisphere than vermis, but no empty baskets were seen. There was an increase in GFAP in Bergmann glia. The parietal, frontal and cingulate cortices were thickened in the right cerebral hemisphere, as was the cortex of the superior and middle temporal gyri. The cortex was also unusually cellular. There was an increased

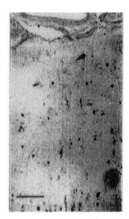

Fig. 7 Case 2. Layer 1 of frontal cortex. Note the increased number of neurons and, in particular, the misorientated pyramidal cell just beneath the pial surface (top). The bar represents 100 μm and lies just above the junction between layers I and II. (Luxol fast blue and cresyl violet.)

number of small neurons in layer 1 of frontal cortex including some inverted pyramidal cells (Fig. 7); these were normal in configuration and neurofilament expression. The corpus callosum was thin, measuring 2.5 mm in thickness just posterior to the genu. Neuronal density appeared to be

146

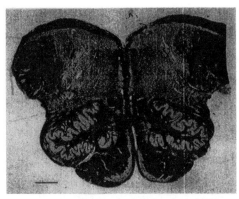

Fig. 8 Case 3. Medulla oblongata. The striae medullares are hypertrophied and the arcuate nuclei appear larger than usual. Compare the regular configuration of the inferior olives with the abnormal outline in Fig. 2. (Luxol fast blue and cresyl violet; bar represents 2 mm.)

increased in the hippocampus. The deep grey nuclei were unremarkable. Electron microscopy of the frontal cortex revealed moderately well-preserved tissue. No abnormalities of synapses, mitochondria, lysosomes or other organelles were identified.

Case 3, age 27 years

The brain weighed 1450 g. The substantia nigra looked pale. In the medulla oblongata the striae medullares were hypertrophied and the arcuate nuclei appeared larger than usual (Fig. 8). The substantia nigra was adequately populated with neurons. There was a bilateral break in the inferior end of the inferomedial olivary ribbon, and small groups of band-like ectopic neurons lay peripheral to the olives. In the cerebellum there was a widespread patchy decrease in the number of Purkinje cells (hemisphere greater than vermis) with an excess of Bergmann glia; the dentate ribbon was discontinuous.

In the cerebral cortex, neuronal density appeared high and there was mild focal disturbance of the laminar pattern in frontal cortex. A group of nerve cells lay deep in the white matter of anterior frontal cortex. There was a small focus of gliosis in the molecular layer of one orbitofrontal gyrus. In the occipital lobe a larger lesion, that involved the whole thickness of the cortex and some of the underlying white matter, extended patchily over two convolutions of the lingual gyrus; the nerve cells had been replaced by large reactive astrocytes. Both lesions were consistent with an old head injury. Neuronal density in the hippocampus appeared increased in all CA areas.

Case 4, age 24

The brain was very large and weighed 1805 g; there was no swelling or herniation. The gyral pattern was normal. There

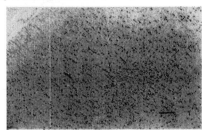

Fig. 9 Case 4. Superior temporal gyrus. The neuronal arrangement is irregular, particularly in lamina 3. Note the pial surface in the top left hand corner. (Luxol fast blue and cresyl violet; bar represents 250 μm.)

was no atrophy of the cerebellar vermis or hemisphere. The brain was soft to touch and contained numerous bacteria that had proliferated post-mortem, but neuronal morphology was generally well preserved. There were small groups of neurons in the inferior cerebellar peduncles. The number of Purkinje cells in the cerebellum appeared reduced in all areas, but there were no empty baskets. There was subpial gliosis in the right cerebral hemisphere. The cortex appeared to be thickened in the main cortical regions and neuronal density looked increased in the frontal and cingulate gyri. In contrast, neuronal density was decreased in the thickened superior temporal gyrus where the laminar pattern was disorganized (Fig. 9). No abnormalities were detected in sections from the hippocampus and deep grey matter.

Case 5, age 20 years

The brain weighed 1405 g and the gyral pattern was normal. The medulla was slightly flattened and the pyramids were

147

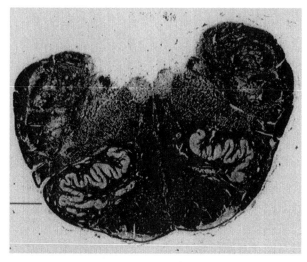

Fig. 10 Case 5. Medulla Oblongata. The medulla is slightly flattened and the pyramids poorly demarcated from each other (Luxol fast blue and cresyl violet, magnification bar represents 2 mm.)

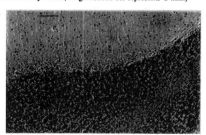

Fig. 11 Case 5. Cerebellar hemisphere. There is a reduced number of Purkinje cells and a mild increase in Bergmann glia. (Haematoxylin and eosin; bar represents 100 μm.)

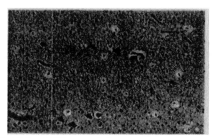

Fig. 12 Case 5. White matter in the superior temporal gyrus. The density of neurons is 40/mm^2 in this field. (Haematoxylin and eosin; bar represents 50 μm.)

poorly demarcated from each other (Fig. 10). There was no atrophy of the cerebellar vermis or hemisphere. Histologically, the external arcuate nuclei and the external arcuate fibres were prominent. The anterior portions of the inferior olivary ribbons were interrupted and asymmetrically bilaterally attenuated. In the cerebellum there was a diffuse decrease in Purkinje cell density in the hemisphere and vermis (Fig. 11). There was a slight increase in Bergmann glia number and a moderate patchy increase in GFAP staining in the molecular layer. In the left cerebral hemisphere the leptomeninges showed sparse perivascular lymphocytic cuffs, and there was widespread capillary engorgement in the grey matter. The white matter of the superior temporal gyrus contained many scattered mature neurons (Fig. 12). There were numerous corpora amylacea within the subpial zone and molecular

layer of the insular cortex. The striatum and internal capsule contained a few lymphocytic cuffs. The hippocampus and parahippocampal gyrus were unremarkable.

Case 6, age 24 years

The brain was unusually large, swollen and weighed 1820 g, but there was no herniation. The gyral pattern was normal. The medulla oblongata had not been completely removed. There was no atrophy of the cerebellar vermis or hemisphere. There was no histological evidence of oedema. The neurons of the locus coeruleus were loosely grouped and there was a slight reduction in the number of nigral neurons. In the cerebellum there was a moderate reduction in the number of Purkinje cells in the hemisphere and vermis, and moderate

Table 2 *Pathological findings in cerebral cortex and underlying white matter*

Case	Cortical dysgenesis	White matter	Other
1	Slightly irregular laminar pattern in superior frontal gyrus with clusters of abnormally orientated pyramidal cells. White matter/layer 6 boundary poorly defined.	Numerous patches of ectopic grey matter and increased numbers of single neurons	
2	Thickened cortex and increased neuronal density. Increased numbers of neurons in lamina 1 of frontal cortex, including inverted pyramidal cells.		
3	Increased neuronal density and mild focal disturbance of laminar pattern in frontal cortex	Patch of nerve cells deep in the deep white matter of anterior frontal cortex. Increased number of single neurons.	Small shallow focus of gliosis in frontal cortex. Larger area of gliosis involving full cortical thickness in one occipital lobe.
4	Thickened cortices and increased neuronal density in frontal cortex and cingulate gyri. Laminar pattern of superior temporal gyrus disorganised.	Subpial gliosis.	
5		Increased number of single neurons in superior temporal gyrus.	Numerous corpora amylacea within subpial zone and molecular layer of insular cortex.
6		Increased number of white matter neurons.	

Table 3 *Pathological findings in the brainstem*

Case	Olivary dysplasia	Neuronal ectopia	Other
1	Dysplastic olives with apparent reduplication of medial accessory olive.	Bilateral groups of neurons lateral to olives and in inferior cerebellar peduncle.	Large medulla oblongata with small pyramids. Aberrant pontine tract bilaterally. Small midbrain.
2		Bilateral groups of neurons lateral to olives. Group of neurons in one inferior cerebellar peduncle.	Unusually small aqueduct.
3	Bilateral break in the inferior end of the inferomedial olives.	Bilateral band-like groups of neurons lateral to olives.	Hypertrophy of striae medullaris and enlarged arcuate nuclei.
4		Small groups of neurons in inferior cerebellar peduncles.	Widely dispersed locus coeruleus.
5	Bilateral break in the anterior portions of the inferior olives.		Slight flattening of medulla anteroposterior. Fissure separating pyramids poorly defined. Prominent external arcuate nuclei and external arcuate fibres.
6	Adequate section not available.		Neurons of locus coeruleus loosely grouped.

patchy increase in GFAP in Bergmann glia, without an obvious increase in cell number. In the right cerebral hemisphere, there were neurons in the white matter, and the deep white matter arteries showed scanty lymphocytic cuffing. The basal ganglia were unremarkable. No obvious abnormality was noted in the hippocampus in a section taken from a cryoprotected block.

The neuropathological findings (in the cerebral cortex and underlying white matter, the brainstem and the cerebellum) are summarized in Tables 2–4.

(During revision of this manuscript the brain and spinal cord of a cachectic, handicapped 41-year-old woman with autism became available for study. She met ADI criteria for autism. The brain weighed 1233 g. There was partial reduplication of the inferior olive at one level. Purkinje cells were irregularly aligned with some lying in the deep molecular layer. The Bergman glia appeared excessively numerous and there was an excess of corpora amylacea in the molecular layer. There were excess numbers of multipolar neurons in the molecular layer of the right cerebral hemisphere. The amygdaloid nucleus contained tightly packed round or elongated clusters of mature large neurons, some within bundles of myelinated fibres that appeared out of place.)

Table 4 *Pathological findings in the cerebellum*

Case	Purkinje cell layer	Other
1	Cytoplasmic inclusions in Purkinje cells in the vermis and hemisphere.	Break in dentate ribbon. Patches of subcortical ectopic grey matter.
2	Decreased numbers of Purkinje cells and increase in GFAP in Bergmann glia.	
3	Patchy decrease in numbers of Purkinje cells and proliferation of Bergmann glia.	Break in dentate ribbon.
4	Decreased numbers of Purkinje cells.	
5	Decreased number of Purkinje cells. Areas of Bergmann glia proliferation and moderate patchy increase in GFAP staining.	
6	Decreased numbers of Purkinje cells and moderate patchy increase in GFAP in Bergmann glia.	

Table 5 *Neuronal density ($10^{-2} \times$ n/mm^3) in superior frontal gyrus*

Case	Autistic subjects			Control subjects		
	Age (years)	Brain (kg)	Count	Age (years)	Brain (kg)	Count
2	22	1.60	330	20	NA	259
4	24	1.81	194	24	1.50	311
5	20	1.40	144	40	1.47	180
6	24	1.82	216	43	1.52	226
IOP average[†]			(221)*			(244)
3	27	1.45	365	35	NA	342
1	4	1.53	336	4	1.18‡	373
				6	1.23‡	395

NA = not available. [†]Figures in brackets are averages for Institute of Psychiatry processed cases. ‡Female. *Exact P = 0.56, Mann–Whitney U, Wilcoxon rank sum test.

Morphometry

Amongst the normal control subjects there was considerable variation in neuronal counts in the frontal cortex and hippocampal sub-fields, but more consistency in the Purkinje cell counts. The range of frontal counts in the brains of autistic individuals was similar to that in the control subjects, although the count in Case 5, who had severe epilepsy, fell below the control range (Table 5). There were no consistent differences between autistic and control subjects in neuronal counts across the different hippocampal sub-fields, although Case 3 had elevated counts in all CA fields compared with his control (Table 6). Purkinje cell counts were consistently lower in the adult autistic cases than in control subjects (Table 7). Statistical comparison of neuronal densities between control and autistic cases from the Institute of Psychiatry (Mann–Whitney U, Wilcoxon rank sum test) only revealed significant differences in the density of Purkinje cells (exact P = 0.02). White matter neuronal densities in the autistic brains were unremarkable in the areas systematically counted (data not shown).

Post-mortem findings in cases where tissue was unavailable for study

Post-mortem findings, but not tissue, were available for a further 14 individuals with a clinical diagnosis of autism. Brain weights were recorded in four young adult males (1530, 1450, 1400 and 1300 g), one young adult female (1400 g) and one 16-year-old female (1330 g). Eleven brains were reportedly macroscopically normal. The meninges were thickened and adherent in one case with a history of meningitis in infancy. In the brain of the 16-year-old girl the cortical ribbon was narrower than expected and subcortical white matter was reduced in amount. The substantia nigra was rather poorly pigmented. Microscopically, the cortex was described as well populated by nerve cells. No microscopic reports were available on any other brains.

Discussion

The identified neuropathology in this series is already more extensive than previously reported. The findings included increased brain size and developmental abnormalities of the cerebral cortex, brainstem and cerebellum; in some cases there was also secondary pathology. Claims of consistently elevated neuronal density in the hippocampus have not been replicated. It seems unlikely that misdiagnosis is responsible for any discrepancies with previous findings. Although only one individual was seen during life (Case 3), all of the cases had received a clinical diagnosis of autism. In addition case notes were reviewed after death and the parents interviewed using the ADI (Le Couteur *et al.*, 1989). Nevertheless, because the cases in this study were all mentally handicapped, the applicability of the findings to more able individuals is uncertain. The heterogeneity of autism is emphasized by Case 1, which stands out because of the severe early motor difficulties, the severity of the malformations and the presence of Purkinje cell inclusions.

Four brains were large with little evidence of significant oedema. In two cases macrocephaly was also noted during childhood. In Case 1 the temporal lobes were enlarged and hyperconvoluted, but there were no gyral abnormalities

Table 6 *Neuronal density ($10^{-2} \times$ n/mm^3) in areas CA1, CA3 and CA4 of the hippocampus*

Case	Autistic subjects				Control subjects			
	Age (years)	CA1	CA3	CA4	Age (years)	CA1	CA3	CA4
2	22	231	156	104	20	167	164	92
4	24	239	168	103	24	145	236	99
5	20	189	208	98	26	186	229	149
					40	197	266	145
					43	216	231	93
IOP average[†]		(220)*	(177)*	(102)(*)		(182)	(225)	(116)
3	27	334	247	154	35	215	180	124
1	4	306	279	306	4	298	322	279
					6	212	237	162

[†]Figures in brackets are averages for Institute of Psychiatry processed cases. *Exact $P = 0.10$ and (*)exact $P = 0.56$, Mann–Whitney U, Wilcoxon rank sum test.

Table 7 *Purkinje cell densities (n/mm^2) of Purkinje cell layer of the cerebellum*

Case	Autistic subjects		Control subjects	
	Age (years)	Count (n/mm^2)	Age (years)	Count (n/mm^2)
2	22	169	20	220
4	24	196	26	241
5	20	128	40	220
6	24	160	43	268
IOP average[†]		(163)*		(237)
3[‡]	27	131		
1	4	251	4	231

[†]Figures in brackets are averages for Institute of Psychiatry processed cases. [‡]No identically processed cerebellar tissue from a young male control was available. *Exact $P = 0.02$, Mann–Whitney U, Wilcoxon rank sum test.

in the other cases. There were also several instances of macroscopically abnormal development of the brainstem, and of the corpus callosum in one brain.

There was microscopic pathology in the cerebral hemispheres, cortex and cerebellum. Abnormalities in cortical development were seen in individual cases, including: areas of increased cortical thickness, high neuronal density, neurons in the molecular layer, neuronal disorganization, poor differentiation of the grey–white matter boundary, neuronal heterotopias and focally increased numbers of single neurons in the white matter (Table 2). In the brainstem (Table 3), the inferior olives were malformed in three brains and ectopic neurons related to the olivary complex were seen in a further two. Olivary dysplasia was associated with enlarged arcuate nuclei in two cases. In one brain there was also a subtle abnormality of the locus coeruleus. Purkinje cell density was decreased in all the adult cases, but inclusions were seen only in Case 1. In two cases there were minor developmental cerebellar abnormalities.

Hippocampal neuronal density looked relatively high in two cases, but only in Case 3 (Table 6) was there any evidence of increased density in all CA subfields. There was no evidence of a statistically significant increase in cell density in the cases processed at the Institute of Psychiatry compared with control subjects (Table 6); however, sampling and number of cases were limited. There was no hippocampal sclerosis or other pathology in any case. Examination of the amygdala has been limited by tissue sampling for neurochemistry but, with the exception of the most recent case, no abnormalities were identified.

In several brains there was also evidence of acquired pathology. The number of Bergmann glia was increased in three cases and there was also increased staining for GFAP, but no empty baskets were seen (the presence of groups of basket cell axons in the absence of the Purkinje cell perikaryon that they normally ensheath is generally interpreted as evidence for acquired Purkinje cell loss). Cerebral subpial gliosis was observed in two cases. There were increased numbers of corpora amylacea in the insular cortex of Case 5 (and in the molecular layer of the cerebellum of the most recently identified case). The two areas of cortical gliosis in Case 3 were probably a consequence of the head injury in childhood.

Comparison with previous studies

The most striking contrast with previous findings is that four of the six brains were unusually large and heavy, although megalencephaly was uncommon amongst the cases unavailable for study. Brain weights were not reported by Ritvo *et al.* (1986) or by Kemper and Bauman (1993); however, in this latter series they were apparently 100–200 g heavier than expected in most subjects aged <12 years, but 100–200 g lighter than expected in the majority of adult subjects (Bauman, 1996). One of the cases in Darby's literature review (1976) had a heavy brain, weighing 1550 g at 5 years of age (case 11 in that review); the brain of one of the two idiopathic cases described by Williams *et al.* (1980) weighed 1520 g (their case 1), and the other weighed 1430 g (their case 3); and the female described by Coleman *et al.* (1985) had a brain weight of 1380 g (Rodier *et al.*, 1996). There are two reports of autistic individuals with unusually small brains; one was associated with premature closure of the cerebral sutures and severe self injury (Hof *et al.*, 1991); the other was also profoundly handicapped and physically disabled (Guerin *et al.*, 1996). The association between autism and increased brain weight contrasts with the finding of microcephaly in many cases of mental handicap unaccompanied by autism (see for instance Cole *et al.*, 1994).

There is some convergent evidence for increased brain size in individuals with autism. Three MRI studies have found increased brain volume in child and adult subjects. Filipek *et al.* (1992) reported increased brain volume in autistic children compared with normal subjects, developmental language disorder and non-autistic mentally handicapped control subjects. Piven *et al.* (1995, 1996) found increased total brain volume in adolescents and adults compared with normal control subjects. Increased head circumference in autistic individuals has been noted in several different samples (Hauser *et al.*, 1975; Bolton *et al.*, 1994; Bailey *et al.*, 1995, Woodhouse *et al.*, 1996; Lainhart *et al.*, 1997). Together these data suggest that the finding of megalencephaly (brain weight > 2.5 SD above the mean) is in keeping with a tendency towards increased brain size in some adults and children with autism.

Cortical dysgenetic lesions have not been a prominent feature of previous studies. They were not highlighted by Kemper and Bauman (1993), with the exception that anterior cingulate cortex was consistently unusually coarse and poorly laminated, and associated with increased cell packing density in one case (Kemper, 1988). Polymicrogyria has been seen in two post-mortem cases (Ritvo *et al.*, 1986; Kemper, 1988) and several MRI studies have observed developmental cortical abnormalities in a small proportion of patients (Gaffney and Tsai, 1987; Piven *et al.*, 1990; Schifter *et al.*, 1994).

In this study there was no significant cerebellar atrophy or apparent granule cell loss; neuronal size in the dentate nucleus and olive appeared unremarkable; and there was no tendency for olivary cells to cluster at the periphery of the convolutions. The extent of the facial nuclei has not yet been assessed. There was, however, clear evidence of developmental brainstem abnormalities that have not been reported previously (Table 3). The MRI findings in the brainstem in autism are largely contradictory, probably reflecting methodological differences and the small size of the relevant structures.

Possible mechanisms

Primary megalencephaly may be associated with increased cell number and increased cell size. Frontal cortical neuronal density appeared to be increased in three cases—including in some areas of thickened cortex—but this is not evident in the limited morphometry. The wide variation in cortical neuronal density in control subjects, and the possibility of cortical neuronal loss secondary to epilepsy, limit the conclusions that can presently be drawn. Nevertheless, there

is no evidence of substantially decreased neuronal density in the megalencephalic brains, suggesting that raised total cell number may contribute to brain enlargement. Increased cell replication and impaired developmental cell death might both lead to an excess of neurons. Programmed cell death is well documented in mammalian postnatal cerebral cortex, but also affects a significant proportion of cells in proliferative and, to a lesser extent, postmitotic regions of murine foetal cerebral cortex (Blaschke *et al.*, 1996).

Different cortical dysgenetic lesions occurred either alone or in combination, but there was no evidence of neuronal cytomegaly, abnormal neuronal configuration or abnormal neurofilament expression. Although focal increases in white matter neuronal density were seen (Table 2 and Fig. 12), limited morphometry did not reveal a generalized increase. The co-occurrence of different patterns of dysgenesis is not uncommon (Prayson and Estes, 1995), and the findings suggest that there may be abnormalities in cortical neuronal proliferation, migration and programmed cell death (Rorke, 1994; Mischel *et al.*, 1995).

Evidence of abnormal neuronal migration, and possibly abnormal control of cell number, was also found in the brainstem and cerebellum. Whether shared mechanisms underlie the cortical and brainstem findings is unclear. Nevertheless olivary anomalies seldom occur in isolation and heterotopias are usually associated with cortical developmental abnormalities, particularly megalencephaly, pachygyria and lissencephaly (Harding and Copp, 1997). Olivary development involves long distance migration from the primary precerebellar neuroepithelium, which is also the source of cells forming the arcuate nuclei and basis pontis (Essick, 1912); the cells forming the dentate nucleus arise from the superior portion of the rhombic lip. A tendency for inferior olivary neurons to cluster at the periphery of the convolutions was not identified, but Kemper and Bauman's (1993) observation may be related to the abnormalities that were observed in this series. In a case of Coffin–Siris syndrome (DeBassio *et al.*, 1985), peripheral clustering of olivary neurons occurred in association with islands of ectopic olivary neurons, a large medial accessory olive, unusually large arcuate nuclei and ectopic neurons in the white matter of the cerebellum at the level of the dentate nucleus.

There is only limited evidence, so far, that abnormal development also affects more rostral brainstem structures. An aberrant pontine tract was identified in Case 1 and there was mild disorganization of the locus coeruleus in Case 6. Kemper and Bauman (1993) observed disorganization of the nucleus locus coeruleus and the nucleus raphe dorsalis in one brain and, in another case, the centrally placed neurons of the basis pontis were apparently more densely packed and enlarged compared with control subjects (Kemper, 1988).

Decreased Purkinje cell density is a relatively consistent observation across the post-mortem studies, although in several cases in this series many stretches of folia were well populated with Purkinje cells. The frequency of developmental medullary abnormalities indirectly supports the hypothesis that the Purkinje cell findings have a developmental basis. Kemper and Bauman (1993) argued that, in the absence of glial cell hyperplasia or retrograde olivary cell loss, decreased Purkinje cell density pointed to a loss occurring at, or before, 30 weeks gestation. Nevertheless, if substantial Purkinje cell loss occurs only early in development, then the apparently normal development of the cerebellar cortex is slightly puzzling. Purkinje cells play a central role in normal cerebellar development and they control proliferation of cells in the murine external granule layer (Feddersen *et al.*, 1992; Smeyne *et al.*, 1995). Postmitotic external granule layer cells migrate to form the internal granule layer (IGL), which increases in thickness in man from the 5–6th prenatal month to the 4–5th postnatal month (Raaf and Kernohan, 1944), being very thin until 32 weeks gestation (Friede, 1973). Consequently, any substantial loss of Purkinje cells prior to 32 weeks gestation could be associated with hypoplastic cerebellar folia. The modest patchy glial cell hyperplasia seen in this series raises the additional possibility of postnatal loss of Purkinje cells, perhaps related to epilepsy (although, as yet, no empty baskets have been identified). Whilst olivary gliosis has not been observed, moderate loss of olivary cells may be difficult to identify, as the cells normally show great variation in density and lie relatively far apart (Brodal, 1940). The Purkinje cell inclusions seen in the only child in this series add a further complication. Such inclusions have not previously been reported and their aetiology is unknown. Purkinje cell density was unremarkable in this case, but we are not aware of any precedent for the complete disappearance of inclusion-bearing cells.

In summary, developmental neuropathology was not localized to the limbic system, cerebellum (Kemper and Bauman, 1993), or derivatives of a single hindbrain rhombomere (Rodier *et al.*, 1996). Although there is evidence of abnormal neuronal migration, other factors influencing neuronal number, survival and orientation also seem to be important. There is clearly a need for further study of the pathological basis of increased brain size. Of course, some developmental pathology may be either a consequence of maldevelopment at remote sites, or epiphenomena of more fundamental abnormalities. Identifying the genes predisposing to autism may help to clarify these relationships. With regard to timing, it would be premature to conclude that a single developmental event led to these findings. Nevertheless, abnormal development had sometimes begun by the time of olivary cell migration, which occurs before the end of the 3rd month.

Relationship to symptomatology

Explanations of developmental cognitive and behavioural dysfunction by neuropathology are precarious, as brain function may not be impaired and inferences based upon localization in adults may not be pertinent. As yet, no single pathology common to all cases of autism has been identified. Of course, autism is a complex behavioural disorder and it would be too much to expect such specificity at this level of analysis.

The finding of cortical dysgenetic lesions and megalencephaly suggests that cerebral dysfunction may underlie some cognitive and behavioural abnormalities, and may provide the pathological substrate of epilepsy. The inconsistency of the neuropathological findings indicates, however, that they are probably imperfect markers of abnormal cortical development and organization. Whilst brainstem abnormalities might cause neurological impairments (Rodier *et al.*, 1996), they seem unlikely to lead directly to high level cognitive deficits, but possibly both types of impairments can occur in more severely affected individuals. No consistent hippocampal abnormalities were identified in this series and systematic examination of the amygdala, medial septal nuclei, mamillary bodies and related structures has yet to be undertaken. Involvement of the amygdala remains an important possibility, but the evidence of cortical and brainstem maldevelopment has removed the imperative to argue that all autistic symptomatology arises from medial temporal and related structures. The relationship of cerebellar abnormalities to symptomatology (if any) remains uncertain. Although cerebellar maldevelopment may prove to be a marker of the disease process, behavioural consequences remain hypothetical until cerebellar dysfunction has been demonstrated unambiguously. In summary, in this study we have found no evidence for a highly localized pathology that seems likely to underlie autism. Instead, the findings raise the possibility that a combination of diverse, but related, neurodevelopmental abnormalities give rise to the characteristic symptomatology, and the associated mental handicap and epilepsy.

Acknowledgements

We are deeply indebted to all the parents and professionals who have helped with this study. We wish to thank Andrew Chadwick and Nigel Cairns of the MRC London Degenerative Brain Bank, Department of Neuropathology, for technical support; and Linda Wilkinson, Marion Gosden and Deborah Gomer for secretarial help.

References

Arin DM, Bauman ML, Kemper TL. The distribution of Purkinje cell loss in the cerebellum in autism [abstract]. Neurology 1991; 41 Suppl 1: 307.

Bachevalier J. Medial temporal lobe structures and autism: a review of clinical and experimental findings. [Review]. Neuropsychologia 1994; 32: 627–48.

Bailey A, Cox T. Neuroimaging in child and developmental psychiatry. In: Lewis S, Higgins JP, editors. Brain imaging in psychiatry. Oxford: Blackwell Scientific, 1996: 301–15.

Bailey A, Luthert P, Bolton P, Le Couteur A, Rutter M, Harding B. Autism and megalencephaly [letter]. Lancet 1993; 341: 1225–6.

Bailey A, Le Couteur A, Gottesman I, Bolton P, Simonoff E, Yuzda

E, et al. Autism as a strongly genetic disorder: evidence from a British twin study. Psychol Med 1995; 25: 63–77.

Bailey A, Phillips W, Rutter M. Autism: towards an integration of clinical, genetic, neuropsychological, and neurobiological perspectives. [Review]. J Child Psychol Psychiatry 1996; 37: 89–126.

Bauman ML. Microscopic neuroanatomic abnormalities in autism. [Review]. Pediatrics 1991; 87 S Pt 2: 791–6.

Bauman ML. Neuroanatomic observations of the brain in pervasive developmental disorders. [Review]. J Autism Dev Disord 1996; 26: 199–203.

Bauman ML, Kemper TL. Histoanatomic observations of the brain in early infantile autism. Neurology 1985; 35: 866–74.

Blaschke A, Staley K, Chun J. Widespread programmed cell death in proliferative and postmitotic regions of the fetal cerebral cortex. Development 1996; 122: 1165–74.

Bolton P, Macdonald H, Pickles A, Rios P, Goode S, Crowson M, et al. A case-control family history study of autism. J Child Psychol Psychiatry 1994; 35: 877–900.

Brodal A. Modification of Gudden method for study of cerebral localization. Arch Neurol Psychiatry 1940; 43: 46–58.

Cole G, Neal JW, Fraser WI, Cowie VA. Autopsy findings in patients with mental handicap. J Intellect Disabil Res 1994; 38: 9–26.

Coleman PD, Romano J, Lapham L, Simon W. Cell counts in cerebral cortex of an autistic patient. J Autism Dev Disord 1985; 15: 245–55.

Courchesne E, Yeung-Courchesne R, Press GA, Hesselink JR, Jernigan TL. Hypoplasia of cerebellar vermal lobules VI and VII in autism. N Engl J Med 1988; 318: 1349–54.

Courchesne C, Townsend J, Saitoh O. The brain in infantile autism: posterior fossa structures are abnormal [see comments]. Neurology 1994; 44: 214–23. Comment in: Neurology 1994; 44: 203–8, Comment in: Neurology 1995; 45: 398–402.

Darby JK. Neuropathologic aspects of psychosis in children. J Autism Child Schizophr 1976; 6: 339–52.

DeBassio WA, Kemper TL, Knoefel JE. Coffin-Siris syndrome: neuropathologic findings. Arch Neurol 1985; 42: 350–3.

Dekaban AS, Sadowsky, D. Changes in brain weights during the span of human life: relation of brain weights to body heights and body weights. Ann Neurol 1978; 4: 345–56.

DeLong GR. Autism, amnesia, hippocampus, and learning. [Review]. Neurosci Biobehav Rev 1992; 16: 63–70.

Essick CR. The development of the nuclei pontis and the nucleus arcuatus in man. Am J Anat 1912: 25–54.

Everall IP, Luthert PJ, Lantos PL. Neuronal loss in the frontal cortex in HIV infection [see comments]. Lancet 1991; 337: 1119–21. Comment in: Lancet 1991; 338: 129–30.

Feddersen RM, Ehlenfeldt R, Yunis WS, Clark HB, Orr HT. Disrupted cerebellar cortical development and progressive degeneration of Purkinje cells in SV40 T antigen transgenic mice. Neuron 1992; 9: 955–66.

Filipek PA, Richelme C, Kennedy DN, Rademacher J, Pitcher DA,

Zidel S, et al. Morphometric analysis of the brain in developmental language disorders and autism [abstract]. Ann Neurol 1992; 32: 475.

Friede RL. Dating the development of human cerebellum. Acta Neuropathol (Berl) 1973; 23: 48–58.

Gaffney GR, Tsai LY. Magnetic resonance imaging of high level autism. J Autism Dev Disord 1987; 17: 433–8.

Gillberg C, Steffenburg S. Outcome and prognostic factors in infantile autism and similar conditions: a population-based study of 46 cases followed through puberty. J Autism Dev Disord 1987; 17: 273–87.

Guerin P, Lyon G, Barthelemy C, Sostak E, Chevrollier V, Garreau B, et al. Neuropathological study of a case of autistic syndrome with severe mental retardation. Dev Med Child Neurol 1996; 38: 203–11.

Harding B, Copp AJ. Malformations. In: Graham DI, Lantos PL, editors. Greenfield's neuropathology. 6th ed. London: Arnold, 1997; 397–533.

Hauser S, DeLong GR, Rosman NP. Pneumographic findings in the infantile autism syndrome: a correlation with temporal lobe disease. Brain 1975; 98: 363–88.

Hof PR, Knabe R, Bovier P, Bouras C. Neuropathological observations in a case of autism presenting with self-injury behavior. Acta Neuropathol (Berl) 1991; 82: 321–6.

Kanner L. Autistic disturbances of affective contact. Nerv Child 1943; 2: 217–50.

Kemper TL. Neuroanatomic studies of dyslexia and autism. In: Swann JW, Messer A, editors. Disorders of the developing nervous system: changing views on their origins, diagnoses and treatments. New York: Alan R. Liss, 1988: 125–54.

Kemper TL, Bauman ML. The contribution of neuropathologic studies to the understanding of autism. Neurol Clin 1993; 11: 175–87.

Lainhart JE, Piven J, Wzorek M, Landa R, Santangelo SL, Coon H, et al. Macrocephaly in children and adults with autism. J Am Acad Child Adolesc Psychiatry 1997; 36: 282–90.

Le Couteur A, Rutter M, Lord C, Rios P, Robertson S, Holdgrafer M, et al. Autism diagnostic interview: a standardized investigator-based instrument. J Autism Dev Disord 1989; 19: 363–87.

Lockyer L, Rutter M. A five- to fifteen-year follow-up study of infantile psychosis. Br J Psychiatry 1969; 115: 865–82.

Minshew NJ. Indices of neural function in autism: clinical and biologic implications. [Review]. Pediatrics 1991; 87: 774–80.

Mischel PS, Nguyen LP, Vinters HV. Cerebral cortical dysplasia associated with pediatric epilepsy. Review of neuropathologic features and proposal for a grading system. [Review]. J Neuropathol Exp Neurol 1995; 54: 137–53.

Piven J, Berthier ML, Starkstein SE, Nehme E, Pearlson G, Folstein S. Magnetic resonance imaging evidence for a defect of cerebral cortical development in autism. Am J Psychiatry 1990; 147: 734–9.

Piven J, Arndt S, Bailey J, Havercamp S, Andreasen N, Palmer P. An MRI study of brain size in autism. Am J Psychiatry 1995; 152: 1145–9.

Piven J, Arndt S, Bailey J, Andreasen N. Regional brain enlargement in autism: a magnetic resonance imaging study. J Am Acad Child Adolesc Psychiatry 1996; 35: 530–6.

Prayson RA, Estes ML. Cortical dysplasia: a histopathologic study of 52 cases of partial lobectomy in patients with epilepsy. Hum Pathol 1995; 26: 493–500.

Raaf J, Kernohan JW. A study of the external granular layer in the cerebellum. Am J Anat 1944; 75: 151–72.

Raymond G, Bauman M, Kemper T. The hippocampus in autism: Golgi analysis [abstract]. Ann Neurol 1989; 26: 483–4.

Ritvo ER, Freeman BJ, Scheibel AB, Duong T, Robinson H, Guthrie D, et al. Lower Purkinje cell counts in the cerebellar of four autistic subjects: initial findings of the UCLA-NSAC Autopsy Research Report. Am J Psychiatry 1986; 143: 862–6.

Rodier PM, Ingram JL, Tisdale B, Nelson S, Romano J. Embryological origin for autism: developmental anomalies of the cranial nerve motor nuclei. J Comp Neurol 1996; 370: 247–61.

Rorke LB. A perspective: the role of disordered genetic control of neurogenesis in the pathogenesis of migration disorders. J Neuropathol Exp Neurol 1994; 53: 105–17.

Rutter M. Autistic children. Infancy to adulthood. Semin Psychiatry; 1970; 2: 435–50.

Rutter M, Bailey A, Bolton P, Le Couteur A. Autism and known

medical conditions: myth and substance. [Review]. J Child Psychol Psychiatry 1994; 35: 311–22.

Saitoh O, Courchesne E, Egaas B, Lincoln AJ, Schreibman L. Cross-sectional area of the posterior hippocampus in autistic patients with cerebellar and corpus callosum abnormalities. Neurology 1995; 45: 317–24.

Schifter T, Hoffman JM, Hatten HP Jr, Hanson MW, Coleman RE, DeLong GR. Neuroimaging in infantile autism. [Review]. J Child Neurol 1994; 9: 155–61.

Smeyne RJ, Chu T, Lewin A, Bian F, S.-Crisman S, Kunsch C, et al. Local control of granule cell generation by cerebellar Purkinje cells. Mol Cell Neurosci 1995; 6: 230–51.

Williams RS, Hauser SL, Purpura DP, DeLong GR, Swisher CM. Autism and mental retardation: neuropathologic studies performed in four retarded persons with autistic behavior. Arch Neurol 1980; 37: 749–53.

Woodhouse W, Bailey A, Rutter M, Bolton P, Baird G, Le Couteur A. Head circumference in autism and other pervasive developmental disorders. J Child Psychol Psychiatry 1996; 37: 665–71.

World Health Organization. ICD-10 classification of mental and behavioural disorders: clinical descriptions and diagnostic guidelines. Geneva: World Health Organization, 1992.

Received June 4, 1997. Accepted January 5, 1998

Appendix
Case histories
Case 1
As a baby he was a poor feeder who disliked being held. A clinical hearing test was failed at 7.5 months but the parents knew that he could hear soft sounds and was sensitive to vibrations. He had persistent difficulties with gross motor control, was clumsy and did not chew. He could be propped to stand at 2 years of age but could not move from this position. He acquired a few sounds but no speech; he screamed frequently, especially if there was an echo. He did not turn to his name or speech, and never followed eye gaze or pointing. He could sometimes follow simple instructions, particularly if context bound. He did not imitate or copy, but would sometimes point to a picture in a book. In infancy he continued to dislike being held and sometimes urinated when picked up. He took no interest in people and would only look at his parents if they jumped and waved their arms. He appeared to focus on parts of people and was more interested in his parents' glasses and earrings than their faces; he was particularly interested in buckles and zips. He could spot small items such as milk bottle tops and paper clips but would ignore large objects in the environment. He would not seek comfort if hurt. He would bite his parents and other children, and appeared to enjoy the chaotic reaction that this provoked. He became increasingly destructive and overactive. He was interested in mechanical things and would spend most of the day in minute examination and manipulation of tiny objects; his fine motor coordination appeared unimpaired, although he acquired few fine motor skills. He liked to fiddle with bunches of keys, and would attempt to put these in locks. He enjoyed watching a spinning top, and would spin wheels for hours; he also liked watching credits at the end of television programmes. He flicked light switches repeatedly. He would often flap his arms and pant, particularly if excited, and this could be accompanied by rocking on his toes. He liked to look at the ceiling and spin, and also enjoyed going on roundabouts. In the 1st year he rubbed his feet together and clenched his hands together in the midline; when older he engaged in hand stereotypies close to his face. He gnawed at his fingers and nails, head-banged and pulled at his penis. He appeared intrigued by pain; he went back repeatedly to an exposed mains socket to get a shock and he cut himself with a razor. He would occasionally cry if he hurt himself but appeared insensitive to temperature. He had marked pica and would drink the water in a paddling pool until sick.

Case 2
He sat at 7 months and walked at 1 year. He was dry and clean by 2 years, but 6 months later developed secondary enuresis. Parental concern was aroused at 24 months by speech delay and by his habit of sitting on a table and spinning a record. There was no pre-speech babble and, although he would repeat 'one, two, three' when climbing steps at 18 months of age, he developed no other speech until the age of 7 years. High tone hearing loss was queried, but was thought to be insufficient to interfere with speech acquisition. He did not react to voices or people although he could hear the rustle of sweet papers. He was able to hum tunes and he had favourite records. He did not imitate or point or use gestures to communicate; as a child he would take his mothers hand and lead her to something he wanted. Later in life he acquired a small vocabulary, but would only talk when pressed; most of the time he was mute. He would usually reply with a single word, but had a

few direct phrases such as 'go away' or 'I want my mummy'. His articulation was poor. As a young child he did not understand even simple instructions, but this improved with intensive teaching. There is no history of echolalia. As a young child he avoided eye contact, but this had been taught by the age of 11 years. He took no interest in his parents and was unconcerned by their absence. He avoided other children, made no social overtures and would not seek or respond to comfort when hurt or upset. He did not cry until the age of 6 years, and had a limited range of facial expression which could be inappropriate. As a child he did not engage in pretend play. He would spend many hours on a swing, fiddling with straws (which mother had to carry with her), watching a spinning top or fiddling with pliable objects or pieces of string. He was good at shapes and completed simple jigsaw puzzles upside down. He liked manipulating small objects and was skilled at spotting small objects that people had lost. Certain aspects of his life were routinized. He disliked changes in the furniture at home; he would usually return pieces to their original place. He avoided going to bed unless accompanied by his mother. When older, walks and his mother's visits (when he was in residential care) had to be conducted in a stereotyped manner. He had many hand mannerisms which were accompanied by swaying, as he frequently looked at his hands and became upset if he was stopped. He liked to spin and bounce and had a dancing routine when music was played; he would rock in stressful situations. He was socially disinhibited and as an adult could attack other residents without provocation. He attended a number of different educational centres until he was 9 years of age when he was transferred to a residential school for autistic children until the age of 14 years. He was then moved to a long-stay hospital where he remained until his death.

Case 3

In infancy, he was inaccessible and detached. He had no language except for the word 'no', but he did make some noises and imitated environmental sounds such as a dog barking. He understood simple instructions. His needs were anticipated by his mother whom he would follow around. He was aloof and would not play with other children; he preferred to line up small articles such as pins and needles in rows. As a child he could be indiscriminately affectionate towards strangers but as an adult he resented the company of others. In childhood he had rigid likes and dislikes concerning food, and had to sit at the same spot and use the same spoon; a crooked table cloth distressed him. He collected matches, pins, knives and bus tickets, and enjoyed breaking up razor blades into little pieces and holding them in his mouth. He also enjoyed music. Later he had an obsession for string, thread and shoelaces which he flicked in front of his eyes and sometimes ate. When older, he flicked his face with the empty end of a sleeve which he watched. He had stereotyped postures and mannerisms when excited; he flicked his fingers and flapped his hands from the elbows. He sometimes walked on his toes. When younger he was constantly active, wringing his hands and slapping his head, but became underactive in adulthood. He showed no' response to pain and sometimes tore out his own hair. He entered a residential facility at the age of 7 years.

Case 4

He sat at 6 months and walked at 16 months. The parents were concerned at 18 months because of a lack of interest in his

mother and her activities, his tendency to wander and the need to wake him for feeding. His first word was yoghurt at 36 months. He subsequently developed a small vocabulary of single words but these were not used between the ages of 5 and 12 years. He did not point or use gestures to communicate and did not attend to speech. He echoed some single words and acquired some stereotyped phrases such as 'cup of tea please' and 'tie my shoelace'; he would say 'goodbye' when he wanted others to leave. Most speech was related to food needs and was poorly articulated. He understood single but not double commands. He liked music, and could hum tunes, sing songs and fill in missing words from songs. He ignored people around him, was unconcerned by his parents absence and disliked people coming too close; however, he could enjoy rough and tumble. He did not make social approaches for either physical needs or comfort, but as an adult would sometimes touch his parents. He was socially disinhibited and could also laugh inappropriately. Between the ages of 2 and 3 years he carried a hairbrush and waved a poker in front of his eyes like a windscreen wiper; similarly, he twiddled with sticks and wire. He also liked to put objects in the fire and watch them burn. He lined up items and enjoyed jigsaws. He would touch velvet, petals and leaves. He had complex hand and finger mannerisms in front of his eyes which were accompanied by a rigid facial expression. He bottom hopped until the age of 16 years and rocked violently, breaking four sofas. He was routinized and disliked change; he objected to his mother not having her legs crossed, a door not being fully closed and new clothes. He would notice if objects were moved. As a child he was overactive and had good balance. He was taught to ride a bicycle over the course of 2 years but could never kick a ball. When older, he chewed objects and could not pass cigarette butts without picking them up and eating them. When upset he would bite the back of his fingers and sometimes head-banged; he was insensitive to cold and pain.

Case 5

His parents were concerned at 14 months because of his unusual language development. At 4 months he did not alert to noises and later did not respond to pointing. First words were acquired at 10 months but were used for a few weeks and disappeared, as did subsequent new words. He sat at 8 months, walked at 16 months and was first assessed at 22 months because he walked with his hands raised. He did not usually respond to voice, and deafness was queried. He retained the ability to say a few single words, but did not speak on a daily basis, and any language usually related to food or drink. He did not use his small vocabulary to communicate, neither did he gesture, point or use eye gaze communicatively. Articulation was poor. There was no imaginative or imitative play and little curiosity. As an adult he could say ~100 words, knew a few signs and understood single words. His parents were also concerned in childhood about hyperactive unpredictable behaviour and lack of awareness of danger. Bladder and bowel control were not acquired until the age of 10 years. As a child he did not raise his arms to be lifted, gaze directly at others or check back; his response to other people was unpredictable and he did not greet his parents, show them objects or direct their attention. Facial expression was limited and often inappropriate. He was relatively insensitive to pain and did not offer others comfort. As a young child he was unaffectionate and even in adulthood socially disinhibited. He had no childhood peer relationships but formed an attachment to a fellow resident in adulthood. He lacked curiosity and as a child played with the doors and wheels of toy cars, and enjoyed the texture of sand and pebbles. He was preoccupied by the Ladybird series of books and knew all the local stockists; he liked to carry a book and if left alone would flick its corners all day. He enjoyed repetitively listening to stories on cassettes. He flapped when running or excited, and in enclosed spaces walked in circles. In childhood chewing was immature, he frequently dribbled and chewed or mouthed most things.

Case 6

The parents sought advice at 24 months because of speech delay. There was no pre-speech babble. First words were acquired at 10 months, numbered <10, were not used communicatively and had disappeared by the age of 4 years. There was no social use of sounds, no gesturing or pointing and no imitation of activities. Usually he did not respond to voice, although he did put his hands over his ears to certain domestic sounds. He learnt a limited number of social gestures, understood single words and in adulthood had five to six signs. In childhood he took little notice of his parents and there was no greeting, showing or sharing. He was aloof and would not come for comfort. Any eye contact was fleeting and facial expressions were sometimes inappropriate and reduced in range. He did not check back and there was no separation anxiety. He could be shy with strangers but also socially disinhibited. He took no interest in other children, but sometimes enjoyed being chased or engaging in rough and tumble with his parents. There was no imaginative play. He was an overactive child. He enjoyed tearing paper and later flicking grass against his ear. He always had to have a 'flicker' of some sort but was not interested in this visually. His parents took efforts to prevent him becoming too routinized. He was obsessed by water and would flush a line of school toilets repeatedly. He would empty anything that was only half full, had to break panes of glass that were cracked and would unravel any clothes with imperfections. He smelt most things and from the age of 14 years compulsively touched objects. He occasionally flapped whilst walking and there was some moderate self injury.

157

Pergamon

0021-9630(95)00115-8

J. Child Psychol. Psychiat. Vol. 37, No. 1, pp. 89–126, 1996
Elsevier Science Ltd
© 1996 Association for Child Psychology and Psychiatry
Printed in Great Britain. All rights reserved
0021-9630/96 $15.00 + 0.00

Autism: Towards an Integration of Clinical, Genetic, Neuropsychological, and Neurobiological Perspectives

Anthony Bailey, Wendy Phillips and Michael Rutter

MRC Child Psychiatry Unit and Centre for Social, Genetic and Developmental
Psychiatry, Institute of Psychiatry, London, U.K.

Autism consitutes one of the best validated child psychiatric disorders. Empirical research
has succeeded in delineating the key clinical phenomena, in demonstrating strong genetic
influences on the underlying liability, and in identifying basic cognitive deficits. A range
of neurobiological abnormalities has also been found, although the replicability of specific
findings has not been high. An understanding of the causal processes leading to autism,
and accounting for the marked variability in its manifestations, requires an integration
across these different levels of enquiry. Although this is not yet possible, a partial
integration provides a useful strategy for identifying key research questions, the
limitations of existing hypotheses, and future research directions that are likely to prove
fruitful. The research findings for each research level are critically reviewed in order to
consider how to move towards an integration across levels.

Keywords: Autism, genetics, neuropsychology, brain imaging, neuropathology, psychopathology

Introduction

Research findings in the 1960s and 1970s clearly
demonstrated that autism was associated with basic, and
persistent, cognitive deficits that were not explicable in
motivational terms (Hermelin & O'Connor, 1970;
Rutter, 1979). The finding that about a fifth of autistic
children without clinically detectable neurological abnormalities develop epilepsy as they grow older, often in
adolescence or early adult life (Rutter, 1970), indicated
that some form of "organic" brain dysfunction was
implicated. It came to be generally accepted that autism
constituted a biologically based neurodevelopmental
disorder. Folstein and Rutter's (Folstein & Rutter,
1977a,b) small scale twin study went on to indicate that
genetic factors probably played a major role in aetiology.
All of these findings have stood the test of time and have
been further specified through systematic research
undertaken during the past two decades. The goal of
this review is to summarize the current state of
knowledge on genetic, neuropsychological, and neurobiological findings in relation to autism; to consider how
these might account for the clinical phenomena; and to
discuss how these various levels of research might be
integrated.

This integration is a general need with respect to any
multifactorial medical condition but it has proved quite
difficult to accomplish, even when quite a lot is known
about the pathophysiology (which is not the case with

autism). That is because often there are multiple
abnormalities at each level and more than one route
between levels. Sing & Reilly (1993) have argued that
there are four basic attributes that characterize all
complex systems: *coherence* and interaction among
biological traits; *emergence*, in that risks act in
probabilistic fashion; *hierarchy* so that the disease
process operates through a network of intermediate
biological traits with each level characterized by fewer
agents than exist at the level below (the bottom level
being genes); and diseases reflect a *dynamic process* that
may change over the course of a lifetime.

Psychiatrists and psychologists have generally been
reluctant to accept such propositions. Thus, Kidd (1991)
has argued that it is necessary to maintain a disbelief in
multigene inheritance and psychologists have sought to
account for autism in terms of a single, modular,
cognitive abnormality (see, e.g. Baron-Cohen et al.,
1993; Frith, 1989; Happé, 1994a,b; Hobson, 1993;
Morton & Frith, 1995). For the most part, different
levels of research into autism and other neurodevelopmental disorders have tended to remain rather separate
from one another, with speculations about implications
for other levels but little attempt to integrate the findings
as a whole (but see Courchesne, Townsend & Chase,
1995 and Rourke, 1995 for ambitious attempts to tie
findings together). In approaching the challenge of
integration, it is important to appreciate that there may
not be any one overarching mechanism (Goodman,
1989); whether or not there is will depend on the means
by which the causal process(es) operate.

In that connection, Courchesne et al., (1995) have
highlighted four cautions that need to be borne in mind.
First, similar neurobehavioural phenotypes do not

Requests for reprints to: Anthony Bailey, MRC Child
Psychiatry Unit, Institute of Psychiatry, De Crespigny Park,
London SE5 8AF, U.K.

necessarily imply a single pathogenesis (see, for example, the diverse causes of dementia). Second, functional abnormalities do not necessarily mark either the developmental timing or the type of pathogenesis (because widespread indirect effects are common). Third, structural abnormalities similarly do not necessarily indicate the site of the pathogenic process; experimental approaches are crucial to test hypotheses on the links between structure and function. Fourth, abnormalities in multiple structures do not necessarily mean that there are multiple sources of pathogenesis (because a single pathogenic process may have widespread effects and because a disruption of early development at one site is likely to have consequent effects on the structure of other sites — as a result of both neuronal migration and interconnection between brain areas).

Morton and Frith (1995) have outlined some of the main varieties of conceptual model that need to be considered. One model is provided by Mendelian disorders, where the cause concerns just the operation of a single gene. Despite this apparently simple causal process, Mendelian disorders, and disorders due to a single chromosomal defect, can have quite diverse clinical manifestations. Thus, the Fragile X anomaly may be accompanied by a normal IQ or by severe mental retardation; similarly, the affected individuals may be behaviourally normal, severely socially anxious, or autistic. Genetic research has moved from being (relatively) content with recognition that a medical condition is due to a single gene operating in Mendelian fashion to an appreciation that the challenge is to understand *how* the variable expression comes about (Simonoff et al., in press). Although there may prove to be several different mechanisms operating together, considerable caution needs to be exercised before putting forward different explanations for each set of phenomena. Thus, for many years people have been aware that Huntington's disease showed "anticipation", meaning that the age of onset tended to drop over the generations. It had also been evident that early onset seemed to be associated with transmission through the father. Just before the trinucleotide repeat mechanism that solved this riddle was discovered, Szatmari and Jones (1991) had suggested that, whereas the disease was due to a single gene, the age of onset was controlled by an independent set of polygenes. As we now know, the trinucleotide repeat (which increases through intergenerational transmission) in fact provides the explanation, at least at the extremes (Trottier et al., 1994; Kieburtz et al., 1994), and there is no need to invoke any other genes.

A second model is one in which there are multiple biological causes, and several different behavioural manifestations but a single defining cognitive deficit. Much of mental retardation might be considered to follow that pattern in that, despite the range of aetiologies and the heterogeneity of associated behaviour, there is a common global intellectual impairment such that the course of intellectual development is broadly similar among individuals with mental retardation (Zigler & Hodcapp, 1986). In many respects, IQ functions in a similar fashion across the whole of the IQ range. Nevertheless, the biological correlates are quite different in the severely retarded range from those in the 50–70 range or within the normal IQ distribution (Scott, 1994; Simonoff et al., in press). Also, there is important heterogeneity in the cognitive and behavioural patterns associated with particular medical syndromes leading to mental retardation. It has not proved helpful in research to treat mental retardation as if it were a homogeneous entity (Medical Research Council, 1994). Rather, progress has come through focusing on specific subgroups that seem to have some important unifying characteristic. Autism has been one example of that kind.

A third type of model is provided by conditions that are defined through some supposedly unifying set of clinical characteristics but where both the neuropsychological patterns and the biological causes are quite diverse. Possibly, the disorders involving disruptive behaviour (oppositional, hyperkinetic and conduct) might fit that pattern.

Accordingly, although undoubtedly there is a great need to integrate empirical findings from the different levels of research (Oades & Eggers, 1994), the attempted integration needs to be undertaken with an awareness of the range of causal models that must be considered. The same issue has been addressed with respect to schizophrenia, where it has been pointed out that integrations across levels first require a thorough appreciation and understanding of the abnormalities found at each level (Frith, 1992; Mortimer & McKenna, 1994). The objective of this review is to consider the findings and concepts in relation to autism as they apply to each level, noting the questions raised by the research findings, going on to consider possible ways forward in the search for an integration. Although, in preparing this review, we have throughout gone back to the original empirical research reports, our task has been made easier by the availability of good authoritative reviews in several of the key areas of research. In order to avoid overburdening this review with an exceedingly lengthy bibliography, we have used previous reviews as citations except where it has been important to draw attention to specific findings. Before proceeding to review the genetic, neuropsychological and neurobiological findings, it is necessary to note briefly the main clinical phenomena that have to be accounted for (we make no attempt to review clinical research findings in detail).

Clinical Features

As Rutter and Bailey (1993) pointed out, the clinical features to be accounted for in autism must include not only those that are pathognomonic (i.e. found only with autism) but also those that appear in some way intrinsic to the syndrome, even though they also occur in other conditions. These comprise: the behavioural characteristics; their age of first manifestation; mental retardation; epilepsy; response to drugs; physical characteristics; sex ratio; and course and outcome.

Behavioural Characteristics

Three main sets of behavioural characteristics define the syndrome of autism: social abnormalities, language abnormalities, and stereotyped repetitive patterns of behaviour (Frith, 1989; Happe, 1994a; Lord, 1993; Lord et al., 1989, 1994; Schopler & Mesibov, 1988; Sigman, 1995). The most characteristic social abnormality is the lack of social reciprocity and the impaired ability to develop loving relationships on the basis of interpersonal interactions. Social signalling and appreciation of other people's social cues are both deficient and there is a poor integration of social, communicative, and emotional features — as, for example, is expected in greeting behaviour. There is little protodeclarative pointing, and apparently little interest in sharing pride or pleasure with other people.

Autistic individuals usually show a delay in language development but it is the deviant communication features that are more characteristic. These include a lack of social chat even when language has developed, pragmatic deficits, pronominal reversal, delayed echolalia, neologisms and idiosyncratic unusual usages of language. Rutter (1987) suggested that many of these features may arise because of the autistic child's impaired ability to make use of feedback. That is, some of these features are seen as brief transient phenomena in normal children but they get rapidly eliminated from the language repertoire, probably as a result of feedback. Accordingly, the question in relation to autism is as much why the features persist as why they arise in the first place. Autistic individuals find it difficult to maintain an ongoing topic of conversation, are poor at building a conversational interchange on what the other person has said, are impaired in adapting their communication to different social contexts, and are limited in their use of prosody to communicate social and affective information. In addition, a lack of spontaneous creative pretend play is especially characteristic.

The third area of abnormality concerns the tendency to exhibit stereotyped, repetitive patterns of behaviour. These include quasi-obsessive routines and rituals, abnormal preoccupations, circumscribed interest patterns, abnormal attachments to objects, particular motor stereotopies, and unusual idiosyncratic responses to sensory stimuli.

Although undoubtedly there is a danger of assuming that clinical features cluster together simply because diagnostic conventions specify that they should do so, that does not seem to be the case with autism. Both epidemiological studies of children (Wing & Gould, 1978, 1979) and surveys of adults in a mental handicap hospital (Shah et al., 1982) have shown that these three domains of abnormalities tend to co-occur in the same individuals. The follow-up studies into adult life (Rutter et al., 1992) also show that verbal deficits predict social outcome and that this interconnection between domains is stronger in autism than it is in severe developmental disorders of receptive language. Family studies of autism, too, (Bolton et al., 1994) show that these three sets of behavioural features cluster together in relatives showing autistic like abnormalities of a kind that are much milder than seen in autism as traditionally diagnosed (see Genetic Influences section below).

Age of First Manifestation

Probably the modal age for parents first to become seriously concerned about their autistic child's development is in the months leading up to the second birthday. There is a failure to progress in language development, imaginative play, and social relationships. The concerns arise at that age, amongst other things, because the features of developmental progress seen in normal children are so strikingly absent in autistic individuals. What is less certain, however, is the age that autistic features are first manifest if attention is paid to the most relevant characteristics. The question has been tackled through the use of three main strategies. First, parents of autistic children have been asked retrospectively about behaviours normally manifest in the first two years of life, such as anticipating being picked up by the caregiver, using eye-to-eye gaze for social signalling, joint attention, reaching for a familiar person, and imitating other people's actions, as in waving goodbye or clapping hands (Dahlgren & Gillberg, 1989; Gillberg et al., 1990; Klin et al., 1992). These studies clearly indicate abnormalities in functions that are evident by 12 months of age. In some cases, parents had noted the abnormalities at that age but often that was not the case. As Rutter and Bailey (1993) pointed out, it cannot be assumed that because features ordinarily manifest in infancy are abnormal in older autistic individuals, these abnormalities would have been manifest in infancy. The point is that there are psychological functions that change over the course of development in what "drives" them and also in the part of the brain that subserves that function (see Aslin et al., 1983; Goldman-Rakic et al., 1983).

Second, there have been follow-up studies examining the predictive validity of health visitor findings. Lister (1992) found that nothing was noted at 12-months that differentiated children who later received a diagnosis of autism. Johnson et al., (1992) found that the contemporaneous infant health screening records of children later diagnosed as autistic showed little at 12 months but rather more at 18 months. Baron-Cohen et al., (1992) used a screening schedule that was probably better designed for detecting autism (the checklist for autism in toddlers—CHAT) to screen 41 18-month-olds who had an older brother or sister with autism. Four of the high risk children failed on at least two of the five target areas of pretend play, joint attention, pointing, social interest, and social play whereas no control child showed problems in more than one of these areas. The four high risk children picked out in this way were later found to have autism.

The third strategy is provided by examination of home movies or videos taken by families of their children before autism was diagnosed and usually before it was suspected. These studies, unlike the health visitor reports, have tended to indicate abnormalities as early as 12 months. The limitation of this finding is that many of the children were also mentally retarded and there was an inevitable uncertainty as to how far the early features reflected the retardation rather than the autism. That does not apply, however, to the most recent study by Osterling and Dawson (1994). Systematic blind analyses of video tapes showed abnormalities by 12 months even in those children who were not retarded.

Putting the findings together, it may be concluded that it is likely that in the majority of cases autism is manifest by 18 months of age and possibly it may be evident as early as 12 months, although the signs at that time are much more subtle and easy to miss. Two qualifiers must be added to this general conclusion. First, it is likely that there is a minority of autistic individuals who do not show abnormalities until approaching the age of 2 years (Volkmar & Cohen, 1989). Possibly, this later manifestation pattern is more common in autistic individuals of normal intelligence. It remains unknown whether early development was indeed truly normal in these cases and it is not known whether this minority pattern is in any way meaningfully different from the rest of autism. So far, there is no indication that it is. Second, although autism may be diagnosable as early as 18 months of age, it is probable that there is also a higher proportion of misdiagnoses at that age.

Mental Retardation

Numerous studies have shown that mental retardation is present in some three-quarters of cases of autism (Rutter, 1979). For the most part, psychological theories of autism have ignored this important finding on the assumption that because mental retardation is not specific to autism, it does not require explanation. That is, however, quite unacceptable for several different reasons. To begin with, it leaves completely unexplained why autism and mental retardation are so strongly associated. The answer cannot be that low IQ as such provides a risk factor because there is no invariant association between IQ and autism (thus, neither Down syndrome nor cerebral palsy associated with mental retardation carries a strong risk of autism). On the other hand, mental retardation cannot be dismissed as merely an epiphenomenon. For example, it is strongly associated with long-term outcome (Gillberg, 1991; Lotter, 1978; Rutter, 1970, 1978a). It may be that the focus should be more on verbal IQ than nonverbal. The former shows a substantial association with the severity of autism symptomatology and with familial loading (Bolton et al., 1994). This seems not to be the case with nonverbal IQ to anything like the same extent, suggesting that verbal and nonverbal intelligence may play rather different roles in autism. It should be added that autism is associated with cognitive skills, as well as with cognitive deficits (see section below on Neuropsychological approaches) and these too require explanation.

Epilepsy

Several systematic studies have shown that epilepsy develops in about a fifth to a third of autistic individuals (Gillberg & Steffenburg, 1987; Goode et al., 1994; Olsson et al., 1988; Rutter, 1970; Volkmar & Nelson, 1990). What is most distinctive about the epilepsy associated with autism, as compared with that found in mentally retarded individuals (Goulden et al., 1991) is the high frequency of an onset of epileptic attacks in late adolescence or early adult life. The significance of the age of onset is not known but it is relatively distinctive (Goode et al., 1994). There does not seem to be anything particularly characteristic about the type of epilepsy in those with a late onset. There is also a substantial group in whom the epilepsy begins during the preschool years and this is perhaps particularly characteristic of autism associated with profound mental retardation. In this earlier onset group, infantile spasms may be particularly associated with autism (Riikonen & Amnell, 1981). Early studies showed that the rate of epilepsy was much higher in autistic individuals who are severely retarded than those of normal intelligence (Bartak & Rutter, 1976). Later studies, however, have shown that the risk of epilepsy is not strongly associated with IQ apart from the fact that epilepsy is probably particularly common in those who are profoundly retarded. Thus, Goode et al., (1994) found that the risk of epilepsy in autistic individuals with a nonverbal IQ of 70 or greater was 18%, compared with 16% in the 50–69 range and 20% in the 35–49 range.

Response to Drugs

Quite a wide range of pharmacological agents have been tried in autism but it is apparent that there is no drug that produces a marked and specific beneficial effect (Gillberg & Coleman, 1992; Lord & Rutter, 1994; McDougle et al., 1994; Sloman, 1991). Modest symptomatic benefits may be obtained but what is striking is the *lack* of major effect on the key features of autism. This provides a sharp contrast with the other neuropsychiatric disorders with an onset in childhood, such as Tourette's syndrome and the hyperkinetic syndrome, and even more of a contrast with later onset disorders such as schizophrenia or major affective disorder.

Physical Characteristics

From the outset, autistic children were described as having a normal physiognomy, and indeed often as appearing attractive. Certainly, it is the case that autistic individuals usually do not show the obvious physical stigmata that characterize many cases of severe mental retardation unassociated with autism. However, recent evidence using three quite different samples, has shown that about a quarter of autistic individuals have a head circumference above the 97th percentile (Bailey et al., 1995; Bolton et al., 1994; Woodhouse et al., 1995). This finding appears to differentiate autism from both mental retardation and developmental disorders of language (other than those involving pragmatic deficits). It is not known as yet whether large head size differentiates a distinctive subgroup of autism but the limited evidence that is available shows no clear differences from the rest of autism.

In their twin study, Bailey et al., (1995) noted that some autistic twins showed subtle mid-facial dysmorphic features. Further studies are required in order to determine the strength and specificity of this association. There is probably also some slight increase in other minor congenital anomalies, as is the case with a wide range of disorders.

Finally, although the evidence is not clear cut

(Ghaziuddin et al., 1992, 1994), motor clumsiness has been particularly associated with Asperger's syndrome (Frith, 1991). If this is considered a milder variety of autism (and it is quite unclear whether or not that is an appropriate assumption), there is the apparent paradox that mildness in all other features is associated with apparently greater impairment in the one domain of motor coordination.

Sex Ratio

Numerous studies have shown that autism is much more common in males, in a ratio of about 4 to 1 (Gillberg & Coleman, 1992). The male excess appears to be greater in the case of those with an IQ in the normal range and least in those who are profoundly retarded. Perhaps, too, the male excess is particularly great in typical cases fitting Kanner's original descriptions and least evident in atypical cases (Wing & Gould, 1979; Gillberg, 1991, 1992).

Course and Outcome

Although there have been a few claims that autistic individuals can achieve normal functioning (McEachin et al., 1993), the great majority of follow-up studies have made it clear that the overall pattern of deficits in the three main domains of abnormality continue into adult life (Gillberg, 1991; Lotter, 1978; Rutter, 1970, 1978a). The two strongest predictive factors for adult outcome are IQ (an IQ below 50 is strongly indicative of poor social adjustment) and the level of language functioning at age 5 (a useful level of spoken language being associated with a good outcome). As already noted, a substantial minority of autistic individuals develop epilepsy in late adolescence or early adult life. Goode et al.'s (1994) long-term follow-up study showed a raised rate of deaths in autistic individuals with profound retardation and epilepsy, but no evidence of an increase in mortality in the remainder. Most of the deaths were sudden and were possibly associated with epilepsy.

Genetic Factors

In the first report describing autism, Kanner (1943) described it as an inborn disorder. Yet, for many years, little attention was paid to possible genetic factors because it was so infrequent to have two autistic children in the same family (some 2% of cases in the literature reviewed by Smalley et al., 1988). Also, early chromosome studies failed to reveal any abnormalities. Three things changed the situation radically. First, an awareness that even a 2% rate of autism in siblings meant a huge increase in relative risk compared to the general population, led to the first systematic, general population-based twin study by Folstein and Rutter (1977a, b). This provided evidence of a strong genetic component. Second, discovery of the Fragile X anomaly led to investigations with findings that suggested that a substantial minority of autistic individuals had this anomaly (Blomquist et al., 1985). Because, at first, it was thought that there was a stronger association between autism and the Fragile X than between mental retardation and the Fragile X, this led to a major research interest in the association, as well as a renewal of interest in other chromosome anomalies that might be associated with autism (Gillberg & Wahlstrom, 1985). Third, clinical investigations brought a growing awareness that some cases of autism were associated with single gene medical disorders showing a Mendelian pattern (see Folstein & Rutter, 1988 and Folstein & Piven, 1991). As discussed below, some of the claims made in these three areas of research have not stood the test of time but what is universally accepted now is that genetic factors play a very major role in autism. Indeed, it is clear that autism is the most strongly genetic of all multifactorial psychiatric disorders (Rutter et al., 1993). Attention has turned, accordingly, to a more detailed consideration of specific issues relating to the role of genetic factors.

Associations with Specific Genetic Disorders

The two conditions for which the strongest case for an association with autism has been put are the Fragile X anomaly and tuberose sclerosis. In both cases, a detailed consideration of the evidence is informative in its broader implications, as well as specific findings.

Fragile X anomaly. The Fragile X occurs with about the same frequency as autism, is associated with mental retardation (both mild and severe), and receives its name from the appearance of a fragile site on the long arm of the X chromosome when cultured in low folate media (Warren & Nelson, 1994). The first reports of the Fragile X anomaly and autism suggested that the anomaly occurred in at least 16% of cases of autism (Gillberg & Wahlström, 1985). When a larger number of studies were pooled a few years later, the estimate dropped to 7% (Bolton & Rutter, 1990; Brown et al., 1986). Current estimates, based on new data, put the true rate at about 2.5%, and almost certainly below 5% (Bailey et al., 1993a; Piven et al., 1991). The first point to consider, therefore, is why the estimate has fallen in the dramatic way that it has.

Rutter et al., (1994) suggested that four main reasons were likely to be responsible. First, there is a publishing bias so that positive associations tend to be published and negative ones not. Second, with a small sample size, typical of these early studies, the proportion of findings that are false positives is higher than occurs with large samples (see Pocock, 1983). Third, the early reports were based on inclusion of very low (1–3%) rates of Fragile X expression, which do not have the same meaning as rates of 4% and above. This was first evident from statistical analyses using latent class methods (Bolton et al., 1992a) but it is no longer necessary to rely on demonstration of a fragile site using low folate media. The demonstration that the Fragile X anomaly is due to a trinucleotide repeat sequence in the region containing the FMR-1 gene (Davies, 1991) means that DNA methods can be used. These have shown that individuals with low rates of Fragile X expression do not have this abnormality (Vincent et al., submitted). Fourth, the initial reports of autism in individuals identified because they had the Fragile X anomaly were mainly based on clinical impression rather than systematic standardized assessment. It is now apparent that, although Fragile X individuals can show typical autism, rather more often their pattern of social and communicative abnormalities takes a different form (Hagerman, 1990). Marked social anxiety, gaze avoidance and an ambivalent social approach combined with a turning away of the face seems to be particularly characteristic (Cohen et al., 1989; Wolff et al., 1989; Sudhalter et al., 1990). The cognitive features associated with the social deficits that accompany the Fragile X anomaly may also be different from those found in autism (Mazzocco et al., 1994).

In view of the evidence that the rate of the Fragile X anomaly in individuals with autism is so much lower than originally thought, it is necessary to reconsider the question of whether or not there is any specific association between the two. Einfeld et al., (1989) compared Fragile X males with controls matched for age and IQ. No differences in autistic symptomatology were found between the two groups and, on this basis, the authors argued for a lack of a meaningful causal association. On the other hand, a 2.5% rate of Fragile X in autism is certainly well above general population figures. The alternative is that the association arises only because both autism and the Fragile X are associated with mental retardation. In other words, the suggestion is that the basic association is between mental retardation and Fragile X and that the association between autism and Fragile X is merely secondary and indirect. That is a possibility because the great majority of autistic individuals with the Fragile X are mentally retarded. On the other hand, there is no direct relationship between IQ and autism. Thus, for example, trisomy 21, although the single commonest cause of mental retardation, is only rarely associated with autism. Probably, it is fair to conclude that there may be some specific association between Fragile X and autism but also that the association is probably too weak for it to constitute a strong pointer to any genetic mechanisms that may be involved in autism. In any case, Hallmayer et al.'s (1994) molecular genetic study of multiplex families appeared to exclude linkage to the FMR-1 gene (the gene associated with Fragile X) in the sample investigated.

Tuberose sclerosis. There have been clinical reports of autistic features in individuals with tuberose sclerosis for many years. This is a single gene, autosomal dominant, neurocutaneous disorder, occurring in about 1 per 7,000 individuals (Osborne et al., 1991). It is characterized by a combination of skin lesions and neurological features but protean abnormalities in other organs of the body also occur. About two thirds of patients develop epileptic seizures and a general learning disability is present in about two fifths. About three quarters of cases derive from new mutations (i.e. there is no family history). The physical manifestations of tuberose sclerosis vary greatly from individual to individual, even within the same family and may be very mild, being manifest only by hypomelanotic macules (Smalley et al., 1994). Gene loci have been discovered on both chromosome 9 (Fryer et al., 1987) and 16 (European Chromosome 16 Tuberous Sclerosis Consortium, 1993) — each accounting for about half of the cases.

Hunt and Dennis (1987) using a checklist approach,

reported that 50% of children with tuberose sclerosis showed autistic behaviour. A later more systematic study (Hunt & Shepherd, 1993) showed that 24% met DSM-III-R criteria for autism and a further 19% showed autistic traits. Smalley, Smith and Tanguay's (Smalley et al., 1991; Smalley et al., 1992) findings are broadly similar and Gillberg et al., (1994) reported that 61% showed autism. There are fewer data the other way round and it has been necessary to make various extrapolations. These have produced figures ranging from 3% (Smalley et al., 1992) to 9% (Gillberg et al., 1994) for the proportion of autistic individuals with tuberose sclerosis. On the basis of currently available data, it is not possible to provide a precise figure, although it is probably nearer the bottom than the top of the range mentioned. Even if that is the case, however, that would still make for a more specific association than that found up to now with any other genetically determined medical condition.

Again, the question must be raised as to what the association means. It is likely to be causal in some way (because of its relative strength) but it is noteworthy that the main association occurs with tuberose sclerosis that is accompanied by both mental retardation and epilepsy. It has been reported in the absence of mental retardation (Gillberg et al., 1987). Nevertheless, it seems that autism is much less common in tuberose sclerosis that is associated with normal intelligence, perhaps especially if in addition epilepsy is not present. The point of that observation is that it suggests that the risk for autism arises through the brain disorder accompanying tuberose sclerosis, rather than because a gene for autism is closely associated with the locus of one of the two genes known to be linked with tuberose sclerosis.

Other genetic conditions and chromosome abnormalities. The literature includes reports of autistic features in individuals with untreated phenylketonuria (see Folstein & Rutter, 1988) but none of the reports were based on standardized assessments of autism and the strength of the association, and perhaps even its reality, must be in some doubt. In any case, untreated phenylketonuria is now a rare occurrence and hence it must be an even rarer cause of autism. Gillberg & Forsell (1984) published case reports of two children with autism and a third with an autistic-like condition who showed neurofibromatosis. There have been a few other reports of similar cases but there are no systematic studies that would allow any estimate of the validity, or strength, of the association. It is possible that the association is real, even if it does not account for many cases; it may be relevant that, like tuberose sclerosis, it involves a combination of skin lesions and neural tumours. A diverse range of other genetically determined medical conditions have been reported from time to time to be associated with autism (see the systematic review by Gillberg & Coleman, 1992) but in no case is there good evidence of a strong association.

It is quite likely that autism is associated with some increase in the rate of chromosome anomalies. Probably the rate is something of the order of 5%, in addition to the Fragile X (Gillberg & Coleman, 1992). That figure is high enough to warrant routine examination of the chromosomes in the clinical assessment of autistic individuals, but the meaning of the association remains in considerable doubt. Many of the abnormalities reported are ones of quite uncertain clinical significance. Thus, some are balanced translocations (i.e. they involve exchange, but not loss, of chromosomal material) and these and other anomalies are known to arise in individuals without handicap. It might be hoped that the particular chromosome abnormalities associated with autism would provide clues to the possible locus of the gene or genes that underlie autism. In the event, they do not because autism has been associated with anomalies involving almost all chromosomes. Perhaps the only chromosome in which there is any suggestion of a stronger specific association is chromosome 15 for which there are reports that autism is sometimes associated with an extra marker chromosome deriving from 15 (Gillberg et al., 1991; Hotopf & Bolton, 1995).

Quantification of Genetic Risk in Idiopathic Cases

The evidence on the strength of the genetic component in cases of autism that are unassociated with a known medical condition derives from both family and twin studies. Clinical reports initially put the rate of autism in siblings at about 2% (Smalley et al., 1988). However, this figure was not based on systematic assessment of all siblings. Bolton et al., (1994) studied the 153 siblings of 99 autistic subjects. Of these, 2.9% showed autism and a further 2.9% showed atypical autism, there being a 0% rate of both in the 65 siblings in the Down's syndrome comparison group. Piven et al., (1990a) found a 3% rate of autism in siblings and a 4% rate of severe social impairment. Szatmari et al., (1993) found a rate of 5.3% PDD in siblings compared with 0% in controls. Jorde et al., (1991), reporting data from a large scale Utah family study, reported a recurrence risk of 3.7% if the first autistic child was male and 7.0% if female. It may be concluded that the rate in siblings is probably in the region of 3–7%. This represents something in the order of a 50–100-fold increase in risk. Although it does not seem likely that this could be environmentally mediated, family studies cannot separate genetic and nongenetic influences and it is necessary to turn to twin data.

There have been three general population-based twin studies of idiopathic autism. Folstein and Rutter (1977a,b) in a British study found a 36% pair-wise concordance rate in MZ twins and a 0% rate in same sex dizygotic twins. Steffenburg et al., (1989) in a Nordic study reported a 91% pair-wise concordance rate for autism in MZ twins and a 0% concordance rate in same sex DZ twins. Bailey et al., (1995) found an MZ pair-wise concordance rate of 69% and, again, 0% in DZ pairs in a further British study. Pooling the two British studies, and using the rate of autism among the siblings of autistic singletons to calculate the DZ rate, Bailey et al., (1995) calculated a heritability of 91–93% for an underlying liability to autism (the variation in estimate stemming from different assumptions about the base rate of autism). Clearly, this represents a very strong genetic component. Several issues need to be tackled before concluding that the genetic effect is as strong as it seems. To begin with, the possibility that the findings could

stem, at least in part, from obstetric complications needs to be considered. This possibility particularly arises because both the original Folstein and Rutter (1977a,b) study as well as the study by Steffenburg et al., (1989) showed that obstetric complications differentiated twins with autism from their nonautistic co-twins. In both studies, this was interpreted as indicating the possible role of environmentally induced brain damage. It now seems unlikely that that is the case. That is because most of the obstetric complications were quite minor; because the association with obstetric complications in singletons is weak, and again it mainly applies to minor complications (Nelson, 1991; Tsai, 1987); because the association in singletons may be a function of maternal parity (Piven et al., 1993) (although Bolton et al., 1995, found that applied only to autism when it was associated with a lack of speech); because within the Bailey et al., (1995) twin sample, obstetric complications were associated with congenital anomalies, most of which were likely to derive from aberrations in early pregnancy; and because in the Bolton et al., (1994), family studies the familial loading was greater in the case of autistic subjects with obstetric complications. It is also relevant that other evidence has shown that genetically abnormal fetuses (e.g. with Down syndrome) may give rise to an increased rate of obstetric and perinatal complications (Bolton & Holland, 1994). The totality of the evidence strongly suggests that it is much more likely that the minor obstetric complications derive from a genetically abnormal foetus than that the complications index an environmental risk process (Bolton et al., 1994). Of course, it is possible that isolated cases of autism may stem from neonatal brain damage associated with serious perinatal complications or with very low birth weight, but such cases seem to be uncommon.

A further approach to the possible role of physical environmental factors is provided by a study of specific infectious risks of various kinds. Probably the best documented is Chess, Korn and Fernandez's (Chess et al., 1971) report that autism was quite common in children with congenital rubella. The significance of this finding, however, was changed by the later follow-up data (Chess, 1977), which indicated that many of the children with congenital rubella ceased to exhibit autism as they grew older. It appeared that in course, as well as to some extent in the details of clinical features, the autism associated with rubella is somewhat atypical. In any case, congenital rubella is rather uncommon these days and it could constitute only a rare cause of autism. Deykin and MacMahon (1979a) undertook a systematic study of possible associations with maternal infections during the pregnancy and the results were essentially negative. Several studies have reported seasonal variations in the births of children with autism and this has been taken to suggest an environmental pathogen operating during the pregnancy (Gillberg & Coleman, 1992). Bolton et al., (1992b) examined the postulated association in detail and concluded that it was far less definite than had been claimed. Certainly, it does not provide strong evidence for an environmental cause. A possible association between autism and the cytomegalovirus has been suggested but it does not seem likely that this is other than a quite infrequent cause of autism

(Gillberg & Coleman, 1992). Occasional cases of autism associated with postnatal encephalitis have also been reported but, again, they appear to be quite rare.

Psychosocial environmental risk factors do not appear to be influential, other than rarely. Early suggestions that autism might derive from parental neglect, rejection, or indifference have long since been abandoned. Numerous studies have failed to show any association between autism and qualities of upbringing or frequency of stress experiences. Accordingly, it seems most unlikely that environmentally mediated psychological experiences play any significant role in autism. An apparent exception to that widely accepted generalization is provided by a report (Rutter, in preparation) that some children adopted from Romanian orphanages into U.K. families exhibited an autistic-like syndrome. Although this was very much a minority pattern, the rate was clearly raised in relation to the general population. Nevertheless, its relevance in relation to the broad run of autism is very doubtful because the clinical pattern was usually atypical in certain important features and, more especially, because the autistic features often faded as the children grew older (a rare occurrence in autism). It should be added that the children had suffered quite exceptional privation of both a physical and a psychological kind and it is not as yet clear which aspect of their early experiences led to the risk for this atypical pattern. Such grossly depriving experiences are not found, other than very exceptionally, in series of autistic individuals. Accordingly, the generalization remains that psychosocial stressors and adversities play no significant role in the aetiology of autism.

Another approach is provided by examination of the concordance rate in monozygotic pairs. The 91% pairwise concordance rate for autism in MZ twins found by Steffenburg et al., (1989) would seem to leave little room for nongenetic influences, but the 69% pair-wise concordance rate found by Bailey et al., (1995) would leave rather more scope for nongenetic influences. However, as discussed below, the great majority of the nonautistic twins in discordant MZ pairs showed cognitive and social deficits of autistic quality, albeit of lesser degree. It may be concluded that genetic influences predominate in the aetiology of autism and, moreover, that this is likely to apply to the great majority of cases of autism.

What is the Phenotype?

The findings discussed so far all apply to autism as traditionally diagnosed. Folstein and Rutter (1977a,b) noted, however, that most of the MZ pairs that were not concordant for autism were concordant for some type of cognitive deficit, usually involving language delay. By contrast, this applied to only 1 in 10 of the discordant DZ pairs. The implication was that it might not be autism as such that was inherited, but rather some broader type of cognitive abnormality including, but not restricted to autism. The more recent British twin study undertaken by Bailey et al., 1995) found the same but also demonstrated that the cognitive deficits were usually associated with a persistent social impairment that continued into adult life. Of the MZ pairs, 76% were

concordant for a *combined* social and cognitive disorder compared with 0% in DZ pairs. Conversely, in only 8% of MZ pairs was the co-twin without either a social or cognitive disorder, compared with 90% of the DZ pairs.

The family studies have also strongly suggested that the genetic liability applies to a range of social and cognitive abnormalities in individuals of normal intelligence, of a kind that is very similar in quality to those found in autism, but very different in degree of handicap (see Bolton et al., 1994; Folstein & Piven, 1991 and Rutter et al., 1993 for reviews). Bolton et al., (1994) found that between 12 and 20% of the siblings of autistic probands compared with 2–3% of the Down siblings exhibited this lesser variant of autism, the exact figures depending on the stringency of definition. Other family studies vary in the extent to which the disorders in relatives have involved social or language/cognitive deficits, and there has been some variability in whether these are mainly evident in parents or siblings, but nearly all have shown a much increased rate of abnormalities (Landa et al., 1991, 1992; Wolff et al., 1988; Narayan et al., 1990; Silliman et al., 1989; Piven et al., 1994). Thus, the social characteristics have included a lack of empathy, rapport and emotional responsiveness, hypersensitivity, and the single-minded pursuit of special interests. Communication difficulties have primarily involved pragmatic difficulties together with mixtures of over-communicativeness and under-communicativeness, excessive guardedness and disinhibition. Language related cognitive deficits have also been a feature but, strikingly, neither mental retardation nor general cognitive impairments have been evident (Fombonne et al., submitted; Freeman et al., 1989; Szatmari et al., 1993). There are only two studies with essentially negative findings. Gillberg et al., (1992) found few differences in a rather small scale study; but over a third of their sample had a known medical syndrome and half were severely retarded. Szatmari et al., (1993) compared the unaffected siblings and parents of 52 probands with pervasive developmental disorder and 33 Down's syndrome and low birth weight controls. No significant differences were found between the groups. It is not clear why the findings are so different from most of the other studies but the probands were clinically more heterogeneous and the findings on siblings were not internally coherent. For example, speech delay was nearly three times as common in the siblings of PDD subjects (16.3% versus 6.8%) but reading problems were far less frequent (3.8% versus 20.5%). Rates of special education were also very high in both groups (10.0% in the PDD and 18.2% in controls).

Although there are some inconsistencies across studies, the twin and family studies taken together strongly suggest that the autism phenotype extends well beyond the traditional diagnosis. The extension involves characteristics that are closely similar to autism in quality but markedly different in degree, and which are found in individuals of normal intelligence.

The clinical picture chiefly differs from autism as traditionally diagnosed in the lack of abnormal nonpragmatic language features (such as pronominal reversal and delayed echolalia), the less striking stereotyped repetitive behavioural pattern, the more subtle social deficits, and the lack of an association with epilepsy or mental handicap. There are three main reasons for confidence in the assumption that it is indeed part of autism: (1) the social abnormalities have been found to persist into adult life; (2) the concordance in MZ pairs for the broader phenotype, even after exclusion of autism and pervasive developmental disorders, is much higher than in DZ pairs (Le Couteur et al., 1995); and (3) family data show a much increased loading for the broader phenotype compared with Down's syndrome families (see, e.g. Bolton et al., 1994).

The definition of the boundaries of the broader phenotype remains to be determined. Thus, questions remain on whether it may be evident in language abnormalities, social deficits or circumscribed interest patterns in isolation or whether its manifestation requires two or more of these. There is also the need to determine the specific qualities of each of this trio of abnormalities that is pathognomonic of autism. Even more basic is the question of whether such features are categorically present or absent or whether they are more appropriately considered in terms of a dimension. This is particularly the case because of the need to differentiate the broader phenotype (or lesser variant) of autism from other forms of social abnormality and especially from the schizotypal personality disorder, which constitutes a quite different disorder associated with schizophrenia rather than autism. Clearly, some means of validation would be hugely helpful. Potentially, this might be provided by patterns of psychological abnormality (with respect, for example, to the "theory of the mind", executive planning, central coherence, or pragmatic aspects of language) but that remains a research task for the future.

Rather surprisingly, several studies (Bolton et al., 1995; DeLong, 1994; DeLong & Nohria, 1994; Piven et al., 1990a). Smalley et al., (1995) have reported an increased familial loading for affective disorder, but it is not yet clear whether this is genetically mediated. They compared 36 families with an autistic child with 21 families with a nonautistic child showing either tuberose sclerosis or epilepsy. Major affective disorder was three times as common in the first degree relatives of autistic individuals. In nearly two thirds of the parents with affective disorder, the onset was before the birth of the autistic child. Social phobia was also much increased in the autism families when the autism was unaccompanied by mental retardation. Bolton et al., (submitted), using both standardized interview (SADS-L) and pedigree methods, showed that the raised rate of major affective disorders in the first and second degree relatives of autistic individuals compared with the relatives of individuals with Down's syndrome was not a function of the broader phenotype as defined in terms of cognitive and social abnormalities. Moreover, unlike the broader phenotype, affective disorder was more frequent in females.

At first sight, it would seem unlikely that autism and affective disorders could constitute different manifestations of the same underlying genotype. Rather, the increased familial loading for depressive disorders might reflect the strains and stresses associated with rearing an autistic child. Nevertheless, despite the apparent implausibility of the association, five findings suggest that it may be real: (1) the increase in affective disorders applies to second degree, as well as first degree, relatives; (2) the increase applies to severe unipolar disorders as much as milder depressive disorders; and (3) the increase applies as much to affective disorders with an onset before the birth of the autistic individual as afterwards; (4) the increase has been noted in studies using quite different samples (see references above); and (5) the raised rate of affective disorders is not just a function of the broader phenotype. Accordingly, although only a few of the investigations included adequate controls, it is clear that the apparent association between autism and affective disorders requires further study. If the association between autism and affective disorders is confirmed, it will be important to examine competing hypotheses on the underlying mechanisms.

In addition, there have been suggestions that the phenotype should be extended to include Tourette's syndrome (Comings & Comings, 1991) and anorexia nervosa (Gillberg, 1992) but in neither case is the evidence particularly convincing.

Given that it seems highly likely that the phenotype does extend beyond autism[1], it is necessary to raise questions about the connections between autism as traditionally diagnosed and the so-called lesser variant. The latter shares a number of features with autism proper; for example, it too is much more common in males than females (although this is less so with the milder degrees of the phenotype) and the features are usually evident from early childhood onwards. On the other hand, there are at least two marked differences. The relatives showing this broader phenotype in the various studies have been of normal intelligence and no association with epilepsy has been found. This could represent simply a lower "dose" of the genetic predisposition but the possibility of some kind of "two-hit" mechanism must also be considered. That is, it could be suggested that one set of causal factors predisposes to the broader phenotype, and a separate set of causal factors is involved in the transition to the handicapping condition of autism "proper". At one time, it was thought that this second step might involve perinatal complications (Folstein & Rutter, 1977a,b; Steffenburg et al., 1989) but for the reasons given above that now seems unlikely. The issue is unresolved but there is an apparent paradox in the fact that most cases of autism occur in individuals who are also mentally retarded and who have a much increased rate of epilepsy, but the familial loading mainly involves qualitatively similar abnormalities in individuals without epilepsy and of normal intelligence.

Genetic Heterogeneity

The history of medical genetics strongly suggests that genetic heterogeneity is to be expected in autism. There are numerous examples of different genetic abnormal-

---

[1] Spiker et al. (1994) argued that it does not but their own data on multiplex families showed a substantial number of individuals who were clearly not normal but whose disorders did not fulfil the usual diagnostic criteria for autism.

ities all leading to what appears to be the same clinical picture. Thus, as already noted, some cases of tuberose sclerosis are associated with a gene locus on chromosome 9 and others with a locus on chromosome 16. Other neurological conditions show even greater genetic heterogeneity (see Simonoff et al., in press). Some genetic heterogeneity has already been demonstrated in so far as autism is associated with the Fragile X anomaly, tuberose sclerosis and various other genetic conditions. Claims have been made that more than a third of cases of autism are associated with such known medical conditions (Gillberg, 1992) but review of the evidence suggests that the true rate of known medical conditions in autism is probably about 10% (Rutter et al., 1994). On the other hand, the rate may be higher in atypical cases of autism and autism associated with profound mental retardation. The question then is whether there are currently any clinical indicators of heterogeneity in the remaining 90% of cases of idiopathic autism. One way of tackling this issue is provided by examination of variabilities in clinical expression within monozygotic pairs, a strategy followed by Le Couteur and her colleagues (Le Couteur et al., in press). Their findings showed that both with respect to autistic symptoms and verbal IQ, there was almost as much variation within pairs as there was between pairs. Differences in verbal and nonverbal IQ within concordant MZ pairs ranged up to more than 50 points. The findings strongly pointed to a wide range of phenotypic expression and provided few pointers on possible clinical indicators of genetic heterogeneity. One possible exception was provided by epilepsy where there was a rather greater tendency for concordance within pairs. On the other hand, the presence of epilepsy was not associated with any other indications of meaningful differences and the Bolton et al., (1994) family study showed no variation in familial loading by epilepsy. Spiker et al., (1994) used a somewhat similar strategy with respect to differences between affected family members in those that were multiplex for autism. Again, substantial variation within pairs of affected family members was found for both clinical features and IQ.

There is some slight suggestion that autism that is associated either with profound mental retardation or with a lack of useful spoken language may be different. Thus, Bolton et al., (1994) found that, although the familial loading was strongly associated with the symptom score in verbal probands, this was not so in those without useful language. August and his colleagues (August et al., 1981; Baird & August, 1985) found a raised rate of severe mental retardation in the siblings of autistic probands who were also severely retarded, something that has not been evident in any of the studies of less retarded subjects. Their findings are based on a very small number of cases and cannot be taken as anything more than an indication of a possibility worth examining further. About a third of autistic individuals have hyperserotoninaemia and there is also some evidence that this may be a familial trait to some extent (Cook, 1990). It is possible, although untested, that this might prove to be a marker of genetic heterogeneity but, again, this is no more than a suggestion worth following up. It may be concluded that genetic heterogeneity is

likely to prove to be the case but, so far, there are no strong leads on how this might be indexed in terms of phenotypic characteristics; and variable expression will make its identification a hard task.

Are the Genetic Influences Autism-Specific?

A somewhat related question is whether the genetic influences are likely to prove autism-specific. Clearly they are not to the extent that autism is secondary to conditions such as tuberose sclerosis or the Fragile X anomaly, but these account for only about 1 in 10 cases. It has been suggested that autism is no more than a final common pathway for a heterogeneous range of aetiological processes and that there is no point in searching for autism-specific causal factors (Coleman, 1990; Gillberg, 1992). The available evidence, however, suggests that this is not so. Four key sets of data are relevant. First, neither brain pathology nor mental retardation carry a consistent risk for autism. Some conditions (such as cerebral palsy or Down syndrome) carry a low risk, whereas others (such as tuberose sclerosis) carry a much higher risk. Second, both the twin and family studies show strong associations with a relatively specific pattern of social/cognitive deficits and not with mental retardation or brain disease more generally. Third, the concordance for the broader phenotype of autism in MZ pairs is very high (over 90%). Fourth, although there is considerable variability of phenotypic expression within MZ pairs (and within multiplex families), the variability is within the range of autistic features and does not extend to other psychiatric manifestations of brain pathology. It may be concluded that, in the great majority of cases, the genetic influences are likely to prove to be autism-specific, even though it is probable that they will be multiple.

Mode of Genetic Transmission

The last issue with respect to genetics concerns the mode of genetic transmission. A segregation analysis undertaken by Ritvo et al., (1985) using families ascertained because they had two or more affected siblings, suggested autosomal recessive inheritance and apparently ruled out a multifactorial model. However, the biased nature of the sample, together with no exclusion of cases due to known medical conditions, and uncertainties about diagnosis (including a failure to take into account the possibility of a broader phenotype) call for caution in accepting the conclusions. Also, a further study by the same research group (Jorde et al., 1990) produced a different set of conclusions. An additional complication may be provided by a tendency for families to stop having children after having an autistic child (Jones & Szatmari, 1988), although this was not found by Bolton et al., (1994). Altogether, the evidence suggests that multiple interacting genes are much more likely than a single gene operating in Mendelian fashion. Three main findings point to that conclusion. First, there is the marked fall-off in rate going from MZ co-twins to DZ co-twins or siblings (Bailey et al., 1995; Folstein & Rutter, 1977a,b;

Steffenburg et al., 1989) combined with the further fall-off in both autism and the broader phenotype going from first degree to second degree relatives (Jorde et al., 1990; Pickles et al., 1995a). Using the Risch (1990) approach, Pickles et al., (1995b) estimated that a three gene model was the most likely, although the range could be anywhere between two and ten. Third, Bolton et al., (1994) found that the familial loading increased with the severity of the autism as measured in terms of the number of autism diagnostic interview algorithm symptoms. The one finding that does not seem consistent with that model is that the familial loading seems only slightly greater in the families of female autistic subjects, the sex difference being nonsignificant in most studies. This is apparently inconsistent because a multifactorial threshold model leads to the expectation that loading should be higher in the less often affected sex, namely females. On the other hand, the statistical power to detect a sex difference was low in all studies and the matter remains unresolved (see Rutter et al., 1993).

Future Directions

The strength of genetic components in the vulnerability to autism makes it an obvious candidate for molecular genetic strategies (Rutter, 1994). However, these need to be based on a recognition that autism is likely to prove to be a complex disorder, with several interacting genes implicated, and genetic heterogeneity probable. In addition, there needs to be an acceptance that there are no strong candidate genes. Accordingly, a genomic search approach of the kind found effective in diabetes (see Goodfellow & Schmitt, 1994), applied to pairs of affected siblings or other relatives with definite autism is the design of choice in the first instance to determine the susceptibility loci (Lander & Schork, 1994). The method simply determines whether affected relatives share alleles at a locus more often than would occur by chance. No model of inheritance has to be specified (unlike linkage methods), and the method is relatively robust even in the presence of incomplete penetrance, phenocopies, genetic heterogeneity and high frequency disease alleles. The focus on extreme cases also much reduces the problems caused by misclassification of uncertain phenotypes. Of course, sibling pair or other allelic-sharing strategies will need to be followed by association strategies in order to determine whether there is a clear correlation between functionally relevant allelic variations and the risk of autism in humans, by positional cloning to identify the susceptibility genes themselves and by transgenic studies to determine the gene products and the mechanisms by which they bring about the clinical manifestations (Lander & Schork, 1994; Rutter, 1994). Nevertheless, this now constitutes a realistic research objective.

Even so, it would be an error to assume that, on its own, this will necessarily provide a solution. Traditional quantitative genetic research can be helpful in providing indices of likely genetic heterogeneity, psychological studies can assist in validating the broader phenotype (see later), and neurobiological studies will be needed to make the connections with brain structure and function.

Neuropsychological Approaches

In the 1950s and 1960s, many believed that the psychological abilities of children with autism were not accessible to measurement, because of difficulties in using standardized tests. Yet, we have now amassed a large body of knowledge about cognitive functioning in autism. This is largely a result of the creative talents of Beate Hermelin and Neil O'Connor and colleagues, who pioneered a style of research that continues to influence neuropsychological investigations into developmental disorders. Since the 1970s, the dominant view has been that autism involves cognitive deficits that are not a consequence of impaired social development. Approximately three-quarters of individuals with autism have IQ levels below 70; the remainder have IQs in the normal range, despite being severely socially-impaired. Follow-up studies show that IQ scores are stable over time, are good predictors of educational attainment and are not enhanced when social functioning improves with maturity or as a result of behavioural treatments (Rutter, 1983). Moreover, unlike the IQs of their unaffected siblings, the IQs of autistic individuals are unrelated to the social class or educational background of their parents (Fombonne et al., 1995). In addition, performance on IQ tests typically shows an uneven profile across different subtests. Further evidence that autism involves basic cognitive dysfunction came from a recent genetic study, which found that familial loading for autism was inversely related to the probands' verbal IQ (Bolton et al., 1994).

The main concern of recent years has been to specify the link between cognitive deficits and other features of autism, in particular social impairment. Precisely how could impaired cognitive capacities lead to the characteristic social and communicative symptoms of autism? This narrow focus has brought about significant advances in the understanding of essential features of autism, but it has been at the expense of accounting for the total syndrome, which includes mental retardation, language delay, behavioural rigidity and isolated skills. It is true that not all individuals with autism show all these features, but they are nevertheless an integral part of the disorder (Rutter & Bailey, 1993). The key questions are these: *Why* do these features cluster together? Can their co-occurrence be explained in terms of one specific cognitive deficit, or should we look for the common thread at a different level of analysis?

In this section, we describe briefly research on the various cognitive impairments found in individuals with autism, and the theories that attempt to link these with other aspects of the disorder. In doing this, we consider the extent to which neuropsychological accounts are helpful in explaining the condition and the ways in which the different cognitive deficits may be related to one another. We suggest certain directions in which neuropsychological research might proceed in order to answer remaining questions about the nature and origins of autism and other developmental disorders. In particular, we propose that it is time to broaden the focus of investigations in order to consider directly the whole constellation of features that defines and characterizes autism.

What Cognitive Deficits are Found in Autism?

The challenge is to identify deficits that are specific to autism, rather than being found in a range of mental disorders, and yet are adequate to explain the array of clinical characteristics. Responses to the dual challenge of specificity and completeness of explanation have been of two kinds. The first proposes that the key cognitive deficits are narrow and highly specific, primarily affecting social-cognitive functioning. The second focuses on broad deficits that affect both social and nonsocial development. The development of ideas about the nature of cognitive dysfunction in autism shows something of an hour-glass shape, moving from broad concepts during the 1970s, such as impaired ability to recode and sequence information, to narrow ones during the 1980s, such as failure to process specifically social cues, and more recently a return to broader notions, including impairments in planning and attention-control. These varied concepts of cognitive dysfunction in autism will be outlined below, but since the research in these areas has been reviewed recently by Happe (1994b) and Bishop (1993), they will not receive detailed treatment here.

The narrow perspective. As mentioned, general cognitive deficits were much investigated during the 1970s. The notion of low-level sensory–perceptual deficits, such as stimulus overselectivity or sensory dominance, was replaced by the concept of a general high-level cognitive dysfunction in deriving meaning from structured or semantic information. In a series of stringently controlled experiments, Hermelin and O'Connor and colleagues compared groups of children with and without autism *closely matched on performance in relevant areas.* They found impairments in recoding, sequencing and abstraction (Frith, 1970a,b; Hermelin & O'Connor, 1970; and see review by Frith & Baron-Cohen, 1987). However, while it is feasible that domain-general cognitive deficits of the kind identified by Hermelin & O'Connor (1970) could account for delays and abnormalities in language development, it is far from clear how they could give rise to social aspects of autism, including socially abnormal *usage* of language. A critical task for the psychological approach to understanding autism is to show the *means* by which cognitive deficits could give rise to social impairment (Rutter, 1983). A way forward appeared to be to look at cognitive processing of specifically social and personal information, such as faces, emotional expressions, and internal mental states of other people. This narrower focus has been the dominant, and highly influential, theme of the past decade.

The importance of social understanding is made clear by the work of Marian Sigman, Peter Mundy and colleagues. These writers have demonstrated that a crucial aspect of autism involves differences in all kinds of behavioural responses that index social understanding (Sigman, 1995). For example, in the preschool years, affected children seem not to look for or attend to the emotional or attentional cues of other people. They seem impaired in all aspects of joint attention (pointing, showing, referential looking, social referencing). At later ages, there are difficulties in understanding emotions and

other subjective experiences, even in individuals without mental retardation. Although social functioning is profoundly impaired, it is not the case that all social interaction is absent or impaired in children with autism (Mundy et al., 1986). Instead, the areas of difficulty seem to be those that involve interpersonal understanding.

Studies of *face processing* have found that children with autism may process facial information in a different way from normal (Hobson et al., 1988; Langdell, 1978; Tantam et al., 1989; Boucher & Lewis, 1992). One interpretation of this evidence is that children with autism employ an atypical processing strategy that involves use of component parts, rather than the overall configuration of the face. Apart from face processing studies, other aspects of social information processing have been studied. Klin (1991) showed that young children with autism may not show the normal preference for speech sounds compared with nonspeech stimuli. There is also some evidence that discrimination of people's gender and age in pictures may be impaired (Hobson, 1987; Hobson et al., 1988), although not every study has shown this to be the case.

An important set of experiments by Hobson and colleagues focused on the role of *socio-affective* information, contained in the bodily expressions of emotion. In an early study, Weeks and Hobson (1987) found that children with autism sorted pictures of people by the criterion of type of hat, in preference to emotional expression. For the verbal MA-matched control subjects, the emotional information seemed more salient than information about hats. A number of further studies pointed to a difficulty in processing affect-related information. Hobson has proposed that the primary psychological deficit in autism is a very early failure of "direct perception" of bodily expressions, including emotions. However, autism-specific differences in affect comprehension have not always been found, particularly when subjects are matched with controls of equivalent verbal MA rather than nonverbal ability. Nevertheless, it seems clear that children with autism do experience difficulties in dealing with emotion information (see Hobson, 1993 for a review of this work). It is also apparent that their own bodily *expressions* of emotion are not like those of normal children (e.g. Macdonald et al., 1989; Yirmiya et al., 1989) and that their use of expressive gesture is impaired (Attwood et al., 1988). The extent to which the *experience* of affect is unusual is so far unknown.

A third set of studies into social cognition are those investigating the ability of children with autism to understand mental states. This body of research, and the theory underpinning it, originates from normal developmental psychology and has come to be known as the *"theory of mind"* hypothesis of autism. Leslie (1987) argued that a cognitive mechanism, coming on line in the second year of life, produces and manipulates second-order representations (metarepresentations). This mechanism is responsible for the onset of pretend play in normal development. Later, it allows for understanding of opaque mental states, such as beliefs and desires. Given that spontaneous creative pretend play[2] is virtually absent in children with autism (Baron-Cohen,

1987; Rutter, 1978b), Leslie predicted that understanding of other mental states should also be impaired. Baron-Cohen et al., (1985) tested this hypothesis, using an experimental task designed to test understanding of beliefs in normal preschool children. In this task, subjects witnessed the unexpected transfer of an object from the location where an actor put it to a different location, unseen by the actor. In spite of having language ability equal to or better than normal 4-year-olds (who pass the test with ease), a large majority of adolescents with autism failed to predict that the actor would search for the object in the original location. Instead, they responded like younger children, and predicted action based on current reality rather than the person's mistaken belief. It was not possible to account for this failure in terms of mental retardation, since a group of children with other forms of mental handicap, with lower verbal MA, were successful in the experimental task.

The striking finding of an apparent "mindblindness" specific to persons with autism is now well-replicated, using a range of different tests, many of them ingeniously designed (see Baron-Cohen, 1993 for a review). The deficit does not appear to be limited to understanding of mistaken belief, but also extends to true belief (Leslie & Frith, 1988), and to some aspects of intention and desire (Phillips, 1993, 1995; Phillips et al., 1995a). It appears that impaired understanding of mental states is a robust finding but is not universal, since in all studies a small proportion of able children and older people with autism pass the tests. The study of social-cognitive and social–perceptual deficits has provided key insights into the nature of autistic symptoms and mechanisms that may underlie them. However, there are indications from genetics research (verbal intelligence is related to genetic liability) and neurobiology (lack of strong evidence for localized lesions) that suggest a less specific primary deficit.

The broad perspective. In contrast to the proposal that specific social or social–cognitive abnormalities underlie the core symptoms of autism, a recent suggestion has been that the disorder is characterized by more general difficulties in the high-level planning and control of behaviour. The impetus for research in this area came from the observation that aspects of autistic behaviour are similar in kind to those seen in neurology patients with known lesions in the frontal lobes (see Damasio & Maurer, 1978; Dennis, 1991). Such patients are known to perform poorly on neuropsychological tests that are believed to tap *executive function.* Executive function has been defined as the *set of abilities* involved in maintaining an appropriate problem-solving framework. Included in this set are the abilities to: disengage from the external context; inhibit inappropriate responses; plan and generate sequences of willed actions; sustain an appropriate cognitive set for staying on-task; monitor own performance and make use of feedback; flexibly shift

attentional set. This list of operations is not exhaustive — there may be other aspects of the executive control of behaviour. The main findings of this research effort (recently reviewed by Ozonoff, 1994) are that children and adults with autism have problems in planning and organization (Hughes et al., 1994; Ozonoff et al., 1991a); in using feedback (Prior & Hoffman, 1990); in switching to a new cognitive set (Hughes et al., 1994; Rumsey & Hamburger, 1988; Ozonoff et al., 1991a); and in disengaging from perceptually salient stimuli (Hughes & Russell, 1993). They may also be impaired in generating novel ideas (Jarrold et al., 1994a; Turner, 1995), although not all evidence supports this (Scott & Baron-Cohen, 1995).

Whereas research into executive dysfunction emphasizes the production of behaviour, or output, a second general cognitive model places more stress on the input side, by suggesting an unusually weak drive for *central coherence* (Frith, 1989). Like executive dysfunction theory, the central coherence hypothesis proposes a cognitive abnormality that influences a broad range of psychological functions, from linguistic and social to perceptual. Frith and Happé (1994) proposed that, normally, humans have a strong tendency to interpret stimuli in a relatively global way, taking account of context. This is how we construct meaning from diverse and complex information, and explains why we tend to remember the gist of events rather than precise details (Bartlett, 1932). Frith and Happé suggested that this usually irresistible "effort after meaning" is relatively weak in autism, leading to a tendency to process information piece-meal, rather than in context. The common finding of relatively unimpaired ability in the Block Design subtest of Weschler Intelligence Scales suggests that people with autism are able to resist the "gestalt" qualities of the overall designs that make the task difficult for other people. General visuo-spatial abilities seem not to account for this strength, since individuals with autism are not advantaged in other tasks involving visuo-spatial perception of geometric designs (Shah & Frith, 1993). Similarly, people with autism have been found to do very well when required to locate hidden figures within a larger picture (the Embedded Figures Test), a task that normal people find difficult, because of the strong tendency to see the "gestalt" of the overall figure (Shah & Frith, 1983). Naturally, an unusually local, or bottom-up, bias is not always helpful. Frequently, understanding the meaning of verbal or nonverbal information relies on processing that information *in context.*

Are the Cognitive Deficits Specific to Autism?

Emotion-perception or expression and face-perception difficulties have been reported to be a feature of a number of conditions, including schizophrenia (Cutting, 1994), prosopagnosia (De Kosky et al., 1980) and mental handicap (Gray et al., 1983). Nevertheless, it may be that the affect-related deficits in autism are of a different kind than those in other conditions.

Deficits in understanding minds have withstood the test of specificity relatively well so far. Comparison groups have included children, adolescents and adults

---

[2] Up to a point, pretend play can be taught (Lewis & Boucher, 1988), but such induced play lacks the spontaneous creative qualities that are so characteristic of the play of normal children.

with mental handicap, with specific language deficits and with Down syndrome. However, other clinical groups have yet to be tested, such as those with attention deficit disorder and hyperactivity, and conduct disorder. In particular, conduct-disordered children have been noted to misinterpret other children's intentions (Dodge, 1980), and, therefore, merit investigation of their theory of mind abilities (Happé & Frith, 1995). There has been a proposal (Frith, 1992) that schizophrenia involves a breakdown in understanding minds, and current research is finding apparent deficits in theory of mind skills in this group (Corcoran et al., 1995). This is not necessarily damaging to the theory of mind hypothesis of autism, since what is being proposed in schizophrenia is a breakdown in existing functioning, rather than a failure to develop a theory of mind initially. Recently, Peterson and Siegal (1995) found that signing, profoundly deaf children failed a standard false belief test. As these children were otherwise neurologically intact, there is no reason to suspect that a cognitive deficit was responsible. Instead, the authors argued that poverty of mental-state related conversational input was the basis of these children's impairment. (It remains to be explored whether lack of relevant conversational experience has any contributory role in "mind-blindness" in autism, but it is hard to see how this could be tested.)

The specificity issue in executive dysfunction has received considerable comment. Problems in executive control of behaviour have been found in a wide range of clinical groups, from conduct disorder (Lueger & Gill, 1990) to treated phenylketonuria (Welsh et al., 1990) in children, and Parkinson's disease and schizophrenia in adults (for example, Morris et al., 1988; Pantelis & Nelson, 1994). The difficulty is that executive function is an umbrella term for a constellation of mental operations, not all of which have yet been delineated. Executive dysfunction theory is in need of more precision, and further work is urgently needed to determine whether the executive deficits seen in autism are of a different kind from those found in other conditions. Ozonoff et al., (1994) recently showed that autism could be distinguished from Tourette's syndrome on the basis of a simple information-processing task that seems to involve cognitive set-shifting. Central coherence theory is currently being tested for specificity to autism (Happé, personal communication), but the evidence from Weschler Intelligence Scales of a highly characteristic peak performance in Block Design suggests some degree of diagnostic specificity.

Are the Cognitive Deficits Found in all Persons with Autism?

Theory of mind impairment has been found in up to 80% of verbal children with autism. However, the remaining 20% or so pass the experimental tasks. A small proportion of these also pass a more complex form of the task, with greater information-processing demands (Bowler, 1992; Happé, 1993). It is still an open question whether "theory of mind passers", who have IQs within the normal range, have developed theory of mind competence or whether they make use of some alternative strategy to solve the experimental tasks.

The latter seems likely, since most of these individuals still seem to suffer profound social impairment in everyday life. Recent studies of the relationship between laboratory test performance and real-life mentalizing ability (Fombonne et al., 1994; Frith et al., 1994) suggest that, among "passers", there is a small subset who may have genuine mentalizing abilities, and a larger subgroup for whom a "strategy" seems a better explanation for task success. Further investigation of these individuals is merited, involving experimental tasks that are both more naturalistic and have a higher ceiling. At the other end of the IQ scale, understanding of other minds has not been tested in children with low verbal MA. However, behaviours considered to be related to theory of mind (pointing, pretend play, gaze monitoring) are abnormal in very young children with autism and those with less language and a greater degree of mental handicap (Baron-Cohen, 1989; Mundy et al., 1986; Phillips et al., 1992, 1995b). Evidence has been found that understanding mental states is related to verbal ability (for example, Prior et al., 1990; and see Happé, 1995). Those subjects who pass theory of mind tests tend to have high verbal mental age. High verbal ability does not appear to guarantee success, since many equally verbally-able children fail the experimental tasks (Frith et al., 1991). Nevertheless, the frequent association of verbal ability and other skills, including theory of mind, is in need of explanation. This issue will be dealt with in more detail later.

In an important study that compared the same subjects on both executive function (EF) and theory of mind (ToM) measures, Ozonoff et al., (1991a) found deficits in EF tasks were more common than theory of mind deficits. They (Ozonoff et al., 1991b) also found that EF deficits, but not ToM impairments, were present in a group of adults with Asperger syndrome. Problems in planning and attention-shifting have also been found among mentally handicapped children with autism (Hughes et al., 1994). Superficially, this implies that executive dysfunction may be "universal" to autism, and therefore, may be the better candidate for a primary deficit. The fact that EF deficits are also common in other clinical groups teaches us that we should be wary of drawing such a conclusion. The combination of more specific EF tests and more advanced ToM tests might clarify this issue. With regard to central coherence theory, direct tests are now being carried out. In a preliminary study, Happé (in press) found that even individuals who passed higher-order ToM tests were impaired in a test requiring use of written context to disambiguate homographs (words that look alike when written but are unrelated in meaning and are pronounced differently).

How Well do these Deficits Explain the Features of Autism?

As suggested above, a number of features are in need of explanation, and the utility of the psychological theories depends on the extent to which they can account for these phenomena. At the psychological level, the main features to be explained are the triad of social, communicative and imaginative impairments (Wing &

Gould, 1979); the insistence on sameness and narrowness of interests; the variability in general cognitive functioning, both between individuals (IQs range from normal to profoundly retarded levels) and within individuals (the uneven profile of ability in different IQ subtests). Although savant skills (super-normal abilities) are neither universal features of autism nor exclusive to people with autism, they are particularly common in autism (Frith, 1989; Goode et al., 1994; Rimland, 1978) and therefore require explanation. Each of the psychological theories of autism discussed above has its own set of explanatory strengths and weaknesses.

Social features. Proposed deficits in the narrow group have much to offer in explaining the Wing triad features, in particular the social impairments. For example, the hypothesis of a failure to engage in affectively-laden intersubjective co-ordination (Hobson, 1993) predicts that children with autism will go through infancy without acquiring a concept of persons as "subjects of experience". Such a profound perceptual-affective deficit would certainly make sense of the social and communicative problems found in autism, but would also seem to predict difficulties in very early social interactive behaviours. As noted earlier, in the section on clinical features, there is reason to believe that autism-specific symptoms may be present by the age of 12–18 months (Osterling & Dawson, 1994), but as yet, there is no clear evidence of abnormalities in the early months of life. Of course, these may be present, but in a form that is not easily detectable by parents and not picked up by retrospective research methods.

The power of the theory of mind hypothesis, and one reason for its great influence on recent thinking about autism, lies in its ability to explain at least two core symptoms of autism in terms of a single deficient cognitive mechanism. Specifically, it suggests that lack of reciprocity in social relations and a deep failure in communication could be expected in the absence of the ability to understand intentions and beliefs. While few dispute the existence of "mentalizing" deficits in autism, it is a different question whether or not the theory provides a sufficient account of the disorder. In particular, the original ToM hypothesis (Leslie, 1987) has difficulty accounting for the early age of manifestation — 12–18 months. It has been suggested that normal infants of 12 months demonstrate some awareness of internal states when they engage in intentional or "ostensive" communication (Bretherton et al., 1981; Leslie & Happé, 1989) and in joint attention (Baron-Cohen, 1993). Some authors have suggested that these behaviours arise from cognitive mechanisms that are precursors of metarepresentational ability, and that these precursor mechanisms are faulty in autism. One problem is an absence of an "acid test" for these earlier skills. Although a number of possible precursor mechanisms have been proposed (for example, by Baron-Cohen, 1995 and see Lewis & Mitchell, 1994), it has not yet been possible to demonstrate a causal relationship between a candidate precursor and later ToM skills. The fact that children with autism show deficits both in precursor behaviours (for example, joint attention or imitation) and in ToM ability does not demonstrate a causal link. Prospective studies will be informative,

although causal relationships will remain hard to prove by this strategy alone. A large scale prospective study of 16,000 normal infants is underway (Baron-Cohen, personal communication), in which joint attention, pretend play and certain other infant behaviours have been assessed by health visitors at the routine 18-month check-up, using the Checklist for Autism in Toddlers (CHAT). This instrument proved valuable within a smaller prospective study of high-risk infants (Baron-Cohen et al., 1992). Follow-ups of the epidemiological sample have shown that a combination of joint attention and pretend play deficits at 18 months may predict autism (Baron-Cohen, personal communication).

With regard to the group of broad theories, the precise causal links between executive dysfunction and impaired reciprocal social interaction are not clear. Similarly, the explanatory power of WCC theory is weak in respect of social impairments. Initially, Frith (1989) suggested that weak central coherence is responsible for ToM failure, which then explains pragmatic and social deficits. A more recent formulation does not see impaired ToM as a consequence of WCC, but as an independent deficit (Frith & Happé, 1994). According to this view, WCC and ToM dysfunction explain different aspects of autism, with WCC being associated with more nonsocial features.

Language and communication impairment. Serious abnormalities in language and communication are a fundamental feature of autism. As well as language delay, there are marked qualitative abnormalities (see earlier section on clinical features). Language deficits appear early and are persistent. Language level is a good predictor of social and educational outcome, and is strongly associated with severity of behavioural symptoms, social and cognitive performance and familial loading. The pivotal role of language features, together with the finding that some half of individuals with autism do not acquire useful language at all, means that language impairment must be accounted for in any psychological theory. Current psychological approaches to autism have attempted to explain the language features as one consequence of a specific cognitive deficit.

Pragmatic impairment characterizes autism at all intellectual levels, even where semantic and syntactic aspects of language are relatively unimpaired (Bishop, 1989; Eales, 1993; Tager-Flusberg, 1993). For example, affected individuals have problems with topic maintenance; with "building" on a topic to produce a conversational exchange; with understanding nonliteral utterances; and with adapting their language to different contexts. The theory of mind hypothesis emphasizes the connections between pragmatic competence and the ability to understand what other people know and intend. However, as pragmatic deficits are apparent in early language development, explaining these in terms of impaired understanding of mental states rests on the notion of ToM precursors in the first year or so of life. The EF account would appear to suggest that difficulties in regulating behaviour underlie the language and communication impairments, but the mapping between these is not specified precisely.

The main problem for specific cognitive deficit

hypotheses, however, does not lie in explaining the pragmatic abnormalities but the general language delay and global language impairment that is characteristic of most cases of autism. It is not at all evident why these should result from either ToM or EF deficits. If these deficits are to be taken seriously as contenders for the basis of autism, it is crucial that the issue be tackled. If ToM or EF deficits underlie the language impairment, variations in the former should relate systematically to variation in the extent of the latter. Furthermore, the type of language impairment associated with ToM or EF deficits should differ from other types of language disorder. To date, there has been little attempt to investigate these important questions.

Within theory of mind research, it has been found that most individuals who pass the tests have a relatively high verbal IQ. Good language is not a sufficient factor, however, since some people with equivalent language levels are not successful in ToM tests (Frith et al., 1991). The associations between language ability and EF and WCC performance have been less well explored. The very strong associations between language skills and other aspects of autism mean that we should look more closely at this area. Language ability is not a unitary phenomenon, and some aspects may be more important than others (see Eisenmajer & Prior, 1991). In that connection, it is relevant that language deficits have been found to be more closely associated with social outcome in autism than in severe developmental disorders of receptive language (Mawhood, 1995; Rutter et al., 1992). Although the language deficit hypothesis of the 1970s was found to be unsatisfactory, concepts of language development have become more sophisticated in the past decade, and it may prove fruitful to consider autism deficits in terms of these new ideas.

Pretend play. Both EF and ToM offer explanations for the marked poverty of spontaneous pretend play in autism. According to Leslie (1987), the problem arises because pretence involves the crucial metarepresentational system that is alleged to be dysfunctional in autism. The finding that understanding and production of pretence is not completely absent in autism (Lewis & Boucher, 1988; Jarrold et al., 1994b) showed that a metarepresentation deficit might not be a full explanation. Harris (1993) proposed that an EF related problem can account for lack of pretence, since treating one object as if it were another requires the child to "ignore" the familiar schema evoked by the object, and instead act according to his or her internal plan. An initial test of this hypothesis failed to find support (Jarrold et al., 1994a), but other aspects of executive dysfunction, such as a generativity deficit, could also account for pretend play impairments. This illustrates once again the need for the EF concept to be refined. It may be the case that object substitution and other basic forms of pretence are not features that are critical to the lack of pretend play in autism. Some children with autism show simple, routine forms of pretence, but these are not elaborated upon. Neither does their play mature into sociodramatic or shared pretence.

Repetitive behaviours, circumscribed interests and resistance to change. Theories in the broad category seem to be stronger in areas in which narrow theories are weak. A major weakness of narrow cognitive theories is that they do not give a convincing account of nonsocial features of autism, such as repetitive activity and behavioural rigidity. Explanations for these features tend to be in terms of secondary consequences of social impairment. Executive function theory finds it easier to explain repetitive and stereotyped behaviours, since these are predicted if behaviour cannot be flexibly controlled by the central executive (Shallice, 1988). However, insistence on sameness and circumscribed interests are frequently pursued with an apparent emotional intensity that is hard to understand in terms of a "default" activity. Central coherence theory offers an account for the ease with which children with autism detect changes in detail, which may be relevant to resistance to change. However, it does not explain why changes frequently cause such profound distress. There has been surprisingly little research into the cognitive correlates of behavioural rigidity and specialized interests. Turner (1995) used parent interview methods to measure repetitive behaviour and obsessions in children and young adults with autism, and direct experimental techniques to explore their mentalizing and executive function abilities. She found little evidence of a link with theory of mind, some correlation with perseveration and planning strategies, but a somewhat stronger association with tests of generativity, such as the FAS word fluency test and a "use of objects" task. The notion that repetitive behaviours may be linked to a generativity problem (rather than, say, to one of social anxiety) received support from the parents' reports that their children performed the behaviours when not directed explicitly to do some alternative activity.

General intellectual impairment, spiky IQ patterns, splinter skills and "idiots savants". Contemporary psychological theories of autism have regarded general mental retardation as not being in need of specific explanation, even though it is present in the overwhelming majority of cases. The argument is that since intellectual impairment occurs in many conditions, it must be a coincidental feature in autism. However, the association is very strong, and there needs to be some way of accounting for this. Furthermore, both genetic loading for autism and severity of symptomatology are strongly associated with intellectual level (Bolton et al., 1994). These findings strongly suggest that intellectual impairment is an intrinsic part of autism, which presents particular difficulties for narrow "social" theories (Rutter & Bailey, 1993). On the other hand, the broader phenotype of autism is *not* associated with mental retardation (see Genetics section above) and it remains a puzzle why that is the case when low IQ is so strongly associated with autism as traditionally diagnosed.

In addition to generally depressed intellectual ability in many individuals, there are unusual features to be found in the *patterns* of performance. So far, neither the broad nor narrow psychological theories have been able to account fully for these, although WCC theory addresses some of the issues. The patterns are extraordinary in three ways. First, within standardized IQ tests such as the Wechsler scales, there are strikingly uneven scores across different subtests. Unlike other disorders involving mental retardation, in which subtest scores tend to be more or less even, the profile in autism is very jagged. It should be noted that not all autistic individuals show exactly the same pattern, but group data show that some patterns are particularly common (low in Comprehension and high in Block Design and Digit Span) (Lockyer & Rutter, 1970; Rumsey, 1992; Venter et al., 1992). Unusual patterns of psychological test performance were also seen in the experimental work of Hermelin and her colleagues, who demonstrated atypical processing of structured or meaningful information (see Hermelin & O'Connor, 1970). Secondly, outside of standardized or experimental measures, there are frequent reports of so-called splinter skills or islets of ability. These talents may be in reading (hyperlexia), spelling, mathematics, music or drawing. These relatively preserved abilities, in the context of overall intellectual disability, do not seem to be especially rare. Goode et al., (1994) found that a quarter of individuals with autism (with an IQ of at least 35) showed a special cognitive skill that was both one standard deviation above the general population mean and two standard deviations above their own overall cognitive level. These measured cognitive skills were closely associated with parental accounts of special talents and both were more common in autistic individuals than in those with a developmental disorder of receptive language (Mawhood, 1995). Thirdly, a small proportion of individuals develop an isolated talent to a level that is in excess of that found in normal people—the "idiot savant" phenomenon (O'Connor & Hermelin, 1988). Although the savant phenomenon is not limited to autism, the great majority are autistic, and their spectacular abilities in memory, music, calculation or drawing sometimes wane as their autistic symptoms improve. Moreover, even in those not diagnosed as autistic, idiot savant skills seem to be associated with unusual preoccupations and repetitive behaviour (O'Connor & Hermelin, 1991). The actual level of the talent, although far higher than overall ability, seems to be associated with IQ. As with the more common splinter skills, savant abilities are usually not used constructively in everyday living.

The questions for psychological theories are how the peak test performances, splinter skills and savant talents are related to each other, and whether they are evidence of preserved cognitive function or signs of cognitive deficit. It is not thought that intensive practice or outstanding memory ability can explain these outstanding talents entirely, although they may be involved. One possibility (Pring, Hermelin & Heavey, 1995) is that autism involves a tendency to segment information (that is, favour parts over wholes) and that, in savant individuals, this tendency is especially strong, leading to enhanced performance in certain domains. This hypothesis is clearly related to Frith and Happé's WCC explanation for spiky IQ profiles. A testable prediction would be, therefore, that the tendency to disregard "gestalt" information is variable: autistic savant individuals should show it more than those with unusual talents of a lesser degree. The latter should show it more strongly than autistic individuals without such splinter skills, who may show it more than nonautistic persons.

In this section about variability in intellectual ability, it is pertinent to mention the severity of autism. Clearly, although autism and PDD are profoundly disabling for all affected people, there is yet a great range of severity. Severity can be considered across more than one dimension—for example, intellectual ability and symptom picture. One can readily conceive of someone without severe mental handicap but with extreme forms of social impairment or stereotypic behaviours. However, recent research has shown that IQ itself (at least, verbal IQ) is related to severity of autism symptoms (Bolton et al., 1994). So it may be that these two dimensions of severity are not as independent as they would seem logically.

How are the Various Cognitive Deficits Related?

At one extreme, any of the specific cognitive deficits might cause all the others. For example, social–perceptual and social–cognitive impairment might be a consequence of a broader problem such as executive dysfunction. The other radical position would be that each of the specific deficits is independent and all of these can appear in autism. Naturally, a number of intermediate positions are also possible (see Happé, 1994b; Bishop, 1993; Ozonoff, 1994; Hughes et al., 1994).

One possibility is that theory of mind impairment causes executive dysfunction. Understanding one's own mind is an important aspect of having a concept of mind, and willed action is highly dependent on being able to monitor one's intentions. Evidence for this causal link demands that individuals who show EF deficits will also fail tests of understanding own intentions, but such investigations have not been done. The only relevant data are those provided by Ozonoff et al. (1991a). They described individuals who passed false belief tasks even though they had problems in planning or set-shifting, which fails to support ToM-to-EF causation. However, the theory of mind tasks used may have had too low a ceiling to show deficits, and in any case were tests of understanding others' false beliefs, not own intentions. It remains a possibility that an understanding of mental states is necessary for adequate executive function.

A more convincing argument perhaps may be made for the converse situation, in which executive dysfunction impairs the development of mentalizing ability. The ToM experimental findings could be artefactual, resulting from failure to cope with the EF demands of the tasks themselves. Alternatively, there could be genuine theory of mind deficits that are caused by EF problems. It is clear that the ability to master ToM tasks involves general cognitive abilities, including working memory, inhibition of prepotent responses and inference. This is especially evident in the early puppet narratives (Baron-Cohen et al., 1985). However, other ToM experiments have included carefully devised control tasks (e.g. Sodian & Frith, 1992), and it is not obvious why executive dysfunction should lead to success in these tasks but failure in ToM tasks. Furthermore, if ToM task failure is artefactual, one could expect to find individuals who fail experimental tasks but apparently can deal with mental states in certain nontest situations. In fact, the reverse situation is sometimes found (Frith et al., 1994).

If the causal direction is EF-to-ToM, it is more likely that executive dysfunction leads to real social–cognitive deficits. Those who argue for this causal direction have suggested that difficulties in cognitive set-shifting could account for joint attention deficits, which many consider to have a precursor relationship to theory of mind impairment. A useful investigation would involve testing autistic toddlers' ability to shift attention between two inanimate objects compared with their ability to control shifts of attention between a person and an object.

A third possible relationship is one in which both broad and narrow deficits exist independently. Goodman (1989) pointed out that autism, like other unitary medical conditions, may involve more than one primary deficit. The common factor may be found at another level of analysis, such as neurobiology. The observed similarities between patients with known frontal lesions and people with autism led to the suggestion that frontal lobe function may be implicated in autism. However, the frontal lobes consist of a number of functionally distinct areas and systems, and it is at least possible that some of these are relevant to social understanding (for example, superior mesial cortex and orbito-frontal cortex) while others are more related to domain-general cognitive operations (dorsolateral cortex). (See Brothers, 1990 and Baron-Cohen & Ring, 1994 for a discussion of these issues.) One possibility is that autism involves both general executive dysfunction caused by problems in distributed neural systems *and* specific social dysfunction deriving from abnormalities in a modular brain system that has evolved to deal specifically with intraspecies interaction. The survival value of a streamlined mechanism for computing the behaviour of conspecifics is easy to imagine (Baron-Cohen, 1995; Whiten & Perner, 1991).

Another possible combination of neuropsychological deficits has been suggested by Frith and Happé (1994). These authors proposed that both weak central coherence (WCC) and theory of mind impairment may exist independently in autism. Happé (in press) found that evidence of WCC could be found even in those high-functioning individuals who could pass theory of mind tests. Frith and Happé suggested that a complete understanding of autism may rest on the notion of two different cognitive systems being impaired, one a modular system dedicated to processing mental state information and the other a more distributed system that determines "cognitive style", or the manner in which information is processed.

Future Prospects for Neuropsychological Research in Autism

Much of this review has focused on the leading cognitive theories of autism. Important next steps include work to refine the concept of executive dysfunction as it applies to autism, to develop and test the hypothesis of weak central coherence and to explore theory of mind abilities in those high-functioning individuals who pass basic laboratory tests but are severely socially impaired in real life. In addition, a number of more general issues require investigation. *Neurological implications of the psychological fin-*

dings. It is clearly vital that neuropsychological and neurobiological research should work together to produce converging evidence about the biological basis of autism. There have been efforts to relate psychological performance to anatomical substrate by extrapolating from the impact of known acquired brain lesions on psychological test performance (for example, Prior, 1979). The executive dysfunction theory itself arose from the observation of similarities between autism and frontal lobe symptomatology (Damasio & Maurer, 1978; Rumsey & Hamburger, 1988). However, it must be borne in mind that there are grave dangers in extrapolating from late-acquired lesions to *developmental* abnormality. Research into the impact of early brain disorders and *early*-acquired lesions shows that effects on psychological functioning can be quite different in children compared with adults (e.g. Vargha-Khadem et al., 1992). Consequently, moving from cognitive test performance to brain structure in developmental disorders requires much caution.

There is reason to suppose that neurobiological abnormality in autism may be at the level of widespread brain systems, rather than discrete lesions (see below). Use of functional imaging technology during neuropsychological testing will be a valuable strategy for exploring this possibility (see section on Towards An Integration below).

Relationships between neuropsychological deficits—a tool for understanding PDD and other disorders. There are three ways in which autism-related neuropsychological test performance can be used as a research tool. First, the notion of co-existing neuropsychological deficits could be a useful way to address the *variability* of the autism syndrome—age of onset, presence of nontriad features, variations in social behaviour, language ability and IQ levels. Patterns of neuropsychological deficits could reveal subgroups that might have aetiological significance. Second, it could help to clarify *boundaries*, or relationships between autism and other disorders in which social functioning is impaired. These disorders include semantic–pragmatic disorder and Asperger syndrome, which some have argued are equivalent to high-functioning or mild autism, while others suggest are distinguishable subgroups of pervasive developmental disorder or even unrelated disorders (see Bishop, 1989). Another developmental disorder, which is not thought to be part of the autism spectrum but is associated with social impairment, is so-called right-hemisphere disorder, or nonverbal learning disability (NLD). A range of cognitive, motor and social perception problems have been reported in children with apparently good verbal intelligence but impaired academic performance (Semrud-Clikeman & Hynd, 1990). Rourke (1993) reported on a group of children with specific difficulties in arithmetic who also showed clumsiness, impaired pragmatics and social functioning, and a failure to benefit from feedback in problem-solving tasks. Whereas in autism and related disorders, there is usually relatively good visuo-spatial ability and poorer verbal ability, in Rourke's NLD group the reverse situation was common. However, in Asperger syndrome, clumsiness and higher verbal IQ than performance IQ is sometimes reported. A recent investigation (Klin et al., 1995) found that individuals with Asperger's syndrome (diagnosed according to ICD-10) had behavioural and psychological profiles that paralleled the NLD syndrome. Individuals with autism, however, had a different profile. Thus, the boundary between autism-related and nonrelated conditions is indistinct. The ambiguity surrounding these disorders could perhaps be resolved by testing NLD children (and those with other symptom patterns) with the range of neuropsychological and social–cognitive tests that have been found to be impaired in autism. One possibility is that some children classified as having RHD or NLD would have test profiles similar to autism, and therefore could be considered to have an autism-spectrum disorder. Others might show a completely different picture. Third, it will be possible to investigate certain medical conditions in which some affected individuals have autism while others do not. Two such disorders are Fragile X syndrome and tuberose sclerosis. It is unclear at present what the relationships are between affected persons with and without autism. Comparison of neuropsychological test patterns could provide a way forward.

Neuropsychological impairment and the "broader phenotype". Another aspect of diagnostic boundaries could be addressed by extending research on executive function, theory of mind and other neuropsychological functions to the relatives of autistic probands. As outlined above, some relatives have been found to show a "lesser variant" of the disorder, involving very mild forms of social interactive, cognitive and repetitive behavioural symptoms (Bolton et al., 1994). At present, the putative broader phenotype is defined in terms of these reported behavioural signs but a more precise definition is desirable. Accurate identification of affected relatives will be an important step forward in the search for mechanisms of genetic transmission.

One question is whether the mildly affected relatives also show neuropsychological deficits that are similar in nature to (but milder than) those found in autism. If cognitive deficits (such as those described in this paper) are truly primary to autism, they should be present in all persons who carry the autism genotype, including those with the lesser variant. If they are not present in the broader phenotype, then our understanding of the role of cognitive deficits in autism will have to be revised. Preliminary research with relatives showed that signs of executive dysfunction, but not theory of mind problems, could be detected in some nonautistic siblings (Ozonoff et al., 1993). However, some of the measures used were inappropriate for the group tested, in that they were developed for preschool children. Clearly, to address this question, it will be necessary to develop ToM, WCC, EF and language pragmatics tests that are sufficiently sensitive to detect very subtle impairments in children and adults with normal IQ levels. For obvious reasons, a broad battery of tests will be needed for this purpose. That is because it is clear that autism is associated with a range of cognitive deficits, no one of which seems to provide a plausible basis for the syndrome as a whole.

A number of other issues concerning the broader autism phenotype remain to be investigated. It is striking that, although most autistic individuals have intellectual impairment, the broader phenotype of milder symptoms is usually found in relatives with a normal IQ level. The familial genetic liability, however, is inversely related to the cognitive level (verbal IQ) of the proband (Bolton et al., 1994). Furthermore, it is unknown what factors might be decisive in whether the full-blown syndrome develops or only the lesser form.

Relationships between neuropsychological functioning and behavioural features. There is a need to map the relationships between cognitive functioning and behavioural symptoms in autism. Preliminary work relating theory of mind abilities to real-life social skills has already been mentioned. This needs to be extended, with particular attention to those individuals who pass ToM tests but have real-life mentalizing problems. The advanced naturalistic ToM tests that are being developed will be useful in this regard. Similarly, the connections between cognitive inflexibility and behavioural rigidity are being explored (Turner, 1995). The area of stereotyped and restricted activities is in urgent need of more investigation, as is the domain of special talents and splinter skills. It is clearly important to be able to see how behavioural features, neuropsychological performance and neurobiological abnormalities are linked. As has been suggested in schizophrenia, different symptom pictures may be associated with different cognitive deficits, and these patterns may be helpful in exploring biological heterogeneity.

It would be useful to investigate these cognitive–behavioural links in individuals who have developmental features that resemble autism, but are also markedly different in some aspects. For example, current research into the development of children adopted into British families from orphanages in Romania is showing that some of them have patterns of behaviour that are very similar to those seen in autism, but may have a different developmental course. Similarly, it will be worthwhile to explore neuropsychological patterns and behavioural features in other disorders, such as severe developmental receptive language disorder and schizophrenia, in order to examine similarities and differences between autism and these conditions.

Conclusion

One of the strengths of autism research at the neuropsychological level has been the hypothesis-driven nature of the investigations. This has meant that research has been clearly focused, rather than diffuse and haphazard, and has led to new understandings of the nature of the disorder. In the history of psychological research into autism, the "searchlight" has moved around to fix on different aspects of the disorder. In recent decades it has highlighted in turn sensory-perceptual abnormalities, language impairment, and most recently, social and pragmatic deficits. The theory of mind hypothesis has been especially helpful in accounting for the latter features. However, autism is crucially a *syndrome*, a constellation of features that cluster together, and we need to know *why* they cluster together. To answer this question, the searchlight beam must now be broadened, so that attention is focused on the totality of the syndrome, rather than on different aspects individually. On the one hand, it may be possible to identify one critical cognitive deficit that can account for cognitive, social and behavioural features, and it is worthwhile continuing to follow up that possibility. In particular, we need to understand how mental retardation and language abilities are related to specific cognitive deficits. On the other hand, it might be the case that autism is a unitary biological disorder that has diverse consequences at the levels of biology and psychology (Goodman, 1989). It may be that several specific cognitive deficits are needed to explain the range of features, and that there are additional emotion-related symptoms. All of these may arise from a single abnormality at the level of neuropathology or genetics. To focus too narrowly on any subset of the features of autism may be to arrive at only a partial understanding of autism.

Neurobiology

In general, neurobiological investigations of autism have been rather less driven by theory than the genetic and psychological studies. Replicable findings have remained elusive and consequently hypothesis driven research has been difficult to establish. The strong claims made recently for the significance of various subtle abnormalities may partially reflect the search for solid "facts" from which to progress. Nevertheless whilst it is relatively easy to construct post hoc arguments linking these empirical findings with autistic symptomatology, there have been few attempts to test their causal role. In considering the significance of the various neurobiological findings three issues are relevant: the symptomatology that requires explanation; the robustness of putative neurobiological abnormalities; and the validity of any hypothesized links between the findings and the symptomatology.

Over the years social and language deficits have each been viewed as primary abnormalities, leading to speculation about the brain basis of the disorder based upon the respective localization of these functions. The genetic findings suggest, however, that such a conceptualization is oversimplified. Thus whilst social and language deficits are usually found together in non-autistic MZ co-twins (Bailey et al., 1995), in a proportion of twins they occur in isolation, suggesting that neither abnormality is a consequence of the other. A similar issue arises with respect to the primacy of particular cognitive deficits (see above). In addition there is a need to account for features, such as low IQ, that are usually present although not pathognomonic of autism. This is particularly so because low IQ is such a strong prognostic factor and because verbal abilities relate to familial loading (see above). It seems prudent at present to consider that both the specific and apparently nonspecific symptomatology merits a neurobiological explanation. While ultimately this may prove to be too stringent a criterion, it does focus attention on the potential generalizability of putative mechanisms and it is a reminder of the likely complexity of the developmental processes underlying the disorder.

Replicability and Meaning of Findings

In contrast to the findings from genetic and psychological studies, the replicability of neurobiological investigations has been relatively poor (Bailey, 1993; Filipek et al., 1992a). One contributory factor is that insufficient care seems to have been paid to methodological issues. Laboratory and technologically based approaches are not intrinsically more reliable than interview or questionnaire methods and as much care is required in biological studies as in clinical research. An additional difficulty is that because many studies have been conducted outside a well developed theoretical framework, it is difficult to identify findings that are internally inconsistent and to control for factors producing artefactual differences between groups of subjects.

A further factor that seems likely to have contributed to poor replicability is subject heterogeneity. Even recent neuroimaging studies have sometimes examined aetiologically heterogeneous groups of subjects leading to difficulties in identifying findings that are specific to autism. The association between autism and certain medical conditions can of course provide convergent evidence for pathological mechanisms, but the appropriate comparisons have to be made. Another form of heterogeneity that merits attention is that related to disease severity. Thus psychological studies usually control for subject's intellectual level and comparisons between studies take IQ into account. Although some biological studies have included only high functioning individuals, frequently subjects with a wide range of intellectual abilities have been studied. As verbal IQ seems to be closely related to disease severity, a correlation between intellectual level and a biological variable would point to the need for further systematic investigation. Finally, unknown heterogeneity has almost certainly contributed to some of the differences between studies. This can arise because of variability in clinical diagnosis and differences in the specificity of individual diagnostic instruments.

Identification of the nature of the links between neurobiological findings and symptomatology in a genetically influenced developmental disorder is a formidable task and some of the complexities merit mention. The first is that disease genes may have pleiotropic effects. Thus, some biological abnormalities may be consequences of a genetically influenced process, but have no causal relationship to the cognitive abnormalities. The specific dysmorphic features associated with particular genetic mental handicap syndromes provide an example of an association of this sort. Other consistent neuroanatomical findings might simply reflect when in development abnormal genetic or environmental influences were active. To determine the significance of any anatomical variations requires convergent evidence from functional studies. A further problem is that much of our knowledge about the brain localization of cognitive operations and inferences about the likely effects of localized abnormalities has come from the study of acquired lesions in adult humans or animals. The evidence for very specific impairments following localized lesions in children is much less strong and some functions may be taken over by other cortical areas. Moreover in autism and related developmental disorders we are concerned with a failure to *acquire* skills; the site and nature of the processes involved in skill acquisition may be very different from their instantiation in the adult. Whilst the study of younger patients is likely to be helpful—although fraught with practical difficulties—a much greater understanding of the neurobiology of normal brain and cognitive development will also be necessary to make inferences about early deviant behaviours. Finally, difficulties can arise in deciding which of the multiple actions of a putative neurobiological abnormality are relevant to developmental symptomatology. An example is provided by the various reports of monoamine abnormalities in autistic individuals. These chemicals are important neurotransmitters but also have the potential to influence brain development (Kalsbeek et al., 1987; Julius, 1991) and both actions may be relevant. In summary it is clear that neurobiological researchers need to be especially careful to consider the various alternative interpretations of their findings.

Two recent reviews have surveyed the neurobiological studies of autism; Gillberg and Coleman (1992) provided a particularly wide-ranging bibliography, whilst Bauman and Kemper's (1994) focus was predominantly North American. In this section the main findings in each area of investigation are briefly summarized and then the significance of the results and future plans discussed.

Neuroanatomical Studies

Mental handicap syndromes are often associated with gross abnormalities in brain development. Frequently, the overall size of the brain is reduced—microcephaly—but qualitative abnormalities are also found, particularly in the cerebral hemispheres and overlying cortex. Understandably, there has been an expectation that autism, too, might be associated with gross abnormalities in brain development and that a consistently localized abnormality might underlie the distinctive symptomatology. There have been a great many structural imaging studies of autism and a much smaller number of postmortem studies. The neuroimaging studies have been the subject of several recent detailed reviews (Courchesne, 1991; Gillberg & Coleman, 1992; Filipek et al., 1992a; Lotspeich & Ciaranello, 1993; Minshew & Dombrowski, 1994). Two articles bring together the findings from the largest postmortem series in which whole brain serial sections were examined (Kemper & Bauman, 1993; Bauman & Kemper, 1994).

Neuroimaging Studies

The strongest claims for a highly localized structural abnormality are those that relate to the involvement of the cerebellar vermis. Courchesne et al., (1987) reported hypoplasia of the posterior cerebellar vermis in an MRI study of a high functioning autistic individual. Subsequently 18 autistic individuals and a group of normal controls were examined; a significant reduction in the size of cerebellar vermal lobules VI–VII was found in

the autistic group, but no difference in the size of vermal lobules I–V (Courchesne et al., 1988). It has been argued that there is concordant evidence that cerebellar abnormalities are the most consistent neuroanatomical lesion in autism (Courchesne et al., 1994a) and that such abnormalities underlie some of the characteristic symptomatology. Nevertheless studies that have used similar imaging protocols have not replicated the vermal findings (Garber & Ritvo, 1992; Holttum et al., 1992; Kleinman et al., 1992; Piven et al., 1992). Courchesne et al., (1994a) suggested that one reason for the failure to replicate is that the autistic population may in fact comprise two subgroups: one with posterior vermal hypoplasia, the other with vermal hyperplasia. Whilst the variance of posterior vermal areas may be increased in autistic individuals, the introduction of an *auxiliary* hypothesis of two subgroups reduces the falsifiability of the original claims. The recent MRI study of Hashimoto et al., (1995) has been cited in support of the cerebellar hypothesis (Courchesne, 1995). Nevertheless, this study is methodologically less rigorous than previous investigations and does not in fact replicate the original claim of specific hypoplasia.

A key question with all findings, even when replicated, is whether they are diagnosis-specific. A preliminary report by Ciesielski and Knight (1994) claimed that both autistic individuals and nonautistic survivors of childhood leukaemia treated by irradiation showed cerebellar hypoplasia on quantitative MRI scans but the cognitive patterns and socio-emotional features of the two groups were quite different. If confirmed, this would cast doubt on the causal hypothesis linking cerebellar abnormalities and autism.

The other strong claim for a consistently localized abnormality relates to abnormalities in the medial temporal lobe and related structures. The postmortem findings are dealt with below, but interest in this region was first aroused by the observation of left temporal horn dilatation in a pneumoencephalographic study (Hauser et al., 1975); abnormalities of the underlying hippocampus and related structures have been hypothesized to underlie autistic symptomatology (Hauser et al., 1975; DeLong, 1992; Bauman & Kemper, 1994). Dilatation of the temporal horns has not been confirmed in subsequent Computerized Tomography (CT) studies and posterior hippocampal volumes were unchanged in the only published MRI study of this structure (Saitoh et al., 1995). The studies of other components of the ventricular system have produced variable findings, but together they suggest that occasional ventricular abnormalities are unlikely to be confined to the temporal horns. Thus some early CT studies, which included a heterogenous group of subjects, reported increased lateral ventricular size in a sub-group (Damasio et al., 1980; Gillberg & Svendsen, 1983); dilatation was also reported in a small proportion of individuals without concomitant neurological disorders (Campbell et al., 1982). Subsequent CT studies failed to confirm this finding (see, for instance, Jacobson et al., 1988). The only MRI study to have examined the lateral ventricular area included two autistic subjects with neurofibromatosis (Gaffney et al., 1989); the significance of the reported increase in that area is consequently unclear. A

179

similarly inconsistent picture emerges with respect to measures of the third ventricle. A subgroup of individuals in the study of Campbell et al., (1982) had enlarged third ventricles and a significant increase in size was noted in the study of Jacobson et al., (1988); no difference in third ventricular measurements was found, however, in the studies of Rosenbloom et al., (1984) or Creasey et al., (1986). In contrast the findings for the fourth ventricle are clear. Only one group (Gaffney et al., 1987) has reported a statistically significant increase in fourth ventricular size (although not consistently across different imaging planes). No significant increase has been found in at least six other studies. A number of groups have examined subcortical structures but the findings are inconsistent. Gaffney et al., (1988), Hashimoto et al., (1993, 1995) reported MRI evidence of brainstem involvement, but this finding has not been confirmed by other investigators (Hsu et al., 1991; Garber & Ritvo, 1992; Piven et al., 1992). Jacobson et al., (1988) reported lower radiodensities of the caudate nuclei compared with controls. Gaffney et al., (1989) reported a decrease in the area of the lenticular nuclei, but there was no significant change using an imaging sequence with better white/grey matter differentiation. Creasey et al., (1986) also found no change in basal ganglia volumes.

Turning next to the cerebral cortex and underlying white matter, several studies have identified relatively circumscribed abnormalities in a small number of subjects. The only report of consistent localization for these abnormalities is from Courchesne et al., (1993). They observed an apparent reduction in parietal lobe volume in a subgroup of autistic individuals. Other studies have noted occasional abnormalities in disparate areas of the cortex and white matter (Damasio et al., 1980; Gillberg & Svendsen, 1983; Gaffney & Tsai, 1987; Piven et al., 1990b; Schifter et al., 1994). As yet there is no clear evidence from structural neuroimaging studies that any cortical abnormalities are consistent in their localization, neither are there published MRI volume data for the different regions of the cerebral hemispheres. The studies of Piven et al., (1990b) and Schifter et al., (1994) found evidence of cortical developmental anomalies in a small number of patients. Such anomalies arise in utero and the most subtle are much more easily identified with MRI than CT.

The findings from two recent neuroimaging studies suggest that brain volume may be increased in autistic individuals compared with controls. Piven et al., (1995) reprted that volume was increased compared to normal controls and Filipek et al., (1992b) reported an increase compared to normal, developmental language disorder and nonautistic mentally handicapped controls. A number of earlier neuroimaging studies failed to find any significant change in various indices of brain size, however, pointing to the need for replication of the recent results. Nevertheless, no studies have found evidence of decreased brain size in autistic individuals. Some support for the recent neuroimaging findings comes from postmortem data (see below) and indirectly from anthropometric data (see Clinical Features section above). Interestingly a number of disorders reported to be associated with autism—Tuberous Sclerosis (Hunt &

Dennis, 1987), Neurofibromatosis (Gillberg & Forsell, 1984), Hypomelanosis of Ito (Akefeldt & Gillberg, 1991) and Sotos syndrome (Zapella, 1990)—are also sometimes associated with increased brain size or head circumference; these syndromes all involve cortical pathology to a greater or lesser extent.

Postmortem Studies

Postmortem material from individuals with a rare disorder is difficult to obtain and only a few studies of autism have been reported. Consequently the few findings have had a considerable impact; for the past 10 years the focus has been predominantly upon claims of microscopic abnormalities localized to the cerebellum and the medial temporal and related structures.

Interest in the cerebellum was initiated by Bauman and Kemper's (Bauman & Kemper, 1985) very detailed report on a mentally handicapped autistic male with epilepsy. Purkinje cell density in the cerebellum was apparently reduced but there was no evidence of gliosis or retrograde cell loss in the inferior olives. They suggested that the finding pointed to an early developmental insult. Williams et al., (1980) had also noted subjective loss of Purkinje cells in a handicapped autistic individual with epilepsy. The significance of the observation in these two cases was unclear because Purkinje cell loss is a recognized complication of epilepsy (Meldrum & Bruton, 1992), which may also lead to proliferation of the Bergmann glia and granule cell loss. Ritvo et al., (1986) found Purkinje cell density to be significantly lower in four autistic brains than controls; none of these subjects had epilepsy although three had unspecified EEG abnormalities. There was, however, a marked age difference between the autistic and control subjects. Detailed counts have not been published for Bauman and Kemper's series of six brains, but the reduction in Purkinje cell number apparently varies in severity (Bauman, 1991). In four of the cases Purkinje cell density was decreased by 50–95% in some areas (Arin et al., 1991), but three of these individuals also had a history of epilepsy (Kemper & Bauman, 1993). Bailey et al., (1995) found decreased Purkinje cell density in three adult autistic brains, but normal density in the brain of a child. Two of the adults had a history of epilepsy and in one case the Purkinje cells were surrounded by Bergmann glia and in the other there was cortical sub-pial gliosis. Bauman's group have also noted an apparent reduction in the number of neurons in the cerebellar granule cell layer (Kemper & Bauman, 1993) and both Bauman and Kemper (1994) and Bailey et al., (submitted) have noted other mild cerebellar changes in some cases.

The other claim of localized microscopic abnormalities relates to the medial temporal structures. Bauman and Kemper's group (Bauman & Kemper, 1994) have reported the relatively consistent finding of abnormally small and densely packed neurons in the hippocampus, subiculum, mamilliary body, septum and amygdala. In the absence of neocortical pathology, these abnormalities have been claimed to underlie autistic symptomatology and comparisons have been drawn with the behavioural effects of medial temporal lesions (Bauman

& Kemper, 1985; DeLong, 1992; Kemper & Bauman, 1993). Quantitative neuronal densities have been published on only one case (Bauman & Kemper, 1985). Pyramidal neuronal size has been measured in hippocampal areas CA1 and CA4 in two cases, but only the neurons in CA4 were significantly smaller than in controls (Raymond et al., 1989). Although the restricted distribution of the microscopic abnormalities has been emphasized, no special attention appears to have been paid to the neocortex. The brains examined by Bailey et al. (submitted) were divided in the midline and the septal nuclei and mamilliary bodies have not been examined. No subjective abnormalities were noted in the amygdala. Hippocampal neuronal density in CA1 was generally at the upper end of the range for normal controls. No medial temporal abnormalities has been observed in the cases reported by Williams et al., (1980) or by Coleman et al., (1985) and only the cerebellae have been examined microscopically in the series reported by Ritvo et al., (1986). Darby's review (1976) of 33 cases found no consistent abnormalities.

Although no gross structural abnormalities were reported in the earlier postmortem studies, four of the six brains in the series of Bailey et al., (1993b, 1995) were megalencephalic. An increase in the cerebral cortex is usually considered to be primarily responsible for the increased brain weight in megalencephaly. The cortex was thickened in some areas in two of the cases and neuronal disorganization was noted in the superior temporal gyrus of one case. Mild olivary abnormalities were noted in most cases; such abnormalities seldom occur in isolation and olivary heterotopias have been reported in association with megalencephaly, pachygyria, lissencephaly, and other disorders (Harding, 1992). Other abnormalities were also noted in the brainstem. Minor developmental cortical abnormalities have been noted in two other brains (Kemper, 1988; Ritvo et al., 1986), but brain weights have only been reported by Williams et al., (1980); one large brain fell within the normal range of weights reported by Blinkov and Glezer (1968) but outside the normal range of Dekaban and Sadowsky (1978). The brains in the series of Bauman and Kemper were also apparently considerably heavier than control brains (Bauman, personal communication). There is one postmortem report of an unusually small brain (Hof et al., 1991) in an individual with premature closure of the cerebral sutures. The suggestion from several independent studies of increased brain weights contrasts with the more usual finding in studies of mental handicap of decreased brain weight (see, for example Cole et al., 1994).

Neurophysiological Studies

Although anatomical studies may provide some clues as to the brain basis of autistic behaviour, functional studies are necessary to determine which anatomical abnormalities have functional sequelae and ultimately to demonstrate involvement in abnormal cognitive processes. The observation that epilepsy developed in about one quarter of individuals with autism (Rutter, 1970) provided the first clear indication of abnormal brain function. Subsequent studies have confirmed the asso-

ciation although the rates of epilepsy have varied between studies. Some studies have found a greater rate of seizures in more handicapped individuals (Rutter, 1984; Volkmar & Nelson, 1990; Bailey et al., 1995), but this was not confirmed in the recent large follow-up study by Goode et al., (1994). Several studies have also noted that although some individuals have an onset of seizures in early childhood, a sizeable group develop seizures in adolescence or early adulthood (Rutter, 1984; Deykin & MacMahon, 1979b; Volkmar & Nelson, 1990; Goode et al., 1994). All types of seizures may occur in autistic individuals, although a high incidence of complex-partial seizures was noted by Olsson et al., (1988) in an aetiologically mixed group. Several reports have noted an association with infantile spasms. Rather strikingly none of the postmortem studies have found evidence of medial temporal sclerosis in autistic subjects with epilepsy.

EEG abnormalities are found in about 50% of autistic individuals although the range varies considerably from study to study (Minshew, 1991). Small (1975) noted that abnormal EEG's were associated with lower IQ. Tsai et al., (1985) reported that in half of the individuals with an abnormal EEG, there was evidence of bilateral diffuse abnormalities. Even when there were unilateral abnormalities, there was no predilection for any particular part of the brain. No EEG pattern appears to be pathognomonic of autism. Nevertheless the epilepsy and EEG data provide clear evidence of abnormal brain function that may possibly be related to the severity of the disorder.

New functional imaging technologies, such as PET and SPET have also been used to measure brain function, usually at rest. These approaches detect brain activity indirectly by measuring changes in metabolism or blood flow. The findings from the relatively small number of studies are rather contradictory. Although there were early claims of diffusely elevated cerebral metabolism (Rumsey et al., 1985; Horwitz et al., 1988), these have not been replicated (Herold et al., 1988); indeed George et al., (1992) reported decreased brain perfusion in a SPET study of four subjects. Only two studies have reported consistently localized areas of metabolic abnormality. Gillberg et al., (1993) observed apparently decreased temporal lobe perfusion in a SPET study of an aetiologically heterogenous group of subjects. George et al., (1992) also reported decreased perfusion in the right lateral temporal region and both frontal lobes. Zilbovicius et al., (1995), using SPET, reported reduced frontal perfusion in five autistic children aged three to four years but no difference from controls three years later.

Rumsey et al., (1985) drew attention to greater variations in the PET findings in autistic subjects than controls, with more autistic individuals showing extreme relative metabolic rates and asymmetries. In fact heterogeneities in regional metabolic rates, in the setting of normal global metabolism, have been a feature of a number of independent studies (De Volder et al., 1987; Siegel et al., 1992; Buchsbaum et al., 1992). Horwitz et al., (1988) went on to examine the correlations between the metabolic rates in different regions and found these to be lower in autistic subjects than controls. Only the study of Schifter et al., (1994) has combined structural and functional imaging. In some cases areas of decreased perfusion coincided with subtle MRI evidence of cortical abnormalities.

Of course functional imaging studies of cognitive tasks are likely to be an increasingly important tool in the investigation of autism. To date, researchers have had to rely on event related potential (ERP) studies to investigate the integrity of information processing pathways in autistic individuals. ERP studies are technically demanding and many of the data are contradictory. There have been many studies of the Auditory Brainstem Evoked Response (ABER) but they do not provide clear evidence for brainstem dysfunction in autism (Klin, 1993). The majority of ERP studies of cortical information processing have examined the P3b component. Several early studies reported P300 abnormalities in small numbers of subjects. Courchesne et al., (1985), however, reported a decreased P300 in response to auditory stimuli in a relatively large sample but Erwin et al., (1991) were recently unable to replicate this finding. In the same study, Courchesne et al., (1985) reported abnormally small auditory P300 responses to novel stimuli and similar findings are found in patients with prefrontal damage. The P300 findings in response to visual stimuli are particularly contradictory.

Courchesne's group have recently used event related potentials to study selective attention and attentional shifting in autistic subjects (Townsend & Courchesne, in press; Courchesne et al., 1994b). They suggested that cerebellar damage is associated with impaired attentional shifting in autism and that parietal damage is associated with a narrowed attentional focus. Wainwright-Sharp and Bryson (1993) have recently noted that autistic individuals have difficulty using visually presented information when constraints are placed upon the time available to process the information.

A number of investigators have used other neurophysiological techniques to infer areas of neurological damage in autistic individuals (see Dawson & Lewy, 1989a,b). The range of studies is very broad and includes examination of heart rate responses (James & Barry, 1980), electrodermal reactivity (Van Engeland et al., 1991), Rapid Eye Movement (REM) sleep abnormalities (Tanguay et al., 1976), vestibular eye movement abnormalities (Ornitz, 1985); saccadic eye movements (Rosenhall et al., 1988), gait (Vilensky et al., 1981; Hallett et al., 1993) and retinal evoked responses (Ritvo et al., 1988). It is difficult to draw firm conclusions from these studies either because only one group has ever undertaken a particular type of study, or because there has been little attempt to pursue findings systematically through further work.

Neurochemical Studies

Interpretation of the findings of chemical studies of autistic individuals is especially problematical. The major reason is that the biological variable being assayed is usually rather remote from either brain function or structure. Thus the majority of studies have examined blood or urine levels of the substance of interest and the relative contribution of the brain to these pools may be

small. A related difficulty is that it is difficult to know whether any differences between subjects and controls are possible aetiological factors or instead consequences of some aspect of autistic behaviour or cognition. The first difficulty can be partially overcome by the use of postmortem brain tissue or PET ligand binding studies (Bailey, 1993) but neither of these approaches has so far been adopted. A further interpretive problem is that the replicability of many of these studies has been low under blind conditions (see Boullin et al., 1982; Le Couteur et al., 1988).

Since the early 1960s investigators have searched for neurotransmitter abnormalities in autism. The motivation for the work has arisen mainly from comparisons between autistic behaviours and the behavioural effects of psychotropic drugs in animals and man. The interest in serotonin arose because of its influence upon perception; the stereotyped behaviours of autistic individuals led to study of the dopaminergic system; whilst self injurious behaviours and reduced sensitivity to pain seemed analogous to the effects of opiates. The findings from many neurotransmitter studies have been extensively reviewed (Cook, 1990; Narayan et al., 1993) and only the key points are noted here. Studies of the dopaminergic, noradrenergic and neuropeptide systems have not produced evidence of consistent abnormalities in autistic individuals. Panksepp (1979) argued that endogenous brain opioids were increased in autism and inhibited the development of social attachments; however, there is little empirical support for the hypothesis (Gillberg, 1995). The findings with respect to serotonin are rather more consistent. Thus, whole blood serotonin is elevated in about one quarter of autistic individuals (Cook, 1990; a consequence of increased amounts of serotonin in platelets. In contrast many studies have shown that CSF concentrations of the breakdown product of serotonin—5-hydroxyindoleacetic acid (5HIAA)—are not elevated in autistic individuals. Although elevated peripheral serotonin levels are also found in severe mental retardation, the observation of hyperserotonemia in the relatives of some autistic individuals suggests that the finding may be more than a nonspecific consequence of abnormal brain development. Early claims of marked improvements in autistic symptomatology following treatment with fenfluramine (Geller et al., 1982), which lowers platelet serotonin levels, were not subsequently substantiated. The significance of hyperserotonemia is at present unclear but several groups have also noted an elevated rate of affective disorder amongst the relatives of autistic individuals (Schifter et al., 1994; Bolton et al., 1995; Smalley et al., 1995). Many authors have drawn attention to the role of serotonin in brain development and it is possible that if abnormality has any causal role, it operates through developmental mechanisms.

Conclusion

The neuroimaging and postmortem studies have not found evidence of acquired lesions, neither do they or the functional imaging studies strongly support the hypothesis of an anatomically localized abnormality. Claims of consistent macroscopic cerebellar abnormalities have not been replicated and diminished posterior vermal area has been found in nonautistic individuals with the Fragile X syndrome (Reiss et al., 1991). Neither does the distribution of decreased Purkinje cell density in the postmortem studies strongly support the hypothesis of macroscopic changes specific to the posterior cerebellar vermis. It appears that in some individuals decreased Purkinje cell density and apparent granule cell loss may be in part a consequence of epileptic seizures. The presence of other developmental brainstem and cerebellar abnormalities in some postmortem cases also suggests that any developmental interference in Purkinje cell number is probably not an isolated abnormality. Whilst it remains a possibility that developmental cerebellar abnormalities have a causal role in autism, it seems more likely that they are but one consequence of abnormal brain development.

The early report of macroscopic abnormalities in the medial temporal lobe (Hauser et al., 1975) has not so far been replicated. Much of the strength of the argument for the pivotal role of microscopic abnormalities in the medial temporal structures has rested upon the absence of neocortical pathology. The neuroimaging, postmortem and EEG data suggest, however, that subtle medial temporal abnormalities sometimes occur in the setting of more pervasive abnormalities in brain development and function. Although abnormalities in the medial temporal structures may have an aetiological role in autism, there appears no reason to argue that they account for all the symptomatology. Indeed it seems unwise to suggest that particular areas of the brain are not affected in autism unless normal structure and function have been un-ambiguously demonstrated.

The preliminary finding of increased brain size in some autistic individuals suggests that autism may be associated with a rather more pervasive abnormality in brain development than had been hitherto supposed. Increased head circumference was noted by Kanner (1943) and, although not commented upon, also occurred amongst the cases studied by Hauser et al., (1975). As so often happens, it is the convergent evidence for an abnormality that has currently directed attention to brain size. The EEG and PET data together also suggest that abnormal brain function is not a highly localized phenomena. There are considerable challenges ahead in understanding how these data relate to the syndrome's very distinctive symptomatology and two possible pitfalls need to be avoided. One is of independently equating diverse abnormalities with specific cognitive difficulties and by so doing to lose sight of the interrelationship between the various features. The other, which has frequently occurred in the past, is of focusing upon abnormalities in one area and arguing that the functional consequences are an adequate explanation for autism as a whole.

What issues should neurobiological studies be tackling in the immediate future? An obvious starting point is to follow up the lead of apparently increased brain size, as this finding is unusual in the bulk of cases of mental handicap. A starting point is to determine precisely the proportion of autistic individuals who are affected and the extent to which the finding is a familial trait. A second issue is to establish the nature of the

underlying pathology. Bailey et al., (submitted) have suggested that increased total neuronal number may be one contributory factor and Coleman et al., (1985) noted a smaller glia/neuron ratio in one case compared to the average for two control brains. The finding of raised levels of glial fibrillary acidic protein (GFAP) in the CSF of autistic children (Rosengren et al., 1992) suggests that glial number might also be increased. Clearly further detailed examination of the available post mortem cases is necessary. Another set of questions concerns the nature of the relationship between increased brain size and autistic symptomatology. Increased brain size alone cannot cause autism as many individuals with macrocephaly are not autistic. One possibility is that megalencepahy is simply a remote and unimportant consequence of the pathological process that produces autism. The history of research into autism suggests that this is an important option that should not be discounted. Another possibility is that megalencephaly does not reflect the upper end of the normal distribution, but is the result of a pathological process that also underlies autistic symptomatology. A final possibility is that increased brain size predisposes to further, as yet unrecognized, abnormalities. There is an outstanding need for further MRI studies to search for localized cortical abnormalities and variations in regional volumes as well as further examination of postmortem material. The aetiological significance, if any, of accompanying abnormalities in the brainstem and cerebellum remains to be determined.

A rather different set of research objectives concerns the underlying basis of the PET, EEG and ERP abnormalities that have been detected in autistic individuals. Are the PET heterogeneities and the EEG abnormalities a consequence of underlying cortical dysplasia or dysfunction—and if so do they show a predilection for any particular area—or are they a consequence of subcortical abnormalities? These questions are probably best tackled by further multimodal imaging studies combining PET, MRI and MEG. Of course neither epilepsy nor EEG abnormalities are specific to autism.

A final set of research objectives concerns the information processing consequences, if any, of the abnormalities that have been detected. The bulk of ERP studies have noted abnormalities at a fairly late stage in the processing chain—approximately 300 msecs—and considerable interactions between cortical and subcortical regions have occurred during this time. Townsend and Courchesne (1995) have also noted abnormally large attentional effects as early as 100 msecs after a visual cue and Wainwright-Sharp and Bryson (1993) observed difficulties in stimulus processing when this had to occur within 100 msecs of cue presentation. It remains to be determined at precisely which stage of the information processing chain ERP abnormalities are first detectable and whether abnormalities first occur in the rostral transmission of electrical impulses, in descending transmissions or in subsequent inter-regional coherent activity. To tackle these questions requires a combination of good spatial and excellent temporal resolution and it seems likely that researchers will need to utilise the superior spatial resolution of MEG rather than scalp electrical recordings.

Towards an Integration

The integration of research findings across different levels of investigation into autism represents both a research goal and a research tool. Integration is a goal because it is required for a full understanding of autism and it is a tool because an attempted partial integration of findings across levels can indicate the phenomena that require explanation at each level of investigation; point to the potential limitations of some hypotheses; and indicate fruitful directions and strategies for future studies.

In the Introduction, we noted that several authors had put forward conceptual causal models that sought to integrate findings across levels and it is appropriate to return to them and consider how far they provide a possible way forward. Morton and Frith (1995) proposed a 4-level system in which unspecified biological factors caused abnormal brain conditions, which in turn caused cognitive malfunction (meaning affective, conative, and cognitive aspects) which then caused behavioural symptoms. So far as autism is concerned, their main claim was that all key features are mediated through a single cognitive deficit (although the biological origins and the behavioural sequelae might both be multiple). There are three major limitations to this model. Perhaps most crucially, it has nothing to say about the biological origins, ignores the need to delineate the causal processes involved in the sequence from gene to gene product to abnormal brain functioning, and provides no specification of what form the last might take. Second, it argued that there is no need for the model to explain the accompanying mental retardation because retardation is not invariant and because it is not appropriate to attempt a single cognitive account of both the behavioural manifestations of the autism and the low IQ. The latter argument is based on the claim that what is unitary about autism is the supposed single basic cognitive deficit, a claim that is possible only if the retardation is ignored. Apart from the tautology of the argument, it does not deal with the genetic evidence (from both the twin and family studies) that low verbal IQ is closely connected with the autism phenotype, but that there is a need to account for the differences between autism "proper" and the broader phenotype. Third, it rather sidesteps the findings on the breadth of the cognitive abnormalities in autism. The model's emphasis on the key role of cognitive deficits in autism is well-based but it provides no useful way forward for integrating the genetic, neurobiological and neuropsychological levels.

Rourke's (1995) model (for Asperger syndrome rather than autism as such) is quite different in that its central feature concerns the proposed links between brain abnormalities and cognitive malfunction. A concept of nonverbal learning disabilities is put forward in which there is a limited capacity to deal with information presenting through the auditory modality, with consequent effects on language functioning. It is argued that this arises on the basis of dysfunction or destruction of the white matter of the brain, interfering with interhemi-spheric communication and with right hemisphere brain systems. The syndrome is said to incorporate a wide range of disorders spanning the fetal alcohol syndrome, Asperger syndrome, Williams syndrome, traumatic brain injury and hydrocephalus. The variations in manifestations are said to be a consequence of the timing, type and amount of white matter dysfunction. At present, the model suffers from both a lack of empirical support for some of its key claims, and undue generality. The attempted integration of brain abnormality and cognitive dysfunction is very ambitious and it includes some interesting specific hypotheses but it is underspecified with respect to what is different about each of the component syndromes and it ignores genetic mechanisms.

Courchesne, Townsend and Chase's (1995) model is different yet again in that it is highly specific concerning the hypothesized links between brain structure, brain function and the behavioural manifestations of autism. Thus, it is argued that abnormalities of the cerebellum and parietal cortex underlie primary dysfunction in attention-related information processing, which then results in the higher-level disorder of social communication that characterizes autism. The model has the great asset of taking into account crucial considerations regarding neural development and functioning but it pays little regard to genetic mechanisms and suffers from inadequate attention to the inconsistencies in the supporting empirical evidence.

A fourth model has been put forward by Bachevalier (1994), using results from animal studies. It is argued that the neural basis of autism resides in damage to the medial temporal lobe and especially to the amygdaloid complex. Two-stage bilateral removals of the amygdaloid complex in newborn rhesus monkeys resulted in distinct patterns of memory loss and persistent socio-emotional abnormalities thought to mimic some features of autism. There is no doubt that experimental animal models can be helpful in testing causal hypotheses about brain-behaviour interconnections. However, there are particular difficulties in this approach when the key features of the disorder involve deficits in high level functions such as social communication and language. There is a paucity of human evidence that there are in fact medial temporal abnormalities in autism, and the model does not indicate whether the amnesia causes the behavioural symptoms of autism or whether both derive independently from disruption of different neural circuits.

In our view, none of these models provides a satisfactory integration across levels, all are very partial in what they focus on, and none deals satisfactorily with the extent to which the empirical research findings support one model over another. The need to test competing models is obvious in view of the radically different causal explanations provided by each. We agree with Pennington and Welsh (1995) on the great value of a neuropsychological perspective for understanding autism, on the rather different developmental concepts that are implicit in the models, on the currently inconclusive evidence, and on the conclusion that the testing of competing models will not be possible without better neurobiological data than available up to now. The need to integrate across levels is clear but it remains a task still to be accomplished. The aim of integration is necessarily long term because it depends so heavily upon understanding normal brain function and the nature of the relationships between brain and cognitive development. As yet, the vast majority of these links remain to be discovered.

In approaching the challenge of how findings across and within levels might be integrated, it is necessary to review the questions of the clinical phenomena to be accounted for and of what sort of integration might be reasonable. It is obvious that the clinical manifestations are extremely diverse, with IQ levels varying from profound retardation to superior intelligence, and with social functioning ranging from complete dependency on others to complete autonomy. Therefore, the first query must be whether the syndrome truly has a unity and coherence, or whether the apparent cohesion is an artifact of prevailing diagnostic conventions. Perhaps surprisingly, the evidence is solidly in favour of cohesion. Not only do the epidemiological findings indicate a clustering of phenomena along the lines of diagnostic conventions but, more importantly, the study of monozygotic twin pairs shows that the diversity within pairs closely parallels that between pairs (Le Couteur et al., in press). The *same* genetic predisposition is associated with a very considerable diversity of clinical manifestations: the diversity cannot be just a function of genetic heterogenity. What is more problematical is the decision on where to draw the boundaries. The genetic evidence indicates that the phenotype clearly extends more widely than the traditional diagnostic criteria, but uncertainty remains on just how wide the extensions should be. The evidence is compatable with an extension into socially maladroit personality traits, and even perhaps a certain form of affective disorder, but that is more arguable. What is clear, however, is that the broader phenotype differs from the traditional autism insofar as it is *not* associated with either low IQ or epilepsy. Any adequate integration of findings must account for that difference, but none of the prevailing theories do so.

The only way the boundaries of the autism syndrome, or phenotype, can be established with any certainty is through the use of some form of diagnosis-specific biological marker. An approach through neuropsychological test findings provides one possibility; the need being for a broad-based battery (probably including the array of theory of mind, central coherence, language pragmatics, and executive planning tests that have been demonstrated to differentiate autism from other disorders) with a range that is sensitive to deficits in individuals of normal intelligence. Such a strategy will succeed only insofar as specific types of cognitive deficit underlie the social, communicative and behavioural phenomena of autism, and that they do so within the range of milder variants of the syndrome. A more direct strategy will become available once the susceptibility genes associated with a liability to autism have been localized, or better still identified. These are most likely to be found using the affected sib strategy because this can focus on the handicapping conditions least subject to diagnostic error, yet avoiding the need to decide on which subjects are unaffected. It has the further advantage of requiring no assumptions about mode of inheritance because it is based only on the nature of allelic sharing between affected relatives that differs from general population expectations (Bishop & Williamson, 1990; Risch, 1990) The method involves no assumption that the true phenotype has the diagnostic boundaries chosen to minimize diagnostic uncertainty and, hence, the next step will be to determine if the same gene loci linked with autism as traditionally diagnosed apply to the hypothesized broader phenotype. This method has been applied in a preliminary fashion, for example, to assess the more subtle easy-to-miss skin manifestations of tuberose sclerosis (Smalley et al., 1995).

Several issues need addressing with respect to integration relating to the neuropsychological level of investigation. Most crucially, the precise nature of the basic deficits has yet to be established. There is no doubt that they involve mentalizing aspects of interpersonal relationships or subjectivity in some way but there is disagreement as to the role of metarepresentation, pragmatics of language, joint attention, affective connectedness and arousal (see Dawson, 1991; Pennington & Welsh, 1995; Rutter & Bailey, 1993; Sigman, 1995). There is also uncertainty regarding the role of central coherence or of broader cognitive skills such as those encompassed by the concept of executive planning. The use of research strategies that involve a crossing of levels provides a possible way forward. Thus, the connection with clinical features *within* autistic groups may be tested. Do, for example, abnormalities in central coherence relate to the presence of unusual cognitive talents; do executive planning deficits relate to the degree or type of repetitive, stereotyped behaviours shown; does the degree of "theory of mind" impairment relate to the extent of language abnormality or the level of verbal skills? Alternatively, comparisons may be made within medically defined groups. Thus, do tuberose sclerosis or Fragile X individuals with autism differ from those without autistic features in terms of "theory of mind" or executive planning skills? In many respects, such comparisons within medical conditions known to be associated with an increased risk of autism provide a better test of cognitive hypotheses than comparisons with heterogeneous groups of nonautistic mentally retarded individuals.

A third approach is available through the use of functional imaging methods, which provide a considerable potential for studying the connection between brain function and cognitive performance by using cognitive task actuation techniques. Two strategies may be mentioned to illustrate how they may be used. First, case–control methods may be employed to determine whether autistic individuals are distinctive with respect to their use of an unusual part of the brain to pass particular cognitive tasks (because the usual part is dysfunctional). Already, two groups have used 'theory of mind' tasks in normal volunteers using SPET (Baron-Cohen et al., 1994) and PET (Fletcher et al., 1995) as a prelude to their study of autistic individuals. Their findings are not the same, possibly in part because they used different tasks, but the difference highlights the

185

need for replication. The Fletcher et al., (1995) paper nicely exemplifies the various controls necessary to demonstrate that a particular cognitive process is responsible for the functional imaging changes associated with task performance. The localization of the brain basis of ToM skills provides the crucial starting point but to apply this knowledge to the study of autism, it will be necessary to study autistic subjects who can pass at least some ToM tasks, and to demonstrate that they use some other part of the brain to do so.

Second, functional imaging may be useful in testing the hypothesis that some hypothesized precursor of ToM (such as joint attention) reflects the same brain function, or to investigate the connections between ToM, executive planning and central coherence. For that purpose, repeat testing over key phases of development is likely to be particularly informative. This is acceptable only with methods, such as MRI, that involve no radiation hazard. A caveat is necessary, however, with regard to what is being measured. Brain localization is possible through quantification of the overall level of brain metabolic activity in specific regions, but the data do not assess specific types of brain function. Of course, pharmacological activation much increases the scope of what can be learned but, in that connection, the lack of a marked and specific drug response in autism together with the lack of consistent neurochemical abnormalities (apart from a raised serotonin level in about a third of cases), are likely to prove important limiting factors.

Functional imaging methods differ in their spatial and temporal resolution. PET and SPET have good spatial resolution (PET better than SPET) but average brain activity over many seconds or even minutes. Functional MRI has the potential to provide similar spatial resolution, and somewhat better temporal resolution, without the hazards of radiation, but it remains to be seen whether the sensitivity will be sufficiently great at the magnetic field strengths that are generally available. It is possible that the use of methods with superior temporal resolution (such as MEG) may carry advantages, particularly in combination with those providing good spatial resolution, but at present it is too early to say more than that such approaches are worth exploring.

There are hypotheses about the possible neurobiological basis of deficits in information-processing, and attention in autism (see Courchesne et al., 1995; Dawson, 1991; Ornitz, 1989). Nevertheless, methodological problems are considerable and replicated findings are thin on the ground. Psychophysical studies are able to investigate parallel processing capacity and the ability to undertake configural analysis. Such an approach might be informative, for example, in determining the biological basis of face-processing deficits in autism. Again, however, the potential of the method remains quite uncertain.

There is also a need to develop, and improve, neurobiological studies that do not have their main rationale in any postulated link with neuropsychological functioning. Charting the way forward is necessarily an uncertain venture given the lack of consistency in the findings so far. Clearly, a certain amount of ground-clearing is still required. Thus, for example, there is still a need for a systematic, and extensive structural MRI

study with an explicit focus on the examination of structure–function connections within autism groups, as well as between autistic and nonautistic samples. On the basis of present knowledge, it does not seem likely that autism will prove to be due to sharply localized lesions but the possibility needs ruling out. The strategy of comparisons within and between medically defined groups, already mentioned in relation to neuropsychological deficits, is also worth considering. Are there, for example, similarities in the scan findings among individuals with the Fragile X and with tuberose sclerosis who also exhibit autism, that differentiate them from nonautistic individuals with the same two medical conditions, both of which carry an increased risk of autism?

Neuropathological studies constitute a priority if only because so few have been undertaken so far and because there are some leads to follow-up. Thus, Bailey et al., (submitted) have suggested that increased cell replication is one possible mechanism underlying the increased brain weight found in some cases. The association between autism and tuberose sclerosis, neurofibromatosis and Sotos syndrome, together with occasional reports of malignancies in autistic individuals (Bauman & Kemper, 1994; Bailey et al., submitted) suggest, too, that the genes involved in the control of cell replication may merit particular attention in molecular genetic studies. The association between autism and abnormal brain development, taken together with the slightly increased rate of minor congenital anomalies, raises the questions, too, of whether developmental abnormalities outside the CNS are a consequence of the timing of developmental mishaps, or possible pointers to specific genetic mechanisms. To take that matter further requires a more detailed examination of physical development and physical anomalies than undertaken thus far.

In this review, we have said little about either neurochemical perspectives or pharmacological research, both of which have proved highly informative with other disorders. However, up to now, neither has given rise to appreciable gains in the understanding of autism. New, hypothesis-driven (rather than 'fishing expedition') approaches are likely to be needed if such gains are to be forthcoming.

Finally, we need to consider molecular genetic research. Its value in identification of the phenotype has already been noted (with respect to both clinical manifestations and the pattern of cognitive deficit). Careful attention will need to be paid to the likely presence of genetic heterogeneity. As already noted, so far there is little indication that it can be identified through variation in the clinical picture. However, the possibility that heterogeneity may be indexed by features such as nonverbal IQ level, epilepsy, increased head size, congenital anomalies, or hyperserotonemia warrant consideration. The identification of susceptibility genes is potentially valuable, not because it matters where the genes are located, but because identification of the gene makes it possible to determine the gene products and thereby, their effects on functions. Identification of specific genetic mechanisms should provide invaluable pointers to the neurobiological processes involved in aetiology (just as knowledge on the pathophysiology provides pointers to candidate genes).

It is not obvious, however, what effects are to be expected for the several interacting genes thought to be operative in the liability to autism. Parallels with other medical conditions might lead to an expectation that each gene should have an identifiable connection with a known risk factor for autism, the combination of genes leading to the syndrome as a whole. Thus, coronary artery disease is associated with risk factors as diverse as high cholesterol level, abnormal haemostasis, hypertension, and smoking and it is quite possible that each of these to some extent reflects different genetic factors (Sing & Reilly, 1993; Sing et al., 1992). In the same way, it is likely that atopy reflects both genes involved in general hyperresponsiveness to allergens and genes that influence specific atopic disease expression (Cookson & Hopkin, 1990). But what might be the autism parallels? Are there multiple interacting, but different, risk pathways? If so, what might they be? Or, is this the wrong model altogether? The MZ within-pair differences and the second degree relative findings do not fit easily with a multiple risk factor model. Rather the implication seems to be that the pattern of interacting genes as a whole leads to the overall clinical picture, encompassing its wide variation in expression. If so, that leaves open several crucial questions. What is the brain abnormality (be it structural, neurochemical, neurophysiological, or whatever) that represents the result of the gene products? What aspects of that abnormality account for the range of clinical expression? If that range does not reflect gene dosage (the MZ pair findings suggest that it does not), what accounts for the marked differences (in, e.g. IQ level and epilepsy) between autism 'proper' and the broader phenotype? Similarly, if the variation is not a function of gene dosage, why does the familial loading vary by severity of autism (on a multifactorial model this implies a dosage effect)? Many genes whose functions are known, such as transcriptional regulators, can influence multiple developmental processes, and the identification of which are the relevant biological mechanisms may be far from straightforward. Moreover an understanding of the consequences of epistatic interactions between genes has so far only been achieved in some simple animal models.

Conclusions

It is probably fair to claim that autism has been the subject of more systematic research, across a wider range of domains, than any other child psychiatric disorder. This research has revolutionized concepts of autism over the past three decades. No longer is it thought of as either a type of psychosis (schizophrenic or otherwise) or as a psychogenically induced condition. Rather it has become accepted that it is a neurodevelopmental disorder, in which specific cognitive deficits play a key role, and for which genetic factors predominate in aetiology. The clinical phenomena that are central to the disorder are also much better understood. The challenge now is to provide a better integration across the different levels of research in order to gain an understanding of the causal mechanisms that lead to autism and the

abnormal processes that underlie the clinical features. The objective is no longer completely out of reach but success will depend on conceptual, as well as technological, advances and on the bringing together of different areas of expertise in order to provide a concerted attack on the problem.

References

Akefeldt, A. & Gillberg, C. (1991). Hypomelanosis of Ito in three cases of autism and autistic-like conditions. *Developmental Medicine and Child Neurology, 33,* 737–743.

Arin, D. M., Bauman, M. L. & Kemper T. L. (1991). The distribution of purkinje cell loss in the cerebellum in autism. *Neurology, 47,* (Suppl. 1), 307.

Aslin, R. N., Pisoni, D. B. & Jusczyk P. W. (1983). Auditory development and speech perception in infancy. In M. H. Haith & J. J. Campos (Eds), *Infancy and developmental psychobiology, Vol.2, Mussen's handbook of child psychology* (4th edn, pp. 573–687). New York: Wiley.

Attwood, A., Frith, U. & Hermelin, B. (1988). The understanding and use of interpersonal gestures by autistic and Down's syndrome children. *Journal of Autism and Developmental Disorders, 18,* 241–257.

August, G. J., Stewart, M. A. & Tsai L. (1981). The incidence of cognitive disabilities in the siblings of autistic children. *British Journal of Psychiatry, 138,* 416–422.

Bachevalier J. (1994). Medial temporal lobe structures and autism: a review of clinical and experimental findings. *Neuropsychologia, 32,* 627–648.

Bailey A. (1993). The biology of autism. *Psychological Medicine, 23,* 7–11.

Bailey, A. J., Bolton, P., Butler, L., Le Couteur, A., Murphy, M., Scott, S., Webb, T. & Rutter, M. (1993a). Prevalence of the Fragile X anomaly amongst autistic twins and singletons. *Journal of Child Psychology and Psychiatry, 34,* 673–688.

Bailey, A., Le Couteur, A., Gottesman, I., Bolton, P., Simonoff, E., Yuzda, E. & Rutter, M. (1995). Autism as a strongly genetic disorder: evidence from a British twin study. *Psychological Medicine, 25,* 63–78.

Bailey, A., Luthert, P., Bolton, P., Le Couteur, A., Rutter, M. & Harding, B. (1993b). Autism is associated with megalencephaly (letter). *Lancet, 341,* 1225–1226.

Bailey, A., Luthert, P., Harding, B., Janota, I., Montgomery, M., Dean, A., Rutter, M. & Lantos, P. (Submitted). A postmortem study of autism.

Baird, T. D. & August, G. J. (1985). Familial heterogeneity in infantile autism. *Journal of Autism and Developmental Disorders, 15,* 315–321.

Baron-Cohen, S. (1987). Autism and symbolic play. *British Journal of Developmental Psychology, 5,* 139–148.

Baron-Cohen, S. (1989). Perceptual role-taking and protodeclarative pointing in autism. *British Journal of Developmental Psychology, 7,* 113–127.

Baron-Cohen, S. (1993). From attention-goal psychology to belief–desire psychology: the development of a theory of mind and its dysfunction. In S. Baron-Cohen, H. Tager-Flusberg & D.J. Cohen (Eds), *Understanding other minds: perspectives from autism* (pp. 59–82). Oxford: Oxford University Press.

Baron-Cohen, S. (1995). *Mindblindness: an essay on autism and theory of mind.* Cambridge, MA: MIT Press.

Baron-Cohen, S., Allen, J. & Gillberg, C. (1992). Can autism be detected at 18 months? The needle, the haystack, and the CHAT. *British Journal of Psychiatry, 161,* 839–843.

Baron-Cohen, S., Leslie, A. M. & Frith, U. (1985). Does the

autistic child have a "theory of mind"? *Cognition, 21*, 37–46.

Baron-Cohen, S. & Ring, H. (1994). A model of the mindreading system: neuropsychological and neurobiological perspectives. In C. Lewis & P. Mitchell (Eds), *Children's early understanding of mind: origins and development* (pp. 183–207). Hove, U.K: Lawrence Erlbaum.

Baron-Cohen, S., Ring, H., Moriarty, J., Schmitz, B., Costa, D. & Ell, P. (1994). Recognition of mental state terms: clinical findings in children with autism, and a functional neuroimaging study of normal adults. *British Journal of Psychiatry, 165*, 640–649.

Baron-Cohen, S., Tager-Flusberg, H. & Cohen, D. (1993). *Understanding other minds: perspectives from autism.* Oxford: Oxford University Press.

Bartak, L. & Rutter, M. (1976). Differences between mentally retarded and normally intelligent autistic children. *Journal of Autism and Childhood Schizophrenia, 6*, 109–120.

Bartlett, F. W. (1932). *Remembering: an experimental and social study.* Cambridge: Cambridge University Press.

Bauman, M. (1991). Microscopic neuroanatomic abnormalities in autism. *Pediatrics, 87* (suppl.), 791–796.

Bauman, M. L. & Kemper, T. L. (1985). Histoanatomic observations of the brain in early infantile autism. *Neurology, 35*, 866–874.

Bauman, M. L. & Kemper, T. L. (1994). *Neurobiology of autism.* Baltimore,MD: Johns Hopkins University Press.

Bishop, D. T. & Williamson, J. A. (1990). The power of identity-by-state methods for linkage analysis. *American Journal of Human Genetics, 46*, 254–265.

Bishop, D. V. M. (1989). Autism, Asperger's Syndrome and semantic-pragmatic disorder: where are the boundaries? *British Journal of Disorders of Communication, 24*, 107–121.

Bishop, D. V. M. (1993). Autism, executive functions and theory of mind: a neuropsychological perspective. *Journal of Child Psychology and Psychiatry, 34*, 79–293.

Blinkov, S. M. & Glezer, I. I. (1968). *The human brain in figures and tables: a quantitative handbook.* Los Angeles, CA: Plenum Press.

Blomquist, H. K., Bohman, M., Edvinsson, S. O., Gillberg, C., Gustavson, K. H., Holmgren, G. & Wahlström, J. (1985). Frequency of the Fragile X syndrome in infantile autism: a Swedish multicenter study. *Clinical Genetics, 27*, 113–117.

Bolton, P. & Holland, A. (1994). Chromosomal abnormalities. In M. Rutter, E. Taylor & L. Hersov (Eds), *Child and adolescent psychiatry: modern approaches* (pp. 152–171). Oxford: Blackwell Scientific.

Bolton, P., Macdonald, H., Pickles, A., Rios, P., Goode, S., Crowson, M., Bailey, A. & Rutter, M. (1994). A case-control family history study of autism. *Journal of Child Psychology and Psychiatry, 35*, 877–900.

Bolton, P., Pickles, A., Butler, L., Summers, S., Webb, T., Lord, C. LeCouteur A., Bailey, A. & Rutter, M, (1992a). Fragile X in families multiplex for autism and autism related phenotypes: prevalence and criteria for cytogenetic diagnosis. *Psychiatric Genetics, 2*, 277–300.

Bolton, P., Pickles, A., Harrington, R., Macdonald, H. & Rutter, M. (1992b). Season of birth issues, approaches and findings for autism. *Journal of Child Psychology and Psychiatry, 33*, 509–531.

Bolton, P., Pickles, A., Murphy, M. & Rutter, M. (Submitted). Autism, affective and other psychiatric disorders: patterns of familial aggregation.

Bolton, P. & Rutter, M. (1990). Genetic influences in autism. *International Review of Psychiatry, 2*, 65–78.

Boucher, J. & Lewis, V. (1992). Unfamiliar face recognition in relatively able autistic children. *Journal of Child Psychology and Psychiatry, 33*, 843–859.

Boullin, D., Freeman, B. J., Geller, E., Ritvo, E., Rutter, M. & Yuwiler, A. (1982). (Letter to Editor) Towards the resolution of conflicting findings. *Journal of Autism and Developmental Disorders, 12*, 97–98.

Bowler, D. (1992). "Theory of mind" in Asperger's syndrome. *Journal of Child Psychology and Psychiatry, 33*, 877–893.

Bretherton, I., McNew, S. & Beeghly-Smith, M. (1981). Early person knowledge as expressed in gestural and verbal communication: when do infants acquire a "theory of mind"? In M. Lamb & L. Sherrod (Eds), *Social cognition in infancy* (pp. 333–373). Hillsdale, NJ: Lawrence Erlbaum.

Brothers, L. (1990). The social brain: a project for integrating primate behaviour and neurophysiology in a new domain. *Concepts in Neuroscience, 1*, 27–51.

Brown, W. T., Jenkins, E. C., Cohen, I. L., Fisch, G. S., Wolf-Schein, E. G., Gross, A., Waterhouse, L., Fein, D., Mason-Brothers, A., Ritvo, E., Ruttenburg, B., Bently, W. & Castells, S. (1986). Fragile X and autism: a multicenter survey. *American Journal of Medical Genetics, 23*, 341–352.

Buchsbaum, M. S., Siegel, B. V., Wu, J. C., Hazlett, E., Sicotte, N., Haier, R., Tanguay, P., Asarnow, R., Cadorette, T., Donoghue, D., Lagunas-Solar, M., Lott, I., Paek, J. & Sabalesky, D. (1992). Brief report: attention performance in autism and regional brain metabolic rate assessed by positron emission tomography. *Journal of Autism and Developmental Disorders, 22*, 115–125.

Campbell, M., Rosenbloom, S., Perry, R., George, A. E., Kricheff, I. I., Anderson, L., Small, A. M. & Jennings, S. J. (1982). Computerized axial tomography in young autistic children. *American Journal of Psychiatry, 139*, 510–512.

Chess S. (1977). Follow-up report on autism in congenital rubella. *Journal of Autism and Childhood Schizophrenia, 7*, 68–81.

Chess, S., Korn, S. J. & Fernandez, P. B. (1971). *Psychiatric disorders of children with congenital rubella.* New York: Brunner/Mazel.

Ciesielski, K. T. & Knight, J. E. (1994). Cerebellar abnormality in autism: a nonspecific effect of early brain damage? *Acta Neurobiologiae Experimentalis, 54*, 151–154.

Cohen, I. L., Vietze, P. M., Sudhalter, V., Jenkins, E. C. & Brown, W. T. (1989). Parent–child dyadic gaze patterns in fragile X males and in non-fragile X males with autistic disorder. *Journal of Child Psychology and Psychiatry, 30*, 845–856.

Cole, G., Neal, J. W., Fraser, W. I. & Cowie, V. A. (1994). Autopsy findings in patients with mental handicap. *Journal of Intellectual Disability Research, 38*, 9–26.

Coleman, M. (1990). Delineation of the subgroups of the autistic syndrome. *Brain Dysfunction, 3*, 208–217.

Coleman, P. D., Romano, J., Lapham, L. & Simon, W. (1985). Cell counts in cerebral cortex of an autistic patient. *Journal of Autism and Developmental Disorders, 15*, 245–255.

Comings, D. E. & Comings, B. G. (1991). Clinical and genetic relationships between autism-pervasive developmental disorder and Tourette syndrome: a study of 19 cases. *American Journal of Medical Genetics, 39*, 180–191.

Cook, E. H. (1990). Autism: review of neurochemical investigation. *Synapse, 6*, 292–308.

Cookson, W. O. C. M. & Hopkin, J. M. (1990). Towards a gene for atopy and atopic asthma. In K. Berg, N. Retterstol & S. Refsum (Eds), *From phenotype to gene in common disorders* (pp. 214–223). Copenhagen: Munksgaard.

Corcoran, R., Frith, C. D. & Mercer, G. (in press). Schizophrenia, symptomatology and social inference: investigating "theory of mind" in people with schizophrenia. *Schizophrenia Research.*

Courchesne, E. (1991). Neuroanatomic imaging in autism. *Pediatrics, 87*, (Pt 2), 781–790.

Courchesne, E. (1995). New evidence of cerebellar and brainstem hypoplasia in autistic infants, children and adolescents: the MRI imaging study by Hashimoto and colleagues. *Journal of Autism and Development Disorders, 25*, 19–22.

Courchesne, E., Hesselink, J. R., Jernigan, T. L. & Yeung-Courchesne, R. (1987). Abnormal neuroanatomy in a nonretarded person with autism. *Archives of Neurology, 44*, 335–341.

Courchesne, E., Lincoln, A. J., Kilman, B. A. & Galambos, R. (1985). Event-related brain potential correlates of the processing of novel visual and auditory information in autism. *Journal of Autism and Developmental Disorders, 15*, 55–76.

Courchesne, E., Press, G. A. & Yeung-Courchesne, R. (1993). Parietal lobe abnormalities detected with MR in patients with infantile autism. *American Journal of Roentgenology, 160*, 387–393.

Courchesne, E., Townsend, J. & Saitoh, O. (1994a). The brain in infantile autism: posterior fossa structures are abnormal. *Neurology, 44*, 214–223.

Courchesne, E., Townsend, J. & Chase, C. (1995). Neurodevelopmental principles guide research on developmental psychopathologies. In D. Cicchetti & D. J. Cohen (Eds), *Manual of developmental psychopathology* (pp. 195–226). New York: John Wiley.

Courchesne, E., Townsend, J., Akshoomoff, N. A., Saitoh, O., Yeung-Courchesne, R., Lincoln, A.J., James, H.E., Haas, R.H., Schriebman, L. & Lau, L. (1994b). Impairment in shifting attention in autistic and cerebellar patients. *Behavioral Neuroscience, 108*, 848–865.

Courchesne, E., Yeung-Courchesne, R., Press, G. A., Hesselink, J. R. & Jernigan, T. L. (1988). Hypoplasia of cerebellar vermal lobules VI and VII in autism. *New England Journal of Medicine, 318*, 1349–1354.

Creasey, H., Rumsey, J., Schwartz, M., Duara, R., Rapoport, J. L. & Rapoport, S.I. (1986). Brain morphometry in autistic men as measured by volumetric computed tomography. *Archives of Neurology, 43*, 669–672.

Cutting, J. C. (1994). Evidence for right hemisphere dysfunction in schizophrenia. In A.S. David & J.C. Cutting (Eds), *The neuropsychology of schizophrenia* (pp. 231–244). Hove, U.K: Lawrence Erlbalm.

Dahlgren, S. O. & Gillberg, C. (1989). Symptoms in the first two years of life: a preliminary population study of infantile autism. *European Archives of Psychiatric and Neurological Science, 283*, 169–174.

Damasio, A. R. & Maurer, R. G. (1978). A neurological model for childhood autism. *Archives of Neurology, 35*, 777–786.

Damasio, H., Maurer, R. G., Damasio, A. R. & Chui, H. C. (1980). Computerized tomographic scan findings in patients with autistic behavior. *Archives of Neurology, 37*, 504–510.

Darby, J. K. (1976). Neuropathologic aspects of psychosis in children. *Journal of Autism and Childhood Schizophrenia, 6*, 339–351.

Davies, K. (1991). Breaking the Fragile-X. *Nature, 351*, 439–440.

Dawson, G. (1991). A psychobiological perspective on the early socio-emotional development of children with autism. In D. Cicchetti & S. L. Toth (Eds), *Rochester Symposium on Developmental Psychopathology* (Vol.3, pp. 207–234). Rochester, NY: University of Rochester Press.

Dawson, G. & Lewy, A. (1989a). Arousal, attention, and the socio-emotional impairments of individuals with autism. In G. Dawson (Ed.), *Autism: nature, diagnosis and treatment* (pp. 49–74). New York: Guildford Press.

Dawson, G. & Lewy, A. (1989b). Reciprocal sub-cortical-cortical influences in autism: the role of attentional mechanisms. In G. Dawson (Ed.), *Autism: Nature, Diag-*

nosis and Treatment (pp. 144–173). New York: Guilford Press.

Dekaban, A. S. & Sadowsky, D. (1978). Changes in brain weights during the span of human life: relation of brain weights to body heights and body weights. *Annals of Neurology, 4*, 345–356.

De Kosky, S., Heilman, K., Bowers, M. & Valenstein, F. (1980). Recognition and discrimination of emotional faces and pictures. *Brain and Language, 9*, 206–214.

DeLong, Γ. G. (1992). Autism, amnesia, hippocampus, and learning. *Neuroscience and Biobehavioral Reviews, 16*, 63–70.

DeLong, R. (1994). Children with autistic spectrum disorder and a family history of affective disorder. *Developmental Medicine and Child Neurology, 36*, 674–687.

DeLong, R. & Nohria, C. (1994). Psychiatric family history and neurological disease in autistic spectrum disorders. *Developmental Medicine and Child Neurology, 36*, 441–448.

Dennis, M. (1991). Frontal lobe function in childhood and adolescence: a heuristic for assessing attention regulation, executive control, and the intentional states important for social discourse. *Developmental Neuropsychology, 7*, 327–358.

Deykin, E. Y. & MacMahon, B. (1979a). Viral exposure and autism. *American Journal of Epidemiology, 109*, 628–638.

Deykin, E. Y. & MacMahon, B. (1979b). The incidence of seizures among children with autistic symptoms. *American Journal of Psychiatry, 136*, 1310–1312.

De Volder, A., Bol, A., Michel, C., Congneau, M. & Goffinet, A. M. (1987). Brain glucose metabolism in children with the autistic syndrome: positron tomography analysis. *Brain Development, 9*, 581–587.

Dodge, K. A. (1980). Social cognition and children's aggressive behavior. *Child Development, 51*, 162–170.

Eales, M. J. (1993). Pragmatic impairments in adults with childhood diagnoses of autism or developmental receptive language disorder. *Journal of Autism and Developmental Disorders, 23*, 593–617.

Einfeld, S., Malony, H. & Hall, W. (1989). Autism is not associated with the Fragile X syndrome. *American Journal of Medical Genetics, 34*, 187–193.

Eisenmajer, R. & Prior, M. (1991). Cognitive linguistic correlates of "theory of mind" ability in autistic children. *British Journal of Developmental Psychology, 9*, 351–364.

Erwin, R., Van Lancker, D., Guthrie, D., Schwafel, J., Tanguay, P. & Buchwald, J. S. (1991). P3 responses to prosodic stimuli in adult autistic subjects. *Electroencephalography and Clinical Neurophysiology, 80*, 561–571.

European Chromosome 16 Tuberous Sclerosis Consortium (1993). Identification and characterization of the tuberous sclerosis gene on chromosome 16. *Cell, 75*, 1305–1315.

Filipek, P. A., Kennedy, D. N. & Caviness, V. S. Jr. (1992a). Neuroimaging in child neuropsychology. In I. Rapin & S.J. Segalowitz (eds), *Handbook of neuropsychology, Vol. 6: Child neuropsychology* (pp. 301–329). Amsterdam: Elsevier Science.

Filipek, P. A., Richelme, C., Kennedy, D. M., Rademacher, J., Pitcher, D. A., Zidel, S. & Caviness, V. S. (1992b). Morphometric analysis of the brain in developmental language disorders and autism. *Annals of Neurology, 32*, 475.

Fletcher, P., Happé, F., Frith, U., Baker, S., Dolan, R., Frackowiak, R. & Frith, C. (1995). Other minds in the brain: a functional imaging study of "theory of mind" in story comprehension. *Cognition 57*, 109–128.

Folstein, S. E. & Piven, J. (1991). Etiology of autism: genetic influences. *Pediatrics, 87*, Supplement to issue no. 5, 767–773.

Folstein, S. & Rutter, M. (1977a). Infantile autism: a genetic study of 21 twin pairs. *Journal of Child Psychology and Psychiatry, 18*, 297–321.

Folstein, S. & Rutter, M. (1977b). Genetic influences and infantile autism. *Nature, 265*, 726–728.

Folstein, S. & Rutter, M. (1988). Autism: familial aggregation and genetic implications. *Journal of Autism and Developmental Disorders, 18*, 3–30.

Fombonne, E., Macdonald, H., Bolton, P., Rutter, M., Prior, J., Jordan, H. & Morgan, O. (submitted). A family study of autism: cognitive patterns and levels in parents and siblings.

Fombonne, E., Siddons, F., Achard, S., Frith, U. & Happé, F. (1994). Adaptive behaviour and theory of mind in autism. *European Child and Adolescent Psychiatry, 3*, 176–186.

Freeman, B. J., Ritvo, E. R., Mason-Brothers, A., Pingree, C., Yokota, A., Jenson, W. R., McMahon, W. M., Petersen, P. B., Mo, A. & Schroth, P. (1989). Psychometric assessment of first-degree relatives of 62 autistic probands in Utah. *American Journal of Psychiatry, 146*, 361–364.

Frith, C. D. (1992). *The cognitive neuropsychology of schizophrenia*. Hove, U.K: Lawrence Erlbaum.

Frith, U. (1970a). Studies in pattern detection in normal and autistic children: I. Immediate recall of auditory sequences. *Journal of Abnormal Psychology, 76*, 413–420.

Frith, U. (1970b). Studies in pattern detection in normal and autistic children: II. Reproduction and production of color sequences. *Journal of Experimental Child Psychology, 10*, 120–135.

Frith, U. (1989). *Autism: explaining the enigma*. Oxford: Basil Blackwell.

Frith, U. (1991). *Autism and Asperger Syndrome*. Cambridge: Cambridge University Press.

Frith, U. & Baron-Cohen, S. (1987). Perception in autistic children. In D. J. Cohen & A. Donnellan (Eds), *Handbook of autism and pervasive developmental disorders* (pp. 85–102). New York: John Wiley and Sons.

Frith, U. & Happé, F. (1994). Autism: beyond "theory of mind". *Cognition, 50*, 115–132.

Frith, U., Happé, F. & Siddons, F. (1994). Autism and theory of mind in everyday life. *Social Development, 3*, 108–124.

Frith, U., Morton, J. & Leslie, A. M. (1991). The cognitive basis of a biological disorder: autism. *Trends in Neuroscience, 14*, 433–438.

Fryer, A. E., Chalmers, A., Connor, J. M., Fraser, I., Povey, S., Yates, A. D., Yates, J. R. & Osborne, J. P. (1987). Evidence that the gene for tuberous sclerosis is on chromosome 9. *Lancet, 21*, 659–661.

Gaffney, G. R., Kuperman, S., Tsai, L. Y. & Minchin, S. (1988). Morphological evidence for brainstem involvement in infantile autism. *Biological Psychiatry, 24*, 578–586.

Gaffney, G. R., Kuperman, S., Tsai, L. Y. & Minchin, S. (1989). Forebrain structure in infantile autism. *Journal of the American Academy of Child and Adolescent Psychiatry, 28*, 534–537.

Gaffney, G. R. & Tsai, L. Y. (1987). Brief report: magnetic resonance imaging of high level autism. *Journal of Autism and Developmental Disorders, 17*, 433–438.

Gaffney, G. R., Tsai, L. Y., Kuperman, S. & Minchin, S. (1987). Cerebellar structure in autism. *American Journal of Diseases in Childhood, 141*, 1330–1332.

Garber, H. J. & Ritvo, E. R. (1992). Magnetic resonance imaging of the posterior fossa in autistic adults. *American Journal of Psychiatry, 149*, 245–247.

Geller, E., Ritvo, E. R., Freeman, B. J. & Yuwiler, A. (1982). Preliminary observations on the effect of fenfluramine on blood serotonin and symptoms in three autistic boys. *New England Journal of Medicine, 307*, 165–169.

George, M., Costa, D. C., Kouris, K., Ring, H. A. & Ell, P. J. (1992). Cerebral blood flow abnormalities in adults with infantile autism. *Journal of Nervous and Mental Disease, 180*, 413–417.

Ghaziuddin, M., Butler, E., Tsai, L. & Ghaziuddin, N. (1994). Is clumsiness a marker for Asperger syndrome? *Journal of Intellectual Disability Research, 38*, 519–527.

Ghaziuddin, M., Tsai, L. Y. & Ghaziuddin, N. (1992). Brief report: a reappraisal of clumsiness as a diagnostic feature of Asperger syndrome. *Journal of Autism and Developmental Disorders, 16*, 369–375.

Gillberg, C. (1991). Outcome in autism and autistic-like conditions. *Journal of the American Academy of Child and Adolescent Psychiatry, 30*, 375–382.

Gillberg, C. (1992). Autism and autism-like conditions: subclasses among disorders of empathy. *Journal of Child Psychology and Psychiatry, 33*, 813–842.

Gillberg, C. (1995). Endogenous opioids and opiate antagonists in autism: brief review of empirical findings and implications for clinicians. *Developmental Medicine and Child Neurology, 37*, 239–245.

Gillberg, C. & Coleman, M. (1992). *The biology of the autistic syndromes* (2nd edn). London: MacKeith Press.

Gillberg, C., Ehlers, S., Schaumann, H., Jakobsson, G., Dahlgren, S., Lindblom, R., Gabenholm, A., Tjuus, R. & Blidner, E. (1990). Autism under age 3 years: a clinical study of 28 cases referred for autistic symptoms in infancy. *Journal of Child Psychology and Psychiatry, 31*, 921–934.

Gillberg, C. & Forsell, C. (1984). Childhood psychosis and neurofibromatosis—more than a coincidence? *Journal of Autism and Developmental Disorders, 14*, 1–8.

Gillberg, C., Gillberg, I.C. & Steffenburg, S. (1992). Siblings and parents of children with autism: a controlled population-based study. *Developmental Medicine and Child Neurology, 34*, 389–398.

Gillberg, C. & Steffenburg, S. (1987). Outcome and prognostic factors in autism and similar conditions: a population-based study of 46 cases followed through puberty. *Journal of Autism and Developmental Disorders, 17*, 273–287.

Gillberg, C., Steffenburg, S. & Jakobsson, G. (1987). Neurobiological findings in 20 relatively gifted children with Kanner-type autism or Asperger syndrome. *Developmental Medicine and Child Neurology, 29*, 641–649.

Gillberg, C., Steffenburg, S., Wahlstrom, J., Sjostedt, A., Gillberg, I. C., Martinsson, T., Liedgren, S. & Eeg-Olofsson, O. (1991). Autism associated with marker chromosome. *Journal of the American Academy of Child and Adolescent Psychiatry, 30*, 489–494.

Gillberg, C. & Svendsen, P. (1983). Childhood psychosis and computed tomographic brain scan findings. *Journal of Autism and Developmental Disorders, 13*, 19–32.

Gillberg, C. & Wahlström, J. (1985). Chromosome abnormalities in infantile autism and other childhood psychoses: a population study of 66 cases. *Developmental Medicine and Child Neurology, 27*, 293–304.

Gillberg, I.C., Bjure, J, Uvebrant, P., Vestergren, E. & Gillberg, C. (1993). SPECT (Single photon emission computed tomography) in 31 children and adolescents with autism and autistic-like conditions. *European Child and Adolescent Psychiatry, 2*, 50–59.

Gillberg, I. C., Gillberg, C. & Ahlsén, G. (1994). Autistic behaviour and attention deficits in tuberous sclerosis: a population-based study. *Developmental Medicine and Child Neurology, 36*, 50–56.

Goldman-Rakic, P. S., Isseroff, A., Scwartz, M. L. & Bugbee, N. M. (1983). The neurobiology of cognitive development. In M.H. Haith & J.J. Campos (Eds), *Infancy and developmental psychobiology, vol.2, Mussen's handbook of child psychology* (4th ed., pp. 281–344). New York: Wiley.

Goode, S., Rutter, M. & Howlin, P. (1994). A twenty-year follow-up of children with autism. Paper presented at the

13th biennial meeting of ISSBD, Amsterdam, The Netherlands.

Goodfellow, P. N. & Schmitt, K. (1994). From the simple to the complex. *Nature, 371*, 104–105.

Goodman, R. (1989). Infantile autism: a syndrome of multiple primary deficits? *Journal of Autism and Developmental Disorders, 19*, 409–424.

Goulden, K. J., Shinnar, S., Koller, H., Katz, M. & Richardson, S. A. (1991). Epilepsy in children with mental retardation: a cohort-study. *Epilepsia, 32*, 690–697.

Gray, J. M., Frazer, W. L. & Leudar, I. (1983). Recognition of emotion from facial expression in mental handicap. *British Journal of Psychiatry, 142*, 566–571.

Hagerman, R. J. (1990). The association between autism and Fragile X syndrome. *Brain Dysfunction, 3*, 219–227.

Hallett, M., Lebiedowska, M. K., Thomas, S. L., Stanhope, S. J., Denckla, M. B. & Rumsey, J. (1993). Locomotion of autistic adults. *Archives of Neurology, 50*, 1304–1308.

Hallmayer, J., Pintado, E., Lotspeich, L., Spiker, D., McMahon, W., Petersen, P. B., Nicholas, P., Pingree, C., Kraemer, H. C., Wong, D. L., Ritvo, E., Lin, A., Hebert, J., Cavalli-Sforza, L. L. & Ciaranello, R. D. (1994). Molecular analysis and test of linkage between the FMR-1 gene and infantile autism in multiplex families. *American Journal of Human Genetics, 55*, 951–959.

Happé, F. G. E. (1993). Communicative competence and theory of mind in autism: a test of relevance theory. *Cognition, 48*, 101–119.

Happé, F. G. E. (1994a). *Autism: an introduction to psychological theory*. London: UCL Press.

Happé, F. G. E. (1994b). Current psychological theories of autism: The "Theory of Mind" account and rival theories. *Journal of Child Psychology and Psychiatry, 35*, 215–230.

Happé, F. G. E. (1995). The role of age and verbal ability in the theory of mind task performance of subjects with autism. *Child Development, 66*, 843–855.

Happé, F. (in press). Central coherence and theory of mind in autism: reading homographs in context. *British Journal of Developmental Psychology*.

Happé, F. & Frith, U. (in press). Theory of mind in conduct disordered children: adaptive and maladaptive behaviour in everyday life. *British Journal of Developmental Psychology*.

Harding, B. N. (1992). Malformations of the nervous system. In J. H. Adams and L. W. Duchan (Eds), *Greenfield's Neuropathology* (5th edn, pp. 521–638). London: Edward Arnold.

Harris, P. (1993). Pretending and planning. In S. Baron-Cohen, H. Tager-Flusberg & D. J. Cohen (Eds), *Understanding other minds: perspectives from autism* (pp. 228–246). Oxford: Medical Publications Oxford.

Hashimoto, T., Tayama, M., Miyazaki, M., Murakawa, K. & Kuroda, Y. (1993). Brainstem and cerebellar vermis involvement in autistic children. *Journal of Child Neurology, 8*, 149–152.

Hashimoto, T., Tayama, M., Murakawa, M., Yoshimoto, T., Miyazaki, M., Harada, M. & Kuroda, Y. (1995). Development of the brainstem and cerebellum in autistic patients. *Journal of Autism and Developmental Disorders, 25*, 1–18.

Hauser, S. L., DeLong, G. R. & Rosman, N. P. (1975). Pneumographic findings in the infantile autism syndrome: a correlation with temporal lobe disease. *Brain, 98*, 667–688.

Hermelin, B. & O'Connor, N. (1970). *Psychological experiments with autistic children*. London: Pergamon Press.

Herold, S., Frackowiak, R. S. J., Le Couteur, A., Rutter, M. & Howlin, P. (1988) Cerebral blood flow and metabolism of oxygen and glucose in young autistic adults. *Psychological Medicine, 18*, 823–831.

Hobson, R. P. (1987). The autistic child's recognition of age-and sex-related characteristics of people. *Journal of Autism and Developmental Disorders, 17*, 63–79.

Hobson, R. P. (1993). *Autism and the development of mind*. Hillsdale, NJ: Lawrence Erlbaum Associates.

Hobson, R. P., Ouston, J. & Lee, A. (1988). What's in a face? The case of autism. *British Journal of Developmental Psychology, 79*, 441–453.

Hof, P. R., Knabe, R., Bovier, P. & Bouras, C. (1991). Neuropathological observations in a case of autism presenting with self-injury behavior. *Acta Neuropathologica, 82*, 321–326.

Holttum, J. R., Minshew, N. J., Sanders, R. S. & Phillips, N.E. (1992). Magnetic resonance imaging of the posterior fossa in autism. *Biological Psychiatry, 32*, 1091–1101.

Horwitz, B., Rumsey, J. M., Grady, C. L. & Rapoport, S. I. (1988). The cerebral metabolic landscape in autism: intercorrelations of regional glucose utilization. *Archives of Neurology, 45*, 749–755.

Hotopf, M. & Bolton, P. (1995). A case of autism associated with partial tetrasomy 15. *Journal of Autism and Developmental Disorders, 25*, 41–49.

Hsu, M., Yeung-Courchesne, R., Courchesne, E. & Press, G. A. (1991). Absence of magnetic resonance imaging evidence of pontine abnormality in infantile autism. *Archives of Neurology, 48*, 1160–1163.

Hughes, C. & Russell, J. (1993). Autistic children's difficulty with disengagement from an object: its implications for theories of autism. *Developmental Psychology, 29*, 498–510.

Hughes, C., Russell, J. & Robbins, T. W. (1994). Evidence for executive dysfunction in autism. *Neuropsychologia, 32*, 477–492.

Hunt, A. & Dennis, J. (1987). Psychiatric disorder among children with tuberous sclerosis. *Developmental Medicine and Child Neurology, 29*, 190–198.

Hunt, A. & Shepherd, C. (1993). A prevalence study of autism in tuberous sclerosis. *Journal of Autism and Developmental Disorders, 23*, 329–339.

Jacobson, R., Le Couteur, A., Howlin, P. & Rutter, M. (1988). Selective subcortical abnormalities in autism. *Psychological Medicine, 18*, 39–48.

James, A. L. & Barry, R. J. (1980). A review of psychophysiology in early onset psychosis. *Schizophrenia Bulletin, 6*, 506–525.

Jarrold, C., Boucher, J. & Smith, P. K. (1994a). Executive function deficits and the pretend play of children with autism: a research note. *Journal of Child Psychology and Psychiatry, 35*, 1473–1482.

Jarrold, C., Smith P. K., Boucher J. & Harris, P. (1994b). Comprehension of pretence in children with autism. *Journal of Autism and Developmental Disorders, 24*, 433–455.

Johnson, M. H., Siddons, F., Frith, U. & Morton, J. (1992). Can autism be predicted on the basis of infant screening tests? *Developmental Medicine and Child Neurology, 34*, 316–320.

Jones, M. B. & Szatmari, P. (1988). Stoppage rules and genetic studies of autism. *Journal of Autism and Developmental Disorders, 18*, 31–40.

Jorde, L. B., Hasstedt, S. J., Ritvo, E. R., Mason-Brothers, A., Freeman, B. J., Pingree, C., McMahon, W. M., Peterson, B., Jenson, W. R. & Moll, A. (1991). Complex segregation analysis of autism. *American Journal of Human Genetics, 49*, 932–938.

Jorde, L. B., Mason-Brothers, A., Waldman, R., Ritvo, E. R., Freeman, B. J., Pingree, C., McMahon, M. W., Petersen, P. B., Jenson, W. R. & Mo, A. (1990). The UCLA-University of Utah epidemiologic survey of autism: genealogical analysis of familial aggregation. *American Journal of Medical Genetics, 36*, 85–88.

Julius, D. (1991). Molecular biology of serotonin receptors. *Annual Review of Neuroscience, 14*, 335–360.

Kalsbeek, A., Buijs, R. M., Hofman, M. A., Matthijssen, M. A. H., Pool, C. W. & Uylings, H. B. M. (1987). Effects of neonatal thermal lesioning of the mesocortical dopaminergic projection on the development of the rat prefrontal cortex. *Developmental Brain Research, 32*, 123–132.

Kanner, L. (1943). Autistic disturbances of affective contact. *Nervous Child, 2*, 217–250.

Kemper, T. L. (1988). Neuroanatomic studies of dyslexia and autism. In J. W. Swann & A. Messer (Eds), *Disorders of the developing nervous system: changing views on their origins, diagnoses and treatments* (pp. 125–154). New York: Alan R Liss.

Kemper, T. L. & Bauman, M. L. (1993). The contribution of neuropathologic studies to the understanding of autism. *Neurologic Clinics, 11*, 175–187.

Kidd, K. K. (1991). Trials and tribulations in the search for genes causing neuropsychiatric disorders. *Social Biology, 38*, 163–196.

Kieburtz, K., Macdonald, M., Shih, C., Feigin, A., Steinberg, K., Bordwell, K., Zimmerman, C., Jayalakshmi S., Sotack, J., Gusella, J., Shoulson, I., (1994). Trinucleotide repeat length and progression of illness in Huntington's Disease. *Journal of Medical Genetics, 31*, 872–874.

Kleinman, M. D., Neff, S. & Rosman, N. P. (1992). The brain in infantile autism: are posterior fossa structures abnormal? *Neurology, 42*, 753–760.

Klin, A. (1991). Young autistic children's listening preferences in regard to speech: a possible characterization of the symptom of social withdrawal. *Journal of Autism and Developmental Disorders, 12*, 29–42.

Klin, A. (1993). Auditory brainstem responses in autism: dysfunction or peripheral hearing loss? *Journal of Autism and Developmental Disorders, 23*, 15–35.

Klin, A., Volkmar, F. R. & Sparrow, S. S. (1992). Autistic social dysfunction: some limitations of the theory of mind hypothesis. *Journal of Child Psychology and Psychiatry, 33*, 861–876.

Klin, A., Volkmar, F., Sparrow, S., Cicchetti, D. & Rourke, B. (1995). Validity and neuropsychological characterization of Asperger Syndrome: convergence with nonverbal learning disabilities syndrome. *Journal of Child Psychology and Psychiatry, 36*, 1127–1140.

Landa, R., Piven, J., Wzorek, M., Gayle, J. O., Chase, G. A. & Folstein, S. E. (1992). Social language use in parents of autistic individuals. *Psychological Medicine, 22*, 245–254.

Landa, R., Wzorek, M., Piven, J., Folstein, S. & Isaacs, C. (1991). Spontaneous narrative discourse characteristics of parents of autistic individuals. *Journal of Speech and Hearing Research, 34*, 1339–1345.

Lander, E. S. & Schork, N. J. (1994). Genetic dissection of complex traits. *Science, 265*, 2037–2048.

Langdell, T. (1978). Recognition of faces: an approach to the study of autism. *Journal of Child Psychology and Psychiatry, 19*, 225–238.

Le Couteur, A., Bailey, A., Goode, S., Robertson, S., Gottesman, I., Schmidt, D. & Rutter, M. (in press). A broader phenotype of autism: the clinical spectrum in twins. *Journal of Child Psychology and Psychiatry.*

Le Couteur, A., Rutter, M., Lord, C., Rios, P., Robertson, S., Holdgrafer, M. & McLennan, J. D. (1989). Autism Diagnostic Interview: a semi-structured interview for parents and caregivers of autistic persons. *Journal of Autism and Developmental Disorders, 19*, 363–387.

Le Couteur, A., Trygstad, O., Evered, C., Gillberg, C. & Rutter, M. (1988). Infantile autism and urinary excretion of peptides and protein-associated peptide complexes. *Journal of Autism and Developmental Disorders. 18*, 677–681.

Leslie, A. M. (1987). Pretense and representation: the origins of "theory of mind". *Psychological Review, 94*, 412–426.

Leslie, A. M. & Frith, U. (1988). Autistic children's understanding of seeing, knowing, and believing. *British Journal of Developmental Psychology, 6*, 315–324.

Leslie, A. M. & Happé, F. (1989). Autism and ostensive communication: the relevance of metarepresentation. *Development and Psychopathology, 1*, 205–212.

Lewis, V. & Boucher, J. (1988). Spontaneous, instructed and elicited play in relatively able autistic children. *British Journal of Developmental Psychology, 6*, 325–339.

Lewis, C. & Mitchell, P. (1994). *Children's early understanding of mind: origins and development.* Hove, U.K: Lawrence Erlbaum.

Lister, S. (1992). *The early detection of social and communication impairments.* PhD thesis, University of London.

Lockyer, L. & Rutter, M. (1970). A five to fifteen year follow-up study of infantile psychosis: IV. Patterns of cognitive ability. *British Journal of Social and Clinical Psychology, 9*, 152–163.

Lord, C. (1993). Complexity of social behavior in autism. In S. Baron-Cohen, H. Tager-Flusberg & D. Cohen (Eds), *Understanding other minds: perspectives from autism* (pp. 292–316). Oxford: Oxford University Press.

Lord, C., Rutter, M., Goode, S., Heemsbergen, J., Jordan, H., Mawhood, L. & Schopler, E. (1989). Autism diagnostic observation schedule: a standardized observation of communicative and social behaviour. *Journal of Autism and Developmental Disorders, 19*, 185–212

Lord, C. & Rutter, M. (1994). Autism and pervasive developmental disorders. In M. Rutter, E. Taylor & L. Hersov (Eds), *Child and adolescent psychiatry: modern approaches* (3rd edn, pp. 569–593). London: Blackwell Scientific.

Lord, C., Rutter, M. & Le Couteur, A. (1994). Autism Diagnostic Interview-Revised: a revised version of a diagnostic interview for caregivers of individuals with possible pervasive developmental disorders. *Journal of Autism and Developmental Disorders, 24*, 659–685

Lotspeich, L. J. & Ciaranello, R. D. (1993). The neurobiology and genetics of infantile autism. *International Review of Neurobiology, 35*, 87–129.

Lotter, V. (1978). Follow-up studies. In M. Rutter & E. Schopler (Eds), *Autism: a reappraisal of concepts and treatment* (pp. 475–495). New York: Plenum Press.

Lueger, R. J. & Gill, K.J. (1990). Frontal lobe cognitive dysfunction in conduct disorder adolescents. *Journal of Clinical Psychology, 46*, 696–706.

Macdonald, H., Rutter, M., Howlin, P., Rios, P., Le Couteur, A., Evered, C. & Folstein, S. (1989). Recognition and expression of emotional cues by autistic and normal adults *Journal of Child Psychology and Psychiatry, 30*, 865–877.

Mawhood, L. (1995). A follow-up comparison of autism and developmental language disorder in early adulthood. Unpublished Ph.D. thesis, University of London.

Mazzocco, M. M. M., Pennington, B. F. & Hagerman, R. J. (1994). Social cognition skills among females with Fragile X. *Journal of Autism and Developmental Disorders, 24*, 473–485.

McDougle, C. J., Price, L. H. & Volkmar, F. R. (1994). Recent advances in the pharmacotherapy of autism and related conditions. *Child and Adolescent Psychiatric Clinics of North America, 3*, 71–89.

McEachin, J. J., Smith, T. & Lovaas, O. I. (1993). Long-term outcome for children with autism who received early intensive behavioral treatment. *American Journal of Mental Retardation, 97*, 359–372.

Medical Research Council (1994). *Mental handicap research: new technologies and approaches.* Report of the MRC workshop held at the University of Warwick on 29/30 July 1993.

Meldrum, B. S. & Bruton, C. J. (1992). Epilepsy. In J. H. Adams & L. W. Duchan (Eds), *Greenfield's Neuropathology*, (5th edn, pp. 1246–1283). London: Edward Arnold.

Minshew, N. (1991). Indices of neural function in autism: clinical and biological implications. *Pediatrics, 31*, 774–780.

Minshew, N. J. & Dombrowski, S. M. (1994). *In vivo* neuroanatomy of autism: neuroimaging studies. In M. L. Bauman & T. L. Kemper (Eds), *Neurobiology of Autism* (pp. 66–85). Baltimore, MD: Johns Hopkins University Press.

Morris, R. G., Downes, J. J., Sahakian, B. J., Evendon, J. L., Heald, A. & Robbins, T. W. (1988). Planning and spatial working memory in Parkinson's disease. *Journal of Neurology, Neurosurgery and Psychiatry, 51*, 757–766.

Mortimer, A. M. & McKenna, P. J. (1994). Levels of explanation—symptoms, neuropsychological deficit and morphological abnormalities in schizophrenia. *Psychological Medicine, 24*, 541–545.

Morton, J. & Frith, U. (1995). Causal modelling: a structural approach to developmental psychopathology. In D. Cicchetti & D. J. Cohen (Eds), *Manual of developmental psychopathology* (pp. 357–390). New York: John Wiley.

Mundy, P., Sigman, M., Ungerer, J. & Sherman, T. (1986). Defining the social deficits in autism: the contribution of nonverbal communication measures. *Journal of Child Psychology and Psychiatry, 27*, 657–669.

Narayan, S., Moyes, B. & Wolff, S. (1990). Family characteristics of autistic children: a further report. *Journal of Autism and Developmental Disorders, 20*, 523–536.

Narayan, M., Srinath, S., Anderson, G. M. & Meundi, D. B. (1993). Cerebrospinal fluid levels of homovanillic acid and 5-hydroxyindoleacetic acid in autism. *Biological Psychiatry, 33*, 630–635.

Nelson, K. (1991). Prenatal and perinatal factors in the etiology of autism. *Pediatrics, 87*, 761–766.

Oades, R. D. & Eggers, C. (1994). Childhood autism: an appeal for an integrative and psychobiological approach. *European Child and Adolescent Psychiatry, 3*, 159–175.

O'Connor, N. & Hermelin, B. (1988). Low intelligence and special abilities. *Journal of Child Psychology and Psychiatry, 29*, 391–396.

O'Connor, N. & Hermelin, B. (1991). Talents and preoccupations in idiots-savants. *Psychological Medicine, 21*, 959–964.

Olsson, I., Steffenburg, S. & Gillberg, C. (1988). Epilepsy in autism and autistic-like conditions: a population-based study. *Archives of Neurology, 45*, 666–668.

Ornitz, E. M. (1985). Neurophysiology of infantile autism. *Journal of the American Academy of Child Psychiatry, 24*, 251–265.

Ornitz, E. M. (1989). Autism at the interface between sensory and information processing. In G. Dawson (Ed.), *Autism: nature, diagnosis and treatment* (pp. 174–207). New York: Guilford Press.

Osborne, J. P., Fryer, A. & Webb, D. (1991). Epidemiology of tuberous sclerosis. *Annals of the New York Academy of Sciences, 615*, 125–127.

Osterling, J. & Dawson, G. (1994). Early recognition of children with autism: a study of first birthday home videotapes. *Journal of Autism and Developmental Disorders, 24*, 247–259.

Ozonoff, S. (1994). Executive functions in autism. In E. Schopler & G. Mesibov (Eds), *Learning and cognition in autism*. New York: Plenum Press.

Ozonoff, S., Pennington, B. & Rogers, S. (1991a). Executive function deficits in high-functioning autistic children:

relationship to theory of mind. *Journal of Child Psychology and Psychiatry, 32*, 1081–1106.

Ozonoff, S., Rogers, S. & Pennington, B. (1991b). Asperger's syndrome: evidence for an empirical distinction from high-functioning autism. *Journal of Child Psychology and Psychiatry, 32*, 1107–1122.

Ozonoff, S., Rogers, S., Farnham, J. & Pennington, B. (1993). Can standard measures identify sub-clinical markers of autism. *Journal of Autism and Developmental Disorders, 23*, 429–441.

Ozonoff, S., Strayer, D. L., McMahon, W. M. & Filloux, F. (1994). Executive function abilities in autism and Tourette syndrome: an information processing approach. *Journal of Child Psychology and Psychiatry, 35*, 1015–1032.

Panksepp, J. (1979). A neurochemical theory of autism. *Trends in Neuroscience, 2*, 174–177.

Pantelis, C. & Nelson, H. E. (1994). Cognitive functioning and symptomatology in schizophrenia: the role of frontal-subcortical systems. In A. S. David & J. C. Cutting (Eds), *The neuropsychology of schizophrenia* (pp. 215–229). Hove: Lawrence Erlbaum Associates.

Peterson, C. C. & Siegal, M. (1995). Deafness, conversation and theory of mind. *Journal of Child Psychology and Psychiatry, 36*, 459–474.

Pennington, B. F. & Welsh, M. (1995). Neuropsychology and developmental psychopathology. In D. Cicchetti & D. J. Cohen (Eds), *Manual of developmental psychopathology* (pp. 254–290). New York: John Wiley.

Phillips, W. L. (1993). Understanding intention and desire by children with autism. Unpublished PhD thesis, University of London.

Phillips, W. (submitted). Understanding intention in normal development and in autism.

Phillips, W., Baron-Cohen, S. & Rutter, M. (1992). The role of eye-contact in the detection of goals: evidence from normal toddlers, and children with autism or mental handicap. *Development and Psychopathology, 4*, 375–383.

Phillips, W. L., Baron-Cohen, S. & Rutter, M. (1995). To what extent do children with autism understand desire? *Development and Psychopathology, 7*, 151–169.

Phillips, W., Gómez, J. C., Baron-Cohen, S., Laa, V. & Rivière, A. (1995). Treating people as objects, agents or "subjects": how young children with and without autism make requests. *Journal of Child Psychology and Psychiatry, 36*, 1383–1397

Pickles, A., Bolton, P., Macdonald, H., Rios, P., Storoschuk, S. & Rutter, M. (submitted). A case control family history study of autism: Further findings from extended pedigrees.

Pickles, A., Bolton, P., Macdonald, H., Bailey, A., Le Couteur, A., Sim, C.-H. & Rutter, M. (1995). Latent class analysis of recurrence risks for complex phenotypes with selection and measurement error: a twin and family history study of autism. *American Journal of Human Genetics, 57*, 717–726.

Piven, J., Berthier, M., Startstein, S., Nehme, E., Pearlson, G. & Folstein, S. (1990b). Magnetic resonance imaging evidence for a defect of cerebral cortical development in autism. *American Journal of Psychiatry, 146*, 734–739.

Piven, J., Chase, G. A., Landa, R., Wzorek, M., Gayle, J., Cloud, D. & Folstein, S. (1991). Psychiatric disorders in the parents of autistic individuals. *Journal of the American Academy of Child and Adolescent Psychiatry, 30*, 471–478.

Piven, J., Gayle, J., Chase, J., Fink, B., Landa, R., Wzorek, M. & Folstein, S. E. (1990a). A family history study of neuropsychiatric disorders in the adult siblings of autistic individuals. *Journal of the American Academy of Child and Adolescent Psychiatry, 29*, 177–183.

Piven, J., Gayle, J., Landa, R., Wzorek, M., & Folstein, S., (1991). The prevalence of the Fragile X in a sample of autistic individuals diagnosed using a standardised interview. *Journal of the American Academy of Child and Adolescent Psychiatry, 30,* 825–830.

Piven, J., Nehme, E., Simon, J., Barta, P., Pearlson, G. & Folstein, S. E. (1992). Magnetic resonance imaging in autism: measurement of the cerebellum, pons and fourth ventricle. *Biological Psychiatry, 31,* 491–504.

Piven, J., Simon, J., Chase, G. A., Wzorek, M., Landa, R., Gayle, J. & Folstein, S. (1993). The etiology of autism: pre-, peri- and neonatal factors. *Journal of the American Academy of Child and Adolescent Psychiatry, 32,* 1256–1263.

Piven, J., Wzorek, M., Landa, R., Lainhart, J., Bolton, P., Chase, G. A. & Folstein, S. (1994). Personality characteristics of the parents of autistic individuals (preliminary communication). *Psychological Medicine, 24,* 783–795.

Piven, J., Arndt, S., Bailey, J., Havercamp, S., Andreasen. N. & Palmer, P. (1995). An MRI study of brain size in autism. *American Journal of Psychiatry, 152,* 1145-1149

Pocock, S. J. (1983). *Clinical trials: a practical approach.* Chichester: Wiley.

Pring, L., Hermelin, B. & Heavey, L. (1995). Savants, segments, art and autism. *Journal of Child Psychology and Psychiatry, 36,* 1065-1076

Prior, M. R. (1979). Cognitive abilities and disabilities in infantile autism: a review. *Journal of Abnormal Child Psychology, 7,* 357–380.

Prior, M. R., Dahlstrom, B. & Squires, T. L. (1990). Autistic children's knowledge of thinking and feeling states in other people. *Journal of Child Psychology and Psychiatry, 31,* 587–602.

Prior, M. R. & Hoffman, W. (1990). Neuropsychological testing of autistic children through an exploration with frontal lobe tests. *Journal of Autism and Developmental Disorders, 20,* 581–590.

Raymond, G., Bauman, M. & Kemper, T. (1989). The hippocampus in autism: Golgi analysis. *Annals of Neurology, 26,* 483–484.

Reiss, A. L., Aylward, E., Freund, L. S., Joshi, P. K. & Brian R. M. (1991). Neuroanatomy of Fragile X syndrome: the posterior fossa. *Annals of Neurology, 29,* 26–32.

Riikonen, R. & Amnell, G. (1981). Psychiatric disorders in children with early infantile spasms. *Developmental Medicine and Child Neurology, 23,* 747–760.

Rimland, B. (1978). Savant capabilities of autistic children and their cognitive implications. In G. Serban (Ed.), *Cognitive defects in the development of mental illness* (pp. 43–65). New York: Brunner/Mazel.

Risch, N. (1990). Linkage strategies for genetically complex traits. *American Journal of Human Genetics, 46,* 222–253.

Ritvo, E. R., Creel, D., Reallmuto, G., Crandall, A. S., Freeman, B. J., Bateman, J. B. B., Barr, R., Pingree, C., Coleman, M. & Purple, M. (1988). Electroretinograms in autism: a pilot study of b-wave amplitudes. *American Journal of Psychiatry, 145,* 229–232.

Ritvo, E. R., Freeman, B. J., Scheibel, A. B., Duong, T., Robinson, H., Guthrie, D. & Ritvo, A. (1986). Lower purkinje cell counts in the cerebella of four autistic subjects: initial findings of the UCLA–NSAC Autopsy Research Report. *American Journal of Psychiatry, 143,* 862–866.

Ritvo, E. R., Spence, M. A., Freeman, B. J., Mason-Brothers, A., Mo, A. & Marazita, M. L. (1985). Evidence for autosomal recessive inheritance in 46 families with multiple incidences of autism. *American Journal of Psychiatry, 142,* 187–192.

Rosenbloom, S., Campbell, M., George, A. E., Kricheff, I. I., Taleporos, E., Anderson, L., Reuben, R. M. & Korein, J. (1984). High resolution CT scanning in infantile autism: a quantitative approach. *Journal of the American Academy of Child Psychiatry, 23,* 72–77.

Rosengren, L. E., Ahlsen, G., Belfrage, M., Gillberg, C., Haglid, K. G. & Hamberger, A. (1992). A sensitive ELISA for glial fibrillary acidic protein: application in CSF of children. *Journal of Neuroscience Methods, 44,* 113–119.

Rosenhall, U., Johansson, E. & Gillberg, C. (1988). Oculomotor findings in autistic children. *Journal of Laryngology and Otology, 102,* 435–439.

Rourke, B. P. (1993). Arithmetic disabilities, specific and otherwise: a neuropsychological perspective. *Journal of Learning Disabilities, 26,* 214–226.

Rourke, B. P. (1995). *Syndrome of nonverbal learning disabilities: Neurodevelopmental manifestations.* New York: Guilford Press.

Rumsey, J. M. (1992). Neuropsychological studies of high-level autism. In E. Schopler & G. Mesibov (Eds), *High-functioning individuals with autism* (pp. 41–64). New York: Plenum Press.

Rumsey, J. M., Duara, R., Grady, C. L., Rapoport, J. L., Margolin, R. A., Rapoport, S. I. & Cutler, N. R. (1985). Brain metabolism in autism: resting cerebral glucose utilization rates as measured with positron emission tomography (PET). *Archives of General Psychiatry, 42,* 448–455.

Rumsey, J. M. & Hamburger, S. D. (1988). Neuropsychological findings in high-functioning men with infantile autism residual state. *Journal of Clinical and Experimental Neuropsychology, 10,* 201–221.

Rutter, M. (1970). Autistic children: infancy to adulthood. *Seminars in Psychiatry, 2,* 435–450.

Rutter, M. (1978a). Language disorder and infantile autism. In M. Rutter & E. Schopler (Eds), *Autism: a reappraisal of concepts and treatment* (pp. 85–104). New York: Plenum Press.

Rutter, M. (1978b). Diagnosis and definition. In M. Rutter & E. Schopler, (Eds), *Autism: a reappraisal of concepts and treatment* (pp. 1–25). New York: Plenum Press.

Rutter, M. (1979). Language, cognition and autism. In R. Katzman (Ed.), *Congenital and acquired cognitive disorders* (pp. 247–264). New York: Raven Press.

Rutter, M. (1983). Cognitive deficits in the pathogenesis of autism. *Journal of Child Psychology and Psychiatry, 24,* 513–531.

Rutter, M. (1984). Autistic children growing up. *Developmental Medicine and Child Neurology, 26,* 122–129.

Rutter, M. (1987). The 'what' and 'how' of language development: a note on some outstanding issues and questions. In W. Yule & M. Rutter (Eds), *Language development and disorders* (pp. 159–170). London: Mac-Keith Press.

Rutter, M. (1994). Psychiatric genetics: research challenges and pathways forward. *American Journal of Medical Genetics (Neuropsychiatric Genetics), 54,* 185–198.

Rutter, M. (in preparation). Autistic-like reactive attachment disorders in severely deprived children.

Rutter, M. & Bailey, A. (1993). Thinking and relationships: mind and brain—some reflections on 'theory of mind' and autism. In S. Baron-Cohen, H. Tager-Flusberg & D. Cohen (Eds), *Understanding other minds: perspectives from autism* (pp. 481–504). Oxford: Oxford University Press.

Rutter, M., Bailey, A., Bolton, P. & Le Couteur, A. (1993). Autism: syndrome definition and possible genetic mechanisms. In R. Plomin & G. E. McClearn (Eds), *Nature, nurture, and psychology* (pp. 269–284). Washington, DC: APA Books.

Rutter, M., Bailey, A., Bolton, P. & Le Couteur, A. (1994). Autism and known medical conditions: myth and substance. *Journal of Child Psychology and Psychiatry, 35,* 311–322.

Rutter, M., Mawhood, L. & Howlin, P. (1992). Language delay and social development. In P. Fletcher & D. Hale

(Eds), *Specific speech and language disorders in children* (pp. 63–78). London: Whurr Publishers.

Saitoh, O., Courchesne, E., Egaas, B., Lincoln, A. J. & Schreibman, L. (1995). Cross-sectional area of the posterior hippocampus in autistic patients with cerebellar and corpus callosum abnormalities. *Neurology, 45,* 317–324.

Schifter, T., Hoffman, J. M., Hatten, H. P., Hanson, M. W., Coleman, R. E. & DeLong, G. R. (1994). Neuroimaging in infantile autism. *Journal of Child Neurology, 9,* 155–161.

Schopler, E. & Mesibov, G. B. (1988). *Diagnosis and assessment in autism.* New York: Plenum Press.

Scott, S. (1994). Mental retardation. In M. Rutter, E. Taylor & L. Hersov (Eds), *Child and adolescent psychiatry: modern approaches* (3rd edn, pp. 616–646). Oxford: Blackwell Scientific.

Scott, F. J. & Baron-Cohen, S. (1995). Imagining real and unreal things: evidence of a dissociation in autism. Paper given at SRCD Biennial Conference, Indianapolis, IN, U.S.A.

Semrud-Clikeman, M. & Hynd, G. W. (1990). Right hemispheric dysfunction in nonverbal learning disabilities: social, academic and adaptive functioning in adults and children. *Psychological Bulletin, 107,* 196–209.

Shah, A. & Frith, U. (1983). An islet of ability in autistic children: a research note. *Journal of Child Psychology and Psychiatry, 24,* 613–620.

Shah, A. & Frith, U. (1993). Why do autistic individuals show superior performance on the block design test? *Journal of Child Psychology and Psychiatry, 34,* 1351–1364.

Shah, A., Holmes, N. & Wing, L. (1982). Prevalence of autism and related conditions in adults in a mental handicap hospital. *Applied Research in Mental Handicap, 3,* 303–317.

Shallice, T. (1988). *From neuropsychology to mental structure.* Cambridge: Cambridge University Press.

Siegel, B. V., Asarnow, R., Tanguay, P., Call, J. D., Abel, L., Ho, A., Lott, I. & Buchsbaum, M. S. (1992). Regional cerebral glucose metabolism and attention in adults with a history of childhood autism. *Journal of Neuropsychiatry and Clinical Neurosciences, 4,* 406–414.

Sigman, M. (1995). Behavioral research in childhood autism. In M. Lenzenweger and J. Haugaard (Eds), *Frontiers of developmental psychopathology* (pp. 190–206). New York: Springer/Verlag.

Silliman, E. R., Campbell, M. & Mitchell, R. S. (1989). Genetic influences in autism and assessment of metalinguistic performance in siblings of autistic children. In G. Dawson (Ed.), *Autism: nurture, diagnosis, and treatment* (pp. 225–259). New York: Guildford Press.

Simonoff, E., Bolton, P. & Rutter, M. (in press). Mental retardation: genetic findings, clinical implications and research agenda. *Journal of Child Psychology and Psychiatry.*

Sing, C. F., Haviland, M. B., Templeton, A. R., Zerba, K. E. & Reilly, S. L. (1992). Biological complexity and strategies for finding DNA variations responsible for inter-individual variations in risk of a common chronic disease, coronary artery disease. *Annals of Medicine, 24,* 539–547.

Sing, C. F. & Reilly, S. L. (1993). Genetics of common diseases that aggregate, but do not segregate in families. In C. F. Sing & C. L. Harris (Eds), *Genetics of cellular, individual, family and population variability* (pp. 140–161). New York: Oxford University Press.

Sloman, L. (1991). Use of medication in pervasive developmental disorders. *Psychiatric Clinics of North America, 14,* 165–182.

Small, J. G. (1975). EEG and neurophysiological studies of early infantile autism. (1975). *Biological Psychiatry, 10,* 385–397.

Smalley, S., Asarnow, R. & Spence, M. (1988). Autism and genetics: a decade of research. *Archives of General Psychiatry, 45,* 953–961.

Smalley S. L., Burger F. & Smith M. (1994). Phenotypic variation of tuberous sclerosis in a single extended kindred. *Journal of Medical Genetics, 31,* 761–765.

Smalley S. L., McCracken J. & Tanguay P. (1995) Autism, affective disorders, and social phobia. *American Journal of Medical Genetics (Neuropsychiatric Genetics), 60,* 19–26.

Smalley, S., Smith, M. & Tanguay, P. (1991). Autism and psychiatric disorders in tuberous sclerosis. *Annals of New York Academy of Science, 615,* 382–383.

Smalley, S. L., Tanguay, P. E., Smith, M. & Gutierrez, G. (1992). Autism and tuberous sclerosis. *Journal of Autism and Developmental Disorders, 22,* 339–355.

Sodian, B. & Frith, U. (1992). Deception and sabotage in autistic, retarded, and normal children. *Journal of Child Psychology and Psychiatry, 33,* 591–606.

Spiker, D., Lotspeich, L., Kraemer, H. C., Hallmayer, J., McMahon, W., Petersen, P. B., Nicholas, P., Pingree, C., Wiese-Slater, S., Chiotti, C., Wong D. L., Dimicelli, S., Ritvo, E., Cavalli-Sforza, L. L. & Ciaranello, R. D. (1994). Genetics of autism: characteristics of affected and unaffected children from 37 multiplex families. *American Journal of Medical Genetics, 54,* 27–35.

Steffenburg, S., Gillberg, C., Helgren, L., Anderson, L., Gillberg, L., Jakobsson, G. & Bohman, M. (1989). A twin study of autism in Denmark, Finland, Iceland, Norway, and Sweden. *Journal of Child Psychology and Psychiatry, 30,* 405–416.

Sudhalter, V., Cohen I. L., Silverman, W. & Wolfschein, E. G. (1990). Conversational analyses of males with Fragile X, Down syndrome, and autism: comparison of the emergence of deviant language. *American Journal of Mental Retardation, 94,* 431–441.

Szatmari, P. & Jones, M. B. (1991). IQ and the genetics of autism. *Journal of Child Psychology and Psychiatry, 35,* 215–229.

Szatmari, P., Jones, M. B., Tuff, L., Bartolucci, G., Fisman, S. & Mahoney, W. (1993). Lack of cognitive impairment in first-degree relatives of children with pervasive developmental disorders. *Journal of the American Academy of Child and Adolescent Psychiatry, 32,* 1264–1273.

Tager-Flusberg, H. (1993). What language reveals about the understanding of minds in children with autism. In S. Baron-Cohen, H. Tager-Flusberg & D. Cohen (Eds) *Understanding other minds: perspectives from autism* (pp. 138–157). Oxford: Oxford University Press.

Tanguay, P. E., Ornitz, E. M., Forsythe, A. B. & Ritvo, E. R. (1976). Rapid eye movement (REM) activity in normal and autistic children during REM sleep. *Journal of Autism and Childhood Schizophrenia, 6,* 275–288.

Tantam, D., Monaghan, L., Nicholson, H., & Stirling, J. (1989). Autistic children's ability to interpret faces: a research note. *Journal of Child Psychology and Psychiatry, 30,* 623–630.

Townsend, J. & Courchesne, E. (in press). Parietal damage and narrow "spotlight" spatial attention. *Journal of Cognitive Neuroscience.*

Trottier, Y., Biancalana, V. & Mandel, J.-L. (1994). Instability of CAG repeats in Huntington's disease: relation to parental transmission and age of onset. *Journal of Medical Genetics, 31,* 377–382.

Tsai, L. (1987). Pre-, peri-, and neonatal factors in autism. In E. Schopler & G. B. Mesibov (Eds), *Neurobiological issues in autism* (pp. 180–189). New York: Plenum Press.

Tsai, L. Y., Tsai, M. C. & August, G. J. (1985). Brief report: implication of EEG diagnoses in the subclassification of infantile autism. *Journal of Autism and Developmental Disorders, 15,* 339–344.

Turner, M. (1995). Repetitive behaviours and generation of ideas in high functioning individuals with autism: is there a link? Paper presented at BPS Annual Conference, University of Warwick, U.K.

Van Engeland, H., Roelofs, J. W., Verbaten, M. N. & Slangen, J. L. (1991). Abnormal electrodermal reactivity to novel visual stimuli in autistic children. *Psychiatry Research, 38,* 27–38.

Vargha-Khadem, F., Isaacs, E., Van Der Werf, S., Robb, S. & Wilson, J. (1992). Development of intelligence and memory in children with hemiplegic cerebral palsy: The deleterious consequences of early seizures. *Brain, 115,* 315–329.

Venter, A., Lord, C. & Schopler, E. (1992). A follow-up study of high-functioning autistic children. *Journal of Child and Adolescent Psychiatry, 33,* 489–507.

Vilensky, J. A., Damasio, A. R. & Maurer, R. G. (1981). Gait disturbances in patients with autistic behavior. *Archives of Neurology, 38,* 646–649.

Vincent, J. B., Konecki, D. S., Munstermann, E., Bolton, P., Poustka, A., Poustka F., Rutter M. & Gurling, H. M. D. (submitted). Point mutation analysis of the Fragile X mental retardation (FMR-1) gene in autism.

Volkmar, F. R. & Cohen, D. J. (1989). Disintegrative disorder or 'late onset' autism. *Journal of Child Psychology and Psychiatry, 30,* 717–724.

Volkmar, F. R. & Nelson, I. (1990). Seizure disorders in autism. *Journal of the American Academy of Child and Adolescent Psychiatry, 29,* 127–129.

Warren, S. T. & Nelson, D. L. (1994). Advances in molecular analysis of Fragile X syndrome. *The Journal of the American Medical Association, 271,* 536–542.

Wainwright-Sharp, J. A. & Bryson, S. E. (1993). Visual orienting deficits in high-functioning people with autism. *Journal of Autism and Developmental Disorders, 23,* 1–13.

Weeks, S. J. & Hobson, R. P. (1987). The salience of facial expression for autistic children. *Journal of Child Psychology and Psychiatry, 28,* 137–152.

Welsh, M. C., Pennington, B., Ozonoff, S., Rouse, B. & McCabe, E. R. (1990). Neuropsychology of early-treated phenylketonurea: specific executive function deficits. *Child Development, 61,* 1697–1713.

Whiten, A. & Perner, J. (1991). Fundamental issues in the multidisciplinary study of mindreading. In A. Whiten (Ed.), *Natural Theories of Mind: Evolution, Development and Simulation of Everyday Mindreading* (pp. 1–17). Oxford: Blackwell.

Williams, R. S., Hauser, S. L., Purpura, D. P., DeLong, G. R. & Swisher, C. M. (1980). Autism and mental retardation: neuropathologic studies performed in four retarded persons with autistic behavior. *Archives of Neurology, 37,* 749–753.

Wing, L. & Gould, J. (1978). Systematic recording of behaviours and skills of retarded and psychotic children. *Journal of Autism and Childhood Schizophrenia, 8,* 79–97.

Wing, L. & Gould, J. (1979). Severe impairments of social interaction and associated abnormalities in children: epidemiology and classification. *Journal of Autism and Developmental Disorders, 9,* 11–29.

Wolff, P. H., Gardner, J., Paccia, J. & Lappen, J. (1989). The greeting behavior of Fragile X males. *American Journal of Mental Retardation, 93,* 406–411.

Wolff, S., Narayan, S. & Moyes, B. (1988). Personality characteristics of parents of autistic children. *Journal of Child Psychology and Psychiatry, 29,* 143–154.

Woodhouse, W., Bailey, A., Bolton, P., Baird, G., Le Couteur, A. & Rutter, M. (in press). Head circumference and pervasive developmental disorder. *Journal of Child Psychology and Psychiatry.*

Yirmiya, N., Kasari, C., Sigman, M. D. & Mundy, P. (1989). Facial expressions of affect in autistic, mentally retarded and normal children. *Journal of Child Psychology and Psychiatry, 30,* 725–735.

Zapella, M. (1990). Autistic features in children affected by cerebral gigantism. *Brain Dysfunction, 3,* 241–244.

Zigler, E. & Hodcapp, R. (1986). *Understanding Mental Retardation.* New York: Cambridge University Press.

Zilbovicius, M., Garreau, B., Samson, Y., Remy, P., Barthelemy, C., Syrota, A. & Lelord, G. (1995). Delayed maturation of the frontal cortex in childhood autism. *American Journal of Psychiatry, 152,* 248–252.

Accepted manuscript received 13 July 1995

HYPOPLASIA OF CEREBELLAR VERMAL LOBULES VI AND VII IN AUTISM

E. Courchesne, Ph.D., R. Yeung-Courchesne, B.A., G.A. Press, M.D., J.R. Hesselink, M.D.,
and T.L. Jernigan, Ph.D.

Abstract Autism is a neurologic disorder that severely impairs social, language, and cognitive development. Whether autism involves maldevelopment of neuroanatomical structures is not known.

The size of the cerebellar vermis in patients with autism was measured on magnetic resonance scans and compared with its size in controls. The neocerebellar vermal lobules VI and VII were found to be significantly smaller in the patients. This appeared to be a result of developmental hypoplasia rather than shrinkage or deterioration after full development had been achieved. In contrast, the adjacent vermal lobules I to V, which are ontogenetically, developmentally, and anatomically distinct from lobules VI and VII, were found to be of normal size. Maldevelopment of the vermal neocerebellum had occurred in both retarded and nonretarded patients with autism. This localized maldevelopment may serve as a temporal marker to identify the events that damage the brain in autism, as well as other neural structures that may be concomitantly damaged.

Our findings suggest that in patients with autism, neocerebellar abnormality may directly impair cognitive functions that some investigators have attributed to the neocerebellum; may indirectly affect, through its connections to the brain stem, hypothalamus, and thalamus, the development and functioning of one or more systems involved in cognitive, sensory, autonomic, and motor activities; or may occur concomitantly with damage to other neural sites whose dysfunction directly underlies the cognitive deficits in autism. (N Engl J Med 1988; 318:1349-54.)

AUTISM is a developmental disorder that results in severe deficits in social, language, and cognitive functioning.[1-4] In 1943, Kanner[1] suggested that autism is a biologic rather than a psychological disorder. Nonetheless, the cause of autism remains unknown, and the possibility that the disorder involves abnormal development of neuroanatomical structures remains unconfirmed.

Several studies[5,6] have reported that lateral ventricles are enlarged in some patients with autism. Enlarged ventricles do not serve as markers of damage to specific neuroanatomical regions, however, nor do they specifically point to an abnormality in early neuroanatomical development, since ventriculomegaly may be the result of a variety of congenital and acquired diseases. CT and postmortem studies of patients have found no appreciable abnormalities in the cerebral cortex.[7-11] However, postmortem studies of patients in whom autism was complicated by seizures, severe mental retardation, or the use of medication showed that the numbers of Purkinje cells in the cerebellum were reduced.[9,10,12] Moreover, we recently reported results of in vivo magnetic resonance scanning in a patient with autism uncomplicated by severe mental retardation, epilepsy, or a history of drug use or neurologic disease,[13] which demonstrated developmental hypoplasia of the neocerebellar hemispheres and vermal lobules VI and VII (i.e., declive, folium, and tuber in the superior posterior vermis). Neighbor-

ing paleocerebellar regions of the hemispheres and vermis (anterior vermal lobules I to V and inferior posterior vermal lobules VIII to X) were relatively unaffected.

To clarify further the relation between cerebellar abnormality and autism, the following questions need to be answered about the cerebellar abnormalities: Are they more closely associated with autism or with the concomitant medical histories? Are they due to maldevelopment or to tissue loss occurring later in life, after the development of the brain is complete? Are they frequently present in the general population with autism, or only in rare cases? To answer these questions, we obtained magnetic resonance scans of 18 patients with autism without superimposed disorders.

METHODS

Study Groups

Patients with Autism

The patient group consisted of 18 subjects with autism that was not complicated by severe mental retardation, cerebral palsy, epilepsy, genetic abnormality, other neurologic disease, or the use of anticonvulsant or antipsychotic medication. The criteria for infantile autism as defined by the *Diagnostic and Statistical Manual of Mental Disorders*[14] were used to identify autistic subjects. Their ages ranged from 6 to 30 years (mean, 20.9); 2 patients were female and 16 male. These 18 subjects were all the patients with autism in whom our laboratory has conducted behavioral and neurophysiologic studies for five years.[15-20]

The verbal IQ of the 18 subjects ranged from 45 to 111 on the Wechsler scale (mean, 77); the Wechsler performance IQ ranged from 70 to 112 (mean, 88). Thirteen subjects had full-scale Wechsler IQs between 73 and 108, of whom 7 held jobs (e.g., gardener's aide, assembler in a bicycle shop, and secretarial aide), attended college, or did both. The other five subjects had full-scale IQs between 55 and 70. They had a much lower level of function and required constant custodial care; three of them could not read or solve simple mathematical problems.

Normal Controls

The control group consisted of 12 subjects whose ages ranged from 9 to 37 years (mean, 24.8), of whom 3 were female and 9 male.

From the Neuropsychology Research Laboratory, Children's Hospital Research Center, San Diego, Calif. (E.C., R.Y.-C.); the Neurosciences Department (E.C.) and the Radiology Department (G.P., J.R.H.), School of Medicine, University of California at San Diego, La Jolla, Calif.; and the Psychiatry Department, Veterans Administration Medical Center, San Diego, Calif. (T.L.J.). Address reprint requests to Dr. Courchesne at the Neuropsychology Research Laboratory, Children's Hospital Research Center, 8001 Frost St., San Diego, CA 92123.

Supported by funds from Children's Hospital Research Center, San Diego, by a grant (5-R01-NS-19855) from the National Institute of Neurological and Communicative Disorders and Stroke, and by a grant (1-R01-MH-36840) from the National Institute of Mental Health to Dr. E. Courchesne.

197

Three subjects had volunteered (all men). The other nine had been selected from patients who had undergone magnetic resonance scanning of the brain at the University of California–San Diego Magnetic Resonance Institute according to the following method. The entire file of scans available at the institute was searched for brain scans that included axial and sagittal images; 90 such scans were found. From the patients represented by these scans, normal controls were selected by using the following criteria: age between 6 and 36 years, no symptoms of cerebellar dysfunction, and no evidence of central nervous system abnormalities on the scan, as reviewed independently by two of us who are neuroradiologists. Among the reasons for referral were head and neck pain, depression, headaches, and neurogenic bladder. Nine patients were identified who satisfied all these criteria.

Although an ideal normal control group would have consisted entirely of normal volunteers, limitations on funding dictated the use of existing scans of nine patients found to be normal. Since the central point of this study was to compare the neuroanatomy of persons with autism with that of persons without autism, the controls selected represent a sample of nonautistic persons with normal magnetic resonance scans.

Patients with Other Neurologic Disorders

We also analyzed the scans of patients with various abnormalities of the hindbrain, including developmental malformations and atrophy with onset in childhood or adulthood. This group comprised six patients with cerebellar atrophy associated with metabolic or seizure disorders, two patients with olivopontocerebellar dysgenesis, six patients with Arnold–Chiari Type I malformation of the cerebellum, one patient with agenesis of the corpus callosum, and one patient with Dandy–Walker malformation.

The scans of seven patients with focal lesions of the cerebral white matter were also evaluated.

Protocol for Magnetic Resonance Scanning

After appropriate informed consent was obtained, magnetic resonance scanning was performed in each patient with autism, by means of a 1.5-tesla imaging system (G.E. Signa). A multisection spin-echo sequence (TR [repetition time], 2000 msec; TE [echo time], 25, 70 msec) was conducted in the axial and coronal planes, and a multisection T₁-weighted sequence (TR, 600; TE, 25) in the sagittal plane centered at the midline. The sections were 5 mm thick, with a gap of 2.5 mm between adjacent sections.

Quantification Procedures

Figure 1 (top panel) shows the location of vermal lobules I to V (the anterior vermis), vermal lobules VI and VII (the superior posterior vermis), and vermal lobule VIII (the inferior posterior vermis). In the midline sagittal plane, the boundary between the anterior vermis (i.e., lobules I to V) and vermal lobules VI and VII was defined as the line joining the anterior aspect of the primary fissure to the apex of the fourth ventricle. The boundary between vermal lobules VI and VII and vermal lobule VIII was defined as the line joining the anterior aspect of the prepyramidal fissure to the apex of the fourth ventricle. The boundary between vermal lobule VIII and lobule IX was defined as the line joining the anterior aspect of the secondary fissure and the apex of the fourth ventricle.

Magnetic resonance images for the group with autism, the control group, and the group with nonautistic neurologic disorders were coded and mixed at random before evaluation by the investigators, who were blinded to the identity and group membership of each subject. Quantification of vermal cross-sectional areas was performed on the sagittal image that showed most clearly the aqueduct of Sylvius and the deepest extent of the primary and prepyramidal fissures. On the midsagittal scan of every subject, the boundaries of vermal lobules I to V, VI and VII, and VIII were independently traced twice, once by one of us who is a neuroradiologist and once by a graduate student in our neurosciences department. Next, four investigators measured the areas of these traced regions planimetrically: two measured the set of tracings from the neuroradiologist,

and two measured the set from the student. All tracings and measurements were done on coded images so that the identities and group memberships of the subjects were unknown to the investigators. The four measures of each of the three regions of interest in each subject were highly correlated with one another. For example, correlations between any two of the four measurements of vermal lobules VI and VII ranged from a low of 0.855 to a high of 0.986. The four planimetric measures were averaged, and the results were used in the statistical analyses.

Vermal lobules IX and X were not measured, because the scans used in this study did not show clearly defined boundaries for them. Furthermore, these lobules are classified as the paleocerebellum and the archicerebellum, respectively, and did not have prime relevance to this study. These regions and the cerebellar hemispheres were intended to be measured in later investigations.

RESULTS

The vermal lobules VI and VII of the patients with autism were found to be significantly smaller than those of the controls ($F_{(1,28)} = 10.83$, $P = 0.003$) (Fig. 1). Of the 18 autistic subjects, 14 had lobule areas that fell between 1.1 and 4.33 SD below normal (Table 1). In these 14 subjects, vermal lobules VI and VII were 25 percent smaller than in the control subjects (mean, 229 vs. 305 mm²). Both the patients with lower functioning and those with higher functioning were among those with the severest vermal hypoplasia.

Figure 1A shows five examples of a normal vermis and five examples of a vermis with hypoplasia. Figure 1B shows superimposed contours of lobules I to V and of lobules VI and VII in the same subjects represented in Figure 1A. Vermal lobules I to V (the anterior vermis) were similar in size in the autistic and normal groups (421 vs. 423 mm²), as was vermal lobule VIII (118 vs. 127 mm²) ($P > 0.55$ for both comparisons) (Fig. 1 and Table 1).

In one patient with autism, lobule VIII also appeared to have developmental hypoplasia (2.58 SD below normal) (Fig. 1A). In other respects, the image of this patient matched the pattern of the patients with autism as a whole: vermal lobules VI and VII had pronounced hypoplasia (4.33 SD below normal), and the anterior vermis was of normal size.

To confirm that the smaller size of vermal lobules VI and VII was regionally localized in the patients with autism and was not due to a possibly smaller brain overall, we created a simple index of regionally localized vermal hypoplasia. This index was the ratio of the total of the combined areas of vermal lobules VI and VII to the total of the combined areas of lobules I to V in each subject, expressed as a percentage. It was 72.4 ± 6.5 percent in the control group, but only 59.1 ± 9.2 percent in the autistic group ($F_{(1,28)} = 18.8$, $P < 0.001$). In the patients with autism, the reduction in the area of vermal lobules VI and VII relative to the anterior vermis is shown in Figure 1, and the index of regionally localized vermal hypoplasia shown in Figure 2. In 14 of the patients, the index of hypoplasia was 1.40 to 4.92 SD below that of the control group (Table 1).

The diminished size of vermal lobules VI and VII did not appear to be the result of parenchymal atro-

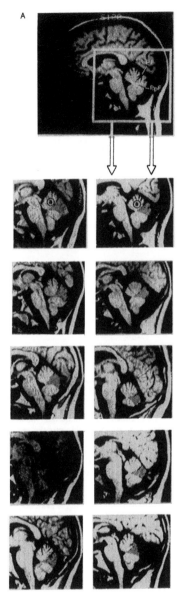

Normal   Autistic

Vermal Lobules I-V
Vermal Lobules VI-VII

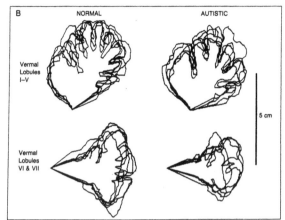

Figure 1. Magnetic Resonance Scans (A) and Tracings (B) of the Vermal Lobules of Five Patients with Autism Who Have Vermal Hypoplasia and Five Controls.

Panel A shows midline sagittal views of the vermis. The patients have vermal hypoplasia, in that their lobules VI and VII are smaller than those in the controls; their lobules I to V and lobule VIII are normal, except for a hypoplastic lobule VIII in the third scan from the bottom. PF denotes primary fissure and PpF prepyramidal fissure.

Panel B shows superimposed outlines of the lobules of five patients and of those of five controls (the same 10 subjects represented in Panel A). Lobules VI and VII of the patients are appreciably smaller than those of the controls; lobules I to V of both groups are similar in area.

phy or encephalomalacia (Fig. 1A). There was no evidence of excessive sulcal widening or abnormal signal intensity within the cerebellar parenchyma. On the contrary, the depth and width of the three major sulci (primary, prepyramidal, and secondary fissures) in the autistic group were similar to those seen in the control group.

Figure 3 shows the difference between the normal mean value for the size of the vermal lobules and the values for the patients with seven neurologic disorders, including autism. The anterior vermis of the group with autism differed from normal by only 2 mm^2; in vermal lobules VI and VII, however, the difference from normal was 56 mm^2. This pattern was not seen in any other group of patients. In the patients with Arnold–Chiari Type I malformation, both the anterior vermis and vermal lobules VI and VII were larger than normal. In contrast, in the patients with Dandy–Walker malformation, olivopontocerebellar dysgenesis, agenesis of the corpus callosum, and cerebellar atrophy, both vermal regions were very much smaller than normal. Finally, in patients with supratentorial abnormalities such as focal lesions in the white matter, both regions were normal (Fig. 3).

DISCUSSION

Our results indicate that autism is strongly associated with anatomical abnormalities in vermal lobules VI and VII of the cerebellum. The abnormalities appear to represent developmental hypoplasia. When the results of magnetic resonance scanning are considered in conjunction with all available postmortem findings regarding the cerebellum of patients with autism,[9,10,12] it appears that abnormalities at the cellular and gross anatomical levels are consistently pres-

199

ent in various neocerebellar regions in the great majority of these patients, with or without superimposed mental retardation or other neurologic disorders. No other part of the nervous system has been shown to be so consistently abnormal in autism.

Nonetheless, our results also show that in some portion of the spectrum of autism, disorders of the cerebellum may have a different expression or may not be involved (for example, in four of the patients with autism the vermal ratio was within 1 SD of normal).

As suggested in recent discussions of the pathophysiologic features of autism,[15,21] neocerebellar maldevelopment could potentially affect cognitive development in autism in two ways. First, damage to the neocerebellum might directly impair cognitive functions and behavioral control attributed to the neocerebellum.[22-26] For instance, since it has been suggested that the neocerebellum is involved in the acquisition and execution of skilled cognitive and motor operations,[27] early damage to this area might hinder the normal, smooth acquisition and execution of sensorimotor schema from which human intellectual growth proceeds.[28] Second, through direct connections to nu-

Table 1. Area of Vermal Lobules and IQ Values in Patients with Autism and Controls.

Group	Vermal Lobules			SD of Ratio from Normal	Age/Sex	Intelligence Quotient		
	Area I–V	Area VI–VII	Area VI–VII: Area I–V			Verbal	Performance	Full-scale
	square millimeters		percent					
Autistic patients								
1	424.2	172.3	40.6	−4.92	22/M	96	112	103
2	395.6	171.0	43.2	−4.51	20/M	80	70	74
3	386.7	194.8	50.4	−3.41	14/M	45	73	55
4	428.3	223.8	52.3	−3.12	30/M	71	78	73
5	367.3	197.1	53.7	−2.90	22/M	105	104	105
6	484.8	270.7	55.8	−2.56	23/M	74	92	80
7	365.8	209.7	57.3	−2.33	22/M	100	112	105
8	452.8	261.7	57.8	−2.26	16/M	81	71	75
9	449.1	260.3	58.0	−2.24	27/M	76	97	83
10	398.6	232.0	58.2	−2.20	20/F	55	87	68
11	394.8	245.4	62.2	−1.59	17/F	55	88	70
12	446.2	277.4	62.2	−1.58	25/M	111	104	108
13	413.4	258.8	62.6	−1.52	20/M	62	71	66
14	468.5	296.7	63.3	−1.40	27/M	89	92	89
15	377.7	259.5	68.7	−0.57	25/M	74	74	73
16	355.4	245.4	69.1	−0.52	6/M	82	92	86
17	499.7	355.4	71.1	−0.20	21/M	70	80	73
18	465.8	356.4	76.5	+0.64	19/M	54	84	68
Mean	420.8	249.4	59.1		20.9	76.7	87.8	80.8
±SD	±43.5*	±52.6†	±9.24†					
Controls								
1	401.6	256.8	64.0	−1.30	30/M			
2	511.6	336.1	65.7	−1.04	31/M			
3	417.1	277.9	66.6	−0.89	29/M			
4‡	404.0	276.0	68.3	−0.63	26/M			
5	386.7	270.7	70.0	−0.37	30/M			
6	459.5	324.2	70.6	−0.28	22/M			
7‡	431.0	306.0	71.0	−0.22	37/M			
8‡	422.0	307.0	72.8	+0.06	33/M			
9	470.6	351.7	74.7	+0.36	13/M			
10	427.8	335.7	78.6	+0.96	19/F			
11	403.3	329.8	81.8	+1.45	19/F			
12	339.8	287.0	84.7	+1.86	9/F			
Mean	422.8	304.9	72.4		24.8			
±SD	±43.8	±30.9	±6.46					

*Not significantly different from control mean.
†Significantly lower than control mean (P<0.003 by analysis of variance).
‡Normal volunteer.

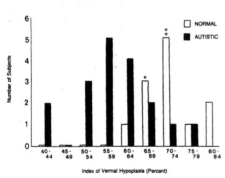

Figure 2. Index of Vermal Hypoplasia in 18 Patients with Autism and 12 Controls.

The index denotes the ratio of the combined area of vermal lobules VI and VII to the combined area of lobules I to V. The values for the three controls who were normal volunteers (stars) fall in the center of the distribution of the values for the nine controls who were patients.

merous sites in the brain stem and thalamus, the neural output of damaged neocerebellar circuits might affect the development and functioning of one or more systems involved in attention, cortical modulation, sensory modulation, regulation of autonomic activity, and motor and behavioral initiation.[29-38] Abnormal functioning in each of these systems has often been proposed in theories and studies of autism.[2,15,39-43] For example, anatomical and physiologic evidence indicates that the neocerebellar cortex is connected, through the deep cerebellar nuclei, with all levels of the reticular activating system, including medullary, pontine, mesencephalic, and intralaminar thalamic segments. Disturbances in the functioning of the reticular activating system were among the first neurobiologic explanations of the cognitive deficits of autism.[2]

Neocerebellar maldevelopment may also point to damage at other neural sites, as follows. First, the same event that damages the neocerebellar vermis may also damage other neural components whose dysfunction underlies the cognitive deficits in autism. Sec-

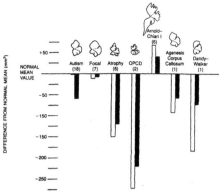

Figure 3. Difference from Normal Value for Combined Area of Vermal Lobules I to V and the Combined Area of Lobules VI and VII in Patients with Seven Neurologic Disorders, Including Autism.

The zero line represents the mean normal value obtained in this study for the midsagittal area of vermal lobules I to V (i.e., 423 mm²), and each white bar represents a difference from this value. The zero line also represents the normal mean in this study for the midsagittal area of vermal lobules VI and VII (i.e., 305 mm²), and each black bar represents a difference from this value.

An example of the midline sagittal view of the vermis is shown above each disorder listed. OPCD denotes olivopontocerebellar dysgenesis, and focal denotes focal lesion in cerebral white matter. Values in parentheses represent the number of patients with the disorder.

ond, the limited range of motor and somatosensory activities in the autistic infant (i.e., "neural deprivation" occurring during development) may lead to reduced growth of dendritic and axonal branches in the neocerebellar vermis, in other neural systems, or in both. Third, neocerebellar damage may represent loss resulting from damage to other neural systems that are closely connected with the vermal neocerebellum. The last explanation is unlikely, since the cerebellum sustains very little secondary loss (less than 3.2 percent) even when large regions of motor or somatosensory cortex are excised.[44] The two other explanations may have some validity not yet established.

The observation that vermal lobules VI and VII are abnormal in the majority of patients with autism, but that the anterior vermis is not, may represent an important first step both in determining the timing of environmentally or genetically mediated events that damage the brain and induce this disorder and in identifying any other neural sites that may be concomitantly damaged. Vermal lobules VI and VII are embryologically and phylogenetically distinct from anterior vermal lobules I to V.[30,45-47] These two regions are derived from different primordial tissue,[47] and the timing of neurogenesis and the migration of Purkinje and granule cells destined for these regions also differ.[46,47] An environmentally mediated event that disturbs the migration of Purkinje cells to the

posterior vermis could also affect neurogenesis that occurs at that time in the subiculum, CA1 and CA3 of the hippocampal formation, portions of the septum, and the amygdalohippocampal area of the corticomedial complex of the amygdala[47,48] — regions involved in memory and emotional behavior. Microscopical abnormalities in these regions have been reported in a postmortem study of one patient with autism.[10] As a second example, very late intrauterine or postnatal disruption of granule-cell migration may render vermal lobules VI and VII hypoplastic in relation to the anterior vermis, since lobules VI and VII receive their final full complement of granule cells after the anterior vermis does.[46] Such a late insult may simultaneously affect the development of hippocampal granule cells, which, like cerebellar granule cells, are among the last neurons to migrate during development.

Studies of families and twins have suggested that genetic factors operate in autism.[2,49] No genetic mutation is known that selectively affects the neocerebellum but not the anterior cerebellum. However, some mouse mutants undergo selective loss of Purkinje or granule cells.[50-53] In particular, the cerebellum of the "nervous" mouse mutant (nr) is hypoplastic because of postnatal Purkinje-cell degeneration (50 percent loss in the vermis and 90 percent in the hemispheres), which is associated with mitochondrial dysfunction; the hippocampus shows maldevelopment of lamina in CA2 and CA3. The most prominent symptoms in affected mice are hypersensitivity to auditory and somatosensory stimulation; hyperactivity when very young, which decreases to hypoactivity later in development and in adulthood; and dysfunctional breeding behavior. These symptoms are similar to symptoms sometimes present in patients with autism. Surprisingly, motor incoordination is mild in the mutant mouse; the most prominent motor symptom is a tendency toward long delay in initiating motor responses under novel situations (e.g., when placed in water for the first time).[51]

The abnormal vermal morphology of our patients with autism differs from that in patients with the developmental and acquired disorders listed in Figure 3, as well as other forms of cerebellar dysgenesis, such as Down's syndrome.[30,54-56] We are investigating several other neurobehavioral disorders (e.g., Rett syndrome) that present with behavior patterns like those of autism, in order to ascertain whether cerebellar abnormalities are present.

Autism has been an enigma for more than four decades. It has been considered by some to be a psychosocial disorder resulting from abnormal parenting. The cerebellar hypoplasia described above, however, supports the view that autism is instead a developmental neurobiologic disorder.

REFERENCES

1. Kanner L. Autistic disturbances of affective contact. Nerv Child 1943; 2:217-50.

2. Rimland B. Infantile autism: the syndrome and its implications for a neural theory of behavior. Englewood Cliffs, N.J.: Prentice-Hall, 1964: 54-8.

3. Rutter M, Schopler E, eds. Autism: a reappraisal of concepts and treatment. New York: Plenum Press, 1978.

4. Schopler E, Mesibov GB, eds. Social behavior in autism. New York: Plenum Press, 1986.

5. Campbell M, Rosenbloom S, Perry R, et al. Computerized axial tomography in young autistic children. Am J Psychiatry 1982; 139:510-2.

6. Damasio M, Maurer RG, Damasio AR, Chui HC. Computerized tomographic scan findings in patients with autistic behavior. Arch Neurol 1980; 37:504-10.

7. Prior MR, Tress B, Hoffman WL, Boldt D. Computed tomographic study of children with classic autism. Arch Neurol 1984; 41:482-4.

8. Creasey H, Rumsey JM, Schwartz M, Duara R, Rapoport JL, Rapoport SI. Brain morphometry in autistic men as measured by volumetric computed tomography. Arch Neurol 1986; 43:669-72.

9. Williams RS, Hauser SL, Purpura DP, DeLong R, Swisher CN. Autism and mental retardation: neuropathologic studies performed in four retarded persons with autistic behavior. Arch Neurol 1980; 37:749-53.

10. Bauman M, Kemper TL. Histoanatomic observations of the brain in early infantile autism. Neurology 1985; 35:866-74.

11. Coleman PD, Romano J, Lapham L, Simon W. Cell counts in cerebral cortex of an autistic patient. J Autism Dev Disord 1985; 15:245-55.

12. Ritvo ER, Freeman BJ, Scheibel AB, et al. Lower Purkinje cell counts in the cerebella of four autistic subjects: initial findings of the UCLA-NSAC autopsy research report. Am J Psychiatry 1986; 143:862-6.

13. Courchesne E, Hesselink JR, Jernigan TL, Yeung-Courchesne R. Abnormal neuroanatomy in a nonretarded person with autism: unusual findings with magnetic resonance imaging. Arch Neurol 1987; 44:335-41.

14. American Psychiatric Association. Diagnostic and statistical manual of mental disorders. 3rd ed. Washington, D.C.: American Psychiatric Association, 1980.

15. Courchesne E. A neurophysiological view of autism. In: Schopler E, Mesibov GB, eds. Neurobiological issues in autism. New York: Plenum Press, 1987:285-324.

16. Courchesne E, Kilman BA, Galambos R, Lincoln AJ. Autism: processing of novel auditory information assessed by event-related brain potentials. Electroencephalogr Clin Neurophysiol 1984; 59:238-48.

17. Courchesne E, Lincoln AJ, Kilman BA, Galambos R. Event-related brain potential correlates of the processing of novel visual and auditory information in autism. J Autism Dev Disord 1985; 15:55-76.

18. Ameli R, Courchesne E, Lincoln AJ, Kaufman AS, Grillon C. Visual memory processes in high-functioning individuals with autism. J Autism Dev Disord (in press).

19. Courchesne E, Courchesne RY, Hicks G, Lincoln AJ. Functioning of the brain-stem auditory pathway in non-retarded autistic individuals. Electroencephalogr Clin Neurophysiol 1985; 61:491-501.

20. Courchesne E, Lincoln AJ, Yeung-Courchesne R, Elmasian R, Grillon C. Pathophysiologic findings in non-retarded autism and receptive developmental language disorder. J Autism Dev Disord (in press).

21. Courchesne E. The missing ingredients in autism. Presented at the Conference on Brain and Behavioral Development: Biosocial Dimensions, Elridge, Md., May 19–22, 1985.

22. Leaton RN, Supple WF. Cerebellar vermis: essential for long-term habituation of the acoustic startle response. Science 1986; 232:513-5.

23. Idem. Long-term habituation of acoustic startle following lesions of the cerebellar vermis or cerebellar hemisphere. Abstr Soc Neurosci 1986; 12:978.

24. Thompson RF. Neuronal substrates of simple associative learning: classical conditioning. Trends Neurosci 1983; 6:270-5.

25. Idem. The neurobiology of learning and memory. Science 1986; 233:941-7.

26. McCormick DA, Thompson RF. Cerebellum: essential involvement in the classically conditioned eyelid response. Science 1984; 223:296-9.

27. Leiner HC, Leiner AL, Dow RS. Does the cerebellum contribute to mental skills? Behav Neurosci 1986; 100:443-54.

28. Piaget J. The origin of intelligence in children. New York: International Universities Press, 1952.

29. Altman J. Morphological and behavioral markers of environmentally induced retardation of brain development: an animal model. Environ Health Perspect 1987; 74:153-68.

30. Gilman S, Bloedel JR, Lechtenberg R. Disorders of the cerebellum. Philadelphia: F.A. Davis, 1981:3-7.

31. Beitz AJ. Structural organization of the fastigial nucleus. In: Palay SL, Chan-Palay V, eds. The cerebellum: new vistas. Berlin: Springer-Verlag, 1982:233-49.

32. Carpenter MB, Batton RR III. Connections of the fastigial nucleus in the cat and monkey. In: Palay SL, Chan-Palay V, eds. The cerebellum: new vistas. Berlin: Springer-Verlag, 1982:250-91.

33. Nieuwenhuys R, Voogd J, van Huijzen C. The human central nervous system. Berlin: Springer-Verlag, 1981.

34. Newman PP, Reza H. Functional relationships between the hippocampus and the cerebellum: an electrophysiological study of the cat. J Physiol (Lond) 1979; 287:405-26.

35. Reis DJ, Doba N, Nathan MA. Predatory attack, grooming, and consummatory behaviors evoked by electrical stimulation of cat cerebellar nuclei. Science 1973; 182:845-7.

36. Haroian AJ, Massopust LC, Young PA. Cerebellothalamic projections in the rat: an autoradiographic and degeneration study. J Comp Neurol 1981; 197:217-36.

37. Haines DE, Dietrichs E. On the organization of interconnections between the cerebellum and hypothalamus. In: King JS, ed. New concepts in cerebellar neurobiology. New York: Alan R. Liss, 1987:113-49.

38. Ryan LJ, Young SJ, Groves PM. Reticular and cerebellar stimulation mimic amphetamine actions on amplitude and timing of frontal cortex evoked neostriatal responses in rats. Abstr Soc Neurosci 1987; 13:978.

39. Ornitz EM. Neurophysiology of infantile autism. J Am Acad Child Psychiatry 1985; 24:251-62.

40. Kootz JP, Cohen DJ. Modulation of sensory intake in autistic children: cardiovascular and behavioral indices. J Am Acad Child Psychiatry 1981; 20:692-701.

41. Damasio AR, Maurer RG. A neurological model for childhood autism. Arch Neurol 1978; 35:777-86.

42. DeMyer MK, Hingtgen JN, Jackson RK. Infantile autism reviewed: a decade of research. Schizophrenia Bull 1981; 7:388-451.

43. Young JG, Cohen DJ, Shaywitz SE, et al. Assessment of brain function in clinical pediatric research: behavioral and biological strategies. Schizophrenia Bull 1982; 8:205-35.

44. Rosenzweig MR, Bennett EL, Alberti M. Multiple effects of lesions on brain structure in young rats. In: Almli CR, Finger S, eds. Early brain damage. Vol. 2. Neurobiology and behavior. New York: Academic Press, 1984:49-70.

45. Fulton JF, Dow RS. The cerebellum: a summary of functional localization. Yale J Biol Med 1937; 10:89-119.

46. Altman J. Autoradiographic and histological studies of postnatal neurogenesis. III. Dating the time of production and onset of differentiation of cerebellar microneurons in rats. J Comp Neurol 1969; 136:269-94.

47. Altman J, Bayer SA. Embryonic development of the rat cerebellum. III. Regional differences in the time of origin, migration, and settling of Purkinje cells. J Comp Neurol 1985; 231:42-65.

48. Bayer SA, Altman J. Directions in neurogenetic gradients and patterns of anatomical connections in the telencephalon. Prog Neurobiol 1987; 29:57-106.

49. Folstein S, Rutter M. Infantile autism: a genetic study of 21 twin pairs. J Child Psychol Psychiatry 1977; 18:297-321.

50. Caviness VS Jr, Rakic P. Mechanisms of cortical development: a view from mutations in mice. Annu Rev Neurosci 1978; 1:297-326.

51. Sidman RL, Green MC. "Nervous," a new mutant mouse with cerebellar disease. In: Sabourdy M, ed. Les mutants pathologiques chez l'animal, leur intérêt pour la recherche biomédicale. Paris: Editions du Centre National de la Recherche Scientifique, 1970:69-79.

52. Mullen RJ, Eicher EM, Sidman RL. Purkinje cell degeneration, a new neurological mutation in the mouse. Proc Natl Acad Sci USA 1976; 73:208-12.

53. Messer A. Cerebellar granule cells in normal and neurological mutants of mice. Adv Cell Neurobiol 1980; 1:179-207.

54. Chaves E, Frank LM. Disorders of basal ganglia, cerebellum, brain stem, and cranial nerves. In: Farmer TW, ed. Pediatric neurology. 3rd ed. Philadelphia: Harper & Row, 1983:605-48.

55. Jervis GA. Early familial cerebellar degeneration (report of three cases in one family). J Nerv Ment Dis 1950; 111:398-407.

56. Sarnat HB, Alcalá H. Human cerebellar hypoplasia: a syndrome of diverse causes. Arch Neurol 1980; 37:300-5.

NeuroReport 8, 197–201 (1996)

THE ability to attribute mental states to others ('theory of mind') pervades normal social interaction and is impaired in autistic individuals. In a previous positron emission tomography scan study of normal volunteers, performing a 'theory of mind' task was associated with activity in left medial prefrontal cortex. We used the same paradigm in five patients with Asperger syndrome, a mild variant of autism with normal intellectual functioning. No task-related activity was found in this region, but normal activity was observed in immediately adjacent areas. This result suggests that a highly circumscribed region of left medial prefrontal cortex is a crucial component of the brain system that underlies the normal understanding of other minds.

'Theory of mind' in the brain. Evidence from a PET scan study of Asperger syndrome

Francesca Happé,[1,2] Stefan Ehlers,[3] Paul Fletcher,[4] Uta Frith,[1,2] Maria Johansson,[3] Christopher Gillberg,[3] Ray Dolan,[4] Richard Frackowiak[4] and Chris Frith[2,4,CA]

[1]MRC Cognitive Development Unit, 4 Taviton Street, London WC1 0BT; [2]Psychology Department, University College London, Gower Street, London WC1E 6BT; [3]Department of Child and Adolescent Psychiatry, University of Goteborg, Sweden; [4]Wellcome Department of Cognitive Neurology, Institute of Neurology, 12 Queen Square, London WC1N 3BG, UK

Key words: Autism; Brain imaging; Brodmann area 8/9; Frontal cortex; Theory of mind

[CA,4] Corresponding Author and Address

Introduction

Theory of mind, a somewhat misleading catch phrase, is used to refer to our everyday ability to attribute mental states to ourselves and others in order to predict and explain behaviour.[1] This ability has become a focus of interest for cognitive scientists, primatologists and philosophers as well as for clinicians dealing with a puzzling mental handicap: autism.[2] Individuals with autism appear to lack the basic ability to construe behaviour in terms of mental states (mentalizing), and have marked difficulty with simple tasks requiring attribution of, for example, a false belief to a story character.[3,4] There is evidence that autism is associated with abnormal brain development,[5–7] and this has prompted the idea that there is an innate brain-based mechanism which underlies the normal development of mentalizing.[8] In addition, since some individuals with autism do well on many cognitive tasks, but still have problems in mentalizing, the brain system that is critically involved in the development of mentalizing may be relatively discreet and vulnerable to selective damage.[9]

In a previous position emission tomography (PET) scan study with normal volunteers[10] we compared the pattern of brain activity while reading stories involving complex mental states with the pattern of activation in two control tasks: reading non-mental stories and unconnected sentences. Using a subtraction technique, where we compare all three conditions, the brain region most specifically associated with mentalizing story comprehension, over and above more general story comprehension, was in the left medial prefrontal cortex, on the border between Brodmann areas 8 and 9. The same region has been identified by another group using a very different story comprehension mentalizing task.[11]

Clearly it would be informative to scan people with autism using the same task. It would be meaningless, however, to scan subjects attempting a task they cannot perform; most individuals with autism cannot think about thoughts and feelings in the way these story tasks require.[12] A small minority, however, do pass standard tests of false belief attribution. Some of these individuals, who tend to be older and more verbal than other autistic subjects[13] show remarkable success across an array of tests that involve mentalizing.[14] These individuals often receive the diagnosis of Asperger syndrome.[15] Their continuing social difficulties in everyday life and their tell-tale slips in more naturalistic mentalizing tests[16] might reflect delay in development of this cognitive component, and suggest that different processes underlie mental state attribution in these individuals.

Subjects and Methods

Subjects were five right-handed males, mean age 24 (range 20–27) years. All had been diagnosed with Asperger syndrome on the basis of developmental history and current presentation (marked social abnormality, good language in the presence of verbal and non-verbal communication difficulties, presence of circumscribed special interests, resistance to change). A history of clumsiness was present in four of the patients, but otherwise clinical examination revealed no neurological abnormalities. The mean WAIS Full Scale IQ for the group was 100 (range 87–112), the mean VIQ was 110 (93–125), mean PIQ

Table 1 Tasks used during scanning and rationale of subtraction design

Condition	Reading	Memory	Integration and inference	Mental state attribution
ToM	+	+	+	+
Phys	+	+	+	–
US	+	+	–	–

Example Mentalizing (ToM) story: A burglar who has just robbed a shop is making his getaway. As he is running home, a policeman on his beat sees him drop his glove. He doesn't know the man is a burglar, he just wants to tell him he dropped his glove. But when the policeman shouts out to the burglar, "Hey, you! Stop!", the burglar turns round, sees the policeman, and gives himself up. He puts his hands up and admits that he did the break-in at the local shop.

Q: Why did the burglar do this?

Example Physical (Phys) story: A burglar is about to break into a jewellers' shop. He skillfully picks the lock on the shop door. Carefully he crawls under the electronic detector beam. If he breaks this beam it will set off the alarm. Quietly he opens the door of the store-room and sees the gems glittering. As he reaches out, however, he steps on something soft. He hears a screech and something small and furry runs out past him towards the shop door. Immediately the alarm sounds.

Q: Why did the alarm go off?

Example Unlinked sentences (US): The four brothers stood aside to make room for their sister, Stella. Gill repeated the experiment, several times. The name of the airport has changed. Louise uncorked a little bottle of oil. The two children had to abandon their daily walk. She took a suite in a grand hotel. It was already twenty years since the operation.

Q: Did the children take their walk?

92 (83–100). Magnetic resonance imaging scans showed no evidence of gross morphological abnormalities, and all volunteers were free from epilepsy and were not currently taking any medication. The study was approved by the local hospital ethics committee, and permission to administer radioactive substances was obtained from the Advisory Committee on Radioactive Substances (ARSAC) UK.

We used exactly the same story comprehension paradigm as previously used with normal volunteers.[10] Thus there were physical stories (Phys), stories requiring mentalizing (ToM), and unconnected sentences (US). Examples of the stories are provided in table 1. The task design aimed at separating out the task demands for story integration ((ToM + Phys) US) and mental state attribution (ToM – Phys). The three types of text were presented on a computer monitor. Each of the three conditions was administered four times over the 12 scans in an ABC counterbalanced design. During each scan two stories were presented. Subjects were given practice passages before beginning, and were told before each scan which type of passage they would be shown. Subjects were required to read the passage silently and, when ready, to touch the screen. At this point the passage was removed and a question appeared which was to be answered silently.

Since the stories were Swedish, Swedish translations of the story materials were used, validated with 10 normal Swedish subjects. This validation showed results very similar to data from 60 English subjects tested on the original English versions. Scores for the three conditions were 13.5, 12.8, and 12.4 of a maximum of 16, compared with 12.9, 12.8, 12.2 in the English sample. We therefore conclude that the materials were comparable across the languages, as well as being comparable across conditions.

Scans were obtained using a CTI model 953B PET scanner (CTI, Knoxville, USA) with colimating septa retracted (FWHM 8 mm transaxial, 4 mm axial). Volunteers received a 20 s bolus of $H_2^{15}O$ (55 MBq ml^{-1}, i.v.; flow rate 10 ml min^{-1}) through a forearm cannula. The data were analysed with statistical parametric mapping (SPM95 software from the Wellcome Department of Cognitive Neurology, London) implemented in Matlab (Mathworks, Sherborne, MA). The scans from each subject were realigned using the first as a reference. As a final preprocessing step the image were smoothed using an isotropic Gaussian kernel. The condition, subject and covariate effects (global blood flow) were estimated according to the general linear model at each voxel. To test hypotheses about regionally specific condition effects, the estimates were compared using linear compounds or contrasts.[17]

saggital   coronal   saggital   coronal

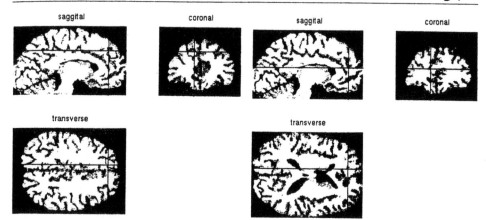

transverse   transverse

FIG. 1. The location of the peak activation in medial prefrontal cortex when theory of mind stories were compared with physical stories. Regions of significantly increased activity as measured by PET are shown superimposed on a standard MRI image that had been normalized into the stereotactic space of Tallairach & Tournoux. Saggital, coronal and horizontal views are shown. The left-hand panel shows the result for six normal volunteers. There was a significant activation on the border between Brodmann areas 8 and 9 (coordinates -12, 36, 36; Z=4.1). The right-hand panel shows the results for five volunteers with Asperger syndrome. There was no increase in activity while reading ToM stories in the area of peak activity in the normal volunteers and this difference between groups was significant. There was, however, an increase in a more inferior region of medial prefrontal cortex (coordinates; -10, 44, 16; Z=2.38).

Table 2. Performance on tasks during scanning'

Condition	Time (s)[a]	Range	Score[b]	Range
Asperger				
ToM	42.2 ± 16.4	28–67	11.4 ± 3.4	8–15
Phys	51.6 ± 23.8	28–85	11.0 ± 3.7	5–14
US	37.7 ± 11.9	25–51	12.4 ± 3.2	8–14
Normal				
ToM	33.7 ± 6.2	21–49	15.4 ± 0.4	15–16
Phys	35.0 ± 5.8	23–44	14.2 ± 0.8	13–15
US	32.2 ± 4.1	23–39	9.6 ± 3.2	6–14

[a]Harmonic mean ± s.d.
[b]Mean ± s.d.; maximum possible = 6.
Column 1 shows the average time taken to read a passage; column 3 shows the total scores obtained for answers to questions about the passages. Scores for each answer were between 0 and 2.

Table 3. Results of scanning: Areas of significant activation in patients with Asperger Syndrome

Brain region	Coordinates	z	p
ToM *vs* US			
Medial prefrontal (9/10)	2,50,20	2.86	0.002
Temporal pole (left 21)	−52,0,−16	3.09	0.001
Temporal pole (right 21)	44,−8,−16	2.74	0.003
Angular gyrus (left 22/39)	−50,−56,16	2.32	0.010
ToM *vs* Phys			
Medial prefrontal (left 9/10)	−10,44,16	2.38	0.000

Results

Table 2 shows times to read and comprehend each passage and scores for the answers to the test questions which were recorded in between scans. A score of 0 was given for answers of 'don't know' or incorrect answers, 1 for partially correct answers, and 2 for fully correct answers.

The average time taken in each condition by the individuals with Asperger syndrome was more variable but not significantly different from the time taken by the normal volunteers. Scores on ToM stories were significantly worse (F(1,9) = 10.8, $p <$ 0.01). Importantly, there were no significant differences in the scores for the other conditions. The Phys stories tended to be slightly more difficult than the ToM stories, and the patient group had slightly better scores for the unlinked sentences.

Brain regions activated in volunteers with Asperger Syndrome comparing theory of mind task with the control tasks are shown in table 3. With one exception, the same areas were significantly activated in the Asperger subjects as in the normal volunteers. The coordinates show the position for the peak activation. Differences in activation between conditions were significantly smaller in the Asperger group when compared directly with the control group. All activations were in the same location, however, taking into account the spatial resolution of PET.

The notable exception to the above concerns the medial prefrontal cortex. The area activated in the control group (area 8: xyz = -10,40,36) was not activated in the patients with Asperger, and this difference between groups was significant (z = 2.12, p < 0.02). The Asperger patients did, however, show activation of an adjacent, but more ventral area of medial prefrontal cortex, area 9/10.

Figure 1 illustrates the pattern of activation in Asperger syndrome volunteers comparing ToM and Phys conditions. For comparison the portion of area 8/9 which showed peak activation during ToM for normal controls is highlighted in red.

Discussion

The purpose of this study was to examine brain activity in relation to specific cognitive processes associated with theory of mind. We do not have a large enough sample to examine the more general abnormalities of brain structure or function found in autism in previous studies.[6] Performance on the tasks used during scanning was at a similar level for the clinical and the normal control group. The exception was the poorer performance on ToM stories among patients with Asperger syndrome, a result which is expected from the theory of mind deficit hypothesis of autism. Nevertheless it should be noted that all Asperger subjects succeeded in correctly answering most of the test questions of the mentalizing stories and read these stories faster than the physical stories.

The comparison of story reading and unlinked sentences highlights areas involved in story integration and in the drawing of inferences. In our previous study[10] the major difference between story and non-story conditions involved the temporal poles bilaterally and the left superior temporal gyrus. These same areas were also activated in the Asperger volunteers, but for this group the difference between stories and sentences was significantly less pronounced in all regions. This suggests that subjects with Asperger syndrome process meaningful connected narrative and meaningless jumbled sentences in a more similar way than do controls.

Interestingly, our Asperger subjects were at least as good as previously scanned controls with unlinked sentences, but performed slightly worse on both story conditions. These findings fit a current theory suggesting that autism is characterized by a cognitive style of weak central coherence, a failure to integrate information in context to extract higher level meaning or gist.[18] Piecemeal processing of stories, as of unlinked sentences, would be predicted by this account.

The most important comparison, between mentalizing (ToM) and non-mentalizing (Phys) stories, indi-cated a critical difference between the clinical and normal groups: the Asperger group did not show activation of the medial part of left prefrontal area 8/9 during ToM stories. A direct comparison of the groups (the group by condition interaction) confirmed that there was a significant difference in this region. These patients showed significant activation of a neighbouring area of left medial prefrontal cortex, Brodmann's area 9/10, when processing ToM stories, however. Controls also showed activation in this area, but to a far lesser extent than area 8/9. This partial overlap between the results from the two groups suggests that the Asperger subjects' mentalizing performance was subserved by a brain system in which one key component was missing.

One explanation for this abnormal pattern of activation is that the Asperger subjects were using a more general purpose reasoning mechanism in order to infer mental states. Area 9, which covers a large expanse of cortex, has been implicated in a number of brain imaging studies of problem solving and general cognitive ability.[19] The borderline portion of area 9/10, activated in the present study, has not been linked to any specific cognitive function, however. No macroscopic structural abnormalities of medial prefrontal cortex were present in the magnetic resonance imaging scans of the five Asperger volunteers, suggesting the possibility that the abnormal activation in this critical region resulted from structural damage in another part of an extended system or in microscopic abnormalities in intercellular connections. While frontal lobe dysfunction has been suggested for people with autism and Asperger syndrome,[20,21] the present findings suggest the need for more specific task analysis of executive functions and a fractionation of the possible components and brain pathways involved.

Conclusion

This study has provided further evidence for a brain location which may be a key anatomical component of the 'theory of mind' system. It will be important to replicate this result with other appropriate subject groups. Further research will also be necessary to identify the other components of the system and the precise role that each plays. Since the brain areas identified so far are not uniquely human, it should also be possible to specify the precursors and components of 'theory of mind' abilities from studies of these brain regions in animals other than man.

ACKNOWLEDGEMENT: This work was carried out at the MRC Cyclotron Unit, Hammersmith Hospital. We are extremely grateful for the use of these facilities. O.F., R.D., R.F. and C.F. are supported by the Wellcome Trust

**Received 23 August 1996;
accepted 25 September 1996**

References

1. Premack D and Woodruff G. *Behav Brain Sci* **4**, 515–516 (1978).
2. Carruthers P and Smith PK. *Theories of Theories of Mind* Cambridge: Cambridge University Press, 1996.
3. Baron-Cohen S, Leslie A and Frith U. *Cognition* **21**, 37–46 (1985).
4. Baron-Cohen S, Leslie A and Frith U. *Br J Dev Psychol* **4**, 113–125 (1986).
5. Gillberg C and Coleman M. *The Biology of the Autistic Syndromes.* London: MacKeith Press, 1992.
6. Bauman ML and Kemper TL, eds. *The Neurobiology of Autism.* Baltimore: Johns Hopkins University Press, 1994.
7. Bailey A, Phillips W and Rutter M. *J Child Psychol Psychiatry* **37**, 89–126 (1996).
8. Leslie A. *Psychol Rev* **94**, 412–126 (1987).
9. Frith U, Morton J and Leslie A. *Trends Neurosci* **14**, 433–438 (1991).
10. Fletcher P, Happé F, Frith U *et al. Cognition* **57**, 109–128 (1995).
11. Mazoyer BM, Tzourio N, Frak V *et al. J Cogn Neurosci* **5**, 467–469 (1993).
12. Happé F. *J Autism Dev Dis* **24**, 129–154 (1994).
13. Happé F. *Child Dev* **66**, 843–855 (1995).
14. Frith U, ed. *Autism and Asperger Syndrome.* Cambridge: Cambridge University Press, 1991.
15. Frith U, Happé F and Siddons F. *Soc Dev* **3**, 108–124 (1994).
16. Happé F. *Cognition* **48**, 101–119 (1993).
17. Friston KJ, Worsley K, Frackowiak RSJ *et al. Hum Brain Mapp* **1**, 214–220 (1994).
18. Frith U and Happé F. *Cognition* **50**, 115–132 (1994).
19. Dolan RJ, Bench CJ, Brown RG *et al. J Neurol Neurosurg Psychiat* **55**, 768–773 (1992).
20. Ozonoff S, Pennington BF and Rogers SJ. *J Child Psychol Psychiat* **32**, 1081–1106 (1996).
21. Hughes C, Russell J and Robbins TW. *Neuropsychologia* **32**, 477–492 (1994).

207

Journal of Neuropathology and Experimental Neurology
Copyright © 1998 by the American Association of Neuropathologists

Vol. 57, No. 7
July, 1998
pp. 645–652

Neuropathology of Infantile Autism

THOMAS L. KEMPER, MD, AND MARGARET BAUMAN, MD

Key Words: Autism; Cerebellar cortex; Cerebellar nuclei; Limbic system; Memory disorders; Mental retardation.

INTRODUCTION

Infantile autism, a behaviorally defined disorder initially described by Kanner (1), is a syndrome which, by definition, is manifested by 36 months of age and is characterized by disordered language and cognitive skills, impaired social interactions, abnormal responses to sensory stimuli, events and objects, poor eye contact, an insistence on sameness, an unusual capacity for rote memorization, repetitive and stereotypic behavior, and a normal physical appearance (2). Disturbances in elementary motor function, when present, are subtle and motor milestones are usually normal (see 3 for review). The prevalence rates are estimated to be 10–13 per 10,000, and the disorder is more commonly seen in boys than in girls, with a ratio of 2.5–4.0:1 (4–6).

Based on the clinical features of the disorder, a number of possible sites of brain abnormality in autism have been hypothesized. Early investigators speculated on the involvement of the limbic system (7), medial temporal lobe (8–11), thalamus (12), basal ganglia (13), and vestibular system (14). A few Magnetic Resonance Imaging (MRI) studies have reported abnormalities of the cerebellar vermis, but the results have not been uniformly replicated (see 15 for review). Imaging studies have also yielded variable observations in regard to brainstem size and structure (16–19). Although an early pneumoencephalographic study (20) reported abnormalities in the region of the medial temporal lobe, subsequent Computerized Tomographic (CT) and MRI investigations have failed to demonstrate definitive findings in this region (6, 21–23). Initial studies using Positron Emission Tomography (PET) suggested a dysfunction of the frontal and parietal lobes, thalamus, caudate nucleus, lenticular nucleus, and insula in adult autistic subjects (24), and using ³¹P NMR spectroscopy, suggested involvement of the dorsal prefrontal cortex (25). More recent PET investigations have observed reduced volume and metabolic activity in the right anterior cingulate gyrus in 7 high-functioning autistic adults (26), and abnormalities of serotonin synthesis in the dentatothalamicortical pathway in 7 autistic boys

From the Departments of Pathology, Anatomy and Neurobiology, and Neurology, Boston University School of Medicine, Boston, Mass (TLK), and the Department of Neurology, Harvard Medical School, Boston, Mass (MB).

Send correspondence to: Thomas L. Kemper, MD, Department of Anatomy and Neurobiology, Boston University School of Medicine, 80 E. Concord Street, Boston, MA 02118.

(27). Using ³¹P NMR spectroscopy in a study of 11 adolescent and adult autistic males, Minshew et al (25) noted involvement of the dorsal prefrontal cortex, which was unrelated to age or IQ (25). Regional blood flow studies have also implicated frontal lobe involvement, with the findings suggesting a delay in maturation in this area (28). In addition to studies highlighting regional differences, there is evidence from both imaging and pathological investigations suggesting that the brain of autistic individuals may be generally enlarged for age and sex (16, 29, 30). Piven et al (16) have observed that there may be some regional selectivity of brain enlargement with relative sparing of the frontal lobe as well as reduced size of the posterior part of the corpus callosum relative to the total brain size.

Relatively few neuropathological studies have been performed on autistic subjects. Early investigations include Aarkrog's (31) report of a "slight thickening of the arterioles, slight connective tissue increase in the leptomeninges and some cell increase" in a frontal lobe biopsy, and the report of Williams et al (32) indicating a lack of a consistent pathology in the hippocampus, parahippocampal gyrus, thalamus, hypothalamus, striatum, and midbrain tectum from 4 individuals with autistic behavior. Ritvo et al (33) has reported a decrease in the number of Purkinje cells in the vermis and hemispheres of the cerebellum. Coleman et al (34) counted neuronal and glial cells in multiple cortical regions of an autistic brain and in 2 age- and sex-matched controls and found no differences. However, examination of the brainstem from this same patient showed a marked reduction in the number of neurons in the facial nucleus and superior olive, as well as shortening of the brainstem between the trapezoid body and the inferior olive (35). The authors suggested that these findings could indicate that the brain abnormalities associated with autism might have their onset around the time of neural tube closure. In a recent autopsy study, Guerin et al (36) reported slight thickening of the meninges, mild ventricular dilatation, thinning of the corpus callosum, scattered perivascular lymphocyte infiltrates, and a few microglial nodules in the lower brainstem in the brain of a 16-year-old autistic boy with mental retardation.

Our own systematic surveys of the whole brain serial sections of 9 autistic brains and comparable controls have shown selective abnormalities in the forebrain limbic system and in the cerebellum and in its related inferior olive

209

in the brainstem, as well as evidence for a pathological process that extends from the period of fetal development into adulthood. Six of these brains were midsagittally cut, with one hemisphere available for the histological studies. The autistic brains were systematically compared with identically processed age- and sex-matched controls using a comparison microscope in which corresponding areas of the brain were viewed side by side in the same field of view at the same magnification. In areas in which consistent abnormalities were found, quantitative and semiquantitative analysis was performed (37–39). The findings in these brains will be reviewed in relationship to the anatomy of the affected regions, the clinical manifestations of infantile autism, and reported observations using in vivo imaging techniques.

Brain Size and Configuration

Brain weight is available for 19 autistic individuals. Eight of the 11 brains from individuals less than 12 years of age showed a significant increase in weight ås compared with controls. This is in contrast to those of 6 of 8 individuals older than 18 years of age, where brain weight was less than expected (40), but the differences did not reach statistical significance.

Neocortex

No abnormality has been noted in the external configuration of the cerebral cortex. With the comparison microscopic examination, 8 of the 9 brains have shown unusually small and more closely packed neurons and less distinct laminar architecture in the anterior cingulate gyrus; in 1 brain there was a minor malformation of the orbitofrontal cortex in 1 hemisphere. The remainder of the cerebral cortex appeared unremarkable.

Allocortex and Subcortical Forebrain Areas

Systematic survey of the forebrain has shown no abnormalities in the striatum, pallidum, thalamus, hypothalamus, basal forebrain, bed nucleus of the stria terminalis, or in myelination. In all 9 brains, the forebrain abnormalities were confined to the limbic system. The neurons in the hippocampal fields CA1–4, subiculum, entorhinal cortex, mammillary body, amygdala, and medial septal nucleus were unusually small and more densely distributed than in age- and sex-matched controls. With the Golgi method for the demonstration of neuronal processes, the neurons in CA1 and CA4 showed reduced complexity and extent of their dendritic arbors (41). In the amygdala, small neuronal size and increased cell packing density were most pronounced medially in the cortical, medial, and central nuclei, whereas the lateral nucleus appeared to be comparable to controls in 8 of the 9 brains. The basolateral complex of the amygdala showed an intermediate degree of involvement. The single exception to this pattern of involvement of the amyg-

dala was observed in a 12-year-old autistic boy with normal intelligence and significant behavior problems. In this brain the entire amygdala was diffusely abnormal.

Similar to the findings noted in the hippocampus and amygdala, the neurons of the medial septal nucleus also demonstrated reduced cell size and increase cell packing density in all brains. However, the adjacent nucleus of the vertical limb of the diagonal band of Broca showed unusually large, plentiful, but otherwise normal-appearing neurons in all autistic subjects less than 12 years of age. In contrast, these same neurons were noted to be small and markedly reduced in number in all of the autistic patients older than 18 years of age (42). Details of the relative degree of involvement of the hippocampal fields, entorhinal cortex, mammillary body, septum, and amygdala in 6 of the 9 autistic brains is presented in the paper by Bauman and Kemper (38).

Cerebellum and Brainstem

Midsagittal photographs of 11 autistic brains, in which the vermis was cut in the midline, show a variable pattern in the size of the lobules of the vermis and widening of the cerebellar folia in several of the brains (Figure 1). On microscopic examination of the cerebellum, all 9 brains showed a variable reduction in the number of Purkinje cells, and in a few of the brains, pallor of the granule cell layer. Reduced numbers of Purkinje cells were noted, predominantly in the posterolateral neocerebellar cortex and adjacent archicerebellar cortex, while the vermis was spared (43, 44). The extent of this decrease in the number of Purkinje cells was not related to the age or functional level of the patient and there has been no evidence of the reactive gliosis usually seen following Purkinje cell loss in childhood or at older ages. Similar to the findings noted in the neurons in the nucleus of the diagonal band of Broca, the neurons in the globose, emboliform, and fastigial cerebellar nuclei appear to differ with age. In all of the younger autistic brains, these neurons were enlarged in size and present in adequate numbers, and in brains of all the autistic subjects older than 22 years, the neurons were pale and reduced in number. The neurons in the dentate nucleus were enlarged in the brains of younger autistic individuals without the later atrophy and cell loss noted in the other cerebellar nuclei (42). In the brainstem, the only abnormality noted was found in the inferior olive, a change that occurred in the part of the olive that projects to the cerebellar cortex with the most marked decrease in the number of Purkinje cells (45). The neurons in this part of the inferior olive in all of the younger brains were enlarged but otherwise normal in appearance and number. In subjects older than 22 years, these same neurons were present in adequate numbers, but were abnormally small and pale. In all of the autistic brains, some of the neurons of the inferior olivary nucleus tended to cluster at the periphery of the inferior con-

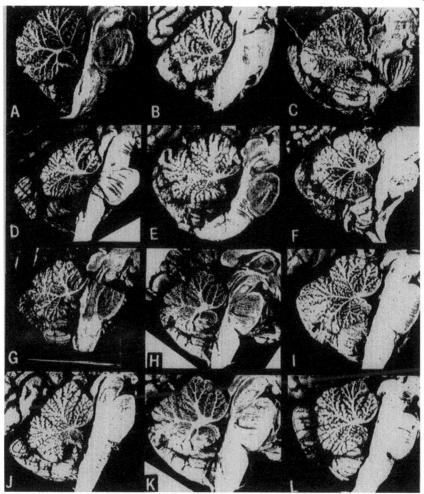

Fig. 1. Identically enlarged photographs of the midsagittal sections of a control 30-year-old male brain (at A) and 11 brains of autistic individuals at 6 years (at B), 8 years (at C), 10 years (at D), 19 years (at E), 20 years (at F), 21 years (at G), 28 years (at H), 35 years (at I), and 54 years of age (at J). In K and L, the brains of autistic individuals with Asperger's syndrome and normal intelligence are shown. The arrows indicate the location of the fissura prima (upper arrow) and fissura praepyramidalis (lower arrow), which divide the vermis into an anterior lobule (lobules I–V), lobules VI and VII, and the posterior vermal lobules VII–X. Note the variability of the size of the different lobules in the autistic brains with a lack of a consistent pattern and the widening of the spaces between the folia of the different lobules in several of the brains (B, D, E, and J).

J Neuropathol Exp Neurol, Vol 57, July, 1998

211

volutions. In 1 brain there was a widened fourth ventricle with a corresponding thinning and elongation of the superior cerebellar peduncle (37).

Nature of the Pathological Changes

There are 3 different neuropathologies in these brains: a curtailment of the normal development of neurons in the forebrain limbic system; an apparent congenital decrease in the number of Purkinje cells; and age-related changes in cell size and number of neurons in the nucleus of the diagonal band of Broca, in the cerebellar nuclei, and in the inferior olive.

The small, densely distributed neurons in the limbic system in the brains of these autistic individuals would be an expected finding during an earlier stage of maturation, a time at which neuronal size and the complexity of the neuropil has not reach adult proportions. In this sense, these changes in the limbic system can be characterized as a curtailment of normal maturation. A curtailment of maturation is the most common finding in the brain of individuals with mental retardation, with the most striking changes occurring in the cerebral cortex (46). This is the neuronal substrate with the most prolonged period of maturation (47). In the autistic individuals, this pattern is different than that found in mental retardation, inasmuch as it appears to be confined to the limbic system, a neuronal substrate with cycles of maturation shorter than that of the cerebral cortex (60).

The decrease in the number of cells in the cerebellar cortex appears to be a congenital lesion. This hypothesis is supported by 2 observations. First, the decrease in cell number occurs without the expected gliosis, suggesting that these abnormalities were acquired early in development. Second, there is a failure of the occurrence of retrograde atrophy in the inferior olivary neurons. Loss of neurons in this nucleus has been regularly observed following cerebellar lesions in the immature postnatal and adult animal (62) and in neonatal and adult humans (45, 48, 49). The occurrence of the retrograde olivary cell loss is believed to be secondary to the tight relationship of the olivary climbing fiber axons to the Purkinje cell dendrites (50). In the fetal monkey, it has been shown that the olivary climbing fibers from the inferior olive initially synapse in a transitory zone located beneath the Purkinje cell, a layer called the lamina dissecans (51). Since this zone is no longer evident in the human fetus after 30 weeks of gestation (52), it is likely that the cerebellar cortical lesion, if it were due to Purkinje cell loss, occurred at or before this time. Another possible explanation for the lack of loss of inferior olivary neurons in these brains is that, rather than a loss of Purkinje cells, there may have been fewer of these cells present from the beginning.

The age-related changes in the neurons of the diagonal band of Broca, in the cerebellar nuclei, and in the inferior

olive are an unusual neuropathology. In the autistic brains, this appears to be a prolonged process that extends from neuronal hypertrophy in childhood to atrophy and, in some of these nuclei, to cell loss in later adult life. As an acute event, neuronal swelling is known to follow transection of an axon (axonal reaction), and is then followed by atrophy and cell loss. Cell swelling followed by atrophy is also known as an anterograde transneuronal event in the inferior olive following lesions of the central tegmental tract or dentate nucleus (53). Thus, the swelling followed by atrophy of some neurons in these autistic brains suggests a disturbance in the synaptic relationships of these nuclei. These hypertrophic and atrophic changes are most marked in the cerebellar circuits in the autistic brains, and occur in association with an apparent congenital decrease in the number of neurons in the cerebellar cortex. The cerebellar nuclear changes appear to be topographically largely independent of the cerebellar cortical changes. The cerebellar nuclear pathology is most marked in the fastigial, globose, and emboliform nuclei, nuclei that receive Purkinje cell projections from the histologically best-preserved cortical areas of the vermis, and paramedian lobes of the cerebellar cortex. The least involved cerebellar nucleus, the dentate, receives its Purkinje cell projection from the most involved cortical area, the lateral lobes of the cerebellum. We have speculated elsewhere (39) that the age-related changes in the cerebellar nuclei may also be understood as a disturbance of the prenatal development of their circuitry, with a timing of the onset of this abnormality similar to that noted for the establishment of the definitive olivocerebellar circuit. At the stage in cerebellar development during which the olivocerebellar fibers are confined to the lamina dissecans, there is already advanced myelination in the olivocerebellar tracts in the inferior cerebellar peduncle. At this stage of development, the myelinated fibers extend to the cerebellar nucleus, but not to the cerebellar cortex, suggesting that a functional circuit between these 2 areas already exists at this time. An abnormality that has an impact on the intimate relationship between the Purkinje cells and the inferior olivary nucleus at this stage or at a later stage of fetal development might favor the persistence of this fetal circuit over the definitive, postnatal olivocerebellar cortical circuit. An abnormal retention of this fetal circuit might account for the presence of "compensatory" postnatal neuronal enlargement of the neurons in the cerebellar nuclei and inferior olive. Since this proposed fetal circuit was not "programmed" to function as the dominant postnatal pathway, it is possible that it will eventually lead to atrophy and loss of neurons in the older autistic individuals. By analogy, the hypertrophy and atrophy of neurons in the nucleus of the vertical limb of the diagonal band of Broca may also be related to a persistence of an abnormal circuit between this nucleus and the heavily involved hippocampal complex.

Relationship to Clinical and Other Features of Infantile Autism

The abnormalities in the anterior cingulate gyrus, hippocampus, subiculum, entorhinal cortex, and mammillary body are in an interrelated forebrain circuit proposed by Papez as a substrate for memory and emotion (54), and in the closely related septal nuclei and amygdala. Experimental lesions in these regions have produced deficits in these and other behaviors, many of which resemble those seen in childhood autism. Hyperactivity, impaired social interaction, hyperexploratory behavior, and the inability to recognize or remember the significance of visually or manually examined objects have been observed following bilateral medial temporal lobe ablations in monkeys (55) and in similar neurosurgical lesions in humans (56). Bilateral removal of the amygdala in monkeys has resulted in indiscriminate examination of objects, loss of fear to normally aversive stimuli, withdrawal from previously rewarding social interactions, poor adaptability to novel situations, and reduced ability to attach meaning to a specific situation based on past experience (57). Murray and Mishkin (58) have also shown that bilateral ablations of the amygdala result in a severe impairment of cross-modal associative memory, suggesting that the amygdala may be important for the integration and generalization of modality specific information by multiple sensory systems in the brain, a task which is frequently difficult for autistic individuals. The strongest support for a role of an early acquired lesion in the amygdala, hippocampus, and adjacent cerebral cortex for the behavioral manifestations of autism is provided by Bachevalier and Merjanian (59). These investigators found striking autistic behavior following bilateral ablation of the amygdala and hippocampus in neonatal monkeys. In a later study, Malkova et al (60) found that the socioemotional behavioral deficits in these monkeys increased with age and remained a profound deficit into adulthood. In contrast, comparable lesions placed in adult monkeys resulted in only a relatively mild deficit in this behavior.

In the forebrain, 2 different memory systems have been recognized. One is declarative or explicit memory that is associated with a rapid, one-trial learning that links different kinds of memories and experiences into "cognitive learning." The other is habit or procedural memory that is not accessible to conscious recollection and is acquired by repeated presentation of the same stimulus (61, 62). Habitual memory is believed to be mediated by the striatum and cerebral cortex (61), areas almost entirely spared in these autistic brains. In contrast, the limbic area abnormalities are in a position to disrupt explicit memory. Although early studies have emphasized the combined role of bilateral lesions in the hippocampus and amygdala for the disruption of declarative memory (63, 64), more recent studies have focused on role of the hippocampus

and entorhinal cortex in this function. In man (65) and in nonhuman primates (66), lesions confined to area CA1 of the hippocampus have been shown to produce declarative memory deficits. Further, in recent monkey experiments, Meunier et al (89) have emphasized the importance of selective lesions in the rhinal cortices (entorhinal and adjacent perirhinal area) in the disruption of these memory processes. All of these areas have been found to be consistently involved in the brain of autistic individuals. Habit or procedural learning appears to be already well developed shortly after birth in both monkeys and humans, whereas explicit memory is more slow to mature (62, 68). While the effect of an early disturbance to the limbic system structures is unknown, it is likely that prenatally acquired lesions in these regions could disrupt or distort the acquisition and interpretation of information. Such a disturbance in information processing could lead to the disordered cognition, language, and social interaction associated with autism. In contrast, the preservation of the habit memory system could account for the need for sameness, preoccupation with a narrow range of interests and activities, and for the unusual capacity for rote memorization observed in some autistic individuals. Further, since there is evidence that representational memory in humans is normally acquired some time after birth, it is possible that a developmental abnormality in this limbic system memory circuit could become clinically evident after birth, accounting for what appears to be a deterioration in social, language, and cognitive abilities, features frequently reported to be part of the early history of childhood autism.

It is also possible that the cerebral cortical abnormalities seen in infantile autism with PET scans (24), ^{31}P NMR spectroscopy (25), or regional blood flow studies (28) could be secondary to the pathological changes in the limbic system, since area CA1 of the hippocampus, the subiculum, the entorhinal cortex, and the amygdala all have substantial afferent and efferent cortical connections (69–70). The one area where there is agreement between imaging studies and pathology is in the cingulate gyrus. In this location Hazendar et al (26) have noted that the right anterior cingulate gyrus appears to be smaller and metabolically less active than in controls.

The relationship of the cerebellar findings to those in the forebrain and to the clinical features of autism are less obvious. Congenital abnormalities of the cerebellum are associated with few if any neurological symptoms (48). Studies in animals have demonstrated the existence of a direct pathway between the fastigial nucleus and the amygdala and septal nuclei, and a reciprocal circuitry between this nucleus and the hippocampus, suggesting that the cerebellum may play a role in the regulation of emotion and higher cortical thought (72, 73).

Recent studies have suggested that the cerebellum may play a role in the perception and control of timing involving both motor and sensory systems (74), that it may be important in mental imagery and anticipatory planning (75), and that it is involved in some aspects of language processing (76). Further, the cerebellum has been implicated in the control of attention, particularly the voluntary shift of selective attention between different sensory modalities (77, 78). It has also been suggested that the cerebellum may play a role in cognitive planning, a function which is independent of memory and which is most significant in novel situations (79). In addition to these functions, the cerebellum also appears to play a role in the regulation of the speed, consistency, and appropriateness of mental and cognitive processes, as well as in the control and integration of motor and sensory information and activity (80). Studies in humans with cerebellar lesions (81) have shown that the cerebellum plays a role in the acquisition of classical conditioned reflex responses.

CONCLUSIONS

At this point, our knowledge of the anatomy of autism is primarily descriptive. The available anatomical evidence indicates that the neuropathology of infantile autism has its origins in the prenatal development of the brain, with an ongoing pathological process that continues into adult life. The consistent abnormalities in the limbic forebrain, although subtle and evident only after comparisons with appropriate controls, have provided the strongest correlation with the clinical features of the disorder. In contrast, the relationship of the more conspicuous neuropathology in the cerebellum to the syndrome of infantile autism has provided an ongoing challenge. Further complicating the clinical correlation of the cerebellar cortical findings to the clinical features of this disorder has been the inconsistencies noted on imaging studies and in gross pathology. We anticipate with interest the results of future studies with more modern techniques and, hopefully, with the development of an appropriate animal model.

REFERENCES

1. Kanner L. Autistic disturbances of affective contact. Nervous Child 1943;2:217–50
2. Diagnostic and Statistical Manual of Mental Disorders, ed 4. Washington, DC: American Psychiatric Association, 1994
3. Bauman ML. Motor dysfunction in autism. In: Joseph AB, Young R, eds. Movement disorders in neurology and neuropsychiatry. Malden, MA: Blackwell Scientific. Forthcoming.
4. Bryson SE, Clark BS, Smith IM. First report of a Canadian epidemiological study of autistic syndromes. J Child Psychol Psychiatry 1988;29:433–45
5. Tanoue Y, Oda S, Asano F, Kawashima K. Epidemiology of infantile autism in southern Ibaraki, Japan: Differences in prevalence in birth cohorts. J Aut Dev Disord 1988;18:155–66
6. Gillberg C, Svendsen P. Childhood psychosis and computed tomographic brain scan findings. J Autism Dev Disord 1983;13:19–32

7. Darby JH. Neuropathological aspects of psychosis in childhood. J Autism Childhood Schizophrenia 1976;6:339–52
8. Boucher J, Warrington EK. Memory deficits in early infantile autism: Some similarities to the amnestic syndrome. Br J Psychol 1976;67:73–87
9. Delong GR. A neuropsychological interpretation of infantile autism. In: Rutter M, Schopler E, eds. Autism. New York: Plenum Press, 1978:207–18
10. Damasio AR, Maurer RG. A neurological model for childhood autism. Arch Neurol 1978;35:777–86
11. Maurer RG, Damasio AR. Childhood autism from the point of view of behavioral neurology. J Aut Dev Disord 1982;12:195–205
12. Coleman M. Studies of the autistic syndromes. In: Katzman R, ed. Congenital and acquired cognitive disorders. New York: Raven Press, 1979:265–303
13. Vilensky JA, Damasio AR, Maurer RG. Gait disturbances in patients with autistic behavior. Arch Neurol 1981;38:646–49
14. Ornitz EM, Ritvo ER. Neurophysiologic mechanisms underlying perceptual inconsistency in autistic and schizophrenic children. Arch Gen Psychiatry 1986;19:22–27
15. Bauman ML, Filipek PA, Kemper TL. Early infantile autism. Int Rev Neurobiol 1997;41:367–86
16. Piven J, Bailey BS, Ranson BJ, Arndt S. An MRI Study of the corpus callosum in autism. Am J Psychiatry 1997;154:1051–56
17. Gaffney GR, Kuperman S, Tsai LY, Minchin S. Morphological evidence for brain stem involvement in infantile autism. Biol Psychiatry 1988;24:578–86
18. Hsu M, Yeung-Courchesne R, Courchesne E, Press GA. Absence of pontine abnormality in infantile autism. Arch Neurol 1991;48: 1160–63
19. Hashimoto T, Tayama M, Murakawa K, Yoshimoto T, Miyazaki M, Harada M, Kuroda Y. Development of the brainstem and cerebellum in autistic patients. J Autism Dev Disord 1995;25:1–18
20. Hauser SL, Delong GR, Rosman NP. Pneumographic findings in the infantile autism syndrome. Brain 1975;98:667–88
21. Hier DB, LeMay M, Rosenberger PB. Autism and unfavorable left-right asymmetries of the brain. J Aut Dev Disord 1979;9:153–59
22. Creasey H, Rumsey JM, Schwartz M, Duara R, Rapoport JL, Rapoport SI. Brain morphometry in autistic men as measured by volumetric computed tomography. Arch Neurol 1986;43:669–72
23. Saitoh O, Courchesne E, Egaas B, Lincoln AJ, Schreibman L. Cross-sectional area of the posterior hippocampus in autistic patients with cerebellar and corpus callosum abnormalities. Neurology 1995;45:317–24
24. Horwitz B, Rumsey JM, Grady CL, Rapoport SI. The cerebral metabolic landscape in autism. Arch Neurol 1988;45:749–55
25. Minshew NJ, Goldstein G, Dombrowski SM, Panchalingam K, Pettegrew JW. A preliminary 31P MRS study of autism: Evidence for undersynthesis and increased degradation of brain membranes. Biol Psychiatry 1993;33:762–73
26. Haznedar MM, Buchsbaum MS, Metzger M, Solimando A, Spiegel-Cohen J, Hollander E. Anterior cingulate gyrus volume and glucose metabolism in autistic disorder. Am J Psychiatry 1997;154: 1047–50
27. Chugani DC, Muzik O, Rothermel R, Behen M, Chakraborty P, Mangner T, da Silva EA, Chugani HT. Altered serotonin synthesis in the dentatothalamocortical pathway in autistic boys. Ann Neurol 1997;42:666–69
28. Zilbovicius M, Garreau B, Samson Y, Remy P, Barthelemy C, Syrota A, Lelord G. Delayed maturation of the frontal cortex in childhood autism. Am J Psychiatry 1995;152:248–52
29. Piven J, Arndt S, Bailey J, Andreasen N. Regional brain enlargement in autism: A magnetic resonance imaging study. J Am Acad Child Adolesc Psychiatry 1996;35:530–36
30. Bailey A, Luthert P, Bolton P, LeCouteur A, Rutter M. Autism and megalencephaly. Lancet 1993;34:1225–26

31. Aarkrog T. Organic factors in infantile psychosis and borderline psychosis. Retrospective study of 45 cases subjected to pneumoencephalography. Dan Med Bull 1968;15:283–88

32. Williams RS, Hauser SL, Purpura DP, Delong GR, Swisher CN. Autism and mental retardation. Arch Neurol 1980;37:749–53

33. Ritvo ER, Freeman BJ, Scheibel AB, Duong T, Robinson H, Guthrie D, Ritvo A. Lower Purkinje cell counts in the cerebella of four autistic subjects: Initial findings of the UCLA-NSAC autopsy research report. Amer J Psychiatry 1986;146:862–66

34. Coleman PD, Romano J, Lapham L, Simon W. Cell counts in cerebral cortex of an autistic patient. J Autism Dev Disord 1985;15: 245–45

35. Rodier PM, Ingram JL, Tisdale B, Nelson S, Roman J. Embryological origins for autism: Developmental anomalies of the cranial nerve nuclei. J Comp Neurol 1996;370:247–61

36. Guerin P, Lyon G, Barthelemy C, Sostak E, Chevrollier V, Garreau B, Lelord G. Neuropathological study of a case of autistic syndrome with severe mental retardation. Dev Med Child Neurol 1996;38: 203–11

37. Bauman ML, Kemper TL. Histoanatomic observations of the brain in early infantile autism. Neurology 1985;35:866–74

38. Bauman ML, Kemper TL. Neuroanatomic observations of the brain in autism. In: Bauman ML, Kemper TL, eds. The neurobiology of autism. Baltimore: Johns Hopkins University Press, 1994:119–45

39. Kemper TL, Bauman ML. The contribution of neuropathological studies to the understanding of autism. Behav Neurol 1993;11:175–87

40. Dekaban AS, Sadowsky BS. Changes in brain weights during the span of human life: Relation of brain weights to body heights and body weights. Ann Neurol 1978;4:345–56

41. Raymond GV, Bauman ML, Kemper TL. Hippocampus in autism: A Golgi analysis. Acta Neuropathol 1996;91:117–19

42. Bauman ML, Kemper TL. Neuroanatomical observations of the brain in autism. In: Panksepp J, ed. Advances in biological psychiatry. New York: JAI Press, 1995:1–26

43. Arin DM, Bauman ML, Kemper TL. The distribution of Purkinje cell loss in the cerebellum in autism (abstract). Neurol 1991;41:307

44. Bauman ML, Kemper TL. Observations on the Purkinje cells in the cerebellar vermis in autism (abstract). J Neuropathol Exp Neurol 1996;55:613

45. Holmes G, Stewart TG. On the connection of the inferior olives with the cerebellum in man. Brain 1908;31:125–37

46. Hammarberg C. Studien über Klinik und Pathologie der Idiotie nebst Untersuchungen über die normale Anatomie der Hirnrinde. Upsula: Nova Acta Regiae Soc Sci Upsula III/17, 1898:1–126

47. Yakovlev PI, Lecours A-R. The myelogenetic cycles of regional maturation of the brain in early life. In: Minkowsi A, ed. Regional development of the brain in early life. Oxford and Edenburgh: Blackwell Scientific Publications, 1964:3–70

48. Norman RM. Cerebellar atrophy associated with etat marbre of the basal ganglia. J Neurol Psychiatry 1940;3:311–18

49. Greenfield JG. The Spino-cerebellar degenerations. Springfield: Charles C. Thomas, 1954:1–126

50. Eccles JC, Ito M, Szentagothai J. The cerebellum as a neuronal machine. New York: Springer, 1967:1–335

51. Rakic P. Neuron-glia relationship during granule cell migration in developing cerebellar cortex. A Golgi and electron microscopic study in macacus rhesus. J Comp Neurol 1971;141:283–312

52. Rakic P, Sidman RL. Histogenesis of cortical layers in human cerebellum particularly the lamina dissecans. J Comp Neurol 1970; 139:473–500

53. Gautier JC, Blackwood W. Enlargement of the inferior olivary nucleus in association with lesions of the central tegmental tract or dentate nucleus. Brain 1961;84:241–64

54. Papez JW. A proposed mechanism of emotion. Arch Neurol Psychiatry 1937;38:725–43

55. Kluver H, Bucy P. Preliminary analysis of functions of the temporal lobes in monkeys. Arch Neurol Psychiatry 1939;42:979–1000

56. Terzian H, Delle-Ore G. Syndrome of Kluver and Bucy reproduced in man by bilateral removal of the temporal lobes. Neurology 1955; 3:373–80

57. Mishkin M, Aggleton JP. Multiple functional contributors of the amygdala in the monkey from the amygdaloid complex. In: Ben-Ari Y, ed. INSERM Symposium, no. 20. Amsterdam: Elsevier North Holland Medical Press, 1981:409–19

58. Murray EA, Mishkin M. Amygdaloidectomy impairs crossmodal association in monkeys. Science 1985;228:604–6

59. Bachevalier J, Merjanian PM. The contribution of medial temporal lobe structures in infantile autism: A neurobehavioral study in primates. In: Bauman ML, Kemper TL, eds. The neurobiology of autism. Baltimore: Johns Hopkins University Press, 1994:146–69

60. Malkova L, Mishkin M, Suomi SJ, Bachevalier J. Socioemotional behavior in adult rhesus monkeys after early versus late lesions of the medial temporal lobe. Ann New York Acad Sci 1977;807:538–40

61. Mishkin M, Appenzeller T. The anatomy of memory. Sci Am 1987; 256:80–89

62. Bachevalier J. Ontogenetic development of habit and memory formation in primates. Ann New York Acad Sci 1990; 608:457–77

63. Mishkin M. Memory in monkeys is severely impaired by combined but not by separate removal of amygdala and hippocampus. Nature 1978;273:297–98

64. Mahut H, Zola-Morgan S, Moss M. Hippocampal resections impair associative learning and recognition memory in the monkey. J Neurosci 1982;2:1214–29

65. Zola-Morgan S, Squire LR, Amaral DG. Human amnesia and the medial temporal region: Enduring memory impairment following bilateral lesions limited to field CA1 of the hippocampus. J Neurosci 1986;6:2950–67

66. Alvarez P, Zola-Morgan S, Squire LR. Damage limited to the hippocampal region produces long-lasting memory impairment in monkeys. J Neurosci 1995;15:3796–807

67. Meunier M, Bachevalier J, Mishkin M, Murray EA. Effects on visual recognition of combined and separate ablations of the entorhinal and perirhinal cortex in rhesus monkeys. J Neurosci 1993; 13:5418–32

68. Overman W, Bachevalier J, Turner M, Peuster A. Object recognition versus object discrimination: Comparison between human infants and infant monkeys. Behav Neurosci 1992;106:15–29

69. Rosene DL, Van Hoesen GW. The hippocampal formation of the primate brain. A review of some comparative aspects of cytoarchitecture and connections. In: Jones EG, Peters A, eds. Cerebral Cortex, Vol. 6. New York and London: Plenum Press, 1987:345–456

70. Amaral DG, Price JL, Pitkänen A, Carmichael ST. Anatomical organization of the primate amygdala complex. In: Aggleton JP, ed. The amygdala: Neurobiological aspects of emotion, memory and mental dysfunction. New York: Wiley-Liss and Sons, 1992:1–66

71. Blatt GJ, Rosene DL. Organization of direct hippocampal efferent projections to the cerebral cortex of the rhesus monkey: Projections from CA1, prosubiculum, and subiculum to the temporal lobe. J Comp Neurol 1998;392:92–114

72. Heath RG, Harper JW. Ascending projections of the cerebellar fastigial nucleus to the hippocampus, amygdala and other temporal lobe sites; evoked potential, and histological studies in monkeys and cats. Exp Neurol 1974;45:268–87

73. Heath RG, Dempsey CW, Fontana CJ, Myers WA. Cerebellar stimulation: Effects on septal region, hippocampus and amygdala of cats and rats. Biol Psychiatry 1978;113:501–29

74. Keele SW, Ivry R. Does the cerebellum provide a common computation for diverse tasks? A timing hypothesis. Ann NY Acad Sci 1990;608:179–207

75. Leiner HC, Leiner AL, Dow RS. Cerebrocerebellar learning loops in apes and humans. Ital J Neurol Sci 1987;8:425–36

215

76. Peterson SF, Fox PT, Posner MI, Mintum MA, Raichle ME. Positron emission tomographic studies in processing of single words. J Cog Neurosci 1989;1:153–70
77. Courchesne E, Akshoomoff NA, Townsend J. Recent advances in autism. In: Naruse H, Ornitz EM, eds. Neurobiology of infantile autism. Amsterdam, London, New York, Tokyo: Excerpta Medica, 1992:111–28
78. Akshoomoff NA, Courchesne E. A new role for the cerebellum in cognitive operations. Behav Neurosci 1992;106:731–38
79. Grafman J, Litvan I, Massaquoi S, Stewart M, Sirigu A, Hallett M. Cognitive planning deficit in patients with cerebellar atrophy. Neurology 1992;42:1493–96
80. Schmahmann JD. An emerging concept. The cerebellar contribution to higher function. Arch Neurol 1991;48:1178–87
81. Brancha V, Zhao L, Wunderlich DA, Morrissy SJ, Bloedel JR. Patients with cerebellar lesions cannot acquire but are able to retain conditioned eyeblink reflexes. Brain 1997;120:1401–13

Received March 11, 1998
Revision received April 3, 1998
Accepted April 6, 1998

216

Neuron, Vol. 28, 355–363, November, 2000, Copyright ©2000 by Cell Press

Autism Spectrum Disorders

Review

Catherine Lord,*‡ Edwin H. Cook,*
Bennett L. Leventhal,* and David G. Amaral†
*Department of Psychiatry
The University of Chicago
5841 South Maryland Avenue
Chicago, Illinois 60637
†Department of Psychiatry
Center for Neuroscience and
  the M.I.N.D. Institute
University of California
Davis, California 95616

Autism is a neurodevelopmental syndrome that is defined by deficits in social reciprocity and communication, and by unusual restricted, repetitive behaviors (American Psychiatric Association, 2000). Autism is a disorder that usually begins in infancy, at the latest, in the first three years of life. Parents often first become concerned because their child is not using words to communicate, even though he or she recites passages from videotapes or says the alphabet. Though social deficits may not be immediately obvious in early years, they become gradually more evident as a child becomes more mobile and as other children become more socially sophisticated. Young children with autism often do not seek out others when they are happy, show or point to objects of interest, or call their parents by name. In preschool years, repetitive behaviors, such as using peripheral vision to look at lines or wheels, or specific hand and finger movements, begin to develop.

Autism is a heterogeneous condition; no two children or adults with autism have exactly the same profile, but difficulties fall into core domains that are reliably measured and usually consistent across time, even though specific behaviors may change with development. A child who may spend a great deal of time spinning objects and watching them out of the corner of her eye at age four, may not show this behavior at all as a teenager, but may be fascinated by sunroofs or bald heads or World War I. A child whose primary method of communicating requests at age two is to lead his mother to whatever he wants, place her hand on it, or use her hand to gesture toward it, may learn to ask for what he wants quite clearly and persistently by the time he is three or four, but continues to show difficulty carrying out back and forth conversations and coordinating eye contact and gestures.

Because of its links to genetics and neural development and the severe abnormalities in social interaction by which it is defined, autism offers the opportunity for scientists to study the neurobiological origins of social communication skills basic to human behavior. For example, even as infants, typically developing children are more adept at catching the eye of other people,

coordinating vocalizations with their intentions, and communicating all but the most extreme emotions with facial expressions than are much older children or adults with autism. Autism is a disorder of contrasts between spared abilities and deficits in areas of social-communicative development that we take for granted: a child with autism who can recite the alphabet and recognize numbers may not turn to his name or follow a pointing gesture. As adults, individuals with autism have a range of outcomes from complete dependence to rare examples of successful employment. However, they almost never marry and only rarely form ordinary, reciprocal friendships. The possibility of identifying links between the acquisition (or failure of acquisition) of basic social behaviors and neurobiology has, in part, fostered the recent surge of interest in the neuroscience of autism.

Issues in Diagnosis and Defining the Phenotype

Over the last 20 years, the conceptualization of a spectrum of autism-related disorders, including Childhood Disintegrative Disorder, Asperger's Disorder, and Pervasive Developmental Disorder-Not Otherwise Specified (PDD-NOS), which all include qualitative deficits in social behavior and communication, has been supported by longitudinal, epidemiological, and family studies (see Filipek et al., 2000 for a general review). However, these disorders vary in pervasiveness, severity, and onset. The umbrella category is termed Pervasive Developmental Disorder in the most common diagnostic systems (American Psychiatric Association, 2000; World Health Organization, 1992). Rett's syndrome has been included in the category of autism spectrum disorders within psychiatric systems because of the overlap in symptoms in toddlers and preschool children but, because of its different course (e.g., loss of purposeful hand use) and neurological characteristics (e.g., deceleration in head circumference), is a more differentiable group than the other syndromes and so generally studied as a distinct disorder. Clear distinctions among the other disorders within the autism spectrum, as listed on Table 1, are possible according to the degree of accompanying language deficit or general cognitive delay (American Psychiatric Association, 1994) or according to the severity of social or behavioral symptoms (Lord et al., 2000). Asperger's disorder involves the presence of autistic social deficits and repetitive, circumscribed interests in individuals who are verbally fluent. It has been of interest to scientists because of the contrast, as discussed earlier, between relatively intact and often verbose qualities of language and limited behaviors. Its prevalence is in dispute because, in controlled studies, it has been difficult to reliably differentiate Asperger's syndrome from autism without mental retardation or language delay, except by neuropsychological profile (which may be tautological).

On the other hand, the appeal of the different categorizations is in part because there is such a range of abilities and patterns of deficits within the autism spectrum that the possibility of finding subcategories related to

‡To whom correspondence should be addressed (e-mail: cathy@
yoda.bsd.uchicago.edu).

Table 1. DSM-IV/ICD-10 Diagnostic Criteria for Autism Spectrum Disorder

	Autistic Disorder	Rett's Disorder	Childhood Disintegrative Disorder	Asperger's Disorder	PDD-NOS
Age of Onset	Delays or abnormal functioning in social interaction, language, or play by age 3.	Apparently normal prenatal development; apparently normal motor development for first 5 months; deceleration of head growth between ages 5 and 48 months.	Apparently normal development for at least the first 2 years of birth; clinically significant loss of previously acquired skills before age 10.	No clinically significant delay in language, cognitive development, or development of age appropriate self-help skills, adaptive behavior, and environment in childhood.	This category is to be used in cases of pervasive impairment in social interaction and communication with presence of stereotyped behaviors of interests when criteria are not met for a specific disorder.
Social Interaction	Qualitative impairment in social interaction, as manifested by at least two of the following: a) marked impairment in the use of multiple nonverbal behaviors, i.e., eye-to-eye gaze; b) failure to develop peer relationships appropriate to developmental level; c) lack of spontaneous seeking to share enjoyment with other people; d) lack of social or emotional reciprocity.	Loss of social engagement early in the course (although often social interaction develops later).	Same as Autistic Disorder along with loss of social skills (previously acquired).	Same as Autistic Disorder.	
Communication	Qualitative impairments of communication as manifested by at least one of the following: a) delay in, or total lack of, the development of spoken language; b) marked impairment in initiating or sustaining a conversation with others, in individuals with adequate speech; c) stereotyped and repetitive use of language or idiosyncratic language; d) lack of varied, spontaneous make-believe or imitative play.	Severely impaired expressive and receptive language development and severe psychomotor retardation	Same as Autistic Disorder, along with loss of expressive or receptive language previously acquired.	No clinically significant delay in language.	
Behavior	Restricted, repetitive, and stereotyped patterns of behavior, as manifested by one of the following: a) preoccupation with one or more stereotyped or restricted patterns of interest; b) adherence to nonfunctional routines or rituals; c) stereotyped and repetitive motor mannerisms; d) persistent preoccupation with parts of objects.	Loss of previously acquired purposeful hand movements; appearance of poorly coordinated gait or trunk movements.	Same as Autistic Disorder, along with loss of bowel or bladder control, play, motor skills previously acquired.	Same as Autistic Disorder.	
Exclusions	Disturbance not better accounted for by Rett's or CDD.		Disturbance not better accounted for by another PDD or schizophrenia.	Criteria are not met for another PDD or Schizophrenia.	

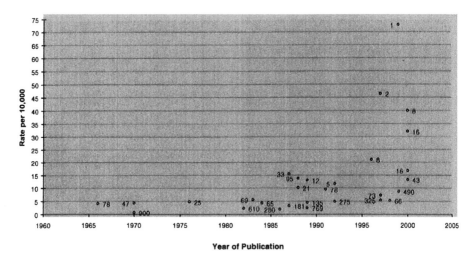

Figure 1. Autism Prevalence in 29 Studies
Numbers indicate thousands in each target population.

etiology or pathophysiology continues to be enticing. In addition, the range of services needed across the autism spectrum is very broad, particularly once children reach elementary school and into adulthood. For example, a child with high functioning autism or Asperger's syndrome may do well academically in a fifth grade program for children gifted in mathematics but need the support of an assistant teacher in order to benefit from social activities and help him as he begins to understand that he is different from other children. Another child the same age whose understanding of language and speech is limited to single words and a few familiar phrases may need continuing speech therapy on vocabulary as well as benefit from the use of a picture system that allows her to understand the schedule for the day and communicate how she would like to spend her free time at school and at home. The value of the spectrum diagnoses is to recognize that both of these children have significant deficits that share similarities as well as differences.

In the last 10 years, standardized measures of autism-related deficits have been developed that reliably measure history and present status, with relative independence from cooccurring language delays or mental retardation. Standard diagnoses of autistic disorder, Childhood Disintegrative Disorder, and PDD-NOS can be made across a wide range of individuals of different ages, language levels, and nonverbal abilities, including young children. Severity of social and communication deficits can be reliably quantified (see Filipek et al., 2000; Lord et al., 2000). Experiments based on developmental cognitive theories have identified increasingly specific points in maturation when "pivotal" behaviors, such as imitation, joint attention, and orienting to social stimuli, fail to develop normally in autism (Osterling and Dawson, 1994). In addition, autism affects not only social behavior

and language but also many other aspects of functioning, including sensory responsiveness, play, and motor activity. Approximately 30% of autistic patients also have an associated seizure disorder.

As shown in Figure 1, adapted from Fombonne (1999), epidemiological studies indicate an increasing prevalence for autism spectrum disorders in the last 15 years. Much of the higher rates may be accounted for by more complete ascertainment and the expansion of diagnostic frameworks to include milder forms of the disorder (Fombonne, 1999). However, it is interesting to note that the highest estimates of prevalence have all occurred in the last 5 years, though in small samples in studies where diagnoses were not always based on standard clinical procedures. These findings and the increases in the numbers of children with autism spectrum disorder referred to school systems (see Baird et al., 2000) and state programs have sparked the interest of many advocacy and scientific groups. The question of rising prevalence is particularly difficult to study because measures and diagnostic systems to establish base rates have changed greatly in the last 10 years, and, though available now, are expensive and time consuming (e.g., require a substantial parent interview and structured observation) if the milder forms of autism spectrum disorder are to be identified.

Many, but not all, individuals with autism, have mental retardation and almost all individuals with autism have a history of language delay. However, there are autism spectrum disorders (e.g., Asperger's disorder) in which neither language delay nor mental retardation is present. Families with children with moderate or mild mental retardation or normal intelligence with autism are no more likely to have children with mental retardation without autism than other families. Thus, the mental retardation appears to be a part, but not a necessary part, of autistic disorders. There is some suggestion that lesser variants of communication difficulties may be familial, not necessarily cooccurring with other features of autism (Folstein et al., 1999). Language delay and milder communication difficulties overlap with many other disorders, however. The relationship between language impairment and autism is an important area of study that requires careful selection of measures and comparison groups because of the variability within normal development, frequent associations with other disorders, and the need to measure the presence of specific social deficits across a range of language levels (e.g., measuring social skills is different in a nonverbal than verbal child). Another approach has been based on the significant minority of individuals with autism who have "islets of ability," usually in skills that require attention to detail, memory, or computations (e.g., such as calendrical calculating or perfect pitch—see Prior and Ozonoff, 1998). Baron-Cohen et al. (1995) have followed up on this notion to suggest that the incidence of autism may be higher in families where a parent has selected a field of interest where imagination and social skills are less emphasized and attention to detail and focus are particularly important, such as engineering or basic science. The question of what are the broader phenotypes of autism and do they extend into differences within the normal population is very complex and just beginning to be studied systematically.

Genetics of Autism

The genetics of autism is an area that has stimulated much recent research (see Cook, 1998, 2000 for recent reviews). Possibly the most significant genetic finding relevant to autism is the recent identification of the gene responsible for Rett's syndrome (Amir et al., 1999). Rett's syndrome is a neurodevelopmental disorder that is associated with mental retardation, loss of communication skills, and autistic features that vary in prominence at different developmental stages. It has been, somewhat controversially, placed within the diagnostic category, pervasive developmental disorders, of which autism is the exemplar. Rett's syndrome is caused by mutations in the methyl-CpG binding protein 2 gene (MECP2). Decreased expression of MECP2 leads to the failure to suppress expression of gene(s) regulated by methylation. When the pathophysiology of MECP2 mutations is further elucidated, it is likely to add to an understanding of autistic disorder.

Autism spectrum disorders are also seen in a substantial minority of patients with full mutations of the Fragile X (FRAXA) gene FMR1. The reverse is not the case, since full FMR1 mutations are seen in less than 1% of recent samples of children with autism. More importantly, analysis of this single gene disorder will contribute to an understanding of the mechanisms by which reduced FMR1 expression leads to mental retardation and to social-communicative symptoms that overlap with those seen in autistic disorders.

Autism is a paradigmatic complex genetic disorder, similar to diabetes, asthma, schizophrenia, Alzheimer's disorder, and many others. The sibling recurrence risk is approximately 4.5%, relative to a population incidence and estimated prevalence of approximately 0.1%–0.5%.

This relative risk to siblings (λ_s) of 9–45 is one of the highest for a complex genetic disorder and is higher than the other disorders listed above. The most compelling evidence for high heritability is the greater than 50% concordance rate for monozygotic twins relative to an ~3% concordance for dizygotic twins. This also suggests multiplicative genetic effects in which more than one and probably more than 2 genes contribute in concert to the high risk for monozygotic twins.

The current focus in molecular genetics of autism is on the identification of molecular genetic variation that contributes to autism susceptibility. Candidate gene findings of interest include a family-based association and linkage finding between the serotonin transporter promoter gene insertion/deletion polymorphism and autistic disorder. Of family-based, controlled studies, one showed preferential transmission of the short arm of the serotonin transporter promoter gene. Two showed transmission of the long arm and two were not significant. Genetic or clinical heterogeneity or multiple tests of candidate genes leading to false positives may have led to this inconsistency. Another candidate gene finding has been one between a microsatellite near the alternative promoters and first 3 exons of the GABA$_A$ β 3 subunit gene (GABRB3), but this has also not been found in all samples.

The chromosomal disorder most frequently found (0%–3%) in recent large samples of autism has been the finding of a maternal duplication of 15q11-q13. This is the same region in which absent maternal gene expression (or mutation) of ubiquitin binding enzyme 3A (UBE3A) leads to Angelman syndrome and in which the absence of paternal chromosomal gene expression leads to Prader-Willi syndrome, two other developmental disorders associated with mental retardation, but that are associated with quite different phenotypes than autistic disorder. Although there may be a convergence of the linkage disequilibrium findings for GABRB3 and the 15q11-q13 duplications, it is also possible that the duplication of 15q11-q13 has distant effects, such as the overexpression of UBE3A, leading to excessive degradation of one or more of its targets.

Several genome-wide screens have been published in autism in the past 3 years (reviewed in Cook, 2000) and more are in progress. Much effort is now focused on confirming the strongest finding from the first published study, i.e., a linkage in a relatively large region (7q32-35). Several other regions of interest have been identified across different genome scans, including 2q, 16p, 19p (e.g., see http://www.agre.org/bnews/scan.cfm).

Neurobiology of Autism

A fundamental goal of neurobiological approaches to the study of autism is the definition of brain regions that are most severely affected. Once affected brain regions are identified and the types of alterations (structural versus neurochemical; failure of development versus degeneration) are better understood, strategies can be developed for prevention, early diagnosis, and treatment. The neurobiology of autism has been hampered, in part, by the heterogeneity inherent in the autism spectrum disorders. It is not currently clear whether autism is a syndrome that varies in severity but nonetheless has a common neural basis or whether the autism spectrum disorders have multiple etiologies and affect various brain systems that nonetheless lead to the core deficits of abnormal social behavior, impaired communication, and stereotypical behavior. Clearly, in this as in every other area of autism research, future progress will depend on better categorization of distinctive subsets of autistic individuals using biochemical, genetic, neuroimaging, behavioral, and other diagnostic tools.

One approach to the neurobiology of autism, the neuropathological approach, employs both postmortem analysis and noninvasive imaging techniques to determine the brain regions involved in autism. A second approach attempts to understand the normal neural substrates of functions, such as social cognition, that are profoundly impaired in autistic disorders. It is a reasonable expectation that one or more components of this system might be altered in autism. Thus, the neurobiology of normal social behavior can potentially narrow the scope of suspect brain regions. A third, but currently more poorly developed approach, is the development of animal models. This effort has been hobbled by a lack of knowledge concerning the etiology(ies) of autism and a paucity of data, which is also highly variable, on the characteristic neuropathology of autism, i.e., it is not quite clear what a successful model of autism would look like.

Neuropathology

Although autopsy studies of autism were begun in the early 1980s, formal reports have only involved about 30 brains. There are a number of reports that the brains of autistic individuals are larger than normal. Bailey et al. (1998), for example, found that four of six postmortem brains that they examined, from individuals ranging in age from 4 to 24 years at time of death, were megalencephalic. Regional neuropathological studies have pointed to possible alterations in the brainstem, cerebellum, and in a set of "limbic" structures, including the hippocampal formation, amygdala, septal nuclei, and anterior cingulate cortex. Cells in various portions of the hippocampal formation, in the medial nuclei of the amygdala, the medial septal nucleus, the mammillary nuclei, and the cortex of the anterior cingulate gyrus tend to be smaller and more densely packed than in normal brains (Kemper and Bauman, 1998). Neurons in the hippocampus of autistic individuals also have reduced complexity of dendritic arbors. Some pathology seems to be age dependent. In the basal forebrain nucleus of the vertical limb of the diagonal band of Broca, for example, neurons were unusually large and numerous but otherwise normal looking in brains of autistic children less than 12 years old but were small and reduced in number in brains of autistic adults older than 18 years. The Bailey et al. (1998) study confirmed qualitative impressions that cell density was higher in the hippocampus of autistic individuals but morphometric analyses did not demonstrate significant differences. They also noted abnormalities in the cytoarchitectonic organization and neuronal density of the superior frontal cortex and superior temporal gyrus of some of their cases but no quantitative differences were found.

Cerebellar abnormality has been a common finding.

Ritvo et al. (1986) noted that there was a loss of Purkinje cells in the brains of four subjects with autism. Kemper and Bauman have generally confirmed the loss of cerebellar Purkinje cells and reported changes in neurons of the deep cerebellar nuclei. Bailey et al. (1998) also observed loss of Purkinje cells but no apparent changes in the number of granule cells or alterations of deep cerebellar nuclei. It is important to note that the loss of Purkinje cells is also a common correlate of seizure disorders (Dam, 1992), and it is essential to determine whether loss of this neuron class also occurs in autistic subjects who are seizure free.

Rodier et al. (1996) found near complete absence of the facial nucleus and superior olive in one postmortem case. Bailey et al. (1998) also found brainstem abnormalities of the superior and inferior olives; however, the organization of the facial nucleus was not evaluated. Kemper and Bauman reported alterations in the portion of the inferior olive that projects to the part of the cerebellar cortex with the most profound loss of Purkinje cells.

The lack of a coherent description of the neuropathology of autism is undoubtedly due, in part, to the relatively small number of brains that have been analyzed and to the use of qualitative methods of assessment. Future progress, both in neuropathological assessment of the autistic brain and in studies of the molecular biology of autism, will require the acquisition of high quality post mortem tissue from well-characterized donors.

Structural Magnetic Resonance Imaging Findings

Given the relatively subtle and variable neuropathological changes that have been described in the autistic brain, it is not surprising that structural magnetic resonance imaging studies have not found consistent changes. Courchesne et al. (1988) reported selective hypotrophy of vermal lobules VI and VII in the cerebellum of autistic subjects. This has proven to be a controversial finding and others have failed to consistently replicate it. One explanation may be that not all subsets of the autistic spectrum demonstrate cerebellar hypoplasia. Holttum et al. (1992) found, for example, that cerebellar hypoplasia does not appear to be associated with high-functioning autism. Saitoh and Courchesne (1998) later found that there were two subgroups of autistic subjects that were characterized either by hypoplasia or hyperplasia of lobules VI and VII. Thus, depending on the composition of a patient population, one might expect to see hypoplasia, hyperplasia, or no change.

Abell et al. (1999) used a voxel-based whole brain analysis and identified gray matter differences in the amygdala and associated brain regions. Decreases of gray matter were found in the right paracingulate sulcus and the left inferior frontal gyrus, whereas increases were found in the amygdaloid complex (particularly the periamygdaloid cortex) the middle temporal and inferior temporal gyrus, as well as in regions of the cerebellum. It is not clear how these changes in MR signal characteristics relate to the increased density of smaller neurons seen in many of these same areas. Aylward et al. (1999) found that the volumes of both the amygdala and the hippocampal formation were reduced in the autistic brain, though neither Piven et al. (1998) nor Saitoh et al.

(1995) observed changes in the hippocampus. Consistent with the neuropathological findings of Kemper and Bauman, Haznedar et al. (1997) observed decreased volume and decreased PET activity in the anterior cingulate gyrus of autistic subjects. Finally, there have been no neuropathological findings in the basal ganglia of autistic patients. However, Sears et al. (1999), using structural MRI, observed an increased volume of the caudate nuclei in autistic subjects that was proportional to compulsions and rituals.

Neurobiology of Social Behavior

Regardless of whether an individual with an autism spectrum disorder is mentally retarded or not and whether the individual has language impairment or obvious stereotypical behaviors, all persons with autism spectrum disorders have some disturbance of normal social behavior. These deficits range from subtle abnormalities in social reciprocity, particularly with peers, to much more obvious difficulties in the use of eye contact, facial expression, and social motivation. A growing body of literature indicates that important aspects of social cognition, such as the salience or interpretation of facial expressions or the appreciation of angle of gaze, are markedly impaired in autistic subjects (Baron-Cohen et al., 2000). Thus, an understanding of the brain systems responsible for social cognition and for interpretation of the social aspects of facial expression might be predictive of regions of brain dysfunction in autism.

Evidence from both human and animal studies indicates that certain brain regions are preferentially involved in social behavior. In the macaque monkey, these would include the amygdala, orbitofrontal cortex, superior temporal gyrus, and temporal polar cortex. Damage to any of these regions in macaque monkeys produces a profound alteration of social behavior. Cortical areas, such as the anterior cingulate gyrus, have also been implicated in the production of species-specific vocalizations. Yet, other cortical regions, such as the inferior temporal gyrus in monkeys and the fusiform gyrus in humans, appear to be preferentially involved in the perception of faces. Neurons ("face cells") that are highly and selectively responsive to the image of faces have been found in the inferior temporal gyrus of macaque monkeys (Perrett et al., 1982). Neurons sensitive to the angle of gaze have been found in the cortex of the superior temporal sulcus (Perrett et al., 1985). Neurons that are attuned to particular facial expressions have also been found in the inferior and superior temporal lobes of macaque monkeys (Hasselmo et al., 1989). Interestingly, cortical areas responsive to faces, facial expressions, and to angle of gaze send direct projections to the primate amygdala (Stefanacci and Amaral, 2000). These functional and neuroanatomical facts have raised the prospect that the amygdala may be important for components of social cognition such as the attention to and interpretation of facial expressions. If this is the case, the amygdala is a prime candidate for dysfunction in autism.

A rare human disorder called Urbach-Wiethe syndrome produces cystic calcifications of the medial temporal lobe. In patient SM, these space-occupying lesions mainly involve the amygdala bilaterally and she is mark-

edly impaired in her ability to judge facial expressions of fear and anger (Adolphs et al., 1995). Even more germane to the pathology of autism, SM is unable to make an accurate judgement of the trustworthiness of an individual from photographic images. Functional imaging studies have demonstrated activation of the amygdala in normal subjects asked to make judgements of facial expressions. Very recently, Baron-Cohen and colleagues (1999) carried out a functional magnetic resonance imaging experiment using a test of judging from the expressions of another person's eyes what that other person might be thinking or feeling. In normal subjects, this test resulted in activation in the superior temporal gyrus and the amygdala with additional activations in the frontal cortex. In the autistic population that they studied, the task produced activations in the temporal lobe and in the frontal cortex but not in the amygdala. These interesting observations will need to be confirmed and extended but raise the prospect that pathology of some sort in the amygdala may play an important role in the defects of social cognition observed in autism. Schultz and colleagues (Schultz et al., 2000) compared activation in the inferior temporal gyri (ITG) during face and object processing in individuals with autism or Asperger's disorder and those with typical development. Individuals with autism spectrum disorders used ITG significantly more during face processing than did normal controls, though the side of the effect varied across an initial and a replication group. Thus, in this study, individuals with autism used strategies typically used in nonface object perception by normal adults in order to discriminate faces. More work on relatively young, homogeneous samples, which balance scientific rigor with ethical restraints, are much needed (Rumsey and Ernst, 2000).

Animal Models

The most successful animal model of autism produced to date involves the bilateral removal of the medial temporal lobe of young macaque monkeys (Bachevalier, 1996). These animals show a variety of socioemotional changes including social isolation and demonstrate some other facets of autistic symptomatology such as stereotypical behaviors. Clearly, the production of large medial temporal lobe lesions does not closely mimic the pathology observed in the autistic brain. It would be interesting if more subtle and more focal dysregulation could be produced in the developing nonhuman primate brain that replicated the autistic behavioral pathology.

Other investigators have attempted to model the neuropathology observed in the brain stem using various teratogens. This work has been motivated by the finding that certain children exposed prenatally to thalidomide developed some symptoms of autism. Rodier and colleagues (1996) have used maternal treatment with valproic acid in rats in an attempt to produce pathology in cranial nerve nuclei (reviewed in Rodier, 2000). The alterations that Rodier and colleagues observed in their patient with autism involved mainly the facial nucleus and the superior olive. In her valproate studies, Rodier observed changes in motor nuclei of V and XII with later treatments affecting the VIth and IIIrd cranial nerve nuclei. None of her treatments affected the facial nucleus (unlike in the postmortem autistic brain). Morever, Rodier et al. (1996) observed that there were no changes of any other brain regions such as the cerebellum, hippocampus, or amygdala. Therefore, even based on the minimal neuropathology available, the valproic acid model would not appear to have much verisimilitude to human autism.

Interventions, Families, and Needs for the Future

Given the limited information available on the etiology(ies) and biology of autism, therapies have generally focused on educational and behavioral interventions. There are increasing efforts to evaluate psychoactive drugs for clinical benefit in autism. For example, a large multisite study is in progress (McDougle et al., 2000) of the effects of risperidone (a serotonin 5HT2A/dopamine D2 receptor blocker), which showed some benefit in a single double-blind placebo-controlled trial in terms of reducing maladaptive behaviors without demonstration of independent effects on core social and communication deficits.

Currently, intensive, structured education forms the core of most treatment approaches, supplemented by positively oriented behavior management, family support, and an emphasis on functional communication. Children and adults with autism can clearly benefit from direct teaching and exposure to developmentally appropriate experiences. Controversy remains, however, as to whether it is possible to alter the trajectory of the development of a child with autism or whether early interventions primarily accelerate development in children who would make good progress in response to many treatments or reduce secondary effects of social isolation and lack of engagement. These issues have been linked, so far without data, to larger questions of neuroplasticity and the degree to which social engagement contributes to basic cognitive functions (Mundy and Neal, 2000).

The variation in outcomes in autism spectrum disorders, from severe behavioral disturbance and profound mental retardation, to uncommon cases of independent, age appropriate functioning, and the limited success of current therapies in completely diminishing the symptoms of autism, has resulted in some parents becoming increasingly experimental in approaches to their child's treatment. This makes parents vulnerable to new claims of remarkable improvements, particularly in response to highly publicized treatments, such as facilitated communication, auditory training, dietary manipulations, and, recently, secretin (Volkmar, 1999). In the last case, a serendipitous finding of behavioral improvement following the administration of secretin during endoscopy (Horvath et al., 1998) led to widespread demand for this "treatment" by parents. Since then, several double blind, placebo-controlled clinical trials of secretin have found it to have no positive effect on autism (e.g., Sandler et al., 1999). Other clinicians and parents have promulgated the practice of controlling the diet of children with autism. Most prominently, gluten-free and casein-free diets have been purported to benefit young children with autism, particularly. Recommendations for such dietary restrictions are based on extremely limited scientific data (Lucarelli et al., 1995), though advocates of such approaches counter that there is little evidence (Sponheim, 1991) against them.

Another issue that has arisen recently is the proposal that at least some cases of autism in which children have had a few words and other social-communicative behaviors that disappear in the second year of life may be linked to vaccinations. This pattern of loss of words often accompanied by increasingly obvious social deficits is described by parents as occurring in about one-fifth of children with autism. The particular vaccinations proposed as causal have varied, but currently the greatest focus has been on combination vaccines for measles, mumps, and rubella (Kawahima et al., 2000; Wakefield et al., 2000). This suggestion, based on research carried out primarily by Wakefield and colleagues, has been extraordinarily controversial. A number of epidemiological studies from countries with comprehensive health registers have appeared not to support a link between MMR vaccines and autism (Taylor et al., 1999; Afzal et al., 2000). Here again, there is a chasm between the visible increase in prevalence of autism as indicated by the need for services, and empirical evidence for the gradual broadening of criteria and improvements in identification, which is felt by some not to be sufficient to account for the increases. It is not surprising that parents and some clinicians and researchers have attempted to account for this gap, with alternative theories.

Parents' societies have traditionally been very important to the field of autism, from the founding of the first autism societies in the US and UK many years ago, to the current research support and advocacy provided by a number of parent-founded, -led, and -supported organizations. These organizations have already begun to be influential in terms of research, especially in funding new investigators and attracting eminent scientists from other fields into studying the disorder. The parents' organizations also have the potential to be extremely helpful in dissemination of scientific information, particularly on the Internet, which, with the hundreds of sources available, provides a tremendous but sometimes overwhelming amount of information.

Sometimes claims for extraordinary outcomes are unwittingly promulgated by scientists unfamiliar with the range of behaviors and developmental course seen in autism spectrum disorders and impatient with standard clinical research procedures such as random assignment, double-blinding, and case-controls. On the other hand, new ideas from diverse perspectives on treatment, prevention, and understanding of the pathophysiology of autism are urgently needed. One of the foremost goals for the next decade will be greater communication between basic scientists, clinical researchers, parents, and persons with autism spectrum disorders so that knowledge from neuroscience and other areas of biology can be more readily applied to autism in ways that yield scientifically valid and effective results.

Acknowledgments

Supported by NIH K05 MH01196, P01 HD35482, K02 MH 01389, R01 MH52223, MH41479, CAN, NAAR, and the M.I.N.D. Institute.

References

Abell, F., Krams, M., Ashburner, J., Passingham, R., Friston, K., Frackowiak, R., Happe, F., Frith, C., and Frith, U. (1999). The neuroanatomy of autism: a voxel-based whole brain analysis of structural scans. Neuroreport 10, 1647–1651.

Adolphs, R., Tranel, D., Damasio, H., and Damasio, A.R. (1995). Fear and the human amygdala. J. Neurosci. 15, 5879–5891.

Afzal, M.A., Minor, P.D., and Schild, G.C. (2000). Clinical safety issues of measles, mumps and rubella vaccines. Bull. World Health Organ. 78, 199–204.

American Psychiatric Association (2000). Diagnostic and Statistical Manual of Mental Disorders DSM-IV-TR (Text Revision) (Washington, D.C.: American Psychiatric Association).

Amir, R.E., Van den Veyver, I.B., Wan, M., Tran, C.Q., Francke, U., and Zoghbi, H.Y. (1999). Rett sydnrome is caused by mutations in X-linked MECP2, encoding methyl-CpG-binding protein 2. Nat. Genet. 23, 185–188.

Aylward, E.H., Minshew, N.J., Goldstein, G., Honeycutt, N.A., Augustine, A.M., Yates, K.O., Barta, P.E., and Pearlson, G.D. (1999). MRI volumes of amygdala and hippocampus in non-mentally retarded autistic adolescents and adults. Neurology 53, 2145–2150.

Bachevalier, J. (1996). Brief report: medial temporal lobe and autism: a putative animal model in primates. J. Aut. Dev. Disord. 26, 217–220.

Bailey, A., Luthert, P., Dean, A., Harding, B., Janota, I., Montgomery, M., Rutter, M., and Lantos, P. (1998). A full genome screen for autism with evidence for linkage to a region on chromosome 7q. Brain 121, 889–905.

Baird, G., Charman, T., Baron-Cohen, S., Cox, A., Swettenham, J., Wheelwright, S., and Drew, A. (2000). A screening instrument for autism at 18 months of age: a 6-year follow-up study. J. Am. Acad. Child Adolesc. Psychiatry 39, 694–702.

Baron-Cohen, S., Bolton, P., Wheliwright, S., Short, L., Mead, G., Smith, A., and Scahill, V. (1995). Autism occurs more often in families of physicists, engineers, and mathematicians. Autism 2, 296–301.

Baron-Cohen, S., Ring, H.A., Wheelwright, S., Bullmore, E.T., Brammer, M.J., Simmons, A., and Williams, S.C. (1999). Social intelligence in the normal and autistic brain: an fMRI study. Eur. J. Neurosci. 11, 1891–1898.

Baron-Cohen, S., Tager-Flusberg, H., and Cohen, D. (2000). Understanding other minds: perspectives from developmental cognitive neuroscience (Oxford: Oxford University Press).

Cook, E. (1998). Genetics of autism. Mental Retard. Dev. Disabil. Res. Rev. 4, 113–120.

Cook, E.H. (2000). Genetics of autism. Child Adolesc. Psychiatric Clin. N. Am., in press.

Courchesne, E., Yeung-Courchesne, R., Press, G.A., Hesselink, J.R., and Jernigan, T.L. (1988). Hypoplasia of cerebellar vermal lobules VI and VII in autism. N. Engl. J. Med. 318, 1349–1354.

Dam, M. (1992). Quantitative neuropathology in epilepsy. Acta Neurol. Scand. 137 (suppl.), 51–54.

Filipek, P.A., Accardo, P.J., Ashwal, S., Baranek, G.T., Cook, E.H., Jr., Dawson, G., Gordon, B., Gravel, J.S., Johnson, C.P., Kallen, R.J., et al. (2000). Practice parameters: screening and diagnosis of autism: report of the Quality Standards Subcommitte of the American Academy of Neurology and the Child Neurology Society. Neurology 55, 468–479.

Folstein, S.E., Santangelo, S.L., Gilman, G.E., Piven, J., Landa, R., Lainhart, J., Hein, J., and Wzorek, M. (1999). Predictors of cognitive test patterns in autism families. J. Child Psychol. Psychiatry 40, 117–128.

Fombonne, E. (1999). The epidemiology of autism: a review. Psychol. Med. 29, 769–786.

Hasselmo, M.E., Rolls, E.T., and Baylis, G.C. (1989). The role of expression and identity in the face-selective responses of neurons in the temporal visual cortex of the monkey. Behav. Brain Res. 32, 203–218.

Haznedar, M.M., Buchsbaum, M.S., Metzger, M., Solimando, A., Spiegel-Cohen, J., and Hollander, E. (1997). Anterior cingulate gyrus volume and glucose metabolism in autistic disorder. Am. J. Psychiatry 154, 1047–1050.

Holttum, J.R., Minshew, N.J., Sanders, R.S., and Phillips, N.E. (1992). Magnetic resonance imaging of the posterior fossa in autism. Biol. Psychiatry 32, 1091–1101.

Horvath, K., Stefanatos, G., Sokolski, K.N., Wachtel, R., Nabors, L., and Tildon, J.T. (1998). Improved social and language skills after secretin administration in patients with autisitc spectrum disorders. J. Assoc. Acad. Minor. Phys. 9, 9–15.

Kawahima, H., Mori, T., Kashiwagi, Y., Takekuma, K., Hoshika, A., and Wakefield, A. (2000). Detection and sequencing of measles virus from peripheral mononuclear cells from patients with inflammatory bowel disease and autism. Dig. Dis. Sci. 45, 723–729.

Kemper, T.L., and Bauman, M. (1998). Neuropathology of infantile autism. J. Neuropathol. Exp. Neurol. 57, 645–652.

Lord, C., Risi, S., Lambrecht, L., Cook, E.H., Leventhal, B.L., Pickles, A., and Rutter, M.J. (2000). Autism Diagnostic Observation Schedule-General (ADOS-G). J. Aut. Dev. Disord. 30, 205–223.

Lucarelli, S., Frediani, T., Zingoni, A.M., Ferruzzi, F., Giardini, O., Quintieri, F., Barbato, M., D'Eufemia, P., and Cardi, E. (1995). Food allergy and infantile autism. Panminerva Med. 37, 137–141.

McDougle, C.J., Scahill, L., McCracken, J.T., Aman, M.G., Tierney, E., Arnold, L.E., Freeman, B.J., Martin, A., McGough, J.J., Cronin, P., et al. (2000). Research Units on Pediatric Psyhopharmacology (RUPP) Autism Network. Background and rationale for an initial controlled study of risperidone. Child Adolesc. Psychiatr. Clin. N. Am. 9, 201–224.

Mundy, P., and Neal, R. (2000). Neural plasticity, joint attention and autistic developmental pathology. International Rev. Res. Ment. Ret. 20, 139–168.

Osterling, J., and Dawson, G. (1994). Early recognition of children with autism: a study of first birthday home videotapes. J. Aut. Dev. Disord. 24, 247–257.

Perrett, D.I., Rolls, E.T., and Caan, W. (1982). Visual neurones responsive to faces in the monkey temporal cortex. Exp. Brain Res. 47, 329–342.

Perrett, D.I., Smith, P.A., Potter, D.D., Mistlin, A.J., Head, A.S., Milner, A.D., and Jeeves, M.A. (1985). Visual cells in temporal cortex sensitive to face view and gaze direction. Proc. R. Soc. Lond. B Biol. Sci. 223, 293–317.

Piven, J., Bailey, J., Ranson, B.J., and Arndt, S. (1998). No differences in hippocampus volume detected on magnetic resonance imaging in autistic individuals. J. Aut. Dev. Disord. 28, 105–110.

Prior, M., and Ozonoff, S. (1998). Psychological factors in autism. In Autism and Pervasive Developmental Disorders, F.R. Volkmar, ed. (Cambridge: Cambridge University Press), pp. 64–108.

Ritvo, E.R., Freeman, B.J., Scheibel, A.B., Duong, T., Robinson, H., Guthrie, D., and Ritvo, A. (1986). Lower Purkinje cell counts in the cerebella of four autistic subjects: initial findings of the UCLA-NSAC Autopsy Research Report. Am. J. Psychiatry 143, 862–866.

Rodier, P.M. (2000). The early origins of autism. Sci. Am. 282, 56–63.

Rodier, P.M., Ingram, J.L., Tisdale, B., Nelson, S., and Romano, J. (1996). Embryological origin for autism: developmental anomalies of the cranial nerve motor nuclei. J. Comp. Neurol. 370, 247–261.

Rumsey, J.M., and Ernst, E.M. (2000). Functional neuroimaging of autistic disorders. Ment. Retard. Dev. Disabil. Res. Rev. 6, 171–179.

Saitoh, O., and Courchesne, E. (1998). Magnetic resonance imaging study of the brain in autism. Psychiatry Clin. Neurosci. 52 (suppl.), S219–S222.

Saitoh, O., Courchesne, E., Egaas, B., Lincoln, A.J., and Schreibman, L. (1995). Cross sectional area of posterior hippocampus in autistic patients with cerebellar and corpus-callosum abnormalities. Neurology 45, 317–324.

Sandler, A.D., Sutton, K.A., DeWeese, J., Girardi, M.A., Sheppard, V., and Bodfish, J.W. (1999). Lack of benefit of a single dose of synthetic human secretin in the treatment of autism and pervasive developmental disorder. N. Engl. J. Med. 341, 1801–1806.

Schultz, R.T., Gauthier, I., Klin, A., Fulbright, R.K., Anderson, A.W., Volkmar, F.R., Skudlarski, P., Lacadie, C., Cohen, D.J., and Gore,

J.C. (2000). Abnormal ventral temporal cortical activity during face discrimination among individuals with autism and Asperger syndrome. Arch. Gen. Psychiatry 57, 331–340.

Sears, L.L., Vest, C., Mohamed, S., Bailey, J., Ranson, B.J., and Piven, J. (1999). An MRI study of the basal ganglia in autism. J. Prog. Neuropsychopharmacol. Biol. Psychiatry 23, 613–624.

Sponheim, E. (1991). Gluten-free diet in infantile autism. A therapeutic trial. Tidsskr Nor Laegeforen 111, 704–707.

Stefanacci, L., and Amaral, D.G. (2000). Topographic organization of cortical inputs to the lateral nucleus of the macaque monkey amygdala: a retrograde tracing study. J. Comp. Neurol. 421, 52–79.

Taylor, E.N., Miller, E., Farrington, C.P., Petropoulos, M.C., Favot-Mayaud, I., Li, J., and Waight, P.A. (1999). Autism and measles, mumps, and rubella vaccine: no epidemiological evidence for a causal association. Lancet 353, 2026–2029.

Volkmar, F. (1999). Lessons from secretin. N. Engl. J. Med. 341, 1842–1844.

Wakefield, A.J., Anthony, A., Murch, S.H., Thomson, M., Montgomery, S.M., Davies, S., O'Leary, J.J., Berelowitz, M., and Walker-Smith, J.A. (2000). Enterocolitis in children with developmental disorders. Am. J. Gastroenterol. 95, 2285–2295.

World Health Organization (1992). The ICD 10 Classification of Mental and Behavioral Disorders: Clinical Descriptions and Diagnostic Guidelines (Geneva: World Health Organization).

Frontal Lobe Contributions to Theory of Mind

Valerie E. Stone
University of California, Davis

Simon Baron-Cohen
University of Cambridge

Robert T. Knight
University of California, Davis

Abstract

■ "Theory of mind," the ability to make inferences about others' mental states, seems to be a modular cognitive capacity that underlies humans' ability to engage in complex social interaction. It develops in several distinct stages, which can be measured with social reasoning tests of increasing difficulty. Individuals with Asperger's syndrome, a mild form of autism, perform well on simpler theory of mind tests but show deficits on more developmentally advanced theory of mind tests. We tested patients with bilateral damage to orbito-frontal cortex (*n* = 5) and unilateral damage in left dorsolateral prefrontal cortex (*n* = 5) on a series of theory of mind tasks varying in difficulty. Bilateral orbito-frontal lesion patients performed similarly to individuals with Asperger's syndrome, performing well on simpler tests and showing deficits on tasks requiring more subtle social reasoning, such as the ability to recognize a faux pas. In contrast, no specific theory of mind deficits were evident in the unilateral dorsolateral frontal lesion patients. The dorsolateral lesion patients had difficulty only on versions of the tasks that placed demands on working memory. ■

INTRODUCTION

Humans, like many other species, use a variety of cues (facial expression, body posture, tone of voice) to predict others' behavior. An animal that recognizes another animal's threatening body posture, for example, might produce a defensive response in anticipation of a possible attack. However, humans do not simply respond to others' *behavior*. We also explicitly model and respond to other people's mental states: their knowledge, intentions, beliefs, and desires. This ability to make inferences about others' mental states has been termed *theory of mind* (Premack & Woodruff, 1978; Wellman, 1990). *Theory of mind* is the term most widely used in the literature and is the term we will use here. There has been debate over whether the ability to infer others' mental states is a true implicit "theory" or the result of more general inferential abilities (Astington & Gopnik, 1991; Gopnik & Wellman, 1992) or whether it is best characterized as taking the "intentional stance" (Dennett, 1987). We will not be addressing these controversies here. Rather, our concern is whether particular brain regions may subserve the ability to make mentalistic inferences.

Theory of mind shows evidence of modularity, in the same sense that language does: (1) Theory of mind can be selectively impaired in the developmental disorder of autism, while other aspects of cognition are relatively spared (Baron-Cohen, Leslie, & Frith, 1985; Baron-Cohen, 1989b; Baron-Cohen, 1995). (2) Theory of mind can be selectively spared while other cognitive functions are impaired, as in Down's syndrome and Williams syndrome (Karmiloff-Smith, Klima, Bellugi, Grant, & Baron-Cohen, 1995). (3) Use of theory of mind is also rapid, (4) automatic, requiring no effortful attention (Heider & Simmel, 1944), and (5) universal, as far as is known (Avis & Harris, 1991). (6) Finally, theory of mind has a particular stereotyped developmental sequence.

The structure of the theory of mind mechanism can be elucidated by examining what happens at each developmental stage and what happens when there is a breakdown at particular developmental stages. Theory of mind first manifests itself in joint attention and protodeclarative pointing (Baron-Cohen, 1989a, 1995) at about 18 months. In joint attention, the child is able to understand not only what another individual is looking at but that the child and some other person are looking at the same object. Before 18 months, infants may be able to understand the fact that "Mommy sees the toy," but around 18

© 1998 Massachusetts Institute of Technology

Journal of Cognitive Neuroscience 10:5, pp. 640-656

months, the child begins to understand "Mommy sees the toy that I see." In protodeclarative pointing, the child uses pointing to call adults' attention to objects that the child wants them to attend to. Many children with autism do not show either joint attention or protodeclarative pointing (Baron-Cohen, 1989a, 1995). They do not look at what other people look at nor do they use pointing to draw adults' attention to things. The next stage in the development of theory of mind is pretend play, in which children are able to decouple pretend from reality. Between 18 and 24 months, children begin to understand the mental state of "pretend" (Leslie, 1987). Also, by age 2, children seem to have a firm grasp of the mental state of desire, for example, "John wants a hamburger" (Wellman & Woolley, 1990). Children's understanding of desire precedes their understanding of belief.

Between ages 3 and 4 children develop the ability to understand false belief (Gopnik & Astington, 1988; Johnson & Wellman, 1980; Wellman, 1990; Wimmer & Perner, 1983). Prior to this age, a child does not understand that other people can hold beliefs about the world that differ from the child's own. Thus, children assume that other people know the same things they know. Between ages 3 and 4, however, children begin to understand that other people may not know all the things that they know and therefore that others may hold false beliefs. Tests of false belief measure the ability of children to understand that another person can hold a belief that is mistaken. These tests demonstrate that children are representing others' mental states, others' beliefs, rather then the physical state of the world or their own state of knowledge (Dennett, 1978).

Between ages 6 and 7, children begin to understand that other people can also represent mental states. At this age children begin to be able to understand second-order false belief, "belief about belief" (Perner & Wimmer, 1985). In a typical second-order false belief task the problem might run something like this: A man and a woman are in a room. The woman puts something somewhere, such as putting a book on a shelf. She then leaves the room. The man hides the book in another location. Unbeknownst to him, the woman is peeking back through a keyhole or a window and sees him moving the book. The subject is asked, "When the woman comes back in, where will the man think that she thinks the book is?" To solve this problem, the child needs to be able to represent not only each person's belief state about the location of the object but also the man's mistaken belief about the woman's belief state.

Theory of mind can break down at certain of these developmental stages. Children with autism who do not show joint attention may never develop these theory of mind abilities. Children with autism are impaired in pretend play (Baron-Cohen, 1995). Most children with autism cannot solve false belief tasks or second-order false belief tasks (Baron-Cohen, et al., 1985; Perner, Leekam, & Wimmer, 1987). Some higher-functioning individuals with autism can eventually pass first-order false belief tasks but will fail second-order false belief tasks (Baron-Cohen 1989b; Happé, 1993). In general, autistics' difficulties are with epistemic mental states concerning knowledge or belief. They do seem to understand the mental state of desire (Baron-Cohen, Leslie, & Frith, 1986; Tager-Flusberg, 1989, 1993).

It should be noted that children with autism and young children do not simply lack the ability to do meta-representation. They can pass what is called a false photograph test (Zaitchik, 1990). In this test a Polaroid picture is taken of a toy placed on a table. The toy is then moved and then the photo comes out and is developed. Before the child sees what is in the photograph, the experimenter asks, "What will the picture show?" Young children and children with autism are not fooled into thinking that the photograph will show a table with nothing on it even though the toy has been moved. Thus they can understand physical representations, such as photographs and pictures, but not mental representations (Charman & Baron-Cohen, 1992, 1995; Leekam & Perner, 1991; Leslie & Thaiss, 1992).

Later, between ages 9 and 11, children develop further theory of mind abilities, such as the ability to understand and recognize faux pas. A faux pas occurs when someone says something they should have not have said, not knowing or not realizing that they should not say it. To understand that a faux pas has occurred, one has to represent two mental states: that the person saying it does not know that they should not say it and that the person hearing it would feel insulted or hurt. Thus there is both a cognitive component and empathic affective component. On our new test of faux pas detection, Baron-Cohen, O'Riordan, Stone, Jones, and Plaisted (1997) found that girls could perform well on this test by age 9, boys by age 11. Boys and girls of ages 7 or 8, although they could pass first- and second-order false belief tasks, did not perform well on the faux pas task.

To validate that the faux pas task is indeed a theory of mind test, Baron-Cohen et al. (1997) also tested it on individuals with Asperger's syndrome, a mild form of autism. In these individuals, language develops at a normal time pace, and their IQ is often normal. However, they still have many subtle social deficits. On our new test of faux pas detection, Baron-Cohen et al. (1997) found that, like 7 to 8 year-olds, individuals with Asperger's syndrome could pass first- and second-order false belief tasks, but were impaired on the faux pas task. Their theory of mind performance was comparable to that of 7- to 9-year-old children. The faux pas task is a thus a good measure of subtle theory of mind deficits. Performance on the most developmentally advanced theory of mind tasks is an index of how severe a person's theory of mind deficit is. Subtle theory of mind deficits can only be picked up with the most developmentally advanced tasks.

Little is known about the neurological basis for theory of mind. Such a complex cognitive ability does not seem a likely candidate for localization—a neural network or circuit is more plausible. Recent neuroimaging studies have reported that regions of the frontal lobes appear to be active during theory of mind tasks, suggesting that these may be part of a theory of mind circuit. Baron-Cohen, Ring, Moriarty, Schmitz, Costa and Ell (1994) found orbito-frontal activation during a simple theory of mind task requiring recognition of mental state terms. Fletcher et al. (1995) found activation in Brodmann's areas 8 and 9 in the left medial frontal cortex during a more complex theory of mind task involving deception and belief attribution. Goel, Grafman, Sadato, and Hallett (1995) also found activation in the left medial frontal cortex during a task requiring mental state inferences.

Baron-Cohen et al. (1994) used a task requiring subjects to judge whether each word on a list of words had to do with the mind or was something the mind could do and compared it to a task requiring a judgment of whether each word on another list had to do with the body or was something the body could do. Children with autism performed poorly on this mental state terms task but not on the body terms, indicating that this task was measuring theory of mind. Using single photon emission computerized tomograph (SPECT) imaging on a sample of developmentally normal control subjects, males aged 20 to 30, Baron-Cohen et al. found that right orbito-frontal cortex (OFC) was significantly more active during the mental state term recognition task than during the control task, relative to frontal polar cortex and posterior regions. One limitation of their study, however, is that they only carried out hypothesis-led region-of-interest (ROI) analyses and did not measure activation in the medial or dorsolateral frontal cortex, so it is unknown how active those areas were during their task. The task also has no inference component.

Fletcher et al. (1995) and Goel et al. (1995) used more complex tasks requiring subtle inferences about mental states. In Goel et al.'s study, subjects were asked to make inferences about objects that required either a visual description of the object, memory retrieval, an inference from the object's form to its function, or an inference that required modeling another person's mental state. They found selective activation for the task requiring mentalistic inferences in left medial frontal cortex and the left temporal lobe. In Fletcher et al.'s study, subjects read a story and then answered a question about the story that required a mentalistic inference. They answered the question silently, to themselves, without making any overt response. There were two control tasks for comparison: stories involving subtle physical inferences, but not mentalistic inferences, and paragraphs consisting of unrelated sentences. Subjects were told which type of story they were about to read and then were scanned both while reading and while answering the question.

Using positron emission tomography (PET) imaging, when pixels active during the physical inference stories were subtracted from pixels active during the theory of mind stories, Brodmann's areas 8 and 9 and the anterior cingulate showed up as active only during the theory of mind task. OFC was not specifically active during the theory of mind task. They conclude that their data "pinpointed the medial dorsal region of the left frontal cortex as being critically involved in mentalising". (Fletcher et al., 1995, p. 121).

Results from lesion patients thus far have not provided any conclusive evidence about which areas might be critical for theory of mind computations. Patients with damage to orbito-frontal cortex and with ventromedial damage, that is, damage that includes both orbital and medial frontal cortex, typically have severe deficits in social functioning (Blumer & Benson, 1975; Damasio, Tranel, & Damasio, 1990; Eslinger & Damasio, 1985; Kaczmarek, 1984; Mattson & Levin, 1990; Saver & Damasio, 1991). These patients are able to correctly analyze social situations in the abstract, but when they respond to similar situations in real life, they choose inappropriate courses of action (Eslinger & Damasio, 1985; Saver & Damasio, 1991). These patients can often say what the correct response is but have difficulty changing their behavior to respond appropriately to the social situation or to changing reinforcements in the environment (Rolls, 1996). Orbito-frontal patients often say inappropriate things and appear disinhibited (Mattson & Levin, 1990). Their conversation typically does not respond to signals of whether the other person is interested in what they are saying or whether they are on topic (Kaczmarek, 1984). Based on some similarities between OFC patients and patients with autism—impaired social judgment, increased indifference, and deficits in the pragmatics of conversation—Baron-Cohen and Ring (1994) have suggested that OFC is part of a neural circuit for mindreading, and that the social impairment following OFC damage occurs because part of the theory of mind module is damaged. However, as far as we are aware, no direct test of theory of mind, such as a test of false belief attribution, has been reported with OFC patients.

Only patients with damage in dorsolateral frontal cortex (DFC) have been directly tested on any kind of theory of mind task. Price, Daffner, Stowe, and Mesulam (1990) report two adult patients with bilateral DFC damage early in life who had difficulties with empathy and failed a perspective-taking task. The task was one developed by Flavell, Botkin, Fry, Wright, and Jarvis (1968) and although not explicitly designed as a theory of mind test, does require a theory of mind. The subject is given a map of a town and told that someone at a certain location on the map needs to get to a particular house on the map and is lost. The experimenter then reads a set of directions for getting from where the lost person is to the

228

house. The directions contain four different ambiguities such that a person could make mistakes and end up at the wrong house. After reading the directions, the experimenter asks the subject to identify which parts of the directions were ambiguous and could have led the lost person to make a mistake. This task requires perspective-taking and understanding false belief. However, the task also places considerable demands on working memory because the subject has to keep all of the directions in memory to answer the question. Because DFC patients typically have difficulty with working memory (Stuss, Eskes, & Foster, 1994), these patients could have failed on this task because of working memory limitations rather than because their theory of mind was impaired.

We undertook to test a series of developmentally graded theory of mind tasks in frontal lobe patients to determine if any subtle theory of mind deficits could be picked up in patients with lesions in the frontal lobe. We tested patients with damage in orbito-frontal cortex because they clearly have deficits in social behavior and because Baron-Cohen et al. (1994) found OFC activation with a theory of mind task. We also tested patients with damage to dorsolateral frontal cortex to compare their theory of mind performance to that of the patients tested by Price et al. (1990). We used tasks in which we could control for the working memory demands of the task.

SUBJECTS

We tested five patients with damage to the left lateral frontal cortex, including both dorsal regions of the lateral frontal cortex and more ventrolateral regions. We will refer to these patients as having DFC damage. This does not imply that their damage is restricted to dorsolateral regions of the lateral frontal cortex, only that all five patients have DFC damage. Figure 1 shows computerized axial tomograph (CT) reconstructions for individual patients, and Figure 2 shows the degree of overlap of the patients' lesions in different areas (see Table 1 for patient characteristics). Of the five DFC patients, four had damage to the lateral portion of Brodmann's area 8 and three of these also had damage to lateral area 9. These patients had middle cerebral artery infarcts, so their damage included only the lateral part of areas 8 and 9, sparing the medial portion. All five patients had damage in the middle frontal gyrus and middle frontal sulcus: Brodmann's area 46. Our map of area 46 is based on recent quantitative analysis of cytoarchitectonic features of cells in different areas of the frontal cortex (Rajkowska & Goldman-Rakic, 1995a, 1995b). Area 46 includes "central portions of one or more convolutions of the middle frontal gyrus and extending to the depth of the middle frontal sulcus" (Rajkowska & Goldman-Rakic, 1995b, p. 328). Slices 4 and 5 in our lesion overlap figure, Figure 2, show that all five DFC patients have

damage in the middle frontal gyrus and the depth of the middle frontal sulcus. These patients all had unilateral lesions from middle cerebral artery infarcts. Bilateral lesions in DFC due to stroke are rare.

Three of the DFC patients were aphasic: J.C., W.E., and R.T. All three had difficulty producing speech. A motor speech evaluation characterized these patients as having apraxia and disarthria. W.E.'s score on the Western Aphasia Battery was 96.3; J.C.'s was 91.9. W.E. scored 55 on the Boston Naming Test; J.C. scored 45. Both W.E. and J.C. are characterized as having anomic aphasia. For comparison, O.A., who is not aphasic, scored 99.6 on the W.A.B., and 58 on the Boston Naming Test.

We also tested five patients with bilateral damage to OFC from head trauma. See Table 1 and Figures 3 and 4 for summaries of the areas damaged in each patient and CT and magnetic resonance image (MRI) scans showing the extent of the damage. D.H., R.V., R.M., and R.B. all had extensive bilateral damage in area 11 and no damage to either the lateral frontal cortex or the basal forebrain area. The damage in R.V. and R.B. also included the polar parts of area 10 bilaterally, with minimal damage to area 38 on the left side, the very tip of the left temporal lobe. In addition, R.B. had more extensive damage to the left temporal lobe, including areas 38, 28, 21, and 20, and sparing the left amygdala. R.M.'s damage also included the polar part of area 10 on the left and about 1 cm of the right anterior temporal lobe, area 38, with the right amygdala spared. R.M. also had extensive damage to the left temporal lobe, extending back approximately 5 cm, including areas 38, 27, 28, 21, and 20 and the left amygdala. M.R. was the most unilateral of the OFC lesion patients in our sample, with extensive damage to area 11 on the right and partial damage to area 11 on the left. M.R. also had some lateral frontal damage on the right, both dorsolateral and ventrolateral frontal: areas 47, 45, and 9; some damage to the polar portion of area 10; and some medial frontal damage on the right to the anterior cingulate, area 33. His basal forebrain area was intact on the left and damaged on the right. Strictly unilateral damage to the OFC is rare because it is not a region in which strokes occur.

In addition, we tested one patient with damage restricted to the anterior temporal cortex, patient B.G. He was included in the sample to control for the bilateral temporal damage of R.V., R.B., and R.M. All patients were at least 6 months post-lesion.

We also tested five non-brain-damaged age-matched control subjects, matched for education with the least-educated patients, that is, having only a high school education.

Tasks

The tasks we used were developmentally graded, ranging in difficulty from tasks that normal 4-year-old children

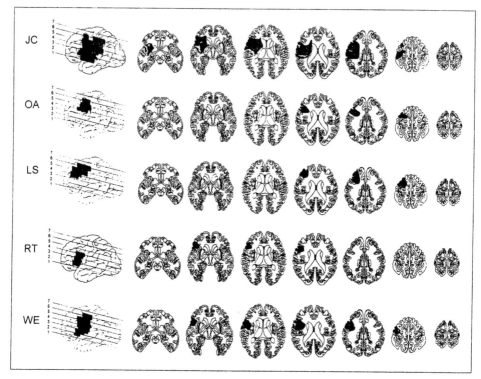

Figure 1. Extent of patients' lesions in the dorsolateral frontal cortex, reconstructed from CT scans.

can do to tasks that children cannot do until ages 9 to 11. We used three tasks altogether:

1. First-order false belief tasks, which develop around 3 to 4 years;
2. Second-order false belief tasks, which develop around 6 to 7 years;
3. Comprehension of social faux pas, which develops around 9 to 11 years (see "Methods").

The logic for this methodology was that deficits in theory of mind should be more evident in the tasks that develop later; therefore, the severity of theory of mind impairment could be estimated by looking at which tasks patients had difficulty with. Other work on deficits in dorsolateral frontal patients has used this kind of methodology to pick up subtle deficits. For instance, Goldstein, Bernard, Fenwick, Burgess, and McNeil (1993) tested a patient with a left frontal lobectomy who performed in the normal range on the Wisconsin Card

Sorting Task (WCST). Using tasks that were similar to the WCST but required more complex planning, these researchers were able to document subtle executive function deficits.

RESULTS

False Belief Tasks

Based on the first- and second-order false belief tasks, neither patient group shows a pronounced theory of mind deficit, such as that seen in autism. Some patients made errors on false belief tasks when they had to remember the stories. However, when the story was in front of the subjects, so that there was no memory load, patients made almost no errors (see Tables 2 and 3 and Figures 5 and 6).[1] Even in the condition with a memory load, it was rare for patients to make errors on the false belief question alone without also making errors on the control questions. The difference in the proportion of

230

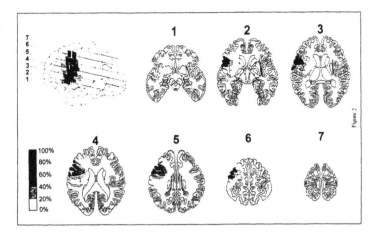

Figure 2. Extent of overlap of DFC patients' lesions, reconstructed from CT scans. The area of 80 to 100% overlap is in area 46, the middle frontal gyrus, and the depth of the middle frontal sulcus.

100%
80%
60%
40%
20%
0%

problems correct between these two conditions on the first-order false belief tasks was statistically significant for four out of five of the DFC patients: L.S. ($z = 2.92, p < 0.01$), R.T. ($z = 4.59, p < 0.00001$), J.C. ($z = 2.66, p < 0.01$, and W.E. ($z = 2.11, p < 0.05$). The difference between Conditions 1 and 2 was significant for L.S. ($z = 2.34, p < 0.01$) and R.T. ($z = 1.88, p < 0.05$) on the second-order false belief tasks. It was also significant for R.V., an OFC

patient, ($z = 3.46, p < 0.001$) on the first-order false belief task. After completing 10 first-order false belief problems in Condition 1, R.V. requested not to be tested in that condition any more because he found it so difficult.

Differences in performance between the false belief task and the true belief task were not significant for any of the frontal patients except J.C. (4/10 vs. 10/10, $z =$

Table 1. Patient Characteristics

Patient	Age	Time Since Lesion Onset	Location of Lesion	Brodmann's Areas Damaged
J.C.	72	9 years	Left lateral frontal, including DFC, superior temporal	Lateral areas 8, 9; areas 44, 45, 46; areas 4, 6
O.A.	64	12 years	Left lateral frontal, including DFC	Lateral areas 8, 9; area 46
W.E.	67	6 months	Left lateral frontal, including DFC	Lateral area 8; areas 44, 45, 46
L.S.	68	22 years	Left lateral frontal, including DFC	Lateral areas 8, 9; area 46
R.T.	80	11 years	Left lateral frontal, including DFC	Areas 45, 46
D.H.	34	16 years	Bilateral OFC	Extensive bilateral area 11
M.R.	42	18 years	Bilateral OFC	Extensive right area 11; partial left area 11; right areas 47, 45, 9, 10, and 33; right basal forebrain area
R.B.	51	22 years	Bilateral OFC & anterior temporal	Extensive bilateral area 11; polar area 10 bilaterally; partial left area 38
R.M.	46	20 years	Bilateral OFC & anterior temporal	Extensive bilateral area 11; polar area 10 bilaterally; partial right area 38; left areas 38, 28, 21, and 20; amygdala spared
R.V.	45	5 years	Bilateral OFC & anterior temporal	Extensive bilateral area 11; left polar area 10; partial right area 38; left area 37, 28, 21, and 20; left amygdala
B.G.	53	4 years	Anterior temporal	Bilateral area 38

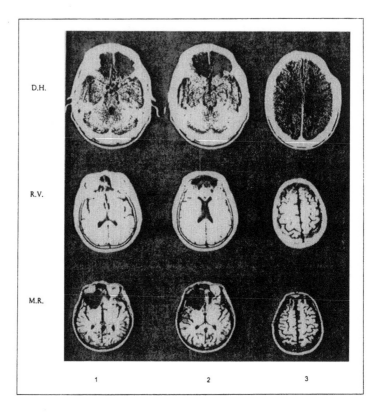

Figure 3. Three patients with bilateral damage to orbito-frontal cortex. CT scans are shown for patient D.H. and MRI scans are shown for patients M.R. and R.V. The images in columns 1 and 2 show the damage to orbito-frontal cortex; column 3 shows that dorsolateral frontal cortex is spared in patients D.H. and R.V., with some right dorsolateral damage in patient M.R. Medial frontal cortex is spared in all patients.

D.H.

R.V.

M.R.

1   2   3

$2.93, p < 0.002$); this was true only in the condition with a memory load.

Because three of the dorsolateral frontal patients were aphasic and had difficulty producing speech, we did not ask subjects to justify their responses on the false belief tasks. However, L.S. spontaneously offered mentalistic justifications on several problems. Even on two problems she got wrong, she provided mental state explanations that made sense of her "errors," for example. "He'll probably think it's on the shelf because he won't see it on the desk where he left it, so that would be the logical place to look."

Order Effects, Practice Effects

There were no effects of prior exposure to a particular story and no practice effects. Subjects' performance did not improve over the course of testing. Subjects were not more likely to give correct answers for false belief tasks they were given in the second session than tasks they were given in the first session, regardless of condition.

Because subjects did not perform significantly better in the second testing session than in the first testing session, familiarity with the stories being used did not seem to help them answer correctly. Only memory load predicts their performance, indicating that working memory limitations may provide the best explanation of their results.

In the condition without a memory load, there was no evidence for a theory of mind deficit at the level of 4- to 7-year-old children in either the orbito-frontal or the dorsolateral frontal patient group.

Faux Pas Task

Control subjects and DFC patients correctly detected all of the faux pas and correctly answered who committed the faux pas. In contrast, almost all of the OFC patients made errors detecting faux pas, answering that nothing awkward had been said in the story. They sometimes answered No to the question, "Did someone say something they shouldn't have said?" The difference between

232

Figure 4. The top two patients, R.M. and R.B., have bilateral damage to the orbito-frontal cortex and additional bilateral damage to the anterior temporal cortex, with more extensive damage on the left. R.M.'s anterior temporal damage is more extensive than R.B.'s and includes one amygdala. The patient in the last row, B.G., has restricted anterior temporal damage. Column 1 shows damage to the temporal lobes; columns 2 and 3 show damage (or, in the case of B.G., lack of damage) to orbito-frontal cortex. All images are T_2 weighted axial MRI slices.

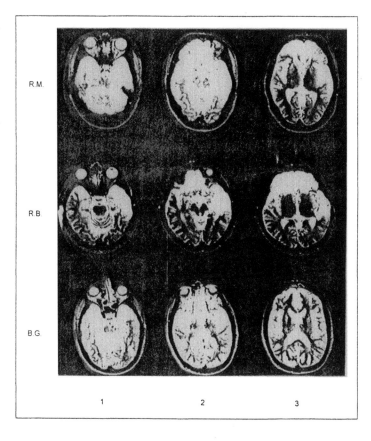

the OFC patients and the control subjects (who were at ceiling) in the detection of faux pas is significant ($t_8 =$ 2.828, $p < 0.02$). All of the OFC patients answered the control questions correctly. Thus, it appears that they understood the stories yet didn't realize that something inappropriate had been said (see Table 4).

In contrast, the DFC patients got confused about the details of the story, and as a consequence all four answered some of the control questions incorrectly. For example, W.E. mixed up who the surprise party was for and therefore made errors on both the control question and the question of who committed the faux pas because he had mixed up the two characters' names. R.T. made a similar mistake on this problem. Although he answered the first two questions correctly, he got mixed up on the later questions and made mistakes. O.A. stated on two of the control questions that he didn't remember what the answer was. All of these errors were made even

though the story was right in front of the patients on the desk and the experimenter told them that they could look back at the stories. They did not always do so even when they got confused.

All of the stories contained a faux pas, that is, someone saying something awkward that should not have been said. There are two possible explanations for why subjects might answer yes to the question of whether something awkward had been said on all 10 stories. One explanation is that they correctly recognized all of the faux pas. Another possible explanation is that they merely had a Yes bias. We can control for the fact that the DFC patients always answered Yes on this question by looking at their responses to the question of who said something they should not have said. If they did not understand that a faux pas had been committed and were merely saying Yes because of a Yes bias, they would have not answered the questions about who committed

Table 2. Proportion of Problems Correct and Types of Errors on False Belief Problems with and without Memory Load (*n* = 20 problems in each condition)

Group tested	Condition 1: Memory Load				Condition 2: No Memory Load			
	% Correct	FB Errors	FB + Control	Control Errors	% Correct	FB Errors	FB + Control	Control Errors
DFC Patients								
L.S.	55	3	4	2	95	0	1	0
R.T.	25	4	7	4	95	0	1	0
O.A.	100	0	0	0	100	0	0	0
J.C.	70	0	4	2	100	0	0	0
W.E.	80	0	2	2	100	0	0	0
Mean	66	1.4	3.4	2	98	0	0.4	0
OFC patients								
D.H.	100	0	0	0	100	0	0	0
M.R.	100	0	0	0	100	0	0	0
R.V.	50	0	5/10	0	100	0	0	0
R.M.	100	0	0	0	not tested			
R.B.	100	0	0	0	100	0	0	0
Mean	100	0	0.5	0	100	0	0	0
Anterior Temporal Control								
B.G.	100	0	0	0	100	0	0	0
Normal Controls								
Mean	100	0	0	0	100	0	0	0

Key to column headings:
FB Errors: Number of problems on which subject made errors on false belief questions only.
FB + Control: Number of problems on which subject made errors on both false belief and control questions.
Control Errors: Number of problems on which subject made errors on control questions only.

the faux pas correctly. However, they all answered these questions correctly if they answered the control questions correctly. They made errors on who committed the faux pas only when they mixed up the two characters and got confused about the story overall. We conclude that the DFC patients did not answer Yes merely because they had a Yes bias but rather were correctly recognizing the faux pas contained in the stories.

For the empathic understanding question, asked in a later session (e.g. "How do you think Jill felt?"), all subjects gave similar answers, and all subjects demonstrated appropriate empathic understanding. For example, in the story about Jill and the curtains, all subjects indicated that Jill would have felt hurt or angry. Even OFC patients who had failed to detect faux pas on particular stories made appropriate empathic inferences about what the characters in those stories would have felt. Their answers did not differ from those of control subjects.

DISCUSSION

The performance of the bilateral OFC patients on these tasks is parallel to what has been found for individuals with Asperger's syndrome. They had no difficulty understanding the stories, as indexed by their performance on the control questions, but they failed to recognize that some faux pas had been committed. Their performance on this task is consistent with their behavior in everyday life, in which they frequently say inappropriate things and inappropriately analyze social situations. Like children who are 7 to 8 years old and individuals with Asperger's syndrome, they can pass first- and second-order theory of mind tasks but make errors on the more difficult faux pas task. Further research with unilateral OFC patients would provide more insight into the effect of bilateral vs. unilateral OFC lesions. However, the one patient, M.R., in our OFC sample whose lesions were mostly unilateral was the most impaired on the faux pas task.

234

Table 3. Proportion of Problems Correct and Types of Errors on Second-Order False Belief Problems with and without Memory Load (n = 10 problems in each condition)

Group tested	Condition 1: Memory Load				Condition 2: No Memory Load			
	% Correct	FB Errors	FB + Control	Control Errors	% Correct	FB Errors	FB + Control	Control Errors
DFC Patients								
L.S.	40	3	2	1	90	0	1	0
R.T.	70	1	2	0	100	0	0	0
O.A.	100	0	0	0	100	0	0	0
J.C.	100	0	0	0	100	0	0	0
W.E.	100	0	0	0	100	0	0	0
Mean	82	0.8	0.8	0.2	99	0	0.2	0
OFC patients								
D.H.	100	0	0	0	100	0	0	0
M.R.	100	0	0	0	100	0	0	0
R.V.	not tested				100	0	0	0
R.M.	100	0	0	0	not tested			
R.B.	100	0	0	0	100	0	0	0
Mean	100	0	0	0	100	0	0	0
Anterior Temporal Control								
B.G.	100	0	0	0	100	0	0	0
Normal Controls								
Mean	100	0	0	0	100	0	0	0

Key to column headings:
FB Errors: Number of problems on which subject made errors on second-order false belief questions only.
FB + Control: Number of problems on which subject made errors on both second-order false belief and control questions.
Control Errors: Number of problems on which subject made errors on control questions only.

Two things are necessary for someone to detect a faux pas. One must understand that one person has knowledge that the other person is unaware of or that one person has a mistaken belief, and one must have the empathic understanding about what kinds of things someone would find upsetting or insulting. Baron-Cohen (1991) found that people with autism could understand others' emotions if those emotions were caused by situations or desires. However, they did not understand emotions that were caused by belief. Their deficit was specifically in integrating empathy with mental state attribution. The OFC patients in this study and the Asperger's subjects in Baron-Cohen et al.'s (1997) study may be exhibiting a more subtle version of this same type of deficit. Because they can pass first- and second-order false belief tasks, we infer that their errors are not due to cognitive limitations in understanding the mental states of the characters in the stories, that is, understanding the levels of false and mistaken belief in the

faux pas stories. Because the OFC patients got all the "empathy" questions right in the faux pas task, performing in the same way as controls, we conclude that their empathic understanding of what another person would find upsetting is intact. Rather, their errors may be due to problems connecting their theory of mind inferences with an understanding of emotion. This interpretation is consistent with Brothers and Ring's (1992) idea that the amygdala and orbito-frontal cortex are essential brain structures for the "hot" aspects of theory of mind, that is, for interpreting the valence and significance of others' actions and intentions. Many other authors, although not investigating theory of mind, have reported the importance of OFC and the amygdala for understanding the significance of others' actions (Adolphs, Tranel, Damasio, & Damasio, 1994; Cahill et al., 1996; Damasio et al., 1990; Franzen & Myers, 1973; Hornak, Rolls, & Wade, 1996; Kling & Steklis, 1976; McGaugh, 1990; Morris et al., 1996; Rolls, 1996; Young et al., 1995).

Figure 5. Patients' performance (% correct) on 20 first-order false belief problems.

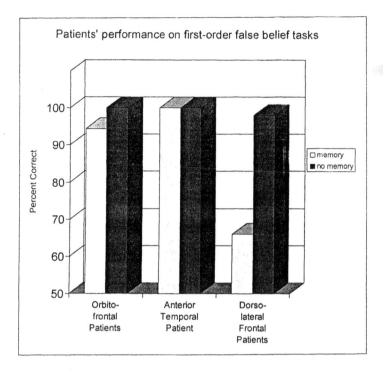

Patients' performance on first-order false belief tasks

Percent Correct

□ memory
■ no memory

Orbito-frontal Patients Anterior Temporal Patient Dorso-lateral Frontal Patients

Saver and Damasio (1991) found that ventromedial patients had no difficulty with "abstract social knowledge," that is, these patients could figure out solutions for interpersonal problems between other people quite well. It was only when they had to make social decisions in their own lives that they showed a deficit. In our study, although the faux pas stories were all about other people, the OFC patients could not always apply abstract social knowledge to tell that something was said that would be awkward or should have not been said. This is consistent with the idea that recognizing a faux pas, even when committed by someone else, requires some affective understanding, in addition to abstract mental state attribution.

We note that we found no evidence that the patients with anterior temporal damage had any difficulty with the short narratives we used. Patients B.G., with only anterior temporal damage, and R.B., with OFC and anterior temporal damage, made no errors on any task. R.M. made only faux pas errors. Mazoyer et al. (1993) and Fletcher et al. (1995) noted that the anterior temporal region was active during tasks that involved narrative but not when subjects were reading unconnected sentences. It appears that the damaged areas in the anterior tempo-

ral cortex in the patients we tested were not crucial for understanding these simple narratives.

The PET imaging results of Fletcher et al. (1995) and Goel et al. (1995) point to Brodmann's areas 8 and 9 in the left medial frontal cortex as being "critically involved in mentalising" (Fletcher et al., 1995, p. 121). Our study supplements theirs by investigating the role of other frontal regions, OFC and DFC, in theory of mind inferences. We found that OFC patients' performance on the faux pas task, in combination with being able to pass simple first- and second-order false belief tasks, is consistent with their having a subtle theory of mind deficit, like Asperger's subjects. We found no similar evidence for theory of mind deficits in unilateral DFC patients. Our patients did not have damage in the areas activated in Fletcher et al.'s study, so we cannot comment on whether these medial areas are critical for theory of mind inferences.

Theory of mind is a complex high-level cognitive ability, developing over the course of many years, and completing its development relatively late. Baron-Cohen (1995) has discussed several components of theory of mind, suggesting that it is not a unitary module but a collection of inferential abilities. Such a complex, multi-

236

Figure 6. Patients' performance (% correct) on 10
second-order false belief
problems.

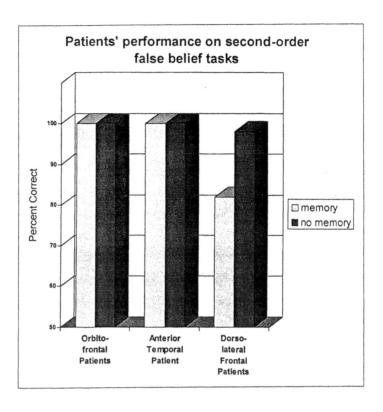

component, cognitive ability is unlikely to be localized in a small region of the cortex. We propose instead that theory of mind is a distributed circuit involving many regions of the cortex, in addition to the limbic system. Based on our results here with bilateral OFC patients, we conclude that OFC is part of this circuit, perhaps particularly involved in theory of mind tasks with an affective component. From previous neuroimaging results, the left medial frontal cortex would appear to be part of this circuit also. The left DFC patients in our study did not show deficits on any of our tasks, so we conclude that the left DFC is not crucial to this theory of mind circuit. Based on our sample, we cannot rule out the possibility that bilateral damage to the DFC would produce theory of mind deficits. Price et al. (1990) did find deficits on a perspective-taking task in patients with bilateral DFC damage, although they did not control for the working memory demands of the task. Further studies investigating the question of how bilateral DFC patients perform on theory of mind tasks are needed, particularly studies that control for working memory. The DFC may be involved in the operation of theory of mind in real time

in social interaction because of the rapid changes of attention required in order to keep up with social interaction. The system may be redundant or plastic so that focal damage in only one region of the theory of mind circuit does not produce strong impairments in the ability to make inferences about another person's mental states. To make an inference as complex as what another person may be thinking, many areas of the brain must work together.

METHODS

First-Order False Belief Tasks

These tasks were designed to test subjects' ability to infer that someone can have a mistaken belief that is different from their own true belief. They were based on Wimmer and Perner (1983) and Baron-Cohen et al. (1985). False belief tasks typically involve one person putting an object somewhere in the presence of another person and then leaving the room. The second person moves the object to another location while the first

Stone et al. 651

237

Table 4. Types of Errors Made on Faux Pas Task ($n = 10$ problems)

Group Tested	Detected Faux Pas	Control Questions	Correctly Named Who Committed Faux Pas	Correct Answer: "Why Shouldn't Have Said?"	Correct Answer: "Why Did They Say It?"	Correct Answer: "How Would X Feel?"
DFC patients						
L.S.	10	8	8	7	8	
R.T.	10	8	10	9	9	
O.A.	10	8	8	10	9	
W.E.	10	9	9	7	9	
Mean	10	8.25	8.75	8.25	8.75	
OFC patients						
D.H.	9	10	9	9	10	10
M.R.	6	10	6	6	10	10
R.V.	7	10	7	7	10	10
R.M.	8	10	8	8	10	10
R.B.	10	10	10	10	10	10
Mean	8	10	8	8	10	10
Anterior Temporal Control						
B.G.	10	10	10	10	10	10
Normal Controls						
Mean	10	10	10	10	10	10

person is away. The first person returns, and the subject is asked three questions: the "belief question," which asks where the first person thinks the object is, and requires an understanding of others' mental states; the "reality question," which asks where the object really is; and the "memory question," which asks where the object was in the beginning. The control questions ensure that the subject knows the real current location of the object and has an accurate memory of where it was before it was moved. Subjects who get these questions wrong in addition to the belief question are assumed to have problems with memory or comprehension, not false belief.

We gave subjects a total of 20 first-order false belief problems, with a series of control conditions to test for working memory problems.

Physical Inference vs. Mentalistic Inference

One possible confound in the standard false belief task is that the belief question is both the only question that asks about mental states and the only question that requires an inference rather than just memory. Thus, we constructed 10 false belief tasks that allowed us to ask another control question that required a physical inference rather than a mentalistic inference. The subject was read a story and shown photographs depicting the ac-

tion in the story. Any reasonable answer was accepted as correct for the physical inference.

For example, one of the stories involved Bill and Jim, standing in their office talking. First we checked that the subjects could correctly identify Bill and Jim in the pictures. Jim puts an open bottle of ink on his desk. As he is doing so, some ink spills. The picture of this scene was a drawing of an ink bottle with ink splashing out and did not show where the ink spilled. None of the subsequent pictures showed the surface of the desk. Jim then leaves the office. Bill moves the ink bottle to a cabinet and closes the cabinet. He goes back over by Jim's desk and Jim comes back in. There is a wall between the door through which Jim comes back in and the desk, so that Jim cannot see the desk as he reenters. The questions asked were:

Belief question: When Jim comes back in, where will he think the ink bottle is? (correct answer: on the desk)
Reality question: Where is the ink bottle? (in the cabinet)
Memory question: Where was the ink bottle in the beginning? (desk or Jim's hand)
Inference question: Where would there be an ink stain? (On the desk or on the floor next to the desk. We also accepted as correct answers such as "on Bill's hand" or "on the shelf," although no subjects gave such answers without also saying "on the desk.")

238

An error is typically scored if the subject says that when the first person comes back in (Jim, in the above example), he thinks the object is in the location it was moved to (the cabinet in the above example).

False Belief vs. True Belief

Another possible confound is the working memory demands of a false belief task. The number of story elements that must be held in mind to answer the false belief question may be difficult for dorsolateral frontal patients. Thus, we constructed 10 more false belief tasks that could be compared to "true belief" tasks, which tell the same story but in which the first person is present and watching while the second person moves the object to another location. Thus, the story elements are the same; the only difference is that the "true belief" tasks do not require attribution of a false belief. Mixing true belief problems in with false belief problems also prevents patients from using a strategy of always answering the belief question with the first location of the object. Both false belief and true belief stories were videotaped, with actors portraying the story. In this task, rather than having to give a verbal answer, subjects were provided with pictures of the two locations and asked to point to one of the two in response to the belief questions and control questions.

For example, one story went as follows in the false belief and true belief versions:

False Belief

Tony puts some Coke in the cabinet. Then he leaves the room. Maria comes along and moves the Coke from the cabinet into the refrigerator to chill. Later, Tony comes back in.

Where does Tony think the Coke is?
Where is the Coke?
Where did Tony put the Coke in the beginning?

True Belief

Tony puts some Coke in the cabinet. Maria comes along and says, "We shouldn't put it there, we should put it over here." She moves the Coke from the cabinet to the refrigerator to chill while Tony watches.

Where does Tony think the Coke is?
Where is the Coke?
Where did Tony put the Coke in the beginning?

Controlling for Memory Load

In order to further control for the working memory demands of these tasks, subjects were tested on each of the above tasks under two conditions, one in which they had to remember the story and one in which they did not. If subjects truly had difficulty with false belief and mentalistic inferences, memory load should not have affected their performance.

Condition 1, Memory Load

The subject was read the story while being shown either photographs or a videotape depicting the story action. If the subject was being shown photos, the photos were shown one at a time and covered up by the next one. The subject had to remember the entire story in order to answer the questions.

Condition 2, No Memory Load

The subject was read the story while being shown pictures depicting the story action. All the pictures remained in front of the subject while he or she answered the questions. The pictures were either the same photographs as in Condition 1 or prints of video stills from the videotape used in Condition 1.

All 20 false belief problems were tested twice, once in Condition 1 and once in Condition 2, counterbalanced between two testing sessions. For example, if a subject saw a particular story in Condition 2 in the first session, he or she would see that story in Condition 1 in the second session. For example, some subjects got the video version (Condition 1) of the false belief/true belief tasks in the first session, and others got the video stills (Condition 2) in the first session. The two testing sessions were separated by at least month.

R.M., one of the OFC patients, completed only Condition 1, the memory load condition, on the false belief tasks because he moved to another state during the study. This was the more difficult condition. He completed Condition 1 on the first- and second-order belief tasks and answered all of the questions on the faux pas task.

Second-Order False Belief Tasks

These tasks were designed to test the ability to understand what someone else thinks about what another person thinks. Second-order false belief is a more subtle test of theory of mind impairment than first-order false belief, but because the task was styled after tasks used on 6 and 7 year olds, it is still not a very complex theory of mind task.

The second-order false belief tasks were adapted from the first-order false belief tasks used above that required subjects to make both mentalistic and physical inferences. In each story, Person 1 puts an object somewhere and leaves the room. Person 2 moves the object. While Person 1 is out of the room, he or she peeks back in and sees the object being moved, but Person 2 does not know that Person 1 has seen this. The subject is asked, "When Person 1 comes back in, where will Person 2 think that Person 1 thinks the object is?" Control ques-

239

tions ask where the object really is and where the object was in the beginning and ask a question requiring a physical inference. Again, the subject was read the story and shown a series of photographs depicting the action described in the story.

As an example, two characters, Martha and Oliver, are sitting in the kitchen talking. Oliver is eating cookies. First we checked that the subjects could correctly identify Martha and Oliver in the pictures. Oliver gets up and leaves the room. Martha closes up the box of cookies and puts them away in a cabinet. While he is outside of the room, Oliver looks back through the keyhole and sees Martha moving the cookies. Martha goes back and sits down. Then Oliver opens the door.

Belief question: Where does Martha think that Oliver thinks the cookies are? (correct answer: on the table)
Reality question: Where are the cookies? (in the cabinet)
Memory question: Where were the cookies in the beginning? (on the table)
Inference question: Where would there be cookie crumbs? (on the table, on the floor)

Subjects were given 10 such problems. Subjects were tested on each problem twice, once in a condition in which they had to remember the story and one in which they did not. Subjects were tested in these two conditions in two separate sessions, counterbalancing which condition was tested in which session.

Condition 1, Memory Load

The subject was read the story while being shown photographs depicting the story action. The photos were shown one at a time and covered up by the next one. The subject had to remember the entire story in order to answer the questions.

Condition 2, No Memory Load

The subject was read the story while being shown pictures depicting the story action. All the pictures remained in front of the subject while he or she answered the questions.

Recognition of Faux Pas Task

Subjects were read a story that told about the occurrence of a faux pas. So that subjects did not have to remember the stories, the page with the story on it was placed in front of the subject while it was being read and while questions were being asked afterward. For example, two of the stories follow:

Jeanette bought her friend Anne a crystal bowl for a wedding gift. Anne had a big wedding and there were a lot of presents to keep track of. About a year later, Jeanette was over one night at Anne's for din-

ner. Jeanette dropped a wine bottle by accident on the crystal bowl, and the bowl shattered. "I'm really sorry, I've broken the bowl," said Jeanette. "Don't worry," said Anne, "I never liked it anyway. Someone gave it to me for my wedding."

Helen's husband was throwing a surprise party for her birthday. He invited Sarah, a friend of Helen's, and said, "Don't tell anyone, especially Helen." The day before the party, Helen was over at Sarah's, and Sarah spilled some coffee on a new dress that was hanging over her chair. "Oh!" said Sarah, "I was going to wear this to your party!" "What party?" said Helen. "Come on," said Sarah, "Let's go see if we can get the stain out."

All of the stories contained a faux pas, someone saying something awkward. In three of the stories, the faux pas was the last thing said in the story, and in seven of them it was not the last thing said.

After the story, subjects were asked a series of questions:

1. Did someone say something they shouldn't have said? (Tests for detection of faux pas.)
2. Who said something they shouldn't have said? (Tests for understanding of faux pas.)
3. Why shouldn't they have said it? (Requires understanding mental state of listener.)
4. Why did they say it? (Requires understanding mental state of speaker.)
5. An example is, What had Jeanette given Anne for her wedding? (Control question that asks about some detail of the story.)

Questions 2 through 4 were only asked if the subject detected the faux pas, that is, answered Yes to Question 1. If the subject answered No to Question 1, the experimenter skipped to 5, the control question. Subjects were given 10 such stories.

Understanding a faux pas requires understanding both a mental state of belief or knowledge and having some empathic understanding of how the person in the story would feel. We wanted to test empathic understanding separately, so in a later session, subjects were given the same faux pas stories and asked how they thought the characters in the stories would feel. For example, one story involved a woman, Lisa, criticizing some curtains in her friend Jill's apartment, not realizing that Jill had just bought them. Subjects were read the story and asked, "How do you think Jill felt?"

Acknowledgments

This research was supported by NINDS grant F32 NS09977 to Valerie E. Stone, NINDS grant P01 NS17778 to Robert T. Knight and Michael S. Gazzaniga, NINDS grant NS21135 to Robert T. Knight, and the McDonnell-Pew Foundation. The authors would like to thank Donatella Scabini for recruiting patients for research, Alison Gopnik and Rich Ivry for helpful methodological suggestions, Clint Glaze for help in preparing the stimulus materials, and Kathy Baynes, Robin Dolan, Jim Eliassen, Jeff Hutsler, Donna Lemongello, Helmi Lutsep, Oliver Miller, Laura Nisenson, Mado Proverbio, Tony Ro, Josh Rubinstein, Doug Walters, and Martha Whitman for acting in the stimulus materials.

Reprint requests should be sent to Valerie Stone, Department of Psychology, University of Denver, 2155 South Race Street, Denver, CO 80208-2478.

Notes

1. After several problems, Patient R.V. asked not to be tested in Condition 1, with a memory load. He said it was too hard, and he found he forgot the stories. Thus, he was not tested on Condition 1 in all problems on the false belief/true belief task or in the second-order false belief task.

REFERENCES

Adolphs, R., Tranel, D., Damasio, H., & Damasio, A. (1994). Impaired recognition of emotion in facial expressions following bilateral damage to the human amygdala. *Nature, 372*, 669-672.

Astington, J. W., & Gopnik, A. (1991). Theoretical explanations of children's understanding of the mind. *British Journal of Developmental Psychology, 9*, 7-31.

Avis, J., & Harris, P. (1991). Belief-desire reasoning among Baka children: Evidence for a universal conception of mind. *Child Development, 62*, 460-467.

Baron-Cohen, S. (1989a). Perceptual role-taking and protodeclarative pointing in autism. *British Journal of Developmental Psychology, 7*, 113-127.

Baron-Cohen, S. (1989b). The autistic child's theory of mind: A case of specific developmental delay. *Journal of Child Psychology and Psychiatry, 30*, 285-297.

Baron-Cohen, S. (1991). Do people with autism understand what causes emotion? *Child Development, 62*, 385-395.

Baron-Cohen, S. (1995). *Mindblindness: An essay on autism and theory of mind.* Cambridge, MA: MIT Press.

Baron-Cohen, S., Leslie, A., & Frith, U. (1985). Does the autistic child have a "theory of mind"? *Cognition, 21*, 37-46.

Baron-Cohen, S., Leslie, A., & Frith, U. (1986). Mechanical, behavioral and intentional understanding of picture stories in autistic children. *British Journal of Developmental Psychology, 4*, 113-125.

Baron-Cohen, S., O'Riordan, M., Stone, V. E., Jones, R., & Plaisted, K. (1997). Recognition of faux pas by normally developing children and children with Asperger syndrome. Unpublished manuscript, University of Cambridge.

Baron-Cohen, S., & Ring, H. (1994). The relationship between EDD and ToMM: Neuropsychological and neurobiological perspectives. In P. Mitchell & C. Lewis (Eds.), *Origins of an understanding of mind* (pp. 183-207). Hillsdale, NJ: Erlbaum.

Baron-Cohen, S., Ring, H., Moriarty, J., Schmitz, B., Costa, D., & Ell, P. (1994). Recognition of mental state terms: Clinical findings in children with autism and a functional neuroimaging study of normal adults. *British Journal of Psychiatry, 165*, 640-649.

Blumer, D., & Benson, D. F. (1975). Personality changes with frontal and temporal lesions. In D. F. Benson & D. Blumer (Eds.), *Psychiatric aspects of neurological disease* (pp. 151-169). New York: Grune & Stratton.

Brothers, L., & Ring, B. (1992). A neuroethological framework

for the representation of minds. *Journal of Cognitive Neuroscience, 4*, 107-118.

Cahill, L., Haier, R. J., Fallon, J., Alkire, M. T., Tang, C., Keator, D., Wu, J., & McGaugh, J. L. (1996). Amygdala activity at encoding correlated with long-term, free recall of emotional information. *Proceedings of the National Academy of Sciences, 93*, 8016-8021.

Charman, T., & Baron-Cohen, S. (1992). Understanding beliefs and drawings: A further test of the metarepresentation theory of autism. *Journal of Child Psychology and Psychiatry, 33*, 1105-1112.

Charman, T., & Baron-Cohen, S. (1995). Understanding photos, models, and beliefs: A test of the modularity thesis of theory of mind. *Cognitive Development, 10*, 287-298.

Damasio, A. R., Tranel, D., & Damasio, H. (1990). Individuals with sociopathic behavior caused by frontal damage fail to respond autonomically to social stimuli. *Behavioral Brain Research, 41*, 81-94.

Dennett, D. (1978). Beliefs about beliefs. *Behavioral & Brain Sciences, 4*, 568-570.

Dennett, D. (1987). *The intentional stance.* Cambridge, MA: MIT Press.

Eslinger, P. J., & Damasio, A. R. (1985). Severe disturbance of higher cognition after bilateral frontal lobe ablation: Patient EVR. *Neurology, 35*, 1731-1741.

Flavell, J. H., Botkin, P., Fry, C., Wright, T., & Jarvis, P. (1968). *The development of role-taking and communication in children.* New York: Wiley.

Fletcher, P. C., Happé, F., Frith, U., Baker, S. C., Dolan, R. J., Frackowiak, R. S. J., & Frith, C. (1995). Other minds in the brain: A functional imaging study of "theory of mind" in story comprehension. *Cognition, 57*, 109-128.

Franzen, E. A., & Myers, R. E. (1973). Neural control of social behavior: Prefrontal and anterior temporal cortex. *Neuropsychologia, 11*, 141-157.

Goel, V., Grafman, J., Sadato, N., & Hallett, M. (1995). Modeling other minds. *Neuroreport, 6*, 1741-1746.

Goldstein, L. H., Bernard, S., Fenwick, P. B. C., Burgess, P. W., & McNeil, J. (1993). Unilateral frontal lobectomy can produce strategy application disorder. *Journal of Neurology, Neurosurgery, and Psychiatry, 56*, 274-276.

Gopnik, A., & Astington, J. W. (1988). Children's understanding of representational change and its relation to the understanding of false belief and the appearance-reality distinction. *Child Development, 59*, 26-37.

Gopnik, A., & Wellman, H. M. (1992). Why the child's theory of mind really is a theory. *Mind & Language, 7*, 145-171.

Happé, F. G. E. (1993). Communicative competence and theory of mind in autism: A test of Relevance Theory. *Cognition, 48*, 101-119.

Heider, F., & Simmel, M. (1944). An experimental study of apparent behavior. *American Journal of Psychology, 57*, 243-259.

Hornak, J., Rolls, E. T., & Wade, D. (1996). Face and voice expression identification in patients with emotional and behavioral changes following ventral frontal lobe damage. *Neuropsychologia, 34*, 247-261.

Johnson, C. N., & Wellman, H. M. (1980). Children's developing understanding of mental verbs: Remember, know and guess. *Child Development, 51*, 1095-1102.

Kaczmarek, B. (1984). Analysis of verbal utterances in patients with focal lesions of frontal lobes. *Brain and Language, 21*, 52-58.

Karmiloff-Smith, A., Klima, E., Bellugi, U., Grant, J., & Baron-Cohen, S. (1995). Is there a social module? Language, face processing and theory of mind in individuals with Williams syndrome. *Journal of Cognitive Neuroscience, 7*, 196-208.

Kling, A., & Steklis, H. D. (1976). A neural substrate for affiliative behavior in nonhuman primates. *Brain, Behavior, & Evolution, 13*, 216-238.

Leekam, S., & Perner, J. (1991). Does the autistic child have a "metarepresentational" deficit? *Cognition, 40*, 203-218.

Leslie, A. M. (1987). Pretense and representation in infancy: The origins of "theory of mind." *Psychological Review, 94*, 412-426.

Leslie, A. M., & Thaiss, L. (1992). Domain specificity in conceptual development: Neuropsychological evidence from autism. *Cognition, 43*, 225-251.

Mattson, A. J., & Levin, H. S. (1990). Frontal lobe dysfunction following closed head injury. *Journal of Nervous and Mental Disease, 178*, 282-291.

Mazoyer, B. M., Tzourio, N., Frak, V., Syrota, A., Murayama, N., Levrier, O., Salamon, G., Dehaene, S., Cohen, L., & Mehler, J. (1993). The cortical representation of speech. *Journal of Cognitive Neuroscience, 5*, 467-479.

McGaugh, J. L. (1990). Significance and remembrance: The role of neuromodulatory systems. *Psychological Science, 1*, 15-25.

Morris, J. S., Frith, C. D., Perrett, D. I., Rowland, D., Young, A. W., Calder, A. J., & Dolan, R. J. (1996). A differential neural response in the human amygdala to fearful and happy facial expressions. *Nature, 383*, 812-815.

Perner, J., Leekam, S. R., & Wimmer, H. (1987). Three-year-old's difficulty with false belief: The case for a conceptual deficit. *British Journal of Developmental Psychology, 5*, 125-137.

Perner, J., & Wimmer, H. (1985). "John thinks that Mary thinks that . . . ": Attribution of second-order false beliefs by 5- to 10-year-old children. *Journal of Experimental Child Psychology, 39*, 437-471.

Premack, D., & Woodruff, G. (1978). Does the chimpanzee have a theory of mind? *Behavioral and Brain Sciences, 1*, 515-526.

Price, B., Daffner, K., Stowe, R., & Mesulam, M. (1990). The comportmental learning disabilities of early frontal lobe damage. *Brain, 113*, 1383-1393.

Rajkowska, G., & Goldman-Rakic, P. S. (1995a). Cytoarchitectonic definition of prefrontal areas in the normal human cortex: I. Remapping of areas 9 and 46 using quantitative criteria. *Cerebral Cortex, 5*, 307-322.

Rajkowska, G., & Goldman-Rakic, P. S. (1995b). Cytoarchitectonic definition of prefrontal areas in the normal human cortex: II. Variability in locations of areas 9 and 46 and relationship to the Talairach coordinate system. *Cerebral Cortex, 5*, 323-337.

Rolls, E. T. (1996). The orbitofrontal cortex. *Philosophical Transactions of the Royal Society, 351*, 1433-1443.

Saver, J. L., & Damasio, A. R. (1991). Preserved access and processing of social knowledge in a patient with acquired sociopathy due to ventromedial frontal damage. *Neuropsychologia, 29*, 1241-1249.

Stuss, D. T., Eskes, G. A., & Foster, J. K. (1994). Experimental neuropsychological studies of frontal lobe functions. In J. Grafman & F. Boller (Eds.), *Handbook of neuropsychology, Vol. 9* (pp. 149-185). Amsterdam: Elsevier.

Tager-Flusberg, H. (1989). A psycholinguistic perspective on language development in the autistic child. In G. Dawson (Ed.), *Autism: Nature, diagnosis and treatment* (pp. 92-115). New York: Guilford Press.

Tager-Flusberg, H. (1993). What language reveals about the understanding of minds in children with autism. In S. Baron-Cohen, H. Tager-Flusberg, & D. J. Cohen (Eds.), *Understanding other minds: Perspectives from autism* (pp. 138-157). Oxford: Oxford University Press.

Wellman, H. M. (1990). *The child's theory of mind.* Cambridge, MA: MIT Press.

Wellman, H. M., & Woolley, J. D. (1990). From simple desires to ordinary beliefs: The early development of everyday psychology. *Cognition, 35*, 245-275.

Wimmer, H., & Perner, J. (1983). Beliefs about beliefs: Representation and constraining function of wrong beliefs in young children's understanding of deception. *Cognition, 13*, 103-128.

Young, A. W., Aggleton, J. P., Hellawell, D. J., Johnson, M., Broks, P., & Hanley, J. R. (1995). Face processing impairments after amygdalotomy. *Brain, 118*, 15-24.

Zaitchik, D. (1990). When representations conflict with reality: The preschooler's problem with false beliefs and "false" photographs. *Cognition, 35*, 41-68.

242

A Double-blind, Placebo-Controlled Study of Risperidone in Adults With Autistic Disorder and Other Pervasive Developmental Disorders

Christopher J. McDougle, MD; Janice P. Holmes, RN, MSN; Derek C. Carlson, MD; Gregory H. Pelton, MD; Donald J. Cohen, MD; Lawrence H. Price, MD

Background: Neurobiological research has implicated the dopamine and serotonin systems in the pathogenesis of autism. Open-label reports suggest that the serotonin$_{2A}$–dopamine D$_2$ antagonist risperidone may be safe and effective in reducing the interfering symptoms of patients with autism.

Methods: Thirty-one adults (age [mean + SD], 28.1 ± 7.3 years) with autistic disorder (n = 17) or pervasive developmental disorder not otherwise specified (n = 14) participated in a 12-week double-blind, placebo-controlled trial of risperidone. Patients treated with placebo subsequently received a 12-week open-label trial of risperidone.

Results: For persons completing the study, 8 (57%) of 14 patients treated with risperidone were categorized as responders (daily dose [mean ± SD], 2.9 ± 1.4 mg) com-

pared with none of 16 in the placebo group ($P<.002$). Risperidone was superior to placebo in reducing repetitive behavior ($P<.001$), aggression ($P<.001$), anxiety or nervousness ($P<.02$), depression ($P<.03$), irritability ($P<.01$), and the overall behavioral symptoms of autism ($P<.02$). Objective, measurable change in social behavior and language did not occur. Nine (60%) of 15 patients who received treatment with open-label risperidone following the double-blind placebo phase responded. Other than mild, transient sedation, risperidone was well tolerated, with no evidence of extrapyramidal effects, cardiac events, or seizures.

Conclusion: Risperidone is more effective than placebo in the short-term treatment of symptoms of autism in adults.

Arch Gen Psychiatry. 1998;55:633-641

From the Department of Psychiatry, Section of Child and Adolescent Psychiatry, Indiana University School of Medicine, Indianapolis (Dr McDougle); the Department of Psychiatry (Ms Holmes and Drs Carlson and Cohen) and the Child Study Center (Dr Cohen), Yale University School of Medicine, New Haven, Conn; the Department of Psychiatry, Columbia University College of Physicians and Surgeons, New York, NY (Dr Pelton); and the Department of Psychiatry and Human Behavior, Brown University School of Medicine, Providence, RI (Dr Price).

THE MOST consistently effective drug treatments for patients with autistic disorder (autism) and related pervasive developmental disorders (PDDs) have been those that have targeted central dopamine and serotonin (5-hydroxytryptamine) systems; these neurotransmitters have been shown to be dysregulated in some patients with autism.[1-4]

The dopamine antagonist haloperidol has been one of the most extensively studied drugs for treating children with autism. Controlled trials have shown haloperidol to be superior to placebo for reducing withdrawal, stereotypy, hyperactivity, abnormal-object relationships, fidgetiness, negativism, angry affect, and lability of affect.[5] A prospective, longitudinal study, however, found that in 40 (33.9%) of 118 autistic children, drug-related dyskinesias developed during longer-term haloperidol administration.[6]

More recently, controlled investigations have demonstrated that for reducing inter-

fering repetitive behavior and aggression and enhancing some elements of social behavior in autistic patients, the potent serotonin reuptake inhibitor clomipramine hydrochloride (for children)[7,8] is more effective than the potent norepinephrine reuptake inhibitor desipramine hydrochloride and placebo, and the selective serotonin reuptake inhibitor fluvoxamine maleate (for adults)[9] is more effective than placebo.

For editorial comment see page 643

Risperidone, an atypical neuroleptic agent, is a highly potent serotonin$_{2A}$–dopamine D$_2$ antagonist[10] that has been shown in controlled studies to be better tolerated and more effective than haloperidol and placebo for reducing the positive and

243

PATIENTS AND METHODS

PATIENTS

Thirty-one adults diagnosed as having autism or PDD NOS and their parent(s) or legal guardian(s) provided voluntary, written informed consent (or assent for patients with cognitive limitations) for participation in this study, which had been approved by the Human Investigation Committee of Yale University School of Medicine, New Haven, Conn. Seventeen of the patients met diagnostic criteria for autistic disorder, and 14 met criteria for PDD NOS; none of the patients met criteria for a diagnosis of Rett disorder, childhood disintegrative disorder, or Asperger disorder. Diagnoses were based on DSM-IV[27] criteria for PDD. Criteria of the Autism Diagnostic Interview[28] and the Autism Diagnostic Observation Schedule[29] were used to aid in the diagnosis. Incorporating this information, the final diagnosis of autism or PDD NOS was determined by consensus agreement of 2 board-certified psychiatrists (C.J.M. and L.H.P.). The patients did not meet criteria for any other formal DSM-IV Axis I or Axis II disorder other than mental retardation (as described later), although many of the patients (n = 16) were difficult to assess fully because they were nonverbal or minimally verbally responsive. The sample consisted of 9 women and 22 men, including 6 African Americans, 24 whites, and 1 Hispanic, aged 18 to 43 years (age [mean ± SD], 28.1 ± 7.3 years), who were referred by schools, the State of Connecticut Departments of Mental Health and Addiction Services and Mental Retardation, group homes for adults with developmental disabilities, community-based psychiatrists, and family members. All subjects were evaluated and treated within the outpatient (n = 24) and inpatient (n = 7) divisions of the Clinical Neuroscience Research Unit at the Connecticut Mental Health Center, New Haven. The study was conducted between June 27, 1994, and February 28, 1997.

Each patient's symptoms were at least "moderate" in severity, as defined by global severity of illness rating on the Clinical Global Impression (CGI) Scale.[30] In addition, each patient met the following entry criteria for symptom severity for the study: a Yale-Brown Obsessive Compulsive Scale (Y-BOCS) compulsion (repetitive behavior) subscale score of greater than 10, a Self-injurious Behavior Questionnaire (SIB-Q) score of 25 or greater, or a Ritvo-Freeman Real-life Rating Scale overall score of 0.20 or greater. Each of these behavioral rating scales is referenced and described in detail in the "Rating Scales" section below. Full-scale IQ was measured with the Wechsler Adult Intelligence Scale–Revised[31] in the 15 verbal patients, and the Leiter International Performance Scale[32] was used to assess IQ in the 16 nonverbal patients. The IQ (mean ± SD) for the entire group of 31 patients was 54.6 ± 23.9. The degree of mental retardation for each patient is presented in the **Table**.

Additional screening procedures included a medical history, physical and neurologic examinations, a complete blood cell count with differential, electrolytes, fasting glucose level, serum urea nitrogen concentration, creatinine level, liver and thyroid function tests, fragile X testing (negative in all subjects), urinalysis, and electrocardiogram. All women had negative serum pregnancy tests. Subjects were excluded if they met DSM-IV criteria for schizophrenia or had psychotic symptoms or if a significant acute medical condition was identified. One man had neurofibromatosis; none of the other patients had a diagnosed genetic, metabolic, or neurologic cause for their syndrome. Twenty-four (77%) of the patients had received previous treatment with psychotropic drugs. Clinical characteristics, prior drug treatment data, and family history are presented in the Table.

STUDY DRUG ASSIGNMENT AND TREATMENT

Subjects had not taken any psychotropic drugs for at least 4 weeks before the start of the trial. After 2 visits during which baseline behavioral ratings were obtained, patients were randomly allocated according to a computer-generated list to 12 weeks of double-blind treatment with risperidone or placebo (lactose) in identical-appearing capsules. To ensure compliance, medication was administered by parents or other primary caregivers. The risperidone or placebo regimen was started at 1 mg every night. Based on telephone contact with either or both the research nurse clinician (J.P.H.) and the prescribing psychiatrist (C.J.M.), the dosage could then be increased by 1 mg daily every 3 to 4 days to a maximum dosage of 10 mg/d, as tolerated, if a maximal clinical response was not obtained. Thus, the maximal dosage of risperidone was attained within 5 weeks, and patients received this dose for at least 7 weeks. The prescribing psychiatrist, the research nurse clinician who performed the behavioral ratings, the patients, and all family and other members of the patients' treatment teams were unaware of the drug assignment (blind). Other than chloral hydrate up to 2 g/d, as needed to help with symptoms of agitation, no other drugs were administered during the study.

Fifteen patients were randomly assigned to receive risperidone and 16 to receive placebo. Fourteen of the 16 placebo-treated patients were subsequently given open-label risperidone for 12 weeks (1 additional patient completed 4 weeks) following completion of the double-blind placebo phase. For those patients, risperidone was prescribed in a manner identical to that described above.

RATING SCALES

Each patient, along with the members of the treatment team (eg, parents, teachers, case workers, group home staff, workshop staff), participated in 2 detailed assessments of behavioral symptoms at baseline and again at the end of weeks 4, 8, and 12 of the controlled trial. Repetitive behavior was rated with a modified version of the Y-BOCS.[33,34] Each of the 10 items on the Y-BOCS is scored on a 5-point scale from 0, indicating "least symptomatic," to 4, indicating "most symptomatic," so that the total Y-BOCS score ranges from 0 to 40. The first 5 items of the Y-BOCS are designed to assess the severity of repetitive thoughts, whereas the last 5 items determine the severity of repetitive behavior. Because 16 (52%) of the patients were nonverbal and thus unable to provide information about repetitive thoughts, we chose to assess only repetitive behavior for each patient; thus, the maximum Y-BOCS score for each patient was 20. Based on previous findings,[35] the ego-dystonicity diagnostic criterion for obsessive-compulsive disorder was eliminated in rating the repetitive behavior of the patients with PDD. Aggression was rated with the SIB-Q, a 25-item clinician-rated instrument that assesses self-injurious behavior, physical aggression toward others,

244

destruction to property, and other maladaptive behavior (T. Gualtieri, MD, unpublished data). Patients could receive a score from 0, indicating "not a problem," to 4, indicating "severe problem," on each of the 25 items (range for total score, 0-100). The Ritvo-Freeman Real-life Rating Scale[36] served as an observational measure (30 minutes during each behavioral rating session) of a variety of symptoms of autism, including subscales for assessing sensory motor behaviors (eg, hand-flapping, rocking, pacing) (subscale I), social relationship to people (eg, appropriate responses to interaction attempts, initiating appropriate interactions) (subscale II), affectual reactions (eg, abrupt changes in affect, crying, temper outbursts) (subscale III), sensory responses (eg, agitated by noises, rubbing surfaces, sniffing self or objects) (subscale IV), and language (eg, communicative use of language, initiating appropriate verbal communication) (subscale V). Each of the 5 subscales contains a number of individual items that are scored on a 4-point scale: 0 indicates "never"; 1, "rarely"; 2, "frequently"; and 3, "almost always." The average score from the mean value of each of the 5 subscale scores was determined to yield an overall score on the Ritvo-Freeman scale (range for overall score, −0.42 to 2.58). The Ritvo-Freeman scale score increases as the number and frequency of symptoms of autism increase. A mathematical sign correction to subtract normal behavior is necessary on subscales II, IV, and V; this results in some scores with a negative value. Different mood states were assessed on 10 clinician-rated visual analog scales,[37] scored on a 100-mm line where 0 indicates "not at all," and 100 indicates "most ever." The 10 items included "anxious or nervous," "calm," "depressed," "eye contact," "happy," "irritable," "restless," "social interaction," "talkative," and "tired." Finally, the CGI global improvement item—7 indicates "very much worse"; 4, "no change"; and 1, "very much improved"[30]—was recorded at the end of weeks 4, 8, and 12 of treatment (compared with the predrug baseline). Global improvement ratings were based on an aggregate assessment of the patient's social behavior and the level of the patient's interfering repetitive and aggressive behavior. For the 15 patients who received treatment for 12 weeks with open-label risperidone following the double-blind placebo phase, the rating scales were administered in a manner identical to that described above.

PHYSIOLOGICAL MEASURES AND ADVERSE EFFECTS ASSESSMENT

Sitting and standing blood pressures and pulse rate, temperature, respiratory rate, and weight were recorded at baseline and at the end of 4, 8, and 12 weeks of the risperidone trial. Each patient was systematically examined for extrapyramidal (abnormal gait, ataxia, dystonia, hyperkinesia, hypertonia, hypokinesia, hyporeflexia, involuntary muscle contractions, oculogyric crisis, and tremor) and other adverse effects (agitation, constipation, coughing, diarrhea, dizziness, dry mouth, dyspepsia, enuresis, gynecomastia, headache, insomnia, menstrual pattern changes [women], nausea, restlessness, rhinitis, sedation, sialorrhea, and vomiting) at baseline and after 4, 8, and 12 weeks of treatment with risperidone or placebo.

STATISTICAL ANALYSIS

Of the 31 patients who entered the controlled phase of the investigation, 24 completed the entire 12-week study. Of the 7 patients who did not complete the entire trial, 1 patient with autism had to be withdrawn from the study after 1 week because of the emergence of notable agitation (active drug), 4 patients (2 with autism, and 2 with PDD NOS) were removed because of interfering agitation after 4 weeks (placebo), 1 patient with PDD NOS had an abnormal gait develop after 4 weeks (active drug), and the remaining patient (with autism) dropped out after 4 weeks because of a lack of significant improvement in symptoms (active drug). Data from the 30 patients who completed at least 4 weeks of the trial were included in the efficacy analysis. For the 6 patients who completed only 4 weeks of double-blind treatment, the last-observation-carried-forward, intention-to-treat method was used in the data analysis.

Baseline ratings were obtained from the mean scores of the 2 initial behavioral assessment sessions. Student t tests were calculated to determine if significant differences existed on baseline rating scale measures between the risperidone and placebo groups; there were no statistically significant baseline differences. Student t tests were used to determine if significant differences existed between groups in age, full-scale IQ, or dose of risperidone vs placebo. The χ^2 test with the Yates correction was used to determine if significant differences existed between groups for sex distribution, diagnostic subtype distribution, or treatment setting.

A 2-way analysis of variance (ANOVA) with repeated measures was calculated for the 12 weeks of risperidone or placebo treatment to assess the significance of main effects of drug, time, and drug × time interactions (only drug × time interactions are reported below). An analysis of covariance (ANCOVA), using the baseline score as a covariate, was used to determine when significant risperidone-placebo differences took place. A 1-way ANOVA with repeated measures was calculated to determine the main effect of time for the 15 patients who received open-label risperidone following the initial placebo randomization phase. The reported P values for all ANOVAs and ANCOVAs used the Huynh-Feldt correction factor. This correction factor decreases the degrees of freedom used in the ANOVA or ANCOVA to reflect a lack of homogeneity in the variance of measures across time points; for clarity, uncorrected degrees of freedom are given. Results from the ANOVAs for both the intent-to-treat sample (n = 30) and the completer sample (n = 24) are presented below.

The χ^2 test with Yates correction was used to compare the 2 groups for the rate of responders vs nonresponders and to determine if response was related to sex, diagnostic subtype, or treatment setting. Point by serial correlation was used to determine if a categorical response was correlated with age, full-scale IQ, or baseline measures of repetitive behavior (Y-BOCS compulsion subscale score), aggression (total SIB-Q score), level of autistic behavior (Ritvo-Freeman scale overall score), or dose of risperidone. Response was determined by scores obtained at the end of the last week of treatment on the CGI global improvement item compared with baseline. Patients with CGI scores of "much improved" or "very much improved" were categorized as responders; all others were considered nonresponders. Data are given as mean ± SD, unless otherwise indicated, and results are reported as significant when $P<.05$ (2 tailed).

245

ARCH GEN PSYCHIATRY/VOL 55, JULY 1998

Clinical Characteristics of Adults With Autism and Pervasive Developmental Disorder (PDD) Not Otherwise Specified (NOS) Treated With

Patient No.	DSM-IV Diagnosis	Age, y/Sex/ Race	Full-Scale IQ	Treatment Setting	Prior Drug Treatment	Daily Dose of Agent, mg
						Risperidone
1	Autistic disorder	18/M/W	40	Outpt	Thioridazine hydrochloride	5
2	Autistic disorder	38/M/W	96	Outpt	Fluvoxamine maleate, haloperidol, clonazepam, pimozide, sertraline hydrochloride	2
3	Autistic disorder	27/M/AA	45	Outpt	Thioridazine	4
4	Autistic disorder	20/M/W	28	Outpt	Phenytoin sodium, phenobarbital	1
5	Autistic disorder	31/M/AA	34	Outpt	Phenytoin	2
6	Autistic disorder	25/F/W	43	Outpt	Phenytoin, perphenazine, valproic acid	3
7	Autistic disorder	21/M/W	50	Inpt	Lorazepam, chlorpromazine hydrochloride	3
8	Autistic disorder	36/M/W	113	Inpt	Clomipramine hydrochloride, lorazepam, buspirone hydrochloride, valproic acid, fluvoxamine, haloperidol, clonazepam, imipramine hydrochloride, perphenazine	4
9	Autistic disorder	22/M/W	58	Inpt	Clonazepam	1
10	PDD NOS	34/M/W	22	Outpt	Haloperidol	6
11	PDD NOS	20/M/AA	74	Outpt	Perphenazine	3
12	PDD NOS	34/F/W	57	Outpt	None	2
13	PDD NOS	23/M/W	85	Outpt	None	4
14	PDD NOS	21/M/W	64	Outpt	Methylphenidate hydrochloride	3
15	PDD NOS	21/M/W	24	Outpt	Methylphenidate	1
Mean (±SD)	...	26.0 (±6.7)	55.5 (±26.8)	...	...	2.9 (±1.4)
						Placebo
16	Autistic disorder	26/M/W	41	Inpt	Hydroxyzine hydrochloride, haloperidol, imipramine, thioridazine, methylphenidate	6
17	Autistic disorder	25/M/W	61	Outpt	Haloperidol, pimozide	6
18	Autistic disorder	24/M/W	42	Outpt	None	4
19	Autistic disorder	31/M/AA	38	Outpt	Trifluoperazine hydrochloride	6
20	Autistic disorder	25/M/AA	25	Outpt	None	4
21	Autistic disorder	35/M/W	68	Outpt	None	2
22	Autistic disorder	25/F/H	22	Outpt	Thioridazine, carbamazepine	2
23	Autistic disorder	20/M/W	84	Outpt	Thioridazine	2
24	PDD NOS	38/M/W	92	Inpt	Clomipramine, lorazepam, buspirone, fluoxetine hydrochloride, haloperidol, clonazepam, thioridazine, nortriptyline hydrochloride, imipramine, perphenazine	3
25	PDD NOS	18/F/W	38	Outpt	None	4
26	PDD NOS	29/F/AA	61	Outpt	Lorazepam, clonazepam, sertraline	6
27	PDD NOS	42/F/W	61	Outpt	Hydroxyzine, thioridazine, phenobarbital, methylphenidate, diazepam	4
28	PDD NOS	34/M/W	70	Outpt	Lorazepam, fluvoxamine, methylphenidate, diazepam	4
29	PDD NOS	39/F/W	50	Outpt	None	4
30	PDD NOS	43/F/W	81	Inpt	Clonazepam, chlorpromazine, chlordiazepoxide hydrochloride, thioridazine, fluphenazine hydrochloride	2
31	PDD NOS	27/F/W	28	Outpt	Nortriptyline, methylphenidate, sertraline	1
Mean (±SD)	...	29.7 (±7.8)	52.0 (±22.1)	...	...	3.9 (±1.5)
Mean (±SD)	...	28.1 (±7.3)	54.6 (±23.9)	...	...	3.3 (±1.6)

*AA indicates African American; H, Hispanic; Outpt, outpatient; Inpt, inpatient; and OCD, obsessive-compulsive disorder.

246

Weeks Completed	Treatment Response	Adverse Effects	Family History
Group			
12	Very much improved	None	Paternal first cousin with Down syndrome; paternal second cousin with Down syndrome
12	Much improved	Sedation, dry mouth	Brother: Asperger disorder; 3 paternal first cousins: mental retardation and seizure disorders
12	Much improved	Agitation	Mother: paranoid schizophrenia; maternal aunt: Down syndrome; brother: mental retardation
12	Much improved	Weight gain, sedation, enuresis	Maternal uncle: Down syndrome
12	Much improved	Sedation	Father: alcohol abuse; brother: mental retardation
12	Minimally improved	Enuresis, sedation	None
12	Minimally worse	Sedation	Paternal uncle: paranoid disorder; maternal uncle: mental retardation
4	Minimally worse	None	Maternal grandmother: chronic vocal tic disorder; maternal first cousin: trichotillomania; maternal first cousin: autistic disorder; maternal first cousin: seizure disorder
1	Much worse	Agitation	Mother: generalized anxiety disorder; maternal great uncle: mental retardation; maternal third cousin: mental retardation
12	Very much improved	Sedation, weight gain	2 Paternal first cousins: mental retardation
12	Much improved	Sedation	Family history of psychosis and learning disabilities
12	Much improved	Dyspepsia, diarrhea, constipation	None
12	Minimally improved	Sedation	None
12	Minimally improved	Sedation	None
4	Minimally improved	Abnormal gait, sialorrhea	None
...	...	...	...
Group			
12	Minimally improved	None	Mother: suicide; maternal grandmother: schizophrenia; paternal side: history of cerebral palsy and mental retardation
12	No change	None	Paternal second cousin: chronic motor tic disorder
12	No change	None	None
12	No change	None	None
12	No change	None	None
12	No change	None	Mother: generalized anxiety disorder, schizoid personality disorder; father: schizoid personality disorder
4	No change	Agitation	None
4	Minimally worse	Agitation	Father: Asperger disorder
12	Minimally improved	None	Father: social phobia and dysthymia; mother: major depression; paternal grandfather: alcohol abuse
12	Minimally improved	None	Mother: dysthymia; maternal family history of OCD; sister: alcohol abuse, major depression, and anorexia nervosa; father: alcohol abuse and suicide
12	No change	None	Paternal first cousin: mental retardation
12	No change	None	None
12	No change	Agitation	Father: alcohol abuse
12	No change	None	None
4	Much worse	Agitation	Paternal grandfather: major depression; nephew: autistic disorder
4	Much worse	Agitation	Brother: spina bifida and major depression; paternal niece: learning disability; father: Asperger disorder
...	...	...	...

247

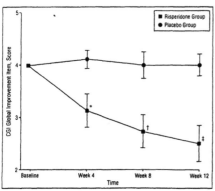

Figure 1. *Global improvement in patients with autism or pervasive developmental disorder not otherwise specified who were given risperidone or placebo for 12 weeks, as measured on the Clinical Global Impression (CGI) Scale global improvement item (see the "Rating Scales" section for an explanation of the scoring). Asterisk indicates $F_{1,27} = 8.93$, $P<.006$; dagger, $F_{1,27} = 9.67$, $P<.004$; and double dagger, $F_{1,27} = 15.07$, $P<.001$ (risperidone vs placebo, analysis of covariance). Variance bars represent SE.*

negative symptoms of schizophrenia.[11,12] Because of its improved profile of extrapyramidal effects and putative mechanism of therapeutic action, the use of risperidone in patients with PDDs has received increasing attention.

Results from the open-label use of risperidone in the treatment of children and adolescents,[13-22] as well as adults[23-26] with PDDs, have been reported. Typically, these studies have described reductions in irritability, impulsivity, hyperactivity, self-injury, aggression, and interfering repetitive behavior, along with improvement in some elements of social function and communication.

To our knowledge, no controlled studies of risperidone treatment of children, adolescents, or adults with PDDs have been published. The present 12-week randomized, double-blind, placebo-controlled investigation was conducted to determine the safety and short-term efficacy of risperidone for the treatment of adults with autistic disorder and PDD not otherwise specified (NOS). It was hypothesized that risperidone would be better than placebo for reducing repetitive behavior and aggression and for improving some aspects of social relatedness. In addition, it was hypothesized that the extrapyramidal and other adverse effects associated with risperidone would be only minimally greater than those of placebo.

RESULTS

Additional clinical characteristics of the risperidone and placebo groups are given in the Table. No significant differences were seen in age, sex distribution, diagnostic subtype distribution, full-scale IQ score, treatment setting, or optimal dose of risperidone between groups.

GLOBAL TREATMENT RESPONSE

Ratings on the CGI global improvement item showed risperidone superior to placebo as evaluated by the drug × time

interaction (mean ± SE, $4.00 ± 0.00$ to $2.54 ± 1.27$ vs $4.00 ± 0.00$ to $4.00 ± 0.79$; $F_{3,84} = 7.80$, $P<.001$, intent-to-treat sample, n = 30 [$F_{3,84} = 6.43$, $P<.002$; completers, n = 24]). Subsequent ANCOVAs determined that risperidone was superior to placebo beginning at week 4 ($F_{1,27} = 8.93$, $P<.006$) and continuing at weeks 8 ($F_{1,27} = 9.67$, $P<.004$) and 12 ($F_{1,27} = 15.07$, $P<.001$) **(Figure 1)**.

Eight (57%) of 14 of the risperidone-treated patients were categorized as responders compared with none of 16 in the placebo group ($\chi^2 = 9.72$, $P<.002$). Treatment response was not related to diagnostic subtype (autistic disorder, 5 of 8; PDD NOS, 3 of 6), sex, or treatment setting or correlated with age, full-scale IQ, baseline measures of repetitive behavior (Y-BOCS compulsion subscale score), aggression (SIB-Q total score), or dose of risperidone. A trend toward a significant correlation was found for treatment response and baseline level of overall autistic behavior (Ritvo-Freeman scale overall score) ($r = 0.31$, $P<.09$).

Nine (60%) of the 15 patients treated with open-label risperidone after completing the double-blind placebo phase were categorized as responders (autistic disorder, 7 of 8; PDD NOS, 2 of 7). Ratings on the CGI Scale showed that risperidone treatment resulted in a statistically significant global improvement in symptoms over time in these patients ($4.00 ± 0.00$ to $2.47 ± 1.06$; $F_{3,42} = 11.60$, $P<.001$).

RESPONSE OF REPETITIVE BEHAVIOR

Risperidone was superior to placebo in the treatment of interfering repetitive behavior ($16.15 ± 3.58$ to $12.77 ± 3.63$ vs $14.29 ± 3.50$ to $14.35 ± 3.02$; $F_{3,84} = 8.73$, $P<.001$ [$F_{3,84} = 7.26$, $P<.002$]). This effect began at week 4 ($F_{1,27} = 11.08$, $P<.003$) and continued through weeks 8 ($F_{1,27} = 8.31$, $P<.008$) and 12 ($F_{1,27} = 6.77$, $P<.02$). For the 15 patients who received treatment with open-label risperidone, the drug also resulted in a significant reduction in Y-BOCS scores over time ($14.27 ± 2.92$ to $11.47 ± 3.64$; $F_{3,42} = 4.41$, $P<.03$).

RESPONSE OF AGGRESSIVE BEHAVIOR

As measured by the total score on the SIB-Q, risperidone was superior to placebo in reducing self-injurious behavior, physical aggression toward others, and property destruction ($47.8 ± 19.5$ to $24.2 ± 9.5$ vs $37.7 ± 11.9$ to $32.8 ± 15.0$; $F_{3,84} = 9.22$, $P<.001$ [$F_{3,84} = 6.51$, $P<.005$]). This effect began at week 4 ($F_{1,27} = 5.61$, $P<.02$) and continued through weeks 8 ($F_{1,27} = 7.92$, $P<.009$) and 12 ($F_{1,27} = 7.16$, $P<.01$). For the 15 patients who were given open-label risperidone, the drug treatment also resulted in a significant reduction in aggressive behavior over time ($32.43 ± 15.89$ to $23.07 ± 13.45$; $F_{3,42} = 3.07$, $P<.05$).

RESPONSE ON RITVO-FREEMAN REAL-LIFE RATING SCALE

Subscale I: Sensory Motor Behaviors

Risperidone resulted in a statistically significant improvement in subscale I scores compared with placebo ($0.79 ± 0.65$ to $0.38 ± 0.38$ vs $0.71 ± 0.58$ to $0.64 ± 0.49$; $F_{3,84} = 5.92$, $P<.004$ [$F_{3,84} = 4.16$, $P<.02$]). This effect be-

248

gan at week 4 ($F_{1,27} = 17.66$, $P<.001$) and continued through weeks 8 ($F_{1,27} = 10.19$, $P<.004$) and 12 ($F_{1,27} = 8.69$, $P<.007$). For the 15 patients who received treatment with open-label risperidone, a significant reduction in subscale I scores over time also occurred (0.68 ± 0.48 to 0.44 ± 0.31; $F_{3,42} = 3.21$, $P<.04$).

Subscale II: Social Relationship to People

Risperidone treatment did not result in a statistically significant improvement in subscale II scores compared with placebo. Similarly, for the 15 patients who received treatment with open-label risperidone, no statistically significant change in subscale II scores over time occurred.

Subscale III: Affectual Reactions

Symptoms within subscale III were significantly reduced by risperidone treatment compared with placebo (1.02 ± 0.39 to 0.35 ± 0.37 vs 0.78 ± 0.49 to 0.82 ± 0.57; $F_{3,84} = 8.78$, $P<.001$ [$F_{3,84} = 7.48$, $P<.001$]). This effect was present at week 4 ($F_{1,27} = 10.17$, $P<.004$) and continued through weeks 8 ($F_{1,27} = 8.55$, $P<.007$) and 12 ($F_{1,27} = 10.40$, $P<.003$). For the 15 patients who were administered open-label risperidone, a statistically significant improvement in subscale III scores over time also occurred (0.75 ± 0.53 to 0.33 ± 0.28; $F_{3,42} = 5.95$, $P<.007$).

Subscale IV: Sensory Responses

Risperidone treatment did not result in a statistically significant improvement in subscale IV scores compared with placebo for the intent-to-treat sample. In the analysis of the 24 completers, however, risperidone was found to be superior to placebo on this measure ($F_{3,66} = 3.48$, $P<.02$). For the 15 patients who were treated with open-label risperidone, a statistically significant improvement in subscale IV scores over time occurred (0.70 ± 0.38 to 0.44 ± 0.36; $F_{3,42} = 5.67$, $P<.004$).

Subscale V: Language

Treatment with risperidone did not result in a statistically significant improvement in language usage compared with placebo as measured by subscale V. Similarly, no statistically significant improvement in subscale V scores over time occurred in the 15 patients treated with open-label risperidone.

Ritvo-Freeman Scale Overall Score

Risperidone treatment resulted in a significant improvement in the overall behavioral symptoms of autism as measured by the overall score on the Ritvo-Freeman scale compared with placebo (0.60 ± 0.44 to 0.32 ± 0.27 vs 0.53 ± 0.41 to 0.45 ± 0.41; $F_{3,84} = 4.19$, $P<.02$ [$F_{3,84} = 4.42$, $P<.01$]). This effect first became evident at week 4 ($F_{1,27} = 10.51$, $P<.003$) and remained significant at weeks 8 ($F_{1,27} = 4.54$, $P<.04$) and 12 ($F_{1,27} = 4.03$, $P<.05$)

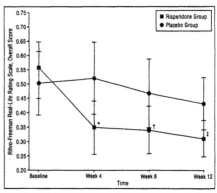

Figure 2. *Change in severity of the overall behavioral symptoms of autism in patients with autism or pervasive developmental disorder not otherwise specified who were given risperidone or placebo for 12 weeks, as measured by the overall score on the Ritvo-Freeman Real-Life Rating Scale (range, −0.42 to 2.58). Asterisk indicates $F_{1,27} = 10.51$, $P<.003$; dagger, $F_{1,27} = 4.54$, $P<.04$; and double dagger, $F_{1,27} = 4.03$, $P<.05$ (risperidone vs placebo, analysis of covariance). Variance bars represent SE.*

(**Figure 2**). For the 15 patients treated with open-label risperidone, a significant improvement in the Ritvo-Freeman scale overall score over time also occurred (0.50 ± 0.38 to 0.27 ± 0.33; $F_{3,42} = 5.50$, $P<.003$).

RESPONSE ON CLINICIAN-RATED VISUAL ANALOG SCALES

On the 10 clinician-rated visual analog scales, risperidone treatment resulted in significant changes in measures of "anxious or nervous" (decreased) (70.4 ± 16.4 to 42.3 ± 28.0 vs 66.6 ± 22.1 to 60.0 ± 28.5; $F_{3,84} = 4.14$, $P<.02$ [$F_{3,84} = 3.57$, $P<.03$]), "depressed" (decreased) (23.8 ± 17.6 to 8.5 ± 11.4 vs 23.1 ± 28.1 to 19.4 ± 25.4; $F_{3,84} = 3.38$, $P<.03$ [$F_{3,84} = 2.58$, $P<.08$]), and "irritable" (decreased) (51.8 ± 23.2 to 21.8 ± 20.4 vs 31.5 ± 24.4-22.3 ± 24.9; $F_{3,84} = 4.33$, $P<.01$ [$F_{3,84} = 4.47$, $P<.01$]), as evaluated by the drug × time interaction. No statistically significant differences over time were identified for the measures of "calm," "eye contact," "happy," "restless," "social interaction," "talkative," or "tired." For the 15 patients who received open-label risperidone, statistically significant changes over time occurred in measures of "anxious or nervous" (decreased) (62.67 ± 26.04 to 37.93 ± 29.95; $F_{3,42} = 3.91$, $P<.02$), "calm" (increased) (26.67 ± 22.25 to 46.60 ± 24.01; $F_{3,42} = 4.37$, $P<.01$), "irritable" (decreased) (27.33 ± 23.75 to 14.13 ± 16.27; $F_{3,42} = 3.03$, $P<.05$), and "restless" (decreased) (54.67 ± 28.25 to 27.00 ± 22.82; $F_{3,42} = 3.69$, $P<.03$). No statistically significant changes over time occurred in measures of "depressed," "eye contact," "happy," "social interaction," "talkative," or "tired."

ADVERSE EFFECTS

Adverse effects associated with risperidone administration are presented in the Table. No clinically significant

249

changes in blood pressure, heart rate, respiratory rate, or temperature were recorded, and no acute extrapyramidal effects (other than possibly the development of an abnormal gait in 1 patient), seizures, or cardiac events occurred. In general, risperidone was well tolerated, with the most prominent adverse effect being mild transient sedation during the initial phase of drug administration.

COMMENT

Risperidone was significantly more effective than placebo for decreasing many of the interfering behavioral symptoms of adults with autism and PDD NOS. Specifically, risperidone was effective in reducing interfering repetitive behavior, as well as aggression toward self, others, and property. While risperidone was more effective than placebo for decreasing the overall behavioral symptoms of autism, as measured by the Ritvo-Freeman scale overall score, this finding was largely accounted for by significant changes in sensory motor behaviors, affectual reactions, and to some extent, sensory responses. Significant differences between risperidone and placebo were not captured on subscales II and V of the Ritvo-Freeman scale, which measure social relationships to people and language, respectively. For many patients, however, clinicians, parents, and other members of the treatment team had the impression that anxiety associated with social interactions was reduced, allowing for enhanced social function. It may be that the rating scales used to assess social relatedness in this study were not sensitive enough to detect changes in this complex aspect of behavior.

In general, risperidone was well tolerated. Thirteen (87%) of 15 patients randomly allocated to risperidone treatment had at least 1 adverse effect—although this included only mild, transient sedation in 5 patients—compared with 5 (31%) of 16 patients given placebo (agitation in all 5 cases). Importantly, the weight gain observed with risperidone in the treatment of some children and adolescents with autism and other PDDs[21] did not occur to the same degree in this study of adult patients.

The pattern of symptomatic change in this study of adults with autism is similar to that observed in a previous systematic investigation of open-label risperidone use in children and adolescents with autism and other PDDs.[21] That risperidone is effective in both children and adolescents, as well as adults with autism, contrasts with controlled studies of the use of fluvoxamine that demonstrated efficacy and tolerability for autistic adults[9] but significant increases in agitation, aggression, insomnia, and other forms of behavioral activation and limited efficacy in the pediatric sample (C.J.M., J.P.H., D.J.C., L.H.P., unpublished data, 1998). These disparate results may be due to different influences of brain development on serotonin$_2$ receptors and the serotonin transporter protein, respectively.

Because of recent reports of possible tardive dyskinesia in children treated with risperidone,[38] continued close monitoring of the drug and longer-term follow-up

studies are warranted. Double-blind, placebo-controlled studies are needed to determine the safety and efficacy of risperidone in adults with other subtypes of PDD, such as Asperger disorder, as well as in children and adolescents with the broad range of these profound disorders.

Accepted for publication February 12, 1998.

This study was supported in part by grants MH-30929 and HD-03008 from the Public Health Service, Bethesda, Md; by a Young Investigator Award (Dr Pelton) and an Independent Investigator Award (Dr McDougle) from the National Alliance for Research in Schizophrenia and Depression, Chicago, Ill; by the Theodore and Vada Stanley Foundation Research Awards Program, Arlington, Va (Drs McDougle and Price); by the State of Connecticut, Department of Mental Health and Addiction Services, Hartford; and by a Research Unit on Pediatric Psychopharmacology (RUPP): Autism and Other Pervasive Disorders contract to Indiana University (Dr McDougle) from the National Institute of Mental Health, Rockville, Md.

Elizabeth Kyle, AS, prepared the manuscript; Sally Vegso, MS, performed the statistical analyses; and Elizabeth Ruff constructed the graphics.

Reprints: Christopher J. McDougle, MD, Indiana University School of Medicine, Section of Child and Adolescent Psychiatry, James Whitcomb Riley Hospital for Children, 702 Barnhill Dr, Room 3701, Indianapolis, IN 46202-5200 (e-mail: cmcdougl@iumc.iupui.edu).

REFERENCES

1. McDougle CJ. Psychopharmacology. In: Cohen DJ, Volkmar FV, eds. *Handbook of Autism and Pervasive Developmental Disorders.* 2nd ed. New York, NY: John Wiley & Sons Inc; 1997:707-729.
2. Gillberg C, Svennerholm L, Hamilton-Hellberg C. Childhood psychosis and monoamine metabolites in spinal fluid. *J Autism Dev Disord.* 1983;13:383-396.
3. McDougle CJ, Naylor ST, Cohen DJ, Aghajanian GK, Heninger GR, Price LH. Effects of tryptophan depletion in drug-free adults with autistic disorder. *Arch Gen Psychiatry.* 1996;53:993-1000.
4. Cook EH, Leventhal BL. The serotonin system in autism. *Curr Opin Pediatr.* 1996; 8:348-354.
5. Anderson LT, Campbell M, Grega DM, Perry R, Small AM, Green WH. Haloperidol in the treatment of infantile autism: effects on learning and behavioral symptoms. *Am J Psychiatry.* 1984;141:1195-1202.
6. Campbell M, Armenteros JL, Malone RP, Adams PB, Eisenberg ZW, Overall JE. Neuroleptic-related dyskinesias in autistic children: a prospective, longitudinal study. *J Am Acad Child Adolesc Psychiatry.* 1997;36:835-843.
7. Gordon CT, Rapoport JL, Hamburger SD, State RC, Mannheim GB. Differential response of seven subjects with autistic disorder to clomipramine and desipramine. *Am J Psychiatry.* 1992;149:363-366.
8. Gordon CT, State RC, Nelson JE, Hamburger SD, Rapoport JL. A double-blind comparison of clomipramine, desipramine, and placebo in the treatment of autistic disorder. *Arch Gen Psychiatry.* 1993;50:441-447.
9. McDougle CJ, Naylor ST, Cohen DJ, Volkmar FV, Heninger GR, Price LH. A double-blind, placebo-controlled study of fluvoxamine in adults with autistic disorder. *Arch Gen Psychiatry.* 1996;53:1001-1008.
10. Leysen JE, Janssen PMF, Megens AAHP, Schotte A. Risperidone: a novel antipsychotic with balanced serotonin-dopamine antagonism, receptor occupancy profile, and pharmacologic activity. *J Clin Psychiatry.* 1994;55(suppl 5): 5-12.
11. Chouinard G, Jones B, Remington G, Bloom D, Addington D, MacEwan GW, Labelle A, Beauclair L, Arnott W. A Canadian multicenter placebo-controlled study of fixed doses of risperidone and haloperidol in the treatment of chronic schizophrenic patients. *J Clin Psychopharmacol.* 1993;13:25-40.
12. Marder SR, Meibach RC. Risperidone in the treatment of schizophrenia. *Am J Psychiatry.* 1994;151:825-835.

13. Simeon JG, Carrey NJ, Wiggins DM, Milin RP, Hosendocus SN. Risperidone effects in treatment-resistant adolescents: preliminary case reports. *J Child Adolesc Psychopharmacol.* 1995;5:69-79.
14. Demb H. Risperidone: maybe this shouldn't be the last resort. In: Antanitus D, ed. *Success Stories in Developmental Disabilities.* Vol 4. Waltham, Mass: Liberty Healthcare Corp; 1995:11-14.
15. Demb HB. Risperidone in young children with pervasive developmental disorders and other developmental disabilities. *J Child Adolesc Psychopharmacol.* 1996; 6:79-80.
16. Fisman S, Steele M. Use of risperidone in pervasive developmental disorders: a case series. *J Child Adolesc Psychopharmacol.* 1996;6:177-190.
17. Fisman S, Steele M, Short J, Byrne T, Lavallee C. Case study: anorexia nervosa and autistic disorder in an adolescent girl. *J Am Acad Child Adolesc Psychiatry.* 1996;35:937-940.
18. Hardan A, Johnson K, Johnson C, Hrecznyj B. Case study: risperidone treatment of children and adolescents with developmental disorders. *J Am Acad Child Adolesc Psychiatry.* 1996;35:1551-1556.
19. Perry RI, Pataki CS, Munoz-Silva DM, Armenteros J, Silva RR. Risperidone in children and adolescents with pervasive developmental disorder: pilot trial and follow-up. *J Child Adolesc Psychopharmacol.* 1997;7:167-179.
20. Frischauf E. Drug therapy in autism. *J Am Acad Child Adolesc Psychiatry.* 1997; 36:577.
21. McDougle CJ, Holmes JP, Bronson MR, Anderson GM, Volkmar FR, Price LH, Cohen DJ. Risperidone treatment of children and adolescents with pervasive developmental disorders: a prospective open-label study. *J Am Acad Child Adolesc Psychiatry.* 1997;36:685-693.
22. Rubin M. Use of atypical antipsychotics in children with mental retardation, autism, and other developmental disabilities. *Psychiatr Ann.* 1997;27:219-221.
23. Purdon SE, Lit W, Labelle A, Jones BD. Risperidone in the treatment of pervasive developmental disorder. *Can J Psychiatry.* 1994;39:400-405.
24. McDougle CJ, Brodkin ES, Yeung PP, Naylor ST, Cohen DJ, Price LH. Risperidone in adults with autism or pervasive developmental disorder. *J Child Adolesc Psychopharmacol.* 1995;5:273-282.
25. Lott RS, Kerrick JM, Cohen SA. Clinical and economic aspects of risperidone treatment in adults with mental retardation and behavioral disturbance. *Psychopharmacol Bull.* 1996;32:721-729.
26. Horrigan JP, Barnhill LJ. Risperidone and explosive aggressive autism. *J Autism Dev Disord.* 1997;27:313-323.
27. American Psychiatric Association. *Diagnostic and Statistical Manual of Mental Disorders, Fourth Edition.* Washington, DC: American Psychiatric Association; 1994.
28. Le Couteur A, Rutter M, Lord C, Rios P, Robertson S, Holdgrafer M, McLennan J. Autism Diagnostic Interview: a standardized investigator-based instrument. *J Autism Dev Disord.* 1989;19:363-387.
29. Lord C, Rutter M, Goode S, Heemsbergen J, Jordan H, Mawhood L, Schopler E. Autism Diagnostic Observation Schedule: a standardized observation of communicative and social behavior. *J Autism Dev Disord.* 1989;19:185-212.
30. Guy W. *ECDEU Assessment Manual for Psychopharmacology.* Washington, DC: National Institute of Mental Health, US Dept of Health, Education, and Welfare; 1976. Publication 76-338.
31. Wechsler D. *Manual for the Wechsler Adult Intelligence Scale-Revised.* San Antonio, Tex: Psychological Corp; 1981.
32. Leiter RG. *Leiter International Performance Scale.* Chicago, Ill: Stoelting Co; 1948.
33. Goodman WK, Price LH, Rasmussen SA, Mazure C, Fleischmann R, Hill C, Heninger GR, Charney DS. The Yale-Brown Obsessive Compulsive Scale (Y-BOCS), I: development, use, and reliability. *Arch Gen Psychiatry.* 1989;46: 1006-1011.
34. Goodman WK, Price LH, Rasmussen SA, Mazure C, Delgado P, Heninger GR, Charney DS. The Yale-Brown Obsessive Compulsive Scale (Y-BOCS), II: validity. *Arch Gen Psychiatry.* 1989;46:1012-1016.
35. McDougle CJ, Kresch LE, Goodman WK, Naylor ST, Volkmar FR, Cohen DJ, Price LH. A case-controlled study of repetitive thoughts and behavior in adults with autistic disorder and obsessive-compulsive disorder. *Am J Psychiatry.* 1995; 152:772-777.
36. Freeman BJ, Ritvo ER, Yokota A, Ritvo A. A scale for rating symptoms of patients with the syndrome of autism in real life settings. *J Am Acad Child Adolesc Psychiatry.* 1986;25:130-136.
37. McDougle CJ, Naylor ST, Goodman WK, Volkmar FR, Cohen DJ, Price LH. Acute tryptophan depletion in autistic disorder: a controlled case study. *Biol Psychiatry.* 1993;33:547-550.
38. Feeney DJ, Klykylo W. Risperidone and tardive dyskinesia. *J Am Acad Child Adolesc Psychiatry.* 1996;35:1421-1422.

ARCHIVES Circulation

The ARCHIVES is available by request to nonfederal physicians in the United States (50 states and Washington, DC) whose official American Medical Association masterfile record shows a primary specialty of psychiatry or child psychiatry in an office- or hospital-based practice as a staff physician, resident in training beyond the first year, or clinical fellow.

If you meet the above qualification criteria and are not currently receiving the ARCHIVES and would like to receive it each month, you must complete a free subscription request card. To receive a request card, please write to Kathryn Osten, American Medical Association, Circulation Processing Department, 515 N State St, Chicago, IL 60610 (fax 312-464-5831). A subscription request card will be sent to you in response. If you are a resident or fellow, please include verification of your training program and a complete mailing address.

251

American Journal on Mental Retardation
1993, Vol. 97, No. 4, 359-372
© 1993 American Association on Mental Retardation

Long-Term Outcome for Children With Autism Who Received Early Intensive Behavioral Treatment

John J. McEachin, Tristram Smith, and O. Ivar Lovaas
University of California, Los Angeles

After a very intensive behavioral intervention, an experimental group of 19 preschool-age children with autism achieved less restrictive school placements and higher IQs than did a control group of 19 similar children by age 7 (Lovaas, 1987). The present study followed-up this finding by assessing subjects at a mean age of 11.5 years. Results showed that the experimental group preserved its gains over the control group. The 9 experimental subjects who had achieved the best outcomes at age 7 received particularly extensive evaluations indicating that 8 of them were indistinguishable from average children on tests of intelligence and adaptive behavior. Thus, behavioral treatment may produce long-lasting and significant gains for many young children with autism.

Infantile autism is a condition marked by severe impairment in intellectual, social, and emotional functioning. Its onset occurs in infancy, and the prognosis appears

This study was supported by Grant No. MH-11440 from the National Institute of Mental Health. The study was based on a dissertation submitted to the University of California, Los Angeles, Department of Psychology, in partial fulfillment of the requirements for the doctoral degree. The authors express their deep appreciation to the many students at UCLA who served as therapists and helped to make this study possible. Special thanks to Bruce Baker and Duane Buhrmester, who helped in the design of this study. Requests for reprints of this article, copies of the Clinical Rating Scale, or additional information about this study should be sent to O. Ivar Lovaas, 405 Hilgard Ave., UCLA, Department of Psychology, Los Angeles, CA 90024-1563.

to be extremely poor (Lotter, 1978). For example, in the longest prospective follow-up study with a sound methodological design, Rutter (1970) found that only 1 of 64 subjects with autism (fewer than 2%) could be considered free of clinically significant problems by adulthood, as evidenced by holding a job, living independently, and maintaining an active and age-appropriate social life. The remaining subjects showed numerous dysfunctions, such as marked oddities in behavior, social isolation, and florid psychopathology. The majority of subjects required supervised living conditions.

Professionals have attempted a wide variety of interventions in an effort to help children with autism. For many years, no scientific evidence showed that any of these interventions brightened the children's long-term prognosis (DeMyer et al., 1981). However, since the 1960s, one of these interventions, behavioral treatment, has appeared promising. Behavioral treatment has been found to increase adaptive behaviors such as language and social skills, while decreasing disruptive behaviors such as aggression (DeMyer, Hingtgen, & Jackson, 1981; Newsom & Rincover, 1989; Rutter, 1985). Furthermore, behavioral treatment has been continuously refined and improved as a result of ongoing research efforts at a number of sites (Lovaas & Smith, 1988).

Some recent evidence has indicated that behavioral treatment has developed to the point that it can produce substantial improvements in the overall functioning of young children with autism (Simeonnson, Olley, & Rosenthal, 1987). Lovaas (1987) provided approximately 40 hours per week of one-on-one behavioral treatment for a period of 2 years or more to an experimental group of 19 children with autism who were under 4 years of age. This intervention also included parent training and mainstreaming into regular preschool environments. When re-evaluated at a mean age of 7 years, subjects in the experimental group had gained an average of 20 IQ points and had made major advances in educational achievement. Nine of the 19 subjects completed first grade in regular (nonspecial education) classes entirely on their own and had IQs that increased to the average range. By contrast, two control groups totalling 40 children, also diagnosed as autistic and comparable to the experimental group at intake, did not fare nearly as well. Only one of the control subjects (2.5%) attained normal levels of intellectual and educational functioning.

These data suggest that behavioral treatment is effective. However, the durability of treatment gains is uncertain. In one prior major study, Lovaas, Koegel, Simmons, and Long (1973) found that children with autism regressed following the termination of treatment. Other studies have shown that children with autism may display increased difficulties when they enter adolescence (Kanner, 1971; Waterhouse & Fein, 1984).

Also, as was stated in the first follow-up (Lovaas, 1987), "Certain residual deficits may remain in the normal-functioning group that cannot be detected by teachers and parents and can only be isolated on closer psychological assessment, particularly as these children grow older" (p. 8). This possibility points to the need for a more detailed assessment and for continued follow-ups of the group over time.

The present investigation contained two parts: In the first part we examined whether several years after the evaluation at age 7, the experimental group in Lovaas's (1987) study had maintained its treatment gains. Subjects in the experimental group and one of the control groups completed standardized tests of intellectual and adaptive functioning. The groups were then contrasted with each other, and their current performance was compared to their performance on previous assessments. The second part of the investigation focused on those subjects who had achieved the best outcome at the end of first grade in the Lovaas (1987) study (i.e., the 9 subjects who were classified as normal functioning out of the 19 in the experimental group). We examined the extent to which these best-outcome subjects could be considered free of autistic symptomatology. A test battery was constructed to assess a variety of possible deficits: for example, idiosyncratic thought patterns, mannerisms, and interests; lack of close relationships with family and friends; difficulty in getting along with people; relative weaknesses in certain areas of cognitive functioning, such as abstract reasoning; not working up to ability in school; flatness of affect; absence or peculiarity in sense of humor. Possible strengths to be identified included normal intellectual functioning, good relationships with family members, ability to function independently, appropriate use of leisure time, and adequate socialization with peers. Numerous methodological precautions were taken to ensure objectivity of the follow-up examination.

Method

Subjects and Background

Characteristics of the subjects and their treatment have been described elsewhere (Lovaas, 1987) and will only be summarized here. The initial treatment study contained 38 children who, at the time of intake, were very young (less than 40 months if mute, less than 46 months if echolalic) and had received a diagnosis of autism from a licensed clinical psychologist or psychiatrist not involved in the study. These 38 subjects were divided into an experimental group and a control group. The assignment to groups was made on the basis of staff availability. At the beginning of each academic quarter, treatment teams were formed. The clinic director and staff members then determined whether any opening existed for intensive treatment. If so, the next referral received would enter the experimental group; otherwise, the subject entered the control group. The experimental group contained 19 children who received 40 or more hours per week of one-to-one behavioral treatment for 2 or more years. The control group was comprised of 19 children who received a much less intensive intervention (10 hours a week or less of one-to-one behavioral treatment in addition to a variety of treatments provided by community agencies, such as parent training or special education classes). The initial study also included a second control group, consisting of 21 children with autism who were followed over time by a nearby agency but who were never referred for this study. However, these 21 subjects were not available for the present investigation. On standardized measures of intelligence, the second control group did not differ from either the experimental group or the first control group at intake, nor did it differ from the first control group when evaluated again when the subjects were 7 years old. These findings suggest that, as measured by standardized tests, (a) the children with autism who were referred to us for treatment were comparable to children with autism seen elsewhere and (b) the minimal treatment provided to the first control group did not alter intellectual functioning.

Statistical analysis of an extensive range of pretreatment measures confirmed that the experimental group and control group were comparable at intake and closely matched on such important variables as IQ and severity of disturbance. The mean chronological age (CA) at diagnosis for subjects in the experimental group was 32 months. Their mean IQ was 53 (range 30 to 82; all IQs are given as deviation scores). The mean CA of subjects in the control group was 35 months; their mean IQ was 46 (range 30 to 80). Most of the subjects were mute, all had gross deficiencies in receptive language, none played with peers or showed age-appropriate toy play, all were emotionally withdrawn, most had severe tantrums, and all showed extensive ritualistic and stereotyped (self-stimulatory) behaviors. Thus, they appeared to be a representative sample of children with autism (Lovaas, Smith, & McEachin, 1989). A more complete presentation of the intake data was reported by Lovaas (1987).

The children in the experimental group and control group received their respective treatments from trained student therapists who worked in the child's home. The parents also worked with their child, and they received extensive instruction and supervision on appropriate treatment techniques. Whenever possible, the children were integrated into regular preschools. The treatment focused primarily on developing language, increasing social behavior, and promoting cooperative play with peers along with independent and appropriate toy play. Concurrently, substantial efforts were directed at decreasing excessive rituals, tantrums, and aggressive behavior. (For a more detailed description of the intervention program, see the treatment manual [Lovaas et al., 1980] and instructional videotapes that supplement the manual [Lovaas & Leaf, 1981].)

At the time of the present follow-up (1984–1985), the mean CA of the experimental group children was 13 years (range = 9 to 19 years). All children who had achieved normal functioning by the age of 7 years had ended treatment by that point. *(Normal functioning* was operationally defined as scoring within the normal range on standardized intelligence tests and successfully completing first grade in a regular, nonspecial education class entirely on one's own.) On the other hand, some of the children who had not achieved normal functioning at 7 years of age had, at the request of their parents, remained in treatment. The length of time that experimental subjects had been out of treatment ranged from 0 to 12 years (mean = 5), with the normal-functioning children having been out for 3 to 9 years (mean = 5).

The mean age of subjects in the control group was 10 years (range 6 to 14). The length of time that these children had been out of treatment ranged from 0 to 9 years (mean = 3). Thus, experimental subjects tended to be older and had been out of treatment longer than had control subjects. This difference in age occurred because the first referrals for the study were all assigned to the experimental group due to the fact that referrals came slowly (7 in the first 3.5 years) and therapists were available to treat all of them. (As noted earlier, subjects were assigned to the experimental group if therapists were available to treat them; otherwise, they entered the control group.)

Statistical analyses were conducted to test whether a bias resulted from the tendency for the first referrals to go into the experimental group. For example, it is conceivable that the first referrals could have been higher functioning at intake or could have had a better prognosis than subsequent referrals. If so, the subject assignment procedure could have favored the experimental group. To assess this possibility, we correlated the order of referral with intake IQ and with IQ at the first follow-up (age 7 years). Pearson correlations were computed across both groups and within each group. These analyses indicated that the order in which subjects were referred was not associated with intake IQ or outcome IQ. Consequently, although the tendency for the first referrals to enter the experimental group created a potential bias, the data indicate that this was unlikely.

Procedure

The assessment procedure included ascertaining school placement and administering three standardized tests. Information on school placement was obtained from subjects' parents, who classified them as being in either a regular or a special education class (e.g., a class for children with autism or mental retardation, language delays, multihandicaps, or learning disabilities). The three standardized tests were as follows:

1. *Intelligence test.* The Wechsler Intelligence Scale for Children-Revised (Wechsler, 1974) was administered when subjects were able to provide verbal responses. This included all 9 best-outcome experimental subjects plus 8 of the remaining 10 experimental subjects and 6 of the 19 control subjects. For subjects who were not able to provide verbal responses, the Leiter International Performance Scale (Leiter, 1959) and the Peabody Picture Vocabulary Test-Revised (Dunn, 1981) were administered. All of these tests have been widely used for the assessment of intellectual functioning in children with autism (Short & Marcus, 1986).

2. *The Vineland Adaptive Behavior Scales* (Sparrow, Balla, & Cicchetti, 1984). The Vineland is a structured interview administered to parents assessing the extent to which their child exhibits behaviors that are needed to cope effectively with the everyday environment.

3. *The Personality Inventory for Children* (Wirt, Lachar, Klinedinst, & Seat, 1977). This measure is a 600-item true–false questionnaire filled out by parents that assesses the extent to which their children show various forms of psychological disturbance (e.g., anxiety, depression, hyperactivity, and psychotic behavior).

These three tests were intended to provide a comprehensive evaluation of intellectual, social, and emotional functioning. All of the tests have been standardized on average populations. Hence, they provide an objective basis for comparing subjects to children without handicaps across the various areas that they assess.

Data were obtained on all subjects except one girl in the control group, who was known to be institutionalized and functioning very poorly. The 9 best-outcome subjects (those who had been classified as normal functioning at age 7) received particularly extensive evaluations, as outlined later. Of the 28 remaining subjects, 17 were evaluated by staff members in our treatment program, and 11 received evaluations from outside agencies such as schools or psychology clinics. (In some cases, the outside agencies did not administer all of the measures in this battery.)

Evaluation of Best-Outcome Subjects. To ensure objectivity in the evaluation of the best-outcome subjects, we arranged for blind administration and scoring of all tests for these subjects as follows. A psychologist not associated with the study recruited advanced graduate students in clinical psychology to administer the tests. The examiners were not familiar with the history of the children, and the psychologist told them simply that the testing was part of a research study on assessment of children. The psychologist advised them that the nature of the study necessitated providing only certain standard background information: age, school placement and grade, and parent's name and phone number. To increase the heterogeneity of the sample and to control for any examiner bias, each examiner also tested one or more subjects who were matched in age to the experimental subjects and had no history of behavioral disturbance. The examiners were randomly assigned an approximately equal number of subjects for testing in the experimental group and the comparison group. Two experimental subjects were not living in the local area. Therefore, for each of them, the psychologist recruited a tester from the subject's hometown area as well as an age-matched control subject, and data were collected as just described. In addition, the child's examiner filled out a clinical rating scale following a structured interview that covered a list of standard topics, including friendships, family relations, and school and community activities. The interview was designed both for eliciting content and for sampling interpersonal style. The rating scale consisted of 22 items, each scored 0 (best clinical status) to 3 (marked deviance) points. The items were designed to include likely areas of difficulty for children with autism of average intelligence (e.g., compulsive or ritualistic behavior, empathy for and interest in others, a sense of humor) as well as areas of potential difficulty for the general child population (e.g., depressed mood, anxiety, hyperactivity). (The complete scale and a copy of instructions for the clinical interview can be obtained by writing to the third author).

Results

Experimental Versus Control Group

This first section examines the overall effects of treatment through comparison of the follow-up data from the 19 subjects who received the intensive (experimental) treatment to the data from those who received the minimal (control) treatment. Data were obtained from all subjects on school placement and from all but one subject in the control group on IQ. On the Vineland, scores were obtained for 18 of 19 experimental subjects and 15 of 19 control subjects. The lowest availability of follow-up scores was on the Personality Inventory for Children, with scores for 15 experimental subjects and 12 control subjects.

The subjects in the control group who had Personality Inventory for Children scores did not appear to differ from subjects who were missing these scores, as compared on

257

t tests for differences in intake IQ, IQ at 7 years old, or IQ in the present study.

As noted earlier, 17 of the 29 subjects who were not in the best-outcome group were evaluated by Project staff members, 11 were evaluated by outside agencies, and 1 was not evaluated. To check whether Project staff members were biased in their evaluations or in their selection of which subjects to evaluate, we used *t* tests to compare subjects they evaluated to those evaluated by outside agencies on intake IQ, IQ at age 7 years, and IQ in the present study. No significant differences between subjects evaluated by Project staff members and those evaluated by outside agencies were found.

School Placement. In the experimental group, 1 of the 9 subjects from the best-outcome group who had attended a regular class at age 7 (J. L.) was now in a special education class. However, 1 of the other 10 subjects had gone from a special education class to a regular class and was enrolled in a junior college at the time of this follow-up. The remaining experimental subjects had not changed their classification. Overall, then, the proportion of experimental subjects in regular classes did not change from the age 7 evaluation (9 of 19, or 47%). In the control group, none of the 19 children were in a regular class, as had been true at the age 7 evaluation. The difference in classroom placement between the experimental group and the control group was statistically significant, χ^2 (1, N = 38) = 19.05, p < .05.

Intellectual Functioning. The test scores for the experimental group and control group on intellectual functioning, adaptive and maladaptive behaviors, and personality functioning are summarized in Table 1. As can be seen in the table, the experimental group at follow-up had a significantly higher mean IQ than did the control group. This difference was significant, $t(35)$ = 2.97, p < .01. Eleven subjects (58%) in the experimental group obtained Full-Scale IQs of at least 80; only 3 subjects (17%) in the control group did as well. The scores were similar to those obtained by the experimental group and con-

trol group at age 7 (mean IQs of 83 and 52, respectively), indicating that the experimental group had maintained its gains in intellectual functioning between age 7 and the time of the current evaluation.

Table 1
Mean Scores and *SD*s by Group and Measure at Follow-Up

	Group			
	Experimental		Control	
Measure	Mean	SD	Mean	SD
IQ	84.5	32.4	54.9	29.1
Vineland[a]				
Communication	5.1	28.4	51.9	26.7
Daily Living Skills	73.1	26.9	45.9	25.4
Socialization	75.5	26.8	49.7	19.9
Adaptive Behavior				
Composite	71.6	26.8	45.7	21.3
Maladaptive Behavior	10.6	8.2	17.1	7.2
PIC[b] Scales				
Mean elevation	61.8	10.2	64.8	8.1
Scales > 70	4.0	3.9	6.2	2.8

[a]Vineland Adaptive Behavior Scale. [b]Personality Inventory for Children.

Adaptive and Maladaptive Behavior. On the Vineland, the mean overall or Composite score was 72 in the experimental group and 48 in the control group. (The average score for the general population on this test is 100, with a standard deviation [*SD*] of 15.) On the three subscales—Communication, Daily Living, and Socialization—each score closely paralleled the Composite score. The interaction between the groups and the subscales was not significant, indicating that across the three subscales, the experimental group consistently scored higher than did the control group. As can be seen in Table 1, Maladaptive Behavior was significantly higher in the control group, $t(31)$ = 2.39, p < .05. The mean score for the control group was in the clinically significant range whereas that of the experimental group was not. (Scores of 13 and above are considered to be indicative of clinically significant levels of maladaptive behavior at ages 6 to 9 years; 12 or above, at 12 to 13 years; and 10 or above, at 14 years and older.) Thus, the findings indicate that the experimental group showed more adaptive behaviors and fewer maladaptive behaviors than did the control group.

Personality Functioning. Scores for the experimental group and control group did not differ on overall scale elevation, with mean *t* scores of 62 and 65, respectively. (On this test, the mean *t* score for the general population is approximately 50 [*SD* = 10].) *T* scores above 60 are considered indicative of possible or mild deviance, whereas *t* scores above 70 are viewed as suggesting a clinically significant problem, namely, one that may require professional attention. There was a significant interaction between the groups and the individual scales on this test, $F(15, 390) = 2.36$, $p < .01$. Results of the Tukey test indicated that the most reliable difference between groups occurred on the Psychosis scale, on which the experimental subjects had a mean of 78 and the control subjects had a mean of 104, $F(1, 26) = 8.53$, $p < .01$. Seven subjects in the experimental group scored in the clinically preferred range (below 70), whereas no subjects in the control group scored that low. Only one other scale showed a significant difference, Somatic Concerns, $F(1, 26) = 4.60$, $p < .05$. The control subjects tended to display a below average level of somatic complaints (mean of 45 as compared to 54 for the experimental subjects).

Best-Outcome Versus Nonclinical Comparison Group

A *t* test indicated no significant difference in age between the best-outcome group and the comparison group of children without a history of clinically significant behavioral disturbance. Subjects in the best-outcome group had a mean age of 12.42 years (range 10.0 to 16.25) versus 12.92 years (range 9.0 to 15.17) for the nonclinical comparison group. Scores on the WISC-R and clinical rating scale were obtained for all subjects; 1 experimental subject and 2 nonclinical comparison subjects were missing Vineland scores, and 2 experimental subjects and 1 nonclinical comparison subject were missing Personality Inventory for Children scores. Both the Vineland and Personality Inventory for Children were completed by parents. In cases where these scores were not obtained, the parents had declined to participate.

On the measures that provide standardized scores, the functioning of the best-outcome subjects was measured most precisely by comparing the best-outcome group against the test norms. Therefore, this analysis is of primary interest. Data for the nonclinical comparison group are mainly useful in confirming that the assessment procedures were valid and in providing a contrast group for the one measure without norms, the Clinical Rating Scale. For the nonclinical comparison group, it will suffice to summarize the results as follows: On the WISC-R this group had mean IQs of 116 Verbal, 118 Performance, and 119 Full-Scale. On the Vineland the group obtained mean standard scores of 102 Communication, 100 Daily Living Skills, 102 Socialization, and 101 Composite. The mean scale score on the Personality Inventory for Children was 49. Thus, the nonclinical comparison group displayed above-average or average functioning across all areas that were assessed.

The next section is focused on the functioning of the best-outcome group on IQ, adaptive and maladaptive behavior, and personality measures and contrasts the best-outcome subjects with the comparison subjects on the Clinical Rating Scale.

Intellectual Functioning. Table 2 presents the IQ data for each subject in the best-outcome group and the mean scores for the group. This table shows that, as a whole, the 9 best-outcome subjects performed well on the WISC-R. Their IQs placed them in the high end of the normal range, about two thirds of an *SD* above the mean. Their Full-Scale IQs ranged from 99 to 136.

Subjects' scores were evenly distributed across a range from 80 to 125 on Verbal IQ and from 88 to 138 on Performance IQ. The subjects averaged 3 points higher on Performance IQ than Verbal IQ. Two of them (J. L. and A. G.) had at least a 20-point difference

Table 2
WISC-R Scores of the Best-Outcome Subjects

Subject	Verbal					Performance					WISC-R IQ		
	Infrm	Simil	Arith	Vocab	Compr	PicC	PicA	BlkD	ObjA	Cod	VIQ	PIQ	Full
R.S.	12	12	13	9	11	10	9	13	12	11	106	106	106
M.C.	17	19	11	14	10	12	16	19	19	11	125	138	136
M.M.	14	13	10	14	11	12	11	11	11	8	114	102	109
L.B.	12	16	11	13	15	7	12	17	17	19	119	131	128
J.L.	6	9	7	4	8	18	11	16	14	7	80	123	100
D.E.	9	17	8	10	15	13	9	12	9	17	98	114	105
A.G.	7	14	12	11	13	9	4	8	11	10	108	88	99
B.W.	12	11	10	10	9	7	10	9	11	10	102	95	99
B.R.	11	14	11	13	16	12	10	12	11	10	118	106	114
Mean	11.1	13.9	10.3	10.9	12	11.1	10.2	13	12.8	11.4	108	111	111

Note. Infrm = Information, Simil = Similarities, Arith = Arithmetic, Vocab = Vocabulary, Compr = Comprehension, PicC = Picture Completion, PicA = Picture Arrangement, BlkD = Block Design, ObjA = Object Assembly, Cod = Coding, VIQ = Verbal IQ, PIQ = Performance IQ, and Full = Full-Scale IQ.

between Verbal and Performance IQ.

On each subtest of the WISC-R, the mean for the general population is 10 (SD = 3). It can be seen from Table 2 that the best-outcome subjects scored highest on Similarities, Block Design, and Object Assembly. They scored lowest on Picture Arrangement and Arithmetic. Thus, the subjects consistently scored at or above average.

Adaptive and Maladaptive Behavior. Table 3 presents the data for the best-outcome group on the Vineland Adaptive Behavior Scales. It can be seen that the best-outcome group scored about average on the Composite Scale and on the subscales for Communication, Daily Living, and Socialization. However, Table 3 shows that some of the best-outcome subjects had marginal scores, including J. L., B. W., and M. M. Even so, all of the best-outcome subjects had Composite scores within the normal range.

As can be seen in Table 3, the Maladaptive Behavior Scale (Parts I and II), the mean score for the best-outcome group indicated that, on average, these subjects did not display clinically significant levels of maladaptive behavior. Three of them scored in the clinically significant range versus one subject in the nonclinical comparison group, which had a mean of 7.7 on this scale.

Personality Functioning. The results of the Personality Inventory for Children are summarized in Table 4. The best-outcome subjects obtained valid profiles on the Personality Inventory for Children, as measured by the three validity scales (Lie, Frequency, and Defensiveness). As can be seen from the table, the subjects scored in the normal range across all scales. They tended to score highest on Intellectual-Screening, Psychosis, and Frequency. Intellectual-Screening assesses slow intellectual development, and Psychosis and Frequency assess unusual or strange behaviors. Only Intellectual-Screening was above the normal range, and this scale is affected by subjects' early history. For example, the scale contains statements such as "My child first talked before he (she) was two years old," which would be false for the best-outcome subjects regardless of their current level of functioning.

As Table 4 indicates, 4 best-outcome subjects had a single scale elevated beyond

Table 3
Scores on the Vineland Adaptive Behavior Scale for the Best-Outcome Subjects

Subject	Adaptive behavior				Maladaptive behavior
	Com	DLS	Soc	Comp	
R.S.	83	98	102	92	6
M.C.	119	93	86	98	16
M.M.	119	79	114	105	2
L.B.	107	108	112	108	4
J.L.	77	103	94	88	13
D.E.	93	81	82	80	15
A.G.	101	97	99	98	5
B.W.	83	74	105	83	9
B.R.	—	—	—	—	—
Mean	98	92	99	94	8.8

Note. Com = Communication, DLS = Daily Living Skills, Soc = Socialization, Comp = Adaptive Behavior Composite.

Autism and Early Intervention

Table 4
T Scores on the Personality Inventory for Children for the Best-Outcome Subjects

Subject	*T* score Mean	<70	L	F	Def	Adj	Ach	I-S	Dvl	Som	Dep	Fam	Dlq	Wdr	Anx	Psy	Hyp	Soc
R.S.	56	1	49	54	43	61	53	75	49	44	69	47	46	69	60	65	46	64
M.C.	52	1	48	63	37	43	39	54	38	64	55	54	46	65	51	75	40	55
M.M.	49	0	42	54	43	50	42	64	46	58	48	55	46	47	53	46	54	36
L.B.	51	1	60	50	49	49	37	70	39	55	49	48	51	45	60	51	49	51
J.L.	70	9	42	84	37	85	77	94	65	78	86	65	61	69	78	76	52	72
D.E.	—	—	—	—	—	—	—	—	—	—	—	—	—	—	—	—	—	—
A.G.	51	0	38	45	49	57	48	39	53	51	49	69	40	55	55	55	49	63
B.W.	54	1	45	63	50	59	64	48	55	47	44	57	90	44	45	46	62	44
B.R.	—	—	—	—	—	—	—	—	—	—	—	—	—	—	—	—	—	—
Mean	55	2	46	56	44	58	51	64	49	57	57	56	54	56	57	59	50	55

Note. Mean = mean elevation across all scales. L = Lie scale, F = Frequency, Def = Defensiveness, Adj = Adjustment, Ach = Achievement, I-S = Intellectual-Screening, Dvl = Development, Som = Somatic Concern, Dep = Depression, Fam = Family Relations, Dlq = Delinquency, Wdr = Withdrawal, Anx = Anxiety, Psy = Psychosis, Hyp = Hyperactivity, Soc = Social Skills.

the clinically significant range and a 5th (J. L.) had nine scales elevated, including the highest scores in the best-outcome group on Intellectual-Screening, Psychosis, and Frequency. Thus, this subject appeared to account for much of the elevation in scores on these scales. By comparison, there were 3 subjects in the nonclinical comparison group with at least one scale elevated.

Clinical Rating Scale. On this scale, 8 of the best-outcome subjects scored between 0 and 10, and the 9th (J. L.) scored 42. The mean was 8.8, with a standard deviation of 12.9. The nonclinical comparison subjects all scored between 0 and 5 (mean = 1.7, *SD* = 2.1). Because these *SD*s are unequal, we used a nonparametric statistic, a Mann-Whitney *U* test, revealing a significant difference between groups, $U = 19$, $p < .05$. Thus, the best-outcome subjects displayed more deviance than did the comparison subjects, but most of the deviance appeared to come from one subject, J. L.

Discussion

This study is a later and more extensive follow-up of two groups of young subjects with autism who were previously studied by Lovaas (1987): (a) an experimental group (*n* = 19) that had received very intensive behavioral treatment and (b) a control group (*n* = 19) that had received minimal behavioral treatment. In the present study we have reported data on these children at a mean age of 13 years for subjects in the experimental group and 10 years for those in the control group. The data were obtained from a comprehensive assessment battery.

The main findings from the test battery were as follows: First, subjects in the experimental group had maintained their level of intellectual functioning between their previous assessment at age 7 and the present evaluation at a mean age of 13, as measured by standardized intelligence tests. Their mean IQ was about 30 points higher than that of control subjects. Second, experimental subjects also displayed significantly higher levels of functioning than did control subjects on measures of adaptive behavior and personality. Third, in a particularly rigorous evaluation of the 9 subjects in the experimental group who had been classified as best-outcome (normal-functioning) in the earlier study (Lovaas, 1987), the test results consistently indicated that the subjects exhibited average intelligence and average levels of adaptive functioning. Some deviance from average was found on the personality test and the clinical ratings. However, this deviance appeared to derive from the extreme scores of one subject, J. L. (see Table 2, 3, and 4). This subject also had been removed from nonspecial education classes and placed in a class for children with language delays, and he obtained relatively

261

low scores (about 80) on the Verbal section of the intelligence test and the Communication section of the measure of adaptive behavior. Thus, he no longer appeared to be normal-functioning. However, the remaining 8 subjects who had previously been classified as normal-functioning demonstrated average IQ, with intellectual performance evenly distributed across subtests, were able to hold their own in regular classes, did not show signs of emotional disturbance, and demonstrated adequate development of adaptive and social skills within the normal range. In addition, subjective clinical impressions of blind examiners did not discriminate them from children with no history of behavioral disturbance. These 8 subjects (42% of the experimental group) may be judged to have made major and enduring gains and may be described as "normal-functioning." By contrast, none of the control group subjects achieved such a favorable outcome, consistent with the poor prognosis for children with autism reported by other investigators (Freeman, Ritvo, Needleman, & Yokota, 1985).

In order to evaluate this outcome, we must pay close attention to whether or not our methodology was sound. The adequacy of our methodology is crucial because the outcome in the present study represents a major improvement over outcomes obtained in previous experimental studies on the treatment of children with autism (Rutter, 1985). The only reports of comparable outcomes have come from uncontrolled case studies (e.g., Bettelheim, 1967), and subsequent investigations have indicated that these case studies grossly overestimated the outcomes obtainable with the treatment that was provided. Similarly, reports of major gains in other populations, such as large IQ increases in children from impoverished backgrounds, also have been based on highly questionable evidence (Kamin, 1974; Spitz, 1986). Such reports have the potential to cause a great deal of harm by misleading consumers and professionals.

A detailed description of all the methodological safeguards that should be built into a treatment study is beyond the scope of the present report (see Kazdin, 1980; Kendall & Norton-Ford, 1982; Spitz, 1986). However, we note that we incorporated a large number of methodological safeguards in both the original study (Lovaas, 1987) and the present investigation:

1. The experimental group and the control group received equivalent assessment batteries at intake and were found to be very similar on a multitude of important variables. Moreover, the number of control group subjects who were predicted to achieve normal functioning, had they received intensive treatment, was approximately equal to the number of experimental subjects who actually did achieve normal functioning with intensive treatment (Lovaas & Smith, 1988). Thus, the subject assignment procedure yielded groups that were comparable prior to treatment. This provided a strong indication that the superior functioning of the experimental group after treatment was a result of the treatment itself rather than a biased procedure for assigning subjects to the experimental group.

2. All subjects remained in the groups to which they were assigned at intake. Only 2 subjects dropped out, and they were not replaced. Therefore, the original composition of the groups was essentially preserved.

3. All subjects were independently diagnosed as autistic by PhD or MD clinicians, and there was high agreement on the diagnosis between the independent clinicians. This provided evidence that subjects met criteria for a diagnosis of autism.

4. Prior to treatment, these subjects appeared to be comparable to those diagnosed as having autism in other research investigations. Evidence for this comes from the second control group that was incorporated into the initial treatment study. This group was evaluated by another research team (independent of ours), had similar IQs at intake based on the same measures of intelligence that we used, yet showed similar outcome data to those reported by other investigators. Additional evidence can be

derived from the similarity of our intake data to data reported by other investigators (Lovaas et al., 1989). For example, although Schopler and his associates (Schopler, Short, & Mesibov, 1989) suggested that our sample had a higher mean IQ than did other samples of children with autism, their own data do not appear to differ from ours (Lord & Schopler, 1989). Thus, there is evidence that our subjects were a typical group of preschool-age children with autism rather than a select group of high-level children with autism who would have been expected to achieve normal functioning with little or no treatment.

5. The first control group, which received up to 10 hours a week of one-to-one behavioral treatment, did not differ at posttreatment from the second control group, which received no treatment from us. Both groups achieved substantially less favorable outcomes than did the experimental group. Because all groups were similar at pretreatment, this result confirms that our subjects had problems that responded only to intensive treatment rather than problems such as being noncompliant or holding back (masking an underlying, essentially average intellectual functioning that would respond to smaller-scale interventions).

6. Subjects' families ranged from high to low socioeconomic status, and, on average, they did not differ from the general population (Lovaas, 1987). Thus, although our treatment required extensive family participation, a diverse group of families was apparently able to meet this requirement.

7. The treatment has been described in detail (Lovaas et al., 1980; Lovaas & Leaf, 1981), and the effectiveness of many components of the treatment has been demonstrated experimentally by a large number of investigators over the past 30 years (cf. Newsom & Rincover, 1989). Hence, our treatment may be replicable, a point that is discussed in greater detail later.

8. The results of the present follow-up, which extended several years beyond discharge from treatment for most subjects, are an encouraging sign that treatment gains have been maintained for an extended period of time.

9. A wide range of measures was administered, avoiding overreliance on intelligence tests, which have limitations if used in isolation (e.g., bias resulting from teaching to the test, selecting a test that would yield especially favorable results, failing to assess other aspects of functioning such as social competence or school performance) (Spitz, 1986; Zigler & Trickett, 1978).

10. The use at follow-up of a normal comparison group, standardized testing, and blind rating allowed for an objective, detailed, and quantifiable assessment of treatment effectiveness. A particularly rigorous assessment was given to those subjects who showed the most improvement.

Taken together, these safeguards provide considerable assurance that the favorable outcome of the experimental subjects can be attributed to the treatment they received rather than to extraneous factors such as improvement that would have occurred regardless of treatment, biased procedures for selecting subjects or assigning them to groups, or narrow or inappropriate assessment batteries.

Despite the numerous precautions that we have taken, several concerns may be raised about the validity of the results. Perhaps the most important is that the assignment to the experimental or control group was made on the basis of therapist availability rather than a more arbitrary procedure such as alternating referrals (assigning the first referral to the experimental group, the second to the control group, the third to the experimental group, and so forth). However, it seems unlikely that the assignment was biased in view of the pretreatment data we have presented on the similarity between the experimental and control groups. On the other hand, we do not know as yet whether there exists a pretreatment variable that does predict outcome but was not among the 19 we chose, yet could have discriminated between groups. In an earlier publication (Lovaas et al., 1989), we responded in some detail to the concern about subject assignment as well as other possible problems associated with the original study. There are certain additional questions that may be raised by this follow-up investigation:

1. The experimental group was older than the control group at the time of this follow-up evaluation. We explained this finding earlier and noted that data analyses indicated that it was unlikely that this age difference reflected a bias in subject assignments.

2. The follow-up assessments for 17 of the lower functioning subjects in this study were conducted by staff members from our Project, who could have biased the test results. However, as noted previously, a check revealed no evidence of such a bias.

3. The Clinical Rating Scale, based on an interview with subjects who had been classified as normal-functioning in the original study, has no norms or data on reliability and validity. However, we regard the interview simply as an extra check on whether the examiners detected residual signs of autism or other behavior problems that were somehow overlooked in the three other (well-standardized) measures in the study and their 30 subscales. We do not regard the interview as an instrument that by itself yields conclusive results. No other interview that suited our purposes currently exists. In future investigations, we plan to use an interview that Michael Rutter and his associates are now developing for the purpose of detecting of residual signs of autism in individuals with average intelligence.

4. As in most long-term follow-up studies, we had some missing data. However, there is no evidence that the missing data would have changed the overall results.

5. In our analysis of the best-outcome group, we noted that the group averages deviated from "normal" on one subscale of the Personality Inventory for Children and on the Clinical Rating Scale. We then attributed this deviance to the extreme scores of one subject rather than to general problems within this group. We recognize that group averages are seldom interpreted this way. However, as statisticians and methodologists have pointed out (e.g., Barlow & Hersen, 1984), there are many times when group averages represent the performance of few or no subjects within the group. This was one of those times, as is clearly shown by the data on individual subjects (Tables 2, 3, and 4). Deviance was found almost exclusively in one subject, not evenly distributed across all subjects, and we have presented the results accordingly.

The most important void for research to fill at this time is replication by independent investigators who employ sound methodologies. Given the objective assessment instruments that we used and the detailed description that we have provided of the treatment (Lovaas et al., 1980), such a replication should be possible. However, the treatment is complex and to replicate it properly, an investigator probably needs to possess (a) a strong foundation in learning theory research; (b) a detailed knowledge of the treatment manual we used; (c) a supervised practicum of at least 6 months in one-to-one work with clients who have developmental delays, emphasizing discrimination learning and building complex language; and (d) a commitment to provide 40 hours of one-to-one treatment to client per week, 50 weeks per year, for at least 2 years. Our best-outcome subjects all required a minimum of 2 years of intensive treatment to achieve average levels of functioning (another indication that those subjects had pervasive disabilities and were not merely noncompliant).

A second void to fill concerns the majority of children who did not benefit to the point of achieving normal functioning with intensive treatment. Perhaps an earlier start in treatment would have been all that was needed to obtain favorable outcomes with many of these children. More pessimistically, perhaps such children require new and different interventions that have yet to be discovered and implemented. In any case, it is essential to develop more appropriate services for these children.

Finally, a rather speculative but promising area for research is to determine the extent to which early intervention alters neurological structures in young children with autism. Autism is almost certainly the result of deficits in such neurological structures (Rutter & Schopler, 1987). However, laboratory studies on animals have shown that alterations in neurological structure are quite possible as a result of changes in the environment in the first years of life (Sirevaag & Greenough, 1988), and there is reason to believe that alterations are also possible in young children. For example, children under 3 years of age overproduce neurons, dendrites, axons, and synapses. Huttenlocher (1984) hypothesized that, with appropriate stimulation from the environment, this overproduction might allow infants and preschoolers to compensate for neurological anomalies much more completely than do older children. Caution is needed in generalizing from these findings on average children to early intervention with children with autism, particularly because the exact nature of the neurological anomalies of children with autism is unclear at present (e.g., Rutter & Schopler, 1987). Nevertheless, the findings suggest that intensive early intervention could compensate for neurological anomalies in such children. Finding evidence for such compensation would help explain why the treatment in this study was effective. More generally, it might contribute to an understanding of brain–behavior relations in young children.

References

Barlow, D. H., & Hersen, M. (1984). *Single case experimental design: Strategies for studying behavior change* (2nd ed.). New York: Pergamon Press.

Bettelheim, B. (1967). *The empty fortress.* New York: The Free Press.

DeMyer, M. K., Hingtgen, J. N., & Jackson, R. K. (1981). Infantile autism reviewed: A decade of research. *Schizophrenia Bulletin, 7,* 388–451.

Dunn, L. M. (1981). *Peabody Picture Vocabulary Test-Revised.* Circle River, MN: American Guidance Service.

Freeman, B. J., Ritvo, E. R., Needleman, R., & Yokota, A. (1985). The stability of cognitive and linguistic parameters in autism: A 5-year study. *Journal of the American Academy of Child Psychiatry, 24,* 290–311.

Huttenlocher, P. R. (1984). Synapse elimination and plasticity in developing human cerebral cortex. *American Journal of Mental Deficiency, 88,* 488–496.

Kamin, L. J. (1974). *The science and politics of I.Q.* New York: Wiley.

Kanner, L. (1971). Follow-up study of 11 autistic children originally reported in 1943. *Journal of Autism and Childhood Schizophrenia, 1,* 119–145.

Kazdin, A. (1980). *Research design in clinical psychology.* New York: Harper & Row.

Kendall, P. C., & Norton-Ford, J. D. (1982). Therapy outcome research methods. In P. C. Kendall & J. N. Butcher (Eds.), *Handbook of research methods in clinical psychology* (pp. 429–460). New York: Wiley.

Leiter, R. G. (1959). Part I of the manual for the 1948 revision of the Leiter International Performance Scale: Evidence of the reliability and validity of the Leiter tests. *Psychology Service Center Journal, 11,* 1–72.

Lord, C., & Schopler, E. (1989). The role of age at assessment, developmental level, and test in the stability of intelligence scores in young autistic children. *Journal of Autism and Developmental Disorders, 19,* 483–499.

Lotter, V. (1978). Follow-up studies. In M. Rutter & E. Schopler (Eds.), *Autism: A reappraisal of concepts and treatment.* London: Plenum Press.

Lovaas, O. I. (1987). Behavioral treatment and normal educational and intellectual functioning in young autistic children. *Journal of Consulting and Clinical Psychology, 55,* 3–9.

Lovaas, O. I., Ackerman, A. B., Alexander, D., Firestone, P., Perkins, J., & Young, D. (1980). *Teaching developmentally disabled children: The me book.* Austin, TX: Pro-Ed.

Lovaas, O. I., Koegel, R. L., Simmons, J. Q., & Long, J. S. (1973). Some generalization and follow-up measures on autistic children in behavior therapy. *Journal of Applied Behavior Analysis, 6,* 131–166.

Lovaas, O. I., & Leaf, R. L. (1981). *Five video*

tapes for teaching developmentally disabled children. Baltimore: University Park Press.

Lovaas, O. I., & Smith, T. (1988). Intensive behavioral treatment with young autistic children. In B. B. Lahey & A. E. Kazdin (Eds.), *Advances in clinical child psychology*(Vol. 11, pp. 285–324). New York: Plenum Press.

Lovaas, O. I., Smith, T., & McEachin, J. J. (1989). Clarifying comments on the young autism study: Reply to Schopler, Short and Mesibov. *Journal of Consulting and Clinical Psychology, 57,* 165–167.

McEachin, J. J. (1987). *Outcome of autistic children receiving intensive behavioral treatment: Psychological status 3 to 12 years later.* Unpublished doctoral dissertation, University of California, Los Angeles.

Newsom, C., & Rincover, A. (1989). Autism. In E. J. Mash & R. A. Barkley (Eds.), *Treatment of childhood disorders*(pp. 286–346). New York: Guilford Press.

Rutter, M. (1970). Autistic children: Infancy to adulthood. *Seminars in Psychiatry, 2,* 435–450.

Rutter, M. (1985). The treatment of autistic children. *Journal of Child Psychology & Psychiatry, 26,* 193–214.

Rutter, M., & Schopler, E. (1987). Autism and pervasive developmental disorders: Concepts and diagnostic issues. *Journal of Autism and Developmental Disorders, 17,* 159–186.

Schopler, E., Short, A., & Mesibov, G. (1989). Relation of behavioral treatment to "normal functioning": Comment on Lovaas. *Journal of Consulting and Clinical Psychology, 57,* 162–164.

Short, A., & Marcus, L. (1986). Psychoeducational evaluation of autistic children and adolescents. In S. S. Strichart & P. Lazarus (Eds.),

Psychoeducational evaluation of school-aged children with low-incidence disorders (pp. 155–180). Orlando, FL: Grune & Stratton.

Simeonnson, R. J., Olley, J. G., & Rosenthal, S. L. (1987). Early intervention for children with autism. In M. J. Guralnick & F. C. Bennett (Eds.), *The effectiveness of early intervention for at-risk and handicapped children* (pp. 275–296). Orlando, FL: Academic Press.

Sirevaag, A. M., & Greenough, W. T. (1988). A multivariate statistical summary of synaptic plasticity measures in rats exposed to complex, social and individual environments. *Brain Research, 441,* 386–392.

Sparrow, S. S., Balla, D. A., & Cicchetti, D. V. (1984). *Interview Edition Survey Form Manual.* Circle Pines, MN: American Guidance Service.

Spitz, H. H. (1986). *The raising of intelligence.* Hillsdale, NJ: Erlbaum.

Waterhouse, L., & Fein, D. (1984). Developmental trends in cognitive skills for children diagnosed as autistic and schizophrenic. *Child Development, 55,* 236–248.

Wechsler, D. (1974). *Manual for the Wechsler Intelligence Scale for Children-Revised.* New York: Psychological Corp.

Wirt, R. D., Lachar, D., Klinedinst, J. K., & Seat, P. D. (1977). *Multidimensional descriptions of child personality: A manual for the Personality Inventory for Children.* Los Angeles: Western Psychological Services.

Zigler, E., & Trickett, P. K. (1978). IQ, social competence, and evaluation of early childhood intervention programs. *American Psychologist, 33,* 789–798.

Received: 5/15/91; first decision: 10/16/91; accepted: 1/23/92.

Journal of Clinical Child Psychology
1998, Vol. 27, No. 2, 168–179

Empirically Supported Comprehensive Treatments for Young Children With Autism

Sally J. Rogers

School of Medicine, University of Colorado Health Sciences Center

Describes treatment of autism, a severe, chronic developmental disorder that results in significant lifelong disability for most persons, with few persons ever functioning in an independent and typical lifestyle. Within the past decade, a number of studies have reported significant changes in the outcomes of very young children with autism following intensive comprehensive treatment. The criteria for empirically supported treatments, as described by Lonigan, Elbert, and Johnson (this issue), were applied to reports of eight treatment efficacy studies published in peer-reviewed journals. Whereas positive outcomes are reported in every case, the field does not yet have a treatment that meets the present criteria for well-established or probably efficacious treatment. Hypothesized variables affecting outcomes that need to be rigorously tested include age at start of treatment, type of treatment used, intensity of treatment, and IQ and language levels at the start of treatment.

In 1943, Leo Kanner published a paper that for the first time described a disorder of severe developmental psychopathology, "autistic disturbance of affective contact," in which there existed multiple, severe impairments that pervaded most aspects of the children's social, cognitive, and communicative functioning (p. 217). His follow-up of this group of children into adulthood revealed persistent severe deficits and, for the majority, a generally poor outcome (Kanner, 1971). Other studies of adult outcomes of children with autism continued to report poor outcomes, with between 61% and 74% unable to function independently and only 5% to 17% leading a fairly normal life (Lotter, 1978). We currently view autism as a severe, chronic disorder that results in significant lifelong disability for most persons.

Children with autism not only face a very high-risk future but also present a number of challenges to the families, school personnel, and therapists who become involved with them due to their difficulties learning ordinary skills and typical social behavior, their sometimes very challenging behavior problems, their difficulty with communication and mastery of the skills of everyday life, their variable learning rates, and their dependence on caretakers for extended periods. Given the high-intensity needs of children with autism and the lifelong costs, both human and financial, associated

with this disability, there has been a continuing search for effective treatments for the various symptoms associated with autism. These treatment approaches can be divided roughly into two types.

The first type involves more focal treatments directed toward specific symptoms or specific learning needs associated with autism, such as reduction of escape behaviors (Lalli, Casey, & Kates, 1995), improvement of sleep disturbance (Durand, Gernert-Dott, & Mapstone, 1997), development of symbolic play skills (Thorp, Stahmer, & Schreibman, 1995), and increasing social interactions with peers (Strain, Kohler, & Goldstein, 1996). The literature on effective focal treatments in autism is plentiful and published in a variety of journals, in the fields of developmental disabilities, applied behavior analysis, and discipline-specific journals. These studies generally consist of single-subject multiple baseline designs or small sample treatment designs. Behavioral treatment approaches are particularly well represented in this body of literature and have been amply demonstrated to be effective in reducing symptom frequency and severity as well as in increasing the development of adaptive skills. There are also examples of effective incidental or naturalistic teaching techniques for working with specific skills (i.e., peer mediated strategies, as in Strain et al., 1996, and communicative approaches, as in Bondy & Frost, 1994). Two sources that provide a compendium of this literature are Schreibman (1988) and Koegel and Koegel (1995).

The second type of approach involves comprehensive programs of treatment that seek to reduce the general level of impairment of persons with autism, or stated in the reverse, treatment that seeks to change the nature of the outcome in autism and improve the overall

This work was supported in part by National Institute of Child Health and Human Development Grant #1 PO1 HD35468–01. I thank the Developmental Psychobiology Research Group for their support.

Requests for reprints should be sent to Sally J. Rogers, Professor of Psychiatry, School of Medicine, University of Colorado Health Sciences Center, Box C–234, 4200 East 9th, Denver, CO 80262. E-mail: sally.rogers@uchsc.edu functioning of persons with autism. Compared to the other treatments represented in this issue, these treatment approaches are extremely large in scope, seeking to address multiple symptoms in children with quite varying levels of severity by applying thousands of hours of treatment across years. Furthermore, carrying out these approaches typically involves a team of individuals of varying levels of training, drawn from educational, clinical, and medical settings within a community. The intersection of clinical and educational services for this group of children has at times resulted in litigation that has required school districts to provide or support one of these treatments for individual children. It has also resulted in qualitatively different systems of financial support for these treatments than most other forms of psychological treatment for children. Insurance reimbursement for psychological services is only one piece of the funding picture.

The focus of this article is on the outcomes of these comprehensive treatment programs of autism rather than the focal treatments for two reasons. First, the comprehensive treatment approaches are trying to change the course of the condition, with the goal of significantly reducing the level of disability associated with long-term outcomes in autism. Given the impairments of most adults with autism, any treatments that can fundamentally alter the course of the condition are of utmost importance for persons with autism and their families. The occurrence rate of autism is currently estimated at 1 per 1,000; this represents a higher frequency than childhood cancer, diabetes, or Down syndrome. Autism can no longer be seen as a rare or low-incidence disorder. Significant numbers of children, families, and communities are affected by autism, and effective treatment needs to be identified and provided.

Second, families are becoming increasingly aware of these programs and of their published promising outcomes. Parents are advocating strongly for their children and are seeking resources for these treatments in their communities. Thus, families, community mental health programs, and educational agencies need information about the empirical basis of comprehensive treatment approaches for autism to make informed decisions about provision of services and allocations of resources.

It is important to note well-known and well-respected comprehensive treatment programs for autism, like the TEACCH program in Chapel Hill, NC. The TEACCH program has not yet published data from their comprehensive preschool treatment model and was, therefore, not included it the latter part of this article. However, a recent controlled study by Ozonoff and Cathcart (1998) demonstrated significant short-term gains in several areas for preschoolers with autism when a daily TEACCH home-teaching session was added to their daily program, compared to a matched control group. It is also worth noting in passing the number of treatments targeted to autism without empirical support. Autism seems to be particularly fertile ground for the proliferation of new ideas concerning potential cures or effective treatments, the majority without an established empirical base (Smith, 1996). It is important to remind ourselves that lack of an empirical demonstration of efficacy does not mean that a treatment is ineffective, but rather that efficacy has not been demonstrated in an objective way. Nonvalidated treatment approaches may be effective, or they may be ineffective but benign. However, as Green (1996) pointed out, a benign but ineffective treatment can be harmful if the ineffective treatment is taking the place of an effective treatment.

In the absence of information about empirically grounded treatment, families of children with autism are at the mercy of providers. Thus, it is the responsibility of psychologists and the rest of the professional community (a) to be knowledgeable about validated effectiveness of the various treatment approaches to autism, (b) to provide families with information that helps them understand the issue of validation and helps them discriminate between validated and unvalidated approaches, and (c) to work toward making effective services available for children (and adults) with autism in every community.

Review of Published Outcome Studies

Over the past 10 years, studies of comprehensive treatment approaches for young children have begun to appear in the peer-reviewed journals. These studies form the basis of this report. At this point in time, eight sets of researchers have published efficacy studies in peer-reviewed journals. The findings from these eight studies, briefly described in Table 1, are reviewed in accordance with the criteria for empirically supported treatments (ESTs), as described by Lonigan, Elbert, and Johnson (this issue). The question to be answered by applying these criteria to these outcome studies is whether evidence exists for a well-established or probably efficacious treatment for autistic disorder.

The Work of Lovaas and Colleagues

The study with the strongest scientific design was carried out by Lovaas and his colleagues and reported in two scientific papers (Lovaas, 1987; McEachlin, Smith, & Lovaas, 1993). The study involved 19 young children with autism treated intensively with behavioral therapy for a 2-year span, compared to two control groups. Children in all three groups were diagnosed by independent clinicians, and virtually all the children came from the same large diagnostic clinic in the Psychiatry Department at the University of California, Los Angeles from faculty members recognized internationally for their expertise in autism. Children in all three groups were of similar chronological age (CA) and

169

Table 1. *Description of Eight Studies Examining the Efficacy of Comprehensive Treatment Programs for Children With Autism*

Study	Treated Sample Description	Mean Age of Treated Children	Type of Comparison Group	Treatment Description, Setting, Length, Follow-Up Period	Outcome Variables	Treatment Outcome Data
Lovaas (1987); McEachlin et al. (1993)	19 children; all diagnosed with autism; mean IQ = 53	32 months	Nontreated control group, not randomly assigned; mean IQ = 46. Received less than 10 hr per week of 1:1 treatment in addition to community services	Manualized behavioral treatment; 40 or more hr/week of 1:1 behavior therapy for 2 yrs or more. 10-year follow-up	IQ, Vineland Adaptive Behavior Scales, personality inventory, school placement	47% of experimental group in regular school compared to none of control group (χ^2 = 19.05, $p < .05$); 30-point difference on IQ tests ($p < .01$); similar differences in adaptive behavior, maladaptive behavior, and clinical cutoff on personality inventory.
Birnbauer & Leach (1993)	9 children (5 boys), met *DSM–III–R* criteria for autism or PDD NOS; mean DQ* = 51	39 months	Nontreated control group of 5 boys, younger but matched on all variables	Lovaas's treatment manual. Mean of 28.7 hr/week of 1:1 behavior therapy at home. Outcome data collected after 24 months of treatment. No follow-up.	IQ, adaptive behavior, language, personality, parental stress.	No group analyses; 4 of 9 treated children had nonverbal IQs of 89 or higher; language levels of treated group ($M = 46$ months) double that of controls.
Sheinkopf & Siegel (in press)	11 children; all diagnosed with autism or PDD NOS; mean IQ = 63	33 months	11 pairwise matched controls (on all variables) receiving regular community services	Lovaas's behavioral treatment in home and regular community treatment; mean 27 hr/week for mean of 21 months. No follow-up.	IQ measure (mainly nonverbal), number of symptoms, severity of symptoms.	Treated group mean IQ 25 points higher than control ($p = .01$); no group differences on number of symptoms; treated group had reduced symptom severity ($p = .01$). All children still in autism spectrum.
Anderson et al. (1987)	14 children (3 girls); with diagnosis of autism or "autistic-like"; mean DQ = 57*	43 months	No comparison group; pre–post design	Lovaas's behavioral treatment in home for 15–25 hr/week for 1 to 2 years. No follow-up.	IQ, language, adaptive behavior, curriculum instrument.	Significant increase in mental age on all measures; increased developmental rates; significant increase in parent teaching skills.

Study	Mean age	Subjects[a]	Design	Treatment	Dependent measures	Results
Harris et al. (1990, 1991)	57 months	10 children (2 girls); all diagnosed with autism; mean IQ = 66	Pre-post design and comparison to group of normally developing peers	Center-based program with individual, small-, and large-group instruction. No follow-up.	IQ and language	67% of younger group achieved positive outcome vs. 11% of older group (χ^2 = 5.86, $p < .02$). Of 5 younger children in public school, 2 of 3 were in regular classes and 1 of 2 was in special classes. Only 1 of 9 younger children were in residential care vs. 4 of 9 older children.
Fenske et al. (1995)	48.9 months	9 children (1 girl); all diagnosed with autism; no IQ data	9 older children (1 girl) M = 101.2 months receiving same treatment; no data on matching variables.	Center-based treatment; 27.5 hr/week; 45.9 months of treatment for preschoolers; 72.4 months of treatment for comparison group; monthly parent training. ABA design. No follow-up.	Positive outcome defined as living at home, enrolled in public school vs. still in center	
Rogers & DiLalla (1991)	45.8 months	49 children (13 girls) with autism or PDD NOS; verbal DQ = 44; nonverbal DQ = 70	27 children (5 girls) with psychiatric and developmental impairments; verbal IQ = 64; performance IQ = 86	22.5 hr of center-based treatment for 6 months or more. Developmental curriculum stressing play, cognition, and social and adaptive behavior in ratios of 1:2. No follow-up. Developmental profiles; standardized language scales	Autistic group demonstrated a greater number of statistically significant gains after treatment than comparison group. Autistic group achieved significant differences in language development after 2 years of treatment.	
Hoyson et al. (1984)	40 months	6 "autistic-like" children; no IQ data reported	Pre-post design; no comparison group	Center-based program: 15 hrs/week in integrated class using developmental behavioral curriculum in ratios of 2.5:1 for 24 months; parent training. Follow-up in fifth grade.	Subscales of curriculum tool (LAP).	Significant increases in developmental rates in all areas. Attainment of normal developmental rates during treatment (i.e.

Note: DQ = developmental quotient; *DSM-III-R* = *Diagnostic and Statistical Manual of Mental Disorders* (3rd ed., Rev.); ABA = Applied Behavior Analysis; PDD NOS = pervasive developmental disorder not otherwise specified; LAP = Learning Accomplished Profile (Le May, 1977); ABA = Applied Behavior Analysis.
[a]IQs or DQs were calculated from data provided in original articles.

mental age (MA) at pretest (MAs were determined by standard infant assessment tools like the Bayley, Cattell, and Stanford–Binet, and a minimum level was required for participation in the study).

The treated children were reported to have received 40 or more hr per week of 1:1 behavioral therapy for 2 or more years delivered largely by university students. The therapy consisted of operant teaching techniques, mostly reinforcement but also some punishment techniques, used to teach a wide range of social, language, cognitive, and self-care skills as well as to reduce inappropriate behaviors. The initial phase of treatment was delivered largely in the homes, with parents also trained and carrying out the treatment. As the children progressed, behavioral teaching was delivered in community settings and typical preschools as well, with considerable focus on generalization and appropriate social behavior. The treatment protocol was written up in a manual (Lovaas et al., 1981), and instructional videotapes were also developed. The students delivering treatment were trained didactically in the principles of applied behavior analysis in college courses and then trained to deliver treatment to the children through advanced trainers. There was tight control of the treatment delivery by those who had developed the treatment program.

The first control group consisted of 19 children with autism referred for treatment but for whom there were not sufficient therapists available. These children received limited amounts of the same therapy as the experimental group, delivered by the same therapy staff, but at much less intense levels, reportedly averaging 10 hr or less per week. These children also participated in typical community interventions (i.e., speech therapy, special preschools). The second control group of 21 children was located essentially through a chart review from the referral source. This group involved children with autism matched on initial CA and MA who received interventions through community systems only with no exposure to the treatment program.

Outcome variables were obtained at two different points in time: after first grade and again in early adolescence. The follow-up study during the age period between 6 and 7 years was based on educational placement and IQ scores from raters blind to the children's histories (Lovaas, 1987). There was a large and statistically significant difference between the groups on both variables, with a mean IQ difference of 25 to 30 points between the experimental group and the two control groups, as well as significant differences in educational functioning. In the experimental group, 47% of children were functioning well in typical first-grade classrooms without any special supports, whereas only 2% of controls were thus placed. Only 10% of the experimental group, but 53% of the combined control groups, were in classes for children with severe disabilities and had IQs in the range of moderate to severe retardation (Lovaas, 1987).

Continued follow-up in late childhood and adolescence (McEachlin et al., 1993) was carried out for the experimental group and the first control group on measures of school placement, IQ, adaptive behavior, and behavioral functioning. At the second follow-up point, 47% of experimental children continued to be educated in regular placements without any evidence of educational handicaps. No control children were in such placements. No data were provided on other educational placements. IQ findings were stable from the earlier follow-up point, with differences of 30 points separating the groups (experimental group IQ, $M = 84.5$; control group $M = 54.9$). Similar levels of difference were reported for all the adaptive behavior scores. There were no group differences on the personality measure overall, with both groups scoring in the range of mild deviance, but there was an interaction of group and the 16 subscale scores, with the most significant group difference occurring on the Psychosis subscale.

There are several methodological strengths of this study. Group sizes, although not large, were not unduly small. There was a treatment manual that outlined both the treatment techniques and the actual content of the treatment. Treatment givers were all trained by the core staff and supervised closely. Children were diagnosed by professionals outside of the treatment team prior to referral and the first set of follow-up data were gathered by outside professionals blind to treatment status. Interrater reliability was reported for pretreatment behavioral measures. Outcome variables at second follow-up included several different kinds of measures, well chosen to document current levels of functioning in areas that are generally significantly affected by autism: IQ, adaptive behavior measures, school placement, and behavioral measures. Follow-up was carried out for many years after the treatment was delivered, so that long-term effect of the treatment could be examined. The two control groups allowed for examination of two different treatment conditions, one of which represented typical community programs and the other representing both typical community treatment and some level of behavioral interventions. Thus, one control group could be considered to be allowing for comparison with nonspecific treatment. A very important finding was that in the treated group, outcome was predicted by pretreatment mental ages.

When applying the criteria for ESTs as described by Lonigan et al. (this issue) to Lovaas's treatment program, several methodological weaknesses also become apparent. The greatest of these is that the assignment to groups was nonrandom. In small sample studies there are inherently greater risks for group inequivalences that cannot be detected through the usual statistical comparisons (Kazdin, 1993). Second, no data documented the amount of treatment that individual children received in any group. There are general statements that experimental children received 40 hr or more per week of treatment and that control group 1 received less than 10, but no substantiation of hours of treatment for any children was provided. There was no indication whether experimental children were receiving any other kinds of treatment (i.e., medications or other therapies). However, given the intensity of the treatment and the length of time that it lasted, it seems evident that behavioral therapy was the main treatment modality. In the second outcome study, many of the assessments were carried out by the research team, and there were missing data on the personality measure for 25% of the experimental children and 33% of the controls. A number of different IQ measures were used in outcome studies. However, the challenges of the participant group require differing batteries, with children ranging in age from 9 to 19 years and ranging in IQ from roughly 25 to 110. This is one small example of the methodological challenges in this type of research. Finally, some have questioned the extent of "recovery" versus very high levels of functioning in persons who still may have autism (Mesibov, 1993; Mundy, 1993). The question of whether the experimental group continued to have any symptoms of autism does not affect the findings of large group differences between the two groups on several important measures of outcome, but it certainly affects public perception of the work.

In summary, according to Lovaas and colleagues, this comprehensive treatment approach, documented in a treatment manual and carried out with strong fidelity to the model, resulted in large sustained improvements in multiple areas of deficit in the experimental group as compared to two control groups, of similar age and functioning levels but not randomly assigned, who received typical levels of intervention available in the community. Follow-up studies conducted years after treatment ended revealed that essentially all of the control group continued to demonstrate impaired levels of functioning, equally divided between mild and severe impairments. Almost half of the treated group appeared to be functioning without impairments in educational, cognitive, or general behavioral areas, and most of the remaining half of the treated group were functioning with mild rather than severe impairments. Given that the criteria for ESTs requires random assignment, this work can not be considered as meeting either criteria for well-established or probably efficacious treatment. However, at this point in time, this is the methodologically strongest study in this literature.

Two other sets of researchers, Birnbrauer and Leach (1993) and Sheinkopf and Siegel (in press), reported controlled studies of outcomes of children treated in adherence to Lovaas's model. Although each article described positive outcomes in the experimental group, each article had problems in methodology or data analysis that limit interpretation of the findings. Birnbrauer and Leach carried out a prospective treatment study with nonrandom assignment of children to experimental and control conditions. They included children with autism or pervasive developmental disorder who had been diagnosed by an outside agency; however, no information regarding the reliability of these diagnoses or the criteria by which they were made was reported. Experimenters excluded children who had IQ scores in the borderline range or above. They accepted 11 children into treatment, but with two families leaving, only 9 children received treatment; the control group consisted of 5 children. Thus, the group sizes were much smaller than Lovaas's.

There are a number of strengths in this study. A comprehensive pretreatment battery was used to measure functioning on standardized measures of IQ, adaptive behavior, and language as well as measures of behavioral functioning. This battery was repeated yearly. Both standardized tests and behavioral ratings were carried out by raters blind to the group status of the children. Interrater reliability was established for behavioral measures. Treatment was based on behavioral principles, including Lovaas's manual, but it was carried out by large groups of volunteers trained and supervised by an experienced staff member. Thus, this study was a community-based study, as compared to Lovaas's university-based study. There were no measures reported of fidelity to the treatment model, and it is reasonable to assume that maintaining consistent teaching methods across as many as 25 people on a child's team per week would be a difficult task. Staff recorded actual hours of treatment for each child, and the mean time in treatment was 18.7 hr per week.

Outcome data were reported after approximately 24 months of treatment. Unfortunately, the outcome data were not presented as group comparisons, and no statistical analyses were reported. All children in both groups continued to demonstrate symptoms of autism after 2 years, and both groups continued to show marked levels of stereotypic behavior and poor toy play. Four out of nine children (44%) of the treated group were considered to have made high improvement, and 56% made moderate to minimal improvement. Of the five controls, one made high improvement and 80% made moderate to minimal improvement. The authors stated that none of the pretreatment variables appeared to predict successful outcomes; however, pretreatment IQ scores were not reported. All of the children in the high-improvement group continued to score below 80 on a language-based IQ test, and two of these four children continued to demonstrate significant deficits in language (including one child with no speech) and adaptive behavior posttreatment.

This article represents an independent replication of Lovaas's model, and reports positive outcomes associated with the treatment. However, some difficulties limit its usefulness as a replication. The children received less than half of the number of treatment

173

273

hours that Lovaas reported. There was no information regarding the fidelity of the treatment model delivered by the therapists. No long-term follow-up data were reported, and there were no statistical analyses of group differences on pre- and posttreatment measures. The high-improvement group was defined by their nonverbal IQ scores in the 85 or above range. However, nonverbal IQ is a problematic outcome measure. Positive changes in nonverbal IQ do not necessarily reflect widespread gains in children with autism because the measures tap an area of strength in autism—visual–perceptual reasoning—and do not measure areas of deficiency related to language, social functioning, or adaptive functioning. There was also a considerable amount of missing IQ data. Two of nine treated children and three of five control children had no IQ data at all, and full IQ protocols were reported on only four of nine treated children and one of five controls. Moreover, the mean developmental rate of the treated group in the area of adaptive behavior was actually below that of the control group.

The other independent replication of Lovaas's approach that used a control group was carried out by Sheinkopf and Siegel (1998). This was a retrospective study, using record reviews from a database of a larger longitudinal study. Within the large sample of the longitudinal study, the author selected the records of 11 children whose parents reported that they had implemented the Lovaas model treatment at some point after the researchers had gathered an initial data set. Initial diagnoses of autism had been made by one of the researchers and a colleague in all cases prior to any data collection. A severity rating scale for symptoms was used in addition to the *Diagnostic and Statistical Manual of Mental Disorders* (3rd ed., Rev.; American Psychiatric Association, 1987) criteria; however, no reliability data were reported for the severity measure. Experimenters formed a control group of 11 children by matching records of serial cases to the treated group on the basis of CA, MA, sex, diagnosis, and test length intervals. Lovaas's manual and the supervision of one of three community therapists formed the basis of the treatment, implemented by paraprofessionals and parents; however, no documentation of treatment fidelity was provided. All children in both groups also received special education services in community preschool classrooms as well as professional therapy such as occupational therapy or speech/language therapy. The two groups did not differ in intensity of these other kinds of therapies. The experimental group received many more hours of treatment than the control group based on the provision of one-to-one instruction. Data on hours of treatment were available for both groups. The control children received a mean of 11 hr of treatment per week and the treated children received 27 hr per week, including a mean of 20 hr per week of one-to-one instruction.

Outcome measures in Sheinkopf and Siegel (1998) were limited to IQ and symptom severity, with a mean 25-point IQ difference between groups (mean of 90 vs. mean of 64, largely using nonverbal measures of IQ). A comparison of mean hours of treatment in the experimental group revealed similar IQ gains in groups receiving 21 hr per week versus 31 hr per week of behavioral teaching. Differences between the treatment and control group on number of autism symptoms posttreatment were not significant, but the treatment group demonstrated modest reductions of statistical significance on scores of symptom severity. Ten of the 11 treated children and 11 of 11 controls continued to receive diagnoses in the autism spectrum at follow-up. No information about language development was provided. Both pre- and posttreatment measures were gathered by the experimenters, who also made the diagnoses (although they were not involved in the treatment). It is not clear whether the raters knew the treatment status of the children prior to the gathering of the outcome measures.

This independent study provides some support for the Lovaas model, but several methodological points arise. The retrospective nature of the study and the lack of central coordination of the treatment raise issues of treatment fidelity. There were no long-term outcome data, and treatment effectiveness was measured in only two areas: IQ and symptoms. The IQ tests used for the majority of children in both groups were nonverbal tests or infant level tests that emphasis visual–spatial skills, an area of strength in autism. Treatment effects on deficits in adaptive behavior, language functioning, academics, and social functioning were not reported. As with the Birnbrauer and Leach (1993) study, there was some evidence of reduced severity of symptoms of autism in the experimental group after 2 years of treatment, but virtually all children continued to meet criteria for autism.

A final published replication of Lovaas's treatment approach was reported by Anderson and colleagues (Anderson, Avery, DiPietro, Edwards, & Christian, 1987). This study, however, used a pre–post design to examine effects of 1 to 2 years of home-based intensive behavioral intervention with 14 young children (*M* age = 43 months) with autism. Children were diagnosed as having autism by a separate agency, although diagnostic criteria were not specified. One therapist plus the parents provided all the treatment, which ranged from 15 to 25 hr per week. The therapists were centrally trained through the May Institute, a well-established agency for children with autism. Outcome data were gathered through use of standardized instruments administered by independent professionals, as well as through a norm-referenced curriculum tool administered by the children's parents and therapists. Information regarding school placement was also gathered. Some evidence of fidelity to the treatment model was

174

274

provided through data concerning parental teaching abilities. Reliability data were provided for virtually all measures that were not standardized: assessments of parental teaching, the norm-referenced tool, descriptive information, socioeconomic rating, and school placement.

A strength of the study by Anderson et al. (1987) involved use of outcome measures that examined the children's functioning in a wide range of areas, involving both developmental functioning and educational placements. Outcome data revealed statistically significant increases in children's functioning in a variety of areas, including mental ages, language functioning, social functioning, and self-care skills. However, in calculating the statistical significance of the changes, the amount of change expected by increasing development without intervention was not taken into account. In further analysis, pretreatment developmental rates of change were compared to developmental rates during treatment, with all children demonstrating elevated rates during treatment, although no tests of statistical significance of these elevations were reported. The authors pointed out that at posttreatment all of the children continued to need special education services and none were "mainstreamed full-time in a regular kindergarten or first grade classroom" (Anderson et al., 1987, p. 363). The two children with the lowest pretreatment performance (developmental levels below 12 months) made virtually no progress in treatment. Finally, although clear gains were demonstrated in the data, only two of the six children receiving 2 years of treatment had any developmental data falling in the normal range. Thus, as with the Birnbrauer and Leach (1993) study, the data do not allow for straightforward comparisons with the Lovaas studies. The children's developmental rates appeared to have been accelerated by the treatment, although all children continued to demonstrate some level of impairment after treatment.

Other Treatment Programs Based on Applied Behavior Analysis

Two other studies of many hours per week of treatment involving the principles of applied behavior analysis in center-based programs used a pre–post design to assess outcome in preschoolers' functioning after 1 to 2 years of such treatment. The treatment delivered by Harris and colleagues (Harris, Handleman, Gordon, Kristoff, & Fuentes, 1991; Harris, Handleman, Kristoff, Bass, & Gordon, 1990) involved a center-based intensive behavioral intervention program using a developmentally oriented curriculum that heavily stressed language development, among other developmental skills. The authors reported a statistically significant 19-point change in verbal IQ and an 8-point change on a standardized language measure after 1 year of treatment for a group of nine higher functioning children with autism. The comparison group, normally developing children with somewhat above-average developmental scores, revealed no changes in test scores after 1 year of participation in the same preschool program. The authors report that all treated children continued to demonstrate impairments after treatment.

Fenske and colleagues (e.g., Fenske, Zalenski, Krantz, & McClannahan, 1985) reported that four of nine preschoolers receiving 2 years or more of treatment at the Princeton Child Development Institute were enrolled in public school regular classes and that two of these nine children were in public school special education classes. The remaining three children, considered to have poor outcomes, remained at the Princeton program. However, no information was given about the children's level of functioning in public school classes or any other outcome variables.

To summarize, a variety of behaviorally based treatment studies of young children have reported positive outcomes. Two independent studies of Lovaas's treatment approach used control groups to provide evidence of positive effects of the treatment, including higher nonverbal IQ scores, improved language functioning, and reduced severity of autistic symptoms. However, these studies did not replicate all aspects of the treatment (particularly in intensity) or the long-term and broad-based approach for assessing outcomes. They did not demonstrate the level of improvement in multiple areas of functioning or the sustained long-term effects of the treatment that Lovaas reported. The field awaits a full independent replication of Lovaas's study.

Possible Variables Affecting Outcome of Comprehensive Treatment of Autism

Age

Fenske et al. (1985) examined the effects of age by comparing outcomes of 9 children younger than 60 months at beginning of treatment ($M = 49$ months) and 9 children older than 60 months enrolled in a center-based behavioral program at Princeton Child Development Institute. The younger group received a mean of 45 months of treatment, and the older group received a mean of 72 months of treatment. No pretreatment data were provided to demonstrate that these groups were matched on any developmental variables. The only outcome variable reported was placement: either living at home and attending public schools, or continuing to receive services at the center. Six of 9 (67%) of the early treated group achieved a positive outcome, whereas only 1 of 9 (11%) of the older group was discharged to

175

the community—a difference that was statistically significant. Of the early treated group who had been discharged, 4 attended regular classes and 2 attended special education classes.

Whereas there were a variety of methodological problems in this study, other converging evidence also speaks to the potential importance of the age variable. First is the fact that every study in the literature that has demonstrated significant changes in the general functioning of groups of children with autism in response to comprehensive treatment has involved children under the age of 5 years. Lovaas and colleagues reported on the lack of sustained treatment effects of his therapy model on older children with autism (Lovaas, Koegel, Simmons, & Long, 1973). This stands in marked contrast to the sustained gains that the same researchers reported using the same treatment with much younger children, as previously reviewed. The hypothesis that age at start of treatment is an important variable in determining outcome has tremendous implications for the field and needs to be tested with methodologically rigorous designs.

IQ and Language Abilities

Given that IQ and language abilities are highly correlated in normal development and in autism, these should probably be thought of as reflections of higher cognitive abilities—hence the grouping of them here. The evidence on relations between pretreatment IQ or language abilities and treatment outcomes is contradictory. In the original Lovaas (1987) article, a discriminate analysis predicted 100% of the nine treated children with the best outcome; pretreatment mental age was the only significant variable. Fenske et al. (1985) mentioned that the presence of language abilities, even abnormal abilities like hyperlexia and echolalia, predicted positive outcomes in the younger group treated, although not in the older group. Although Sheinkopf and Siegel (in press) did not discuss the predictive effects of pretreatment IQ on posttreatment IQ, visual examination of the IQ data for their treated group reveal that in seven of nine cases, ranking by pretreatment IQ corresponds to IQ rank posttreatment. Birnbrauer and Leach (1993) reported that none of their pretreatment measures predicted outcomes in their treated group. Other studies have not reported on possible relations between pretreatment IQ or language measures and posttreatment measures.

An additional variable in this regard involves lower IQ limits for treatment effects. Lovaas (1987) suggested that children with IQs in the severe to profound range of retardation would most likely not respond well to intensive treatment programs, and Anderson et al. (1987) reported this finding in their study. However, Birnbrauer and Leach (1993) found no relation between pretreatment IQ and outcomes. The hypothesis that initial IQ is a predictor of outcome needs to be examined in a controlled fashion.

Intensity of Treatment Provided

All of the treatment studies cited in this article involved approximately 20 or more hours per week of intervention. Although the study with the best outcome also provided the most hours per week of treatment, the only study that specifically examined effect of hours per week on treatment (i.e., Sheinkopf & Siegel, in press) found no difference in gains of children receiving an average of 21 hr compared to children receiving an average of 32 hr per week of treatment. Future studies need to document hours per week of treatment for each participant so that studies and outcomes can be compared on this variable.

Other Treatment Approaches

Are there other models of early comprehensive treatment of young children with autism that have empirical support? Unfortunately, the two studies in this field that have used a significantly different treatment approach than that of Lovaas or applied behavior analysis have been examined using only pre–post designs of treated children. Such designs do not demonstrate causality unambiguously. These studies also have potential problems involving factors such as diagnosis of children, reliability of measures, blindness of raters, psychometric strength of the outcome measures.

Hoyson and colleagues (e.g., Hoyson, Jamieson, & Strain, 1984) described a number of striking gains made by six "autistic-like" children in the Learning Experiences: An Alternative Program for Preschoolers and Parents (LEAP) preschool model, a developmental/behavioral curriculum implemented in an integrated setting. Although IQ was not a factor in selection, children with central nervous system involvement or primary retardation were excluded. The researchers reported a doubling of developmental rates during the intervention period and achievement of normal developmental rates (i.e., 1 month of gain per month of enrollment). They also reported statistically significant gains in all developmental areas, and follow-up in fifth grade revealed three children functioning in regular classrooms. In a chapter describing long-term follow-up, Strain et al. (1996) reported significant reduction in symptoms of autism after 24 months of treatment and placement of 24 out of 51 experimentally treated children in regular public school classes (although there is no mention of supports the children received or their functioning levels).

176

276

Rogers and her colleagues described the effects of a developmentally oriented, 22 hr per week, center-based program in Denver that emphasized play, language, cognition, and social relations in a series of articles. Two studies (Rogers, Herbison, Lewis, Pantone, & Reis, 1986; Rogers & Lewis, 1989) used a pre–post design to assess changes in a large group of children (*n* = 49) over a 6- to 12-month period of intervention in cognition, language, fine and gross motor skills, social and self-care skills, symbolic play skills, and interaction with the mother during free play. Children were not selected by any criterion except diagnoses of autism or Pervasive Developmental Disorder Not Otherwise Specified. Children demonstrated statistically significant increases in developmental rates beyond what would be expected from initial developmental rates in most areas of development, statistically significant changes in symbolic play skills and in positive social interactions with parents, a doubling of developmental rates during treatment, and an achievement of normal developmental rates during the treatment period.

A third study (Rogers & DiLalla, 1991) compared the effects of this treatment model on the progress of a group of children with autism to a group of children with other kinds of behavioral and developmental disorders but without any of the symptoms of autism. The group with autism made proportionally greater gains when compared to their baseline levels in a variety of areas—including cognition and language—than the group without autism. Furthermore, when matched on initial age and developmental level with the comparison group, the group with autism was found to achieve the same rate of progress on various measures of development during intervention as the nonautistic comparison group. The group with autism achieved normal developmental rates (i.e., 1 month of progress for each month of treatment) during the entire period of treatment. This was true both for children with more severe delays and for children with other delays. This study illustrated that children with autism were as likely as children with milder developmental problems to progress rapidly in intensive treatment.

A fourth study (Rogers, Lewis, & Reis, 1987) involved replication of the model by four independent agencies in four rural communities. This study examined both the treatment fidelity of the replication site and the pre–post treatment gains made by the children in those sites in areas of cognition, language, motor skills, and social and self-care skills. Staff members at the replication sites demonstrated treatment fidelity to the model, and children, who had been receiving generic treatment in those sites for 1 year or more, demonstrated considerable acceleration of developmental rates once the Denver treatment model was applied, without any changes in treatment hours, staffing patterns, or any other variable except the application of the treatment model. .

To summarize, the within-group pre–post designs used in the LEAP model and the Denver model of early treatment of young children with autism are considered an acceptable approach to program evaluation in the field of early childhood special education (Fewell & Sandall, 1986). However, these methodologies do not meet criteria for determining empirically supported treatments (see Lonigan et al., this issue). The pre–post methodology should probably be likened to the open trials of a new medication. In medication trials, preliminary positive results obtained from open trials lead to methodologically more rigorous double-blind placebo-controlled trials. In early intervention models, preliminary positive data from pre–post designs should lead to the application of methodologically rigorous controlled designs. These two models await the application of methodologies involving control groups of matched children, random assignment, blind raters, numerous outcome measures, and long-term follow-up before the effectiveness of the models can be evaluated according to the EST criteria.

Summary

The treatment of autism in very young children is a high-profile issue across the United States, with great excitement and many questions generated by the studies just reviewed. These findings have brought about new hope but also great stress for parents, while creating new pressures on school districts and treatment settings to provide intensified intervention programs for these children. In the process, many questions are being asked about the elements of successful intervention approaches and the implementation of effective models by public agencies.

The public wants answers from the scientific community about the effectiveness of various models. Are there multiple effective approaches to intervention in autism? Are the outcomes similar or different in different approaches? Along this line, it is interesting that the positive effects on developmental rates, IQ, and language function are so similar across several of the different treatment models (comparing results across all the studies, those with control groups as well as those with pre–post designs). Dawson and Osterling (1996) suggested that the source of positive outcomes across these different treatment models may be due to common elements involved rather than to program philosophy, and they have provided a helpful analysis of these potential common elements. Only methodologically rigorous continued research will provide sound answers to questions concerning the specific elements, if any, required for effective comprehensive treatment of autism.

Given the dimensions of these intervention approaches, the design and implementation of methodol-

177

ogically rigorous treatment effectiveness studies in this area is a huge undertaking. Other areas of childhood psychopathology can apply a specific treatment carried out in a proscribed way over a few weeks or months and involving a few hours per week at most, resulting in measurable changes in target symptoms. To test the efficacy of one of the comprehensive treatment approaches for autism for an estimated 25 experimental children, treatment must be provided for 20 to 30 hr per week, across at least 24 months, targeting multiple symptoms, with multiple measures of functioning both pre- and posttreatment. Mounting the interventions and gathering the pre- and postoutcome data can involve thousands of treatment hours and more than 100 adults over the course of the study—a massive undertaking in terms of personnel, organization, and funding. The issues of control groups and of method of assignment to them are fraught with difficulty, both ethical and practical.

The next generation of treatment studies focused on young children with autism should focus on applying rigorous methodologies to (a) independent replication of the behavior therapy models in order to determine what range of outcomes can be expected; (b) models that have demonstrated positive effects in "open trials" involving pre–post designs; and finally, (c) direct comparison of different treatment approaches. This could take a decade to accomplish. In the meantime, it would be most helpful if treatment programs for young children with autism could develop a common database. We need a uniform set of procedures that would allow for comparison across programs. At minimum, this would include uniform ways of describing children by diagnosis; uniform measurement protocols; uniform schedules for assessment; and uniform ways of monitoring amount of treatment, type of treatment, and fidelity to treatment models. Leadership in the field is needed to set up such a system, and commitment and collaboration across treatment givers and families will be crucial to such an endeavor.

The hope of significant improvement in the symptoms of autism has been raised by the studies just reviewed. Given the cost of autism to individuals, families, and communities, we need to answer the questions that have been raised about possible outcomes in autism through the application of our science. An appropriate summary of our present state of knowledge has been well stated by Sheinkopf and Siegel (1998):

> [While these studies suggest] that home-based behavioral therapy is a *good* option for children with autism, [they do] not indicate whether such a treatment approach is *better* than other treatments of similar intensity and/or structure. In fact, this limitation mirrors a serious gap in the literature on treatments for young children with autism. There are few controlled trials of

therapy for very young autistic children reported in peer-reviewed journals, and there are fewer (if any) controlled trials comparing various treatment approaches. Future research needs to not only compare treatment modalities but also examine the effects of treatment intensity and setting. (p. 22)

References

American Psychiatric Association. (1987). *Diagnostic and statistical manual of mental disorders* (3rd ed., Rev.). Washington, DC: Author.

Anderson, S. R., Avery, D. L., DiPietro, E. K., Edwards, G. L., & Christian, W. P. (1987). Intensive home-based early intervention with autistic children. *Education and Treatment of Children, 10,* 352–366.

Birnbrauer, J. S., & Leach, D. J. (1993). The Murdoch early intervention program after 2 years. *Behavior Change, 10,* 63–74.

Bondy, A. S., & Frost, L. A. (1994). The picture exchange communication system. *Focus on Autistic Behavior, 9,* 1–19.

Dawson, G., & Osterling, J. (1996). Early intervention in autism: Effectiveness and common elements of current approaches. In M. J. Guralnick (Ed.), *The effectiveness of early intervention: Second generation research* (pp. 307–326). Baltimore: Brookes.

Durand, V. M., Gernert-Dott, P., & Mapstone, E. (1997). Treatment of sleep disorders in children with developmental disabilities. *The Journal of The Association for Persons with Severe Handicaps, 21,* 114–123.

Fenske, E. C., Zalenski, S., Krantz, P. J., & McClannahan, L. E. (1985). Age at intervention and treatment outcome for autistic children in a comprehensive intervention program. *Analysis and Intervention in Developmental Disabilities, 5,* 49–58.

Fewell, R. R., & Sandall, S. R. (1986). Developmental testing of handicapped infants. *Topics in Early Childhood Special Education, 6,* 86–100.

Green, G. (1996). Evaluating claims about treatments for autism. In C. Maurice, G. Green, & S. C. Luce (Eds.), *Behavioral intervention for young children with autism: A manual for parents and professionals* (pp. 15–27). Austin, TX: PRO-ED.

Harris, S. L., Handleman, J. S., Gordon, R., Kristoff, B., & Fuentes, F. (1991). Changes in cognitive and language functioning of preschool children with autism. *Journal of Autism and Developmental Disorders, 21,* 281–290.

Harris, S. L., Handleman, J. S., Kristoff, B., Bass, L., & Gordon, R. (1990). Changes in language development among autistic and peer children in segregated and integrated preschool settings. *Journal of Autism and Developmental Disorders, 20,* 23–31.

Hoyson, M., Jamieson, B., & Strain, P. S. (1984). Individualized group instruction of normally developing and autistic-like children: The LEAP curriculum model. *Journal of the Division of Early Childhood, 8,* 157–172.

Kanner, L. (1943). Autistic disturbances of affective contact. *Nervous Child, 2,* 217–250.

Kanner, L. (1971). Follow-up study of 11 autistic children originally reported in 1943. *Journal of Autism and Childhood Schizophrenia, 1,* 119–145.

Kazdin, A. E. (1993). Commentary: Replication and extension of behavioral treatment of autistic disorder. *American Journal on Mental Retardation, 97,* 377–379.

Koegel, R. L., & Koegel, L. K. (1995). *Teaching children with autism.* Baltimore: Brookes.

Lalli, J. S., Casey, S., & Kates, K. (1995). Reducing escape behavior and increasing task completion with functional communication training, extinction, and response chaining. *Journal of Applied Behavior Analysis, 28,* 261–268.

178

Le May, D., Griffin, P., & Sanford, A. (1977). *Learning Accomplishment Profile–Diagnostic Edition*. Chapel Hill, NC: Chapel Hill Training-Outreach Project.

Lotter, V. (1978). Follow-up studies. In M. Rutter & E. Schopler (Eds.), *Autism: A reappraisal of concepts and treatment* (pp. 475–495). New York: Plenum.

Lovaas, O. I., Koegel, R. L., Simmons, J. Q., & Long, J. S. (1973). Some generalization and follow-up measures on autistic children in behavior therapy. *Journal of Applied Behavior Analysis, 6,* 131–166.

Lovaas, O. I. (1987). Behavioral treatment and normal educational and intellectual functioning in young autistic children. *Journal of Consulting and Clinical Psychology, 55,* 3–9.

Lovaas, O. I., Ackerman, A. B., Alexander, D., Firestone, P., Perkins, J., & Young, D. (1981). *Teaching developmentally disabled children: The me book.* Baltimore: University Park Press.

McEachlin, J. J., Smith, T., & Lovaas, O. I. (1993). Long-term outcome for children with autism who received early intensive behavioral treatment. *American Journal on Mental Retardation, 97,* 359–372.

Mesibov, G. B. (1993). Commentary: Treatment outcome is encouraging. *American Journal on Mental Retardation, 97,* 379–380.

Mundy, P. (1993). Commentary: Normal versus high-functioning status in children with autism. *American Journal on Mental Retardation, 97,* 381–384.

Ozonoff, S., & Cathcart, K. (1998). Effectiveness of a home program intervention for young children with autism. *Journal of Autism and Developmental Disorder, 28,* 25–32.

Rogers, S. J., & DiLalla, D. (1991). A comparative study of a developmentally based preschool curriculum on young children with autism and young children with other disorders of behavior and development. *Topics in Early Childhood Special Education, 11,* 29–48.

Rogers, S. J., Herbison, J., Lewis, H., Pantone, J., & Reis, K. (1986). An approach for enhancing the symbolic, communicative, and interpersonal functioning of young children with autism and severe emotional handicaps. *Journal of the Division of Early Childhood, 10,* 135–148.

Rogers, S. J., & Lewis, H. (1989). An effective day treatment model for young children with pervasive developmental disorders. *Journal of the American Academy of Child and Adolescent Psychiatry, 28,* 207–214.

Rogers, S. J., Lewis, H. C., & Reis, K. (1987). An effective procedure for training early special education teams to implement a model program. *Journal of the Division of Early Childhood, 11,* 180–188.

Schreibman, L. (1988). *Autism.* Newbury Park, CA: Sage.

Sheinkopf, S. J., & Siegel, B. (1998). Home based behavioral treatment of young autistic children. *Journal of Autism and Developmental Disorders, 28,* 15–24.

Smith, T. (1996). Are other treatments effective? In C. Maurice, G. Green, & S. C. Luce (Eds.), *Behavioral intervention for young children with autism: A manual for parents and professionals* (pp. 45–59). Austin, TX: PRO-ED.

Strain, P. S., Kohler, F. W., & Goldstein, H. (1996). Learning experiences ... An alternative program: Peer-mediated interventions for young children with autism. In E. Hibbs & P. Jensen (Eds.), *Psychosocial treatments for child and adolescent disorders: Empirically based strategies for clinical practice* (pp. 573–586). Washington, DC: American Psychological Association.

Thorp, D. M., Stahmer, A. C., & Schreibman, L. (1995). Effects of sociodramatic play training on children with autism. *Journal of Autism and Developmental Disorders, 25,* 265–282.

Received April 2, 1997
Revision received October 23, 1997
Accepted December 10, 1997

179

Acknowledgments

Rapin, I. "An 8-Year-Old Boy with Autism." *JAMA* 285 (2001): 1749–1757. Copyright 2001. The American Medical Association.

Filipek, P.A., Accardo, P.J., Baranek, G.T., Cook, E.H., Jr., Dawson, G., Gordon, B., Gravel, J.S., Johnson, C.P., Kallen, R.J., Levy, S.E., Minshew, N.J., Ozonoff, S., Prizant, B.M., Rapin, I., Rogers, S.J., Stone, W.L., Teplin, S., Tuchman, R.F., and Volkmar, F.R. "The Screening and Diagnosis of Autistic Spectrum Disorders." *J Autism Dev Disord* 29 (1999): 439–484.

Bryson, W.E., and Smith, I.M. "Epidemiology of Autism: Prevalence, Associated Characteristics, and Implications for Research and Service Delivery." *Ment Retard Dev Disabil Res Rev* 4 (1998): 97–103. Reprinted with the permission of Kluwer Academic-Plenum Publishers, Plenum Press.

Fombonne, E. "The Epidemiology of Autism: A Review." *Psychol Med* 29 (1999): 769–786. Reprinted with the permission of Cambridge University Press.

Tuchman, R.F., Rapin, I., and Shinnar, S. "Autistic and Dysphasic Children, II Epilepsy." *Pediatrics* 88 (1991): 1219–1225. Reprinted by permission Pediatrics.

Bailey, A., Le Couteur, A., Gottesman, I., Bolton, P., Simonoff, E., Yuzda, E., and Rutter, M. "Autism as a Strongly Genetic Disorder: Evidence from a British Twin Study." *Psychol Med* 25 (1995): 63–77. Reprinted with the permission of Cambridge University Press.

Spiker, D., Lotspeich, L., Kraemer, H.C., et al. "Genetics of Autism: Characteristics of Affected and Unaffected Children from 37 Multiplex Families." *Am J Med Genet* 54 (1994): 27–35. Copyright © 1994. Reprinted by permission of Wiley-Liss, Inc., a subsidiary of John Wiley & Sons, Inc.

Wassink, T.H., Piven, J., Vieland, V.J., Huang, J., Swiderski, R.E., Pietila, J., Braun, T., Beck, G., Folstein, S.E., Haines, J.L., and Sheffield, V.C. "Evidence Supporting WNT2 as an Autism Susceptibility Gene." *Am J Med Genet* 105, 5 (2001): 406–413. Copyright © 2001. Reprinted by permission of Wiley-Liss, Inc., a subsidiary of John Wiley & Sons, Inc.

Abell, F., Krams, M., Ashburner, J., Passingham, R., Friston, K., et al. "The Neuroanatomy of Autism: A Voxel-Based Whole Brain Analysis of Structural Scans." *Neuroreport* 10 (1999): 1647–1651. Reprinted with the permission of Lippincott Williams & Wilkins.

Adolphs, R., Sears, L., and Piven, J. "Abnormal Processing of Social Information from Faces in Autism." *Journal of Cognitive Neuroscience* 13 (2001): 232–240. Reprinted with the permission of MIT Press.

Adolphs, R., Tranel, D., and Damasio, A.R. "The Human Amygdala in Social Judgment." *Nature* 393 (1998): 470–474. Reprinted by permission from Nature Vol. 393 pp. 470–474. Copyright © 1998 Macmillan Magazines Ltd.

Bailey, A., Luthbert, P., Dean, A., Harding, B., Janota, I., Montgomery, M., Rutter, M., and Lantos, P. "A Clinicopathological Study of Autism." *Brain* 121 (1998): 889–905. Reprinted with the permission of Oxford University Press.

Bailey, A., Phillips, W., and Rutter, M. "Autism: Towards an Integration of Clinical, Genetic, Neuropsychological, and Neurobiological Perspectives." *J Child Psychol Psychiatry* 37 (1996): 89–126. Reprinted with the permission of Cambridge University Press.

Courchesne, E., Yeung-Courchesne, R., Press, G.A., Hesselink, J.R., and Jernigan, T.L. "Hypoplasia of Cerebellar Vermal Lobules VI and VII in Autism." *N Engl J Med* 1998. Copyright © 1998 Massachusetts Medical Society. All rights reserved.

Happe, F., Ehlers, S., Fletcher, P., Frith, U., Johansson, M., Gillberg, C., Dolan, R., Frackowiak, R., and Frith, C. "'Theory of Mind' in the Brain. Evidence from a PET Scan Study of Asperger Syndrome." *Neuroreport* 8 (1996): 197–201.

Kemper, T.L., and Bauman, M. "Neuropathology of Infantile Autism." *J Neuropathol Exp Neurol* 57 (1998): 645–652.

Lord, C., Cook, E.H., Leventhal, B.L., and Amaral, D.G. "Autism Spectrum Disorders." *Neuron* 28 (2000): 355–363. Copyright 2000, with permission from Elsevier Science.

Stone, V.E., Baron-Cohen, S., and Knight, R.T. "Frontal Lobe Contributions to Theory of Mind." *J Cogn Neurosci* 10 (1998): 640–656. Reprinted with the permission of MIT Press.

McDougle, C.J., Holmes, J.P., Carlson, D.C., et al. "A Double-Blind, Placebo-Controlled Study of Risperidone in Adults with Autistic Disorder and Other Pervasive Developmental Disorders." *Arch Gen Psychiatry* 55 (1999): 633–641. Reprinted with the permission of American Medical Association.

McEachern, J.J., Smith, T., and Lovaas, O.I. "Long-Term Outcome for Children with Autism Who Received Early Intensive Behavioral Treatment." *Am J Ment Retard* 97 (1993): 359–372. Reprinted with the permission of American Association on Mental Retardation.

Rogers, S.J. "Empirically Supported Comprehensive Treatment of Young Children with Autism." *J Clin Child Psychol* 27 (1998): 168–179. Reprinted with the permission of Lawrence Erlbaum Associates Inc.

For Product Safety Concerns and Information please contact our EU
representative GPSR@taylorandfrancis.com
Taylor & Francis Verlag GmbH, Kaufingerstraße 24, 80331 München, Germany

www.ingramcontent.com/pod-product-compliance
Ingram Content Group UK Ltd.
Pitfield, Milton Keynes, MK11 3LW, UK
UKHW021113180425
457613UK00005B/67